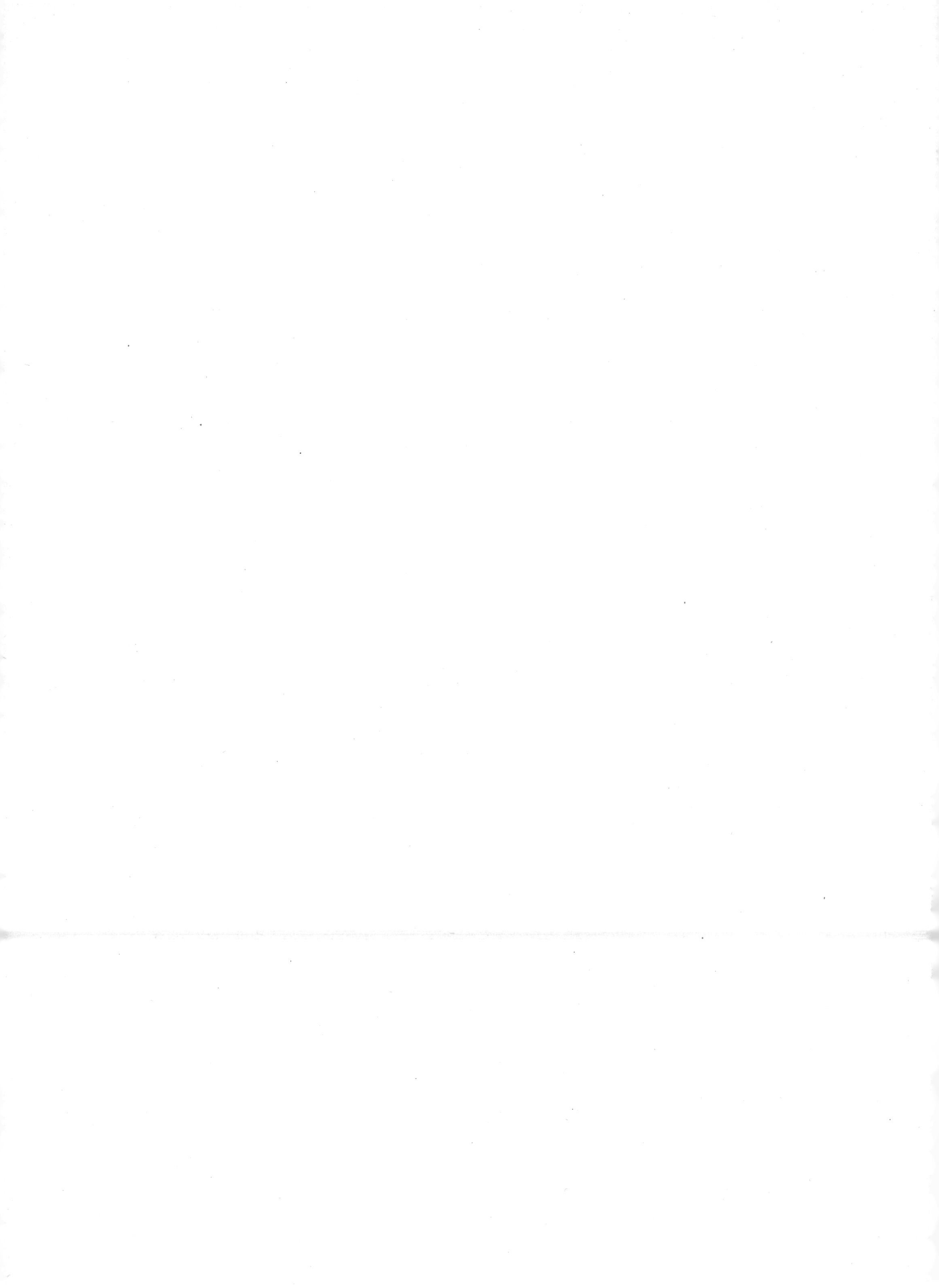

ATLAS OF OPERATIVE OTORHINOLARYNGOLOGY AND HEAD & NECK SURGERY

Vol. 3

FACIAL PLASTICS, COSMETICS AND RECONSTRUCTIVE SURGERY

ATLAS OF OPERATIVE OTORHINOLARYNGOLOGY AND HEAD & NECK SURGERY

Vol. 3

FACIAL PLASTICS, COSMETICS AND RECONSTRUCTIVE SURGERY

Editors

Bachi T Hathiram
Professor and Head
Department of ENT and Head and Neck Surgery
Topiwala National Medical College and
BYL Nair Charitable Hospital
Mumbai, Maharashtra, India

Vicky S Khattar
Assistant Professor
Department of ENT and Head and Neck Surgery
Topiwala National Medical College and
BYL Nair Charitable Hospital
Mumbai, Maharashtra, India

Forewords

Jatin P Shah
Milind V Kirtane

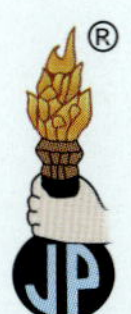

JAYPEE BROTHERS MEDICAL PUBLISHERS (P) LTD

New Delhi • London • Philadelphia • Panama

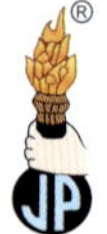

Jaypee Brothers Medical Publishers (P) Ltd

Headquarters

Jaypee Brothers Medical Publishers (P) Ltd
4838/24, Ansari Road, Daryaganj
New Delhi 110 002, India
Phone: +91-11-43574357
Fax: +91-11-43574314
Email: jaypee@jaypeebrothers.com

Overseas Offices

J.P. Medical Ltd
83, Victoria Street, London
SW1H 0HW (UK)
Phone: +44-2031708910
Fax: +02-03-0086180
Email: info@jpmedpub.com

Jaypee-Highlights Medical Publishers Inc.
City of Knowledge, Bld. 237, Clayton
Panama City, Panama
Phone: +507-301-0496
Fax: +507-301-0499
Email: cservice@jphmedical.com

Jaypee Brothers Medical Publishers Ltd
The Bourse
111 South Independence Mall East
Suite 835, Philadelphia, Pennsylvania, USA
19106, USA
Phone: + 267-519-9789
Email: joe.rusko@jaypeebrothers.com

Jaypee Brothers
Medical Publishers (P) Ltd
17/1-B Babar Road, Block-B
Shaymali, Mohammadpur
Dhaka-1207, Bangladesh
Mobile: +08801912003485
Email: jaypeedhaka@gmail.com

Jaypee Brothers
Medical Publishers (P) Ltd
Shorakhute, Kathmandu
Nepal
Phone: +00977-9841528578
Email: jaypee.nepal@gmail.com

Website: www.jaypeebrothers.com
Website: www.jaypeedigital.com

Inquiries for bulk sales may be solicited at: jaypee@jaypeebrothers.com

Atlas of Operative Otorhinolaryngology and Head & Neck Surgery:
Facial Plastics, Cosmetics and Reconstructive Surgery (Vol. 3)

First Edition: **2013**

ISBN 978-93-5090-481-7

Printed at : Ajanta Offset & Packagings Ltd., New Delhi

Dedicated to

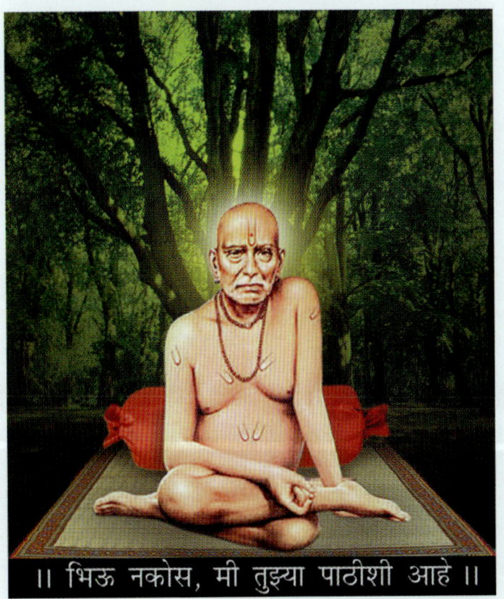

Shri Swami Samarth

My father, Adi Dinshaw Mistry—Who taught me the value of hard work and loyalty
My mother, Viloo Adi Mistry—For her selfless love and caring
Both my parents and mamma—For their blessings and encouragement
My husband, Tempton—Always loving, caring and encouraging
My miracle and happiness, Karishma and Khushi—For making life worthwhile
Rustom, Khushru, Firozee, Sharon, Jenaifer, Zenia,
Travis and Hazel—For believing in me and being with me

Bachi T Hathiram

My father, Subhash Chandra Gyanchand Khattar—My support
My mother, Veena Subhash Khattar—My encouragement
My grandparents, Gyanchand Khattar, Mohandevi Khattar,
Vas Dev Pawa, Tulsidevi Pawa—Who indulged me
Shalu, Sameer, Sehar and Sia—My indulgence
My family, friends, teachers and students

Vicky S Khattar

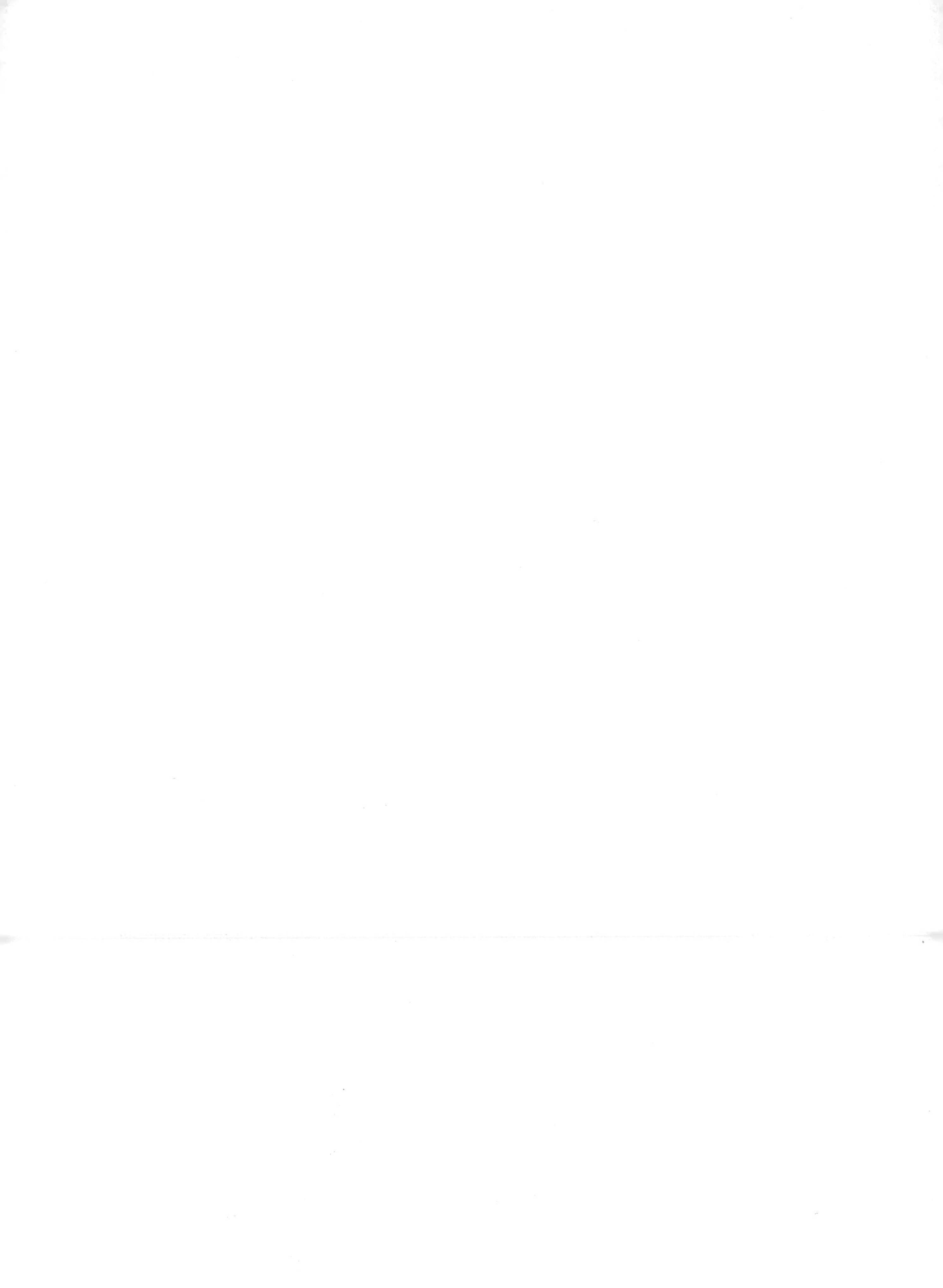

Contributors

Ahmad Abu-Omar DOHNS MRCS
Educational Fellow in Otolaryngology
Whipps Cross University Hospital
London, UK

Bashar Abuzayed MD
Attending Neurosurgeron
Department of Neurosurgery
Cerrahpasa Medical Faculty
Istanbul University Istanbul, Turkey

Rahul Agrawal
Department of ENT and Skull Base Surgery
Dr Balabhai Nanavati Hospital
Mumbai, Maharashtra
India

Vikas Agrawal MS FCPS DORL
Consultant ENT Surgeon
Speciality ENT Hospital, Kandivli
Asian Heart Institue, Bandra
Sevenhills Hospital, Andheri
BSES MG Hospital, Andheri
Mumbai, Maharashtra
India

RG Aiyer
Professor and Head
Department of ENT and Head and Neck Surgery
Govt Medical College and SSG Hospital
Vadodara, Gujarat, India

KM Ajith
Department of ENT
SS Institute of Medical Sciences and Research Center
Davangere, Karnataka
India

Lynzee N Alworth PhD AuD CCC-A F/AAA
Assistant Professor of Audiology
University Audiology Associates
University of Louisville
Kentucky, USA

Danic Hadzibegovic Ana MD
Department of Otorhinolaryngology and Maxillofacial Surgery
Medical School Osijek, University Josip Juraj Strossmayer of Osijek
Croatia

Miroslav Andrić DDS Msc
Clinic of Oral Surgery
School of Dentistry
University of Belgrade
Belgrade, Serbia

Nebil Ark
Fatih University, Faculty of Medicine
Department of Otorhinolaryngology
Head and Neck Surgery
Ankara, Turkey

V Arora
Associate Professor
Department of ENT and Head Neck Surgery
University College of Medical Sciences and GTB Hospital
New Delhi, India

Katie L Austin AuD CCC-A F/AAA
Audiologist
Heuser Hearing Institute, and Heuser Speech and Language Academy
Louisville
Kentucky, USA

Luca Autelitano MD
Maxillo-Facial Surgeon
Smile House, San Paolo Hospital
University of Milan, via A. di Rudinì
Milan, Italy

Gregor Bachmann-Harildstad MD PhD
Akershus University Hospital/UIO
Otorhinolaryngology
Nordbyhagen, Norway

Vincent Bachy
Departement de Chirurgie
ORL et Chirurgie Cervico-Faciale
Site Mont-Godinne: Avenue Docteur G Thérasse
Yvoir, Belgium

Mohamed Badr-El-Dine MD
Professor of Otolaryngology
Consultant Otology Neurotology and Skull Base Surgery
Faculty of Medicine
University of Alexandria, Egypt
President of the Egyptian Society of Skull Base Surgery
Egypt

Yogesh Bajaj MS MD FRCS (ORL HNS)
Consultant ENT
Barts Children's Hospital and Royal London Hospitals
Honorary Lecturer
Anglia Ruskin University
London, UK

Karthikeyan Balasubramanian
Department of Surgical Oncology
Prince Aly Khan Hospital
Mumbai, Maharashtra, India

Maurizio Barbara
ENT Clinic, Sant'Andrea Hospital
Sapienza University
Rome, Italy

Brajendra Baser MS (AIIMS) DNB
Professor and Head of ENT
Shri Aurbindo Institute of
Medical Sciences (SAIMS Medical College)
Director Akash Hospital
Indore, Madhya Pradesh
India

BP Belaldavar
Department of ENT, KLE University's
JN Medical College and
Consultant ENT Surgeon, KLES
Dr Prabhakar Kore Hospital
Belgaum, Karnataka, India

Michael S Benninger MD
Chairman, Head and Neck Institute
The Cleveland Clinic
Professor of Surgery
The Learner School of
Medicine of Case Western
Reserve University
Euclid Avenue
Cleveland, Ohio, USA

Abir K Bhattacharyya MS DNB FRCS FRCS(ORL) FACS
Consultant Otolaryngologist and
Head and Neck Surgeon
Associate Director of
Medical Education (Surgery) and
Royal College Surgical Tutor
Whipps Cross University Hospital
London, UK

Merill Biel
Department of Otolaryngology
University of Minnesota
Minneapolis
Minnesota, USA

Kofi DO Boahene
Assistant Professor
Facial Plastic and
Reconstructive Surgery
Johns Hopkins Facial Plastic and
Reconstructive Surgery Center
Minimally Invasive Skullbase Surgery
Microvascular Surgery
Department of Otolaryngology
Head and Neck Surgery
Johns Hopkins Medical Institute, USA

Miriam Boenisch MD PhD
Medicent Linz, Untere
Donaulände
Linz, Austria

Mariano M Boglione MD
Pediatric Surgeon
General Pediatric Surgery Division
Chief of Lung Transplant Program
Hospital de Pediatría
Prof Dr Juan P Garrahan
Buenos Aires, Argentina

Luis A B Borba MD PhD
Professor
Chief of the Neurosurgical
Department
Evangelic Universitary Hospital
Curitiba, Paraná, Brazil.
Neurosurgeon of the Brain and
Heart Institute
Curitiba, Paraná, Brazil

Jennings R Boyette MD
Department of Otolaryngology—
Head and Neck Surgery
University of Arkansas for
Medical Sciences
Arkansas Children's Hospital
Little Rock, Arkansas, USA

Ryan F Brown MD
Department of Head and Neck
Surgery Kaiser Permanente
Denver Colorado, USA

James A Burns
Massachusetts General Hospital
Division of Laryngeal Surgery
Boston, Massachusetts, USA

Giulia Carnevali MD
Maxillo-Facial Surgeon
Department of Traumatology and
Maxillo Facial Surgery
AOUC Hospital and University of
Florence Largo Palagi
Florence, Italy

Giorgio Carrabba MD PhD
Neurosurgery
Fondazione IRCCS Ca' Granda
Ospedale Maggiore Policlinico
University of Milano
Milano, Italy

Ricardo L Carrau MD FACS
Professor
Department of Otolaryngology
Head and Neck Surgery
The Ohio State University
Medical Center
West 10th Avenue
Cramblett Hall, Columbus
Ohio, USA

Ali Diaz Castillejos
Fellow of Cranial Base Surgery
Evangelic Universitary Hospital
Curitiba, Paraná - Brazil

CW David Chang MD
Associate Clinical Professor, Facial
Plastic and Reconstructive Surgery
Residency Program Director
Department of Otolaryngology
Head and Neck Surgery
University of Missouri
One Hospital Drive
Columbia
Missouri, USA

Dinesh K Chhetri MD
University of California—Los Angeles
Department of Head and Neck Surgery
CHS 62-132, UCLA
School of Medicine
Los Angeles
California, USA

Chi-Yee Choi
Division of Head and Neck Reconstruction Surgery
Department of Surgery
United Christian Hospital
Hong Kong
SAR, China

Tam-Lin Chow
Division of Head and Neck Reconstruction Surgery
Department of Surgery
United Christian Hospital
Hong Kong
SAR, China

Yakup Cil MD
Plastic Surgeon
Eskisehir Military Hospital
Department of Plastic Surgery
Eskisehir, Turkey

Joseph Curry
Department of Otolaryngology
Head and Neck Surgery
University of Miami Miller School of Medicine, Miami
Florida, USA

Sanket Dani
Resident—Department of ENT and Head and Neck Surgery
TN Medical College and
BYL Nair Charitable Hospital
Mumbai, Maharashtra, India

Rajib Dasgupta
London, UK

Danic Davorin MD PhD
Department of Otorhinolaryngology and Maxillofacial Surgery
Medical School Osijek
University Josip Juraj Strossmayer of Osijek, Croatia

Matteo de Notaris MD PhD
Department of Neurosurgery
Hospital Clinic, Faculty of Medicine
Universitat de Barcelona
Laboratory of Surgical Neuroanatomy (LSNA)
Faculty of Medicine
Universitat de Barcelona
Barcelona, Spain

Alberto Deganello MD PhD
Head and Neck Surgeon
Assistant Professor in Otolaryngology
SOD Otolaryngology 1
Department of Surgical Sciences
AOU-Careggi, University of Florence
Vle Morgagni, Florence, Italy

Amir R Dehdashti MD FACS
Geisinger Clinic
Department of Neurosurgery, USA

C E Deopujari
Department of Neurosurgery
Bombay Hospital
Mumbai, Maharashtra, India

Daniel G Deschler
Director
Division of Head and Neck Surgery
Department of Otology and Laryngology
Massachusetts Eye and Ear Infirmary
Associate Professor
Harvard Medical School
Boston, Massachusetts, USA

Akshay P Deshpande
Resident, Department of Plastic Surgery TN Medical College and BYL Nair Charitable Hospital
Mumbai, Maharashtra, India

Snigdha Devane
Resident—Department of ENT and Head and Neck Surgery, TN Medical College and BYL Nair Charitable Hospital
Mumbai, Maharashtra, India

PV Dhond MS (ENT) DORL
Honorary Consultant
Bhagwati Hospital
Mumbai, Maharashtra, India

Sara R Dickie MD
Section of Plastic and Reconstructive Surgery
University of Chicago
Department of Surgery
Chicago, Illinois, USA

J Dings
Department of Neurosurgery
Maastricht University Medical Center
The Netherlands

Gilles Dolivet MD PhD
Head and Neck Surgeon
Otolaryngologist
Head of the Surgical Oncology Department
National Cancer Institute "Alexis Vautrin"
Av. de Bourgogne
Vandoeuvre-Les-Nancy
University of Nancy
France

Adam Donne
Consultant in Paediatric Otolaryngology Alder Hey Children's Hospital
Liverpool, UK

Mark Domanski
Department of Otolaryngology—Head and Neck Surgery
The George Washington University
USA

Prgomet Drago
Clinics of Otorhinolaryngology
Head and Neck Surgery
Clinical Hospital Centar Zagreb
Medical School Zagreb
University of Zagreb, Croatia

Yadranko Ducic MD FACS FRCS
Clinical Professor
Department of Otolaryngology—Head and Neck Surgery at the University of Texas Southwestern Medical Center, Dallas Texas
Baylor Neuroscience Skullbase Program Dallas Fort Worth Texas
Otolaryngology and Facial Plastic Surgery Associates Fort Worth Texas, USA

Jason Durel
Resident Physician
Department of Otolaryngology—Head and Neck Surgery
Louisiana State University Health Sciences Center
New Orleans, Louisiana, USA

Philippe Eloy
Department of Otorhinolaryngology
University of Louvain (Belgium)
Cliniques de Mont Godinne (Yvoir)
Av Therasse
Yvoir, Belgium

Joaquim Enseñat MD PhD
Department of Neurosurgery
Hospital Clinic, Faculty of Medicine
Universitat de Barcelona
Barcelona, Spain

Audrey B Erman
Department of Otology and Laryngology
Massachusetts Eye and Ear Infirmary
Harvard Medical School
Boston, Massachusetts, USA

Waleed F Ezzat
Professor of Otolaryngology Head and Neck Surgery
Ain- Shams University
Cairo, Egypt

Leo FS Ditzel Filho
Research Fellows
Department of Neurological Surgery
The Ohio State University
Columbus, USA

Dan M Fliss MD
Professor and Chairman
Department
Otolaryngology
Head and Neck Surgery
and Maxillofacial Surgery
Tel-Aviv Sourasky Medical Center
6 Weizmann St, Tel-Aviv, Israel

Hossam MT Foda MD
Professor and Chief of Facial Plastic Surgery
Otolaryngology Department
Alexandria Medical School, Egypt

Arun K Gadre MD FACS MS(Bom) DORL
HHI Professor of Otology and Neurotology
Director of Otology, Neurotology and Skull Base Surgery
Associate Professor of Otolaryngology—Head and Neck Surgery
Department of Surgery
University of Louisville
Kentucky, USA

Lorenzo Gaini
Department of Otorhinolaryngology
IRCCS Policlinico
University of Milano-Statale
Milano, Italy

Oreste Gallo MD
Associate Professor in Otolaryngology
Head of the SOD Otolaryngology
Department of Surgical Sciences
AOU-Careggi
University of Florence
Vle Morgagni
Florence, Italy

Werner Garavello
Department of Otorhinolaryngology
San Gerardo Hospital
University of Milano Bicocca
Monza, Italy

Celeste C Gary MD
Department of Otolaryngology
Head and Neck Surgery
Louisiana State University Health Sciences Center
533 Bolivar Street
New Orleans, Louisiana, USA

Jacques Gaudet
Resident Physician,
Department of Otolaryngology–Head and Neck Surgery,
Louisiana State University
Health Sciences Center
New Orleans, Louisiana, USA

Panagiotis Gerbesiotis MD PhD
Registrar—ENT Surgeon
2nd University Department of Otorhinolaryngology
Head and Neck Surgery
ATTIKON Hospital, Rimini 1
Chaidari, Athens, Greece

Nurperi Gazioglu MD
Professor in Neurosurgery
Department of Neurosurgery
Cerrahpasa Medical Faculty
Istanbul University
Istanbul, Turkey

Gianni Gitti MD PhD
Otolaryngologist
Centro Rieducazione Ortofonica
Piazzale della Porta al Prato
Florence
Italy

Haralampos Gouveris
Department of Otorhinolaryngology
The University of
Mainz Hospitals and Clinics
Langenbeckstr, Mainz, Germany

Cassio Zottis Grapiglia MD
Fellow of Cranial Base Surgery
Evangelic Universitary Hospital
Curitiba, Paraná - Brazil

Jorge Orlando Guerrissi
Head, Department of
Plastic and Reconstructive Surgery
Head and Neck Surgery
Argerich Hospital
Health Ministery of Ciudad
Autonoma de Buenos Aires
Argentina

Anish K Gupta
Sr Consultant
Department of ENT
Fortis Hospital
Mohali
Punjab, India

Anuragini Gupta
Jr Resident
Department of ENT
Resident BSPH
Bhilai
Chattisgarh, India

Arunesh Gupta
Assistant Professor
Department of Plastic Surgery
TN Medical College and
BYL Nair Charitable Hospital
Mumbai, Maharashtra, India

Ashok K Gupta
Professor and Head
Department of Otolaryngology
(Unit II)
PGIMER, Chandigarh, India

Rahul Gupta
Assistant Professor
Department of ENT and
Head and Neck Surgery
Govt. Medical College and
SSG Hospital
Vadodara, Gujarat, India

Mehmet Habesoglu
Department of II-Otolaryngology—
Head and Neck Surgery
Haydarpasa Numune Education and
Research Hospital, Turkey

Tulay Erden Habesoglu
Department of II-Otolaryngology—
Head and Neck Surgery
Haydarpasa Numune Education and
Research Hospital, Turkey

Josef Haik MD MPH
Assistant Professor of Plastic Surgery;
Deputy of the Division of Plastic and
Reconstructive Surgery
Director of the Intensive Care Burn
Unit Sheba Medical Center
Tel-Aviv University
Ramat Gan, Israel

Arsheed Hussain Hakeem
Consultant
Department of Head and Neck
Surgery and Surgical Oncology
Prince Aly Khan Hospital
Mumbai, Maharashtra, India

Imtiyaz Hussain Hakeem
Resident
Department of Internal Medicine
Florida Hospital Medical Center
Orlando, Florida, USA

Bachi T Hathiram
Professor and Head
Department of ENT and
Head and Neck Surgery
TN Medical College and
BYL Nair Charitable Hospital
Mumbai, Maharashtra, India

Biswajyoti Hazarika
Senior Consultant
Department of Surgical Oncology
Max Cancer Center
New Delhi, India

Barbara Henderson
Department of Biophysics/Cell
Stress Biology
Roswell Park Cancer Institute
Buffalo, NY, USA

Patrick T Hennessey MD
PGY-5 Resident
The Johns Hopkins Hospital
Department of Otolaryngology—
Head and Neck Surgery, USA

Björn Herman
Department of Otolaryngology
University of Miami
School of Medicine, USA

Yasuyuki Hinohira
Department of Otorhinolaryngology
Showa University School of Medicine
Hatanodai, Shinagawa, Tokyo, Japan

Steven B Hopping
Department of Otolaryngology—
Head and Neck Surgery
The George Washington University
USA

Takashi Horiguchi
Associate Professor
Department of Neurosurgery
Keio University School of Medicine
Japan

K Hörmann
Head and Chair of the Department of ORL and Head and Neck Surgery
University Hospital of Mannheim
Mannheim, Germany

Gilad Horowitz
Department Otolaryngology
Head and Neck Surgery and
Maxillofacial Surgery
Tel-Aviv Sourasky Medical Center
6 Weizmann St, Tel-Aviv, Israel

Sonna Ifeacho
Department of Otolaryngology
Great Ormond Street Hospital
London, UK

Shabbir Indorewala
Department of Otorhinolaryngology
and The Skull Base Group
Dr Balabhai Nanavati Hospital
Mumbai, Maharashtra, India

Ankit Jain
Resident—Department of ENT and Head and Neck Surgery, TN Medical College and BYL Nair
Charitable Hospital
Mumbai, Maharashtra, India

Yong Ju Jang
Professor
Department of Otolaryngology
Asan Medical Center
University of Ulsan College of Medicine, Seoul, Korea

Sharan C Jayaram
Head and Neck Fellow
Department of Otolaryngology
New Queen Elizabeth Hospital
Birmingham, UK

Narayan Jayashankar
Department of Otorhinolaryngology
and the Skull Base Group
Department of ENT and
Skull Base Surgery
Dr Balabhai Nanavati Hospital
Mumbai, Maharashtra, India

Deya Jourdy
Department of Otolaryngology
University of Miami School of Medicine, USA

Javier Herrero Jover MD PhD
Plastic Surgery Department
Centro Medico TEKNON
Vilana, Barcelona, Spain

Akinobu Kakigi MD
Assistant Professor
Department of Otolaryngology
Head and Neck Surgery
Faculty of Medicine
Tokyo University, Japan

Mohan Kameswaran DSc MS FRCS (Ed) FAMS FICS DLO
Consultant ENT Surgeon
Department of Implant Otology
Madras ENT Research Foundation
Raja Annamalaipuram, Chennai
Tamil Nadu, India

Tolga Kandogan MD
Associate Professor of Otolaryngology Head and Neck Surgery
Izmir Bozyaka Teaching and Research Hospital
Department of Otol Aryngology
Head and Neck Surgery
Izmir Bozyaka, Turkey

Sunita Kanojia
Department of ENT
Bombay Hospital
Mumbai, Maharashtra, India

Gauri Kapre
Consultant ENT surgeon
Neeti Clinics, Nagpur
Clinical Fellow
Bombay Hospital
Mumbai, Maharashtra, India

Madan Kapre
Director Neeti Clinics, Nagpur
Honorary senior surgeon
RST Cancer Hospital Nagpur
Maharashtra, India

Pornthep Kasemsiri
Research Fellows
Department of Otolaryngology and
Head and Neck Surgery
The Ohio State University
Columbus, USA

Amin B Kassam
Professor
Department of Neurological Surgery
University of Ottawa
Ottawa, Canada

Daniel F Kelly MD
Brain Tumor Center and Pituitary Disorders Program
John Wayne Cancer Institute at Saint John's Health Center
Santa Monica, California, USA

Guy Kenyon FRCS
Consultant ENT Surgeon
Whipps Cross University Hospital
NHS Trust
69 Harley Street
London, UK

Vicky S Khattar
Assistant Professor
Department of ENT and
Head and Neck Surgery
TN Medical College and
BYL Nair Charitable Hospital
Mumbai, Maharashtra
India

Sunil Khot
Resident—Department of ENT and Head and Neck Surgery
TN Medical College and BYL Nair Charitable Hospital
Mumbai, Maharashtra, India

Ji Heui Kim
Department of Otolaryngology
Asan Medical Center
University of Ulsan College of Medicine
Seoul, Korea

Milind Kirtane
Professor Emeritus Seth GS Medical College
Hon Surgeon at KEM Hospital
Hon Consulting ENT Surgeon at PD Hinduja National Hospital
Hon ENT Consultant to his Excellency the Governor of Maharashtra
Hon ENT Consultant at Prince Aly Khan Hospital
Mumbai, Maharashtra, India

Janusz Klatka
Department of Otolaryngology and Laryngeal Oncology
Medical University of Lublin
Poland

Masahiro Komori
Department of Otolaryngology Head and Neck Surgery
Kochi Medical School
Okatoyo, Nankoku
Kochi, Japan

Shenal Kothari MS
Associate Professor of ENT
Department of ENT
SAIMS Medical College
Indore, Madhya Pradesh, India

Murat Küçüktaş MD
Departments of Dermatology
Nevşehir State Hospital
Nevşehir, Turkey

Melda Kunduk
Assistant Professor
Department of Otolaryngology—Head and Neck Surgery
Louisiana State University Health Science Center
New Orleans
Louisiana, USA

Daniel B Kuriloff MD FACS
Director
Center for Thyroid and Parathyroid Surgery
New York Head and Neck Institute
Lenox Hill Hospital
Associate Professor
Clinical Otolaryngology
Head and Neck Surgery
Columbia University
110 East 59th Street
New York, NY, USA

Balagopal Kurup
Resident
Department of ENT and Head and Neck Surgery
TN Medical College and BYL Nair Charitable Hospital
Mumbai, Maharashtra, India

Zekayi Kutlubay MD
Departments of Dermatology
İstanbul University Cerrahpaşa Medical Faculty, İstanbul, Turkey

Danielle de Lara
Research Fellows
Department of Neurological Surgery
The Ohio State University
Columbus, USA

Guglielmo Larotonda MD
Resident in Otolaryngology, SOD Otolaryngology 1
Department of Surgical Sciences
AOU-Careggi, University of Florence
Vle Morgagni, Florence, Italy

Georges Lawson
Otolaryngology
Head and Neck Surgery Department
Louvain University Hospital of Mont-Godinne, Yvoir, Belgium

Davide Lazzeri MD
Plastic Surgeon
Plastic and Reconstructive Surgery Unit, Santa Chiara Hospital of Pisa
Via Roma Pisa, Italy

Eugenijus Lesinskas MD PhD
Clinic of Ear, Nose Throat and Eye Diseases
Medical Faculty
Vilnius University, Lithuania

Andreas Leunig
Professor Dr. Med. Andreas Leunig
HNO-Zentrum Starnberg
Prinzenweg 1
Starnberg, Germany

Roman Liscak
Na Homolce Hospital
Prague, Czech Republic

Marco Locatelli MD PhD
Neurosurgery,
Fondazione IRCCS Ca' Granda Ospedale Maggiore Policlinico,
University of Milano,
Milano, Italy

Kevin Lollar MD
Private Practice
Hannibal, Missouri, USA

Jennifer L Long MD PhD
University of California-Los Angeles
Department of Head and Neck Surgery
UCLA School of Medicine
Los Angeles, California, USA

Claudio Macrì
ENT Clinic, Sant'Andrea Hospital
Sapienza University
Rome, Italy

Vishal Madan MBBS (Hons) MD MRCP
Consultant Dermatologist
Laser and Dermatological Surgeon
Salford Royal NHS Foundation Trust Stott Lane
Salford, Manchester, UK

Amit Magadum
Resident—Department of Anatomy
JN Medical College
Belgaum, Karnataka, India

Dipesh J Malviya
Resident—Department of Plastic Surgery, TN Medical College and BYL Nair Charitable Hospital
Mumbai, Maharashtra, India

Jaiganesh Manickavasagam FRCS (ORL-HNS)
Royal Hallamshire Hospital
Sheffield, UK

Gauri Mankekar
ENT Consultant
PD Hinduja Hospital
Mahim, Mumbai, Maharashtra, India

Wolf J Mann
Department of Otorhinolaryngology
The University of Mainz Hospitals and Clinics, Mainz, Germany

Alexander Margulis MD
Senior Lecturer
Hebrew University
School of Medicine
Head—Center for Pediatric and Craniofacial Plastic Surgery
Hadassah Medical Center
Jerusalem, Israel

Nayla Matar
Otolaryngology
Head and Neck Surgery Department
Hôtel Dieu de France
Bellevue Medical Center
Saint-Joseph University
Beirut, Lebanon

Nancy McLaughlin
USA

Andrew J McWhorter
Assistant Professor
Director
Department of Otolaryngology—Head and Neck Surgery
Louisiana State University Health Sciences Center
New Orleans
Louisiana, USA

Madhuri Mehta
Department of Otorhinolaryngology and the Skull Base Group
Dr Balabhai Nanavati Hospital
Mumbai, Maharashtra, India

Jayakumar R Menon
Consultant Laryngologist, Kerala Institute of Medical Sciences
Thiruvananthapuram, Kerala, India

Rajendra B Metgudmath
Consultant, Head and Neck Surgical Oncologist, KLES Dr Prabhakar Kore Hospital and MRC Belgaum
Associate Professor
Surgical Oncology (Head and Neck)
JN Medical College, KLE University
Belgaum, Karnataka, India

Jignesh Mewa
Department of Surgical Oncology
Prince Aly Khan Hospital
Mumbai, Maharashtra, India

Julie A Miller
Department of Surgery
Royal Melbourne Hospital and University of Melbourne, Australia

Sonal Modi
Department of Otorhinolaryngology and the Skull Base Group
Dr Balabhai Nanavati Hospital
Mumbai, Maharashtra, India

Arash Mohebati
Senior Fellow in Head and Neck Surgery
Memorial Sloan Kettering Cancer Center New York, USA

Aliasgar Moiyadi
Associate Professor
Department of Neurosurgery
Tata Memorial Center
Mumbai, Maharashtra, India

Simonetta Monini
ENT Clinic, Sant'Andrea Hospital
Sapienza University
Rome, Italy

Eric J Moore MD
Mayo Clinic Department of Otolaryngology
Head and Neck Surgery
200 First Street SW
Rochester, Minnesota, USA

KP Morwani
Department of ENT and Skull Base Surgery
Dr Balabhai Nanavati Hospital
Mumbai, Maharashtra, India

Fabrizio Moscatiello MD PhD
Plastic Surgery Department,
Centro Medico TEKNON
Vilana, Barcelona, Spain

RS Mudhol
Professor and Head, Department of ENT, KLE University's JN Medical College and
Consultant ENT surgeon, KLES Dr Prabhakar Kore Hospital
Belgaum, Karnataka
India

Rajashekhar Myageri
Assistant Professor
SDM Medical College
Dharwad, Karnataka, India

Lalita Naik
Skull Base Surgery Team,
Dr Balabhai Nanavati Hospital
Mumbai, Maharashtra, India

Haralampos Gouveris
Department of Otorhinolaryngology,
The University of Mainz Hospitals
and Clinics, Mainz, Germany

Deepa Nair
Assistant Professor
Department of Head and Neck
Surgical Oncology
Tata Memorial Center
Mumbai, Maharashtra, India

Amith Naragund
Assistant Professor, Department of
ENT, KLE University's
JN Medical College and
Consultant ENT Surgeon, KLES
Dr Prabhakar Kore Hospital
Belgaum, Karnataka, India

Chitra Nayak
Associate Professor and Head
Department of Dermatology
TN Medical College and
BYL Nair Charitable Hospital
Mumbai, Maharashtra, India

Nupur Kapoor Nerurkar
Laryngologist
Bombay Hospital
Mumbai, Maharashtra, India

Thomas P Nikolopoulos
Associate Professor—ENT Surgeon
2nd University Department of
Otorhinolaryngology
Head and Neck Surgery
ATTIKON Hospital, Rimini 1,
Chaidari Athens, Greece

Jerzy Nyzio MD
Intensive Care Unit
St John Grande's Hospital
Kraków, Poland

Matthew Old
Department of Otolaryngology and
Head and Neck Surgery
The Ohio State University
Columbus, USA

Peter D Oliver
Department of Otolaryngology
Head and Neck Surgery
Louisiana State University Health
Sciences Center
Bolivar Street
New Orleans
Louisiana, USA

Goldan Oren MD
Attending Surgeon, Division of
Plastic and Reconstructive Surgery
Sheba Medical Center
Tel-Aviv University
Ramat Gan, Israel

Bradley A Otto
Assistant Professor,
Department of Otolaryngology and
Head and Neck Surgery
The Ohio State University
Columbus, USA

Sumeet Pahwa
Fellow, Surgical Oncology
Prince Aly Khan Hospital
Mumbai, Maharashtra
India

Prathamesh S Pai
Associate Professor
Department of Head and Neck
Surgical Oncology
Tata Memorial Center
Mumbai, Maharashtra
India

Giampiero Parrinello MD
Otolaryngologist, PhD Student
SOD Otolaryngology
Department of Surgical Sciences
AOU-Careggi, University of Florence
Vle Morgagni
Florence, Italy

Prashant Patil
Associate Professor
JN Medical College
Belgaum, Karnataka
India

Amol Patil
Department of Otorhinolaryngology
and The Skull Base Group
Dr Balabhai Nanavati Hospital
Mumbai, Maharashtra
India

R N Patil
Professor
Department of ENT, KLE University's
JN Medical College and
Consultant ENT surgeon, KLES
Dr Prabhakar Kore Hospital
Belgaum, Karnataka, India

Sultan A Pradhan
Professor and Chief Oncologist
Department of Surgical Oncology
Prince Aly Khan Hospital
Mumbai, Maharashtra, India

Rashmi Prashant
Assistant Professor,
Department of ENT
DY Patil Medical College
Pimpri, Maharashtra, India

Alberto Prats-Galino MD PhD
Laboratory of Surgical
Neuroanatomy (LSNA)
Faculty of Medicine
Universitat de Barcelona
Barcelona, Spain

Daniel M Prevedello
Assistant Professor
Department of Neurological Surgery
The Ohio State University
Columbus, USA

Ashutosh G Pusalkar
Emeritus Professor,
Padmashree Dr DY Patil Medical College, Honorary Consultant
Lilavati Hospital and Medical Research Center
Mumbai, Maharashtra, India

Ullas Raghavan FRCS (ORL-HNS)
Doncaster Royal Infirmary Hospital
Doncaster, UK

S Raghunandhan MS DNB MRCS (Ed) DOHNS
Consultant ENT Surgeon
Department of Implant Otology
Madras ENT Research Foundation
Raja Annamalaipuram
Chennai, Tamil Nadu, India

Kannan Rajan
Senior Oncosurgeon
Department of Surgical Oncology
Prince Aly Khan Hospital
Mumbai, Maharashtra, India

Reema Rai
Resident
Department of ENT and Head and Neck Surgery
TN Medical College and BYL Nair Charitable Hospital
Mumbai Maharashtra, India

Suthee Rattanathummawat MD ENT
Phramongkutklao Hospital
Medical University
Bangkok, Thailand

C Rayappa
Department of Head and Neck and Skull Base Surgery
Apollo Speciality Hospital
Chennai, Tamil Nadu, India

Marc Remacle
Otolaryngology
Head and Neck Surgery Department
Louvain University Hospital of Mont-Godinne, Yvoir, Belgium

Roberta Rehder MD
Resident Program
Evangelic Universitary Hospital
Curitiba
Paraná - Brazil

Gresham T Richter MD
Department of Otolaryngology—Head and Neck Surgery
University of Arkansas for Medical Sciences
Arkansas Children's Hospital
Little Rock, Arkansas, USA

Nestor Rigual
Department of Head and Neck/ Plastic Surgery,
Roswell Park Cancer Institute,
Buffalo, NY, USA

Supriya Rode
Resident - Department of ENT and Head and Neck Surgery
TN Medical College and BYL Nair Charitable Hospital
Mumbai, Maharashtra, India

Philippe Rombaux
Department of Otorhinolaryngology
University of Louvain
Cliniques Saint Luc Brussels
Av Hippocrate, Brussels, Belgium

Sabino Russo MD
Consultant in Otolaryngology
Head and Neck Surgery
Department of Otolaryngology
Head and Neck Surgery
National Cancer Institute
Giovanni Paolo II
Vle Flacco
Bari, Italy

H Sadick
Head and Chair of the Department of ORL and Head and Neck Surgery
University Hospital of Mannheim
Mannheim
Germany

Dariusz Sagan
Department of Thoracic Surgery
Medical University of Lublin
Poland

Lucel E Salvan DA
Secretary
ENT-Voice Center
Yanhee International Hospital
Bangkok
Thailand

Suresh Sankhla
Department of Neurosurgery
Dr Balabhai Nanavati Hospital
Mumbai, Maharashtra
India

Zoukaa Sargi
Department of Otolaryngology,
Head and Neck Surgery,
University of Miami Miller School of Medicine
Miami
Florida, USA

Tamer Seyhan MD
Assoc. Prof. of Plastic Reconstructive and Esthetic Surgery
Adana Numune Education and Teaching Hospital
Cukurova, Adana
Turkey

Nishit J Shah
Department of ENT
Bombay Hospital
Mumbai, Maharashtra
India

Jatin P Shah MD MS (Surg) FACS Hon FRCS (Edin) Hon FDSRCS (London) Hon FRACS
Professor of Surgery
EW Strong Chair in Head and Neck Oncology
Chief
Head and Neck Service
Memorial Sloan
Kettering Cancer Center
New York, USA

Hemant Sharma
Resident
Department of ENT and
Head and Neck Surgery
TN Medical College and
BYL Nair Charitable Hospital
Mumbai, Maharashtra, India

Atsushi Shiraishi
Department of Ophthalmology
Ehime University School of Medicine
Shitsukawa, Toon, Ehime, Japan

A M Shivakumar
Professor and Head
Department of ENT
SS Institute of Medical Sciences and
Research Center, Davangere, India

Shy Stahl MD
Attending Surgeon, Division of
Plastic and Reconstructive Surgery
Sheba Medical Center, Tel-Aviv
University, Ramat Gan, Israel

Michael C Singer MD
Instructor
Department of Otolaryngology—
Head and Neck Surgery
Medical College of Georgia, Georgia

PP Singh
Director-Professor and Head
Department of ENT and Head
Neck Surgery, University College of
Medical Sciences and GTB Hospital
New Delhi, India

Murat Songu
Department of Otorhinolaryngology
—Head and Neck Surgery
Dr Behçet Uz Children's
Hospital, Izmir, Department of
Otorhinolaryngology Head and
Neck Surgery, Izmir Ataturk
Research and Training Hospital
Izmir, Turkey

Jonathan E Sorrel
Department of Otolaryngology
Head and Neck Surgery
Louisiana State University Health
Sciences Center and
School of Medicine
New Orleans, Louisiana, USA

Giuseppe Spinelli MD
Maxillo-Facial Surgeon
Chief of the Department of
Traumatology and
Maxillo-Facial Surgery
AOUC Hospital and
University of Florence Largo Palagi
Florence, Italy

Ornouma Sriwanishvipat MD ENT
Yanhee International Hospital
Bangkok, Thailand

Milan Stankovic MD
Clinic for ORL
Medical Faculty University of NIS
Serbia

Andrzej Stepulak
Department of Biochemistry and
Molecular Biology
Medical University of Lublin
Poland

RJ Stokroos
Department of Otorhinolaryngology
and Head and Neck Surgery
Maastricht University
Medical Center
The Netherlands

Girish Surlikar MS (opthal) DOMS FCPS DNB
Ophthalmologist
Private Practice
Mumbai, Maharashtra
India

Harumi Suzaki
Department of Otorhinolaryngology
Showa University
School of Medicine
Hatanodai, Shinagawa
Tokyo, Japan

Andrew C Swift
Consultant ENT Surgeon and
Rhinologist
Aintree University Hospitals
Foundation NHS Trust
Liverpool, UK

Taizo Takeda MD
Emeritus Professor
Kochi Medical School
Kochi, Japan

Paul A Tennant MD
Resident in Otolaryngology
University of Louisville
Kentucky, USA

David J Terris MD FACS
Porubsky Professor and Chairman
Department of Otolaryngology—
Head and Neck Surgery
Medical College of Georgia, Georgia

Alok Thakar
Department of Otorhinolaryngology
All India Institute of Medical
Sciences (AIIMS)
New Delhi, India

Kiskumar Thankappan
Amrita Institute of Medical Sciences
Elamakkara
Kochi, Kerala, India

C Thomas MS FRCS FACS
Senior Consultant and
Head Plastic Surgery
Service in Oman

Livnat Siman Tov MD
Aesthetic and Reconstructive
Plastic Surgeon, Jerusalem, Israel

Jagadish Tubachi
Fellow
Department of Surgical Oncology
Prince Aly Khan Hospital
Mumbai, Maharashtra, India

Jumroon Tungkeeratichai
Assistant Professor
Facial Plastic and
Reconstructive Surgery
Otolaryngology Head and Neck
Surgery, Faculty of medicine
Ramathibodi Hospital
Mahidol University
Bangkok, Thailand

Prof Tuncay Ulug MD
Department of Otorhinolaryngology
Istanbul University-Istanbul
Medical Faculty
Capa, Istanbul, Turkey

Hirohito Umeno MD
Associate professor
Otolaryngology Head and
Neck Surgery
Kurume University
School of Medicine
Asahi-Machi Kurume, Japan

Abhishek D Vaidya
Fellow, Head and Neck Surgery
Tata Memorial Hospital
Mumbai, Maharashtra, India

Gauri Vaidya
Department of ENT
Bombay Hospital
Mumbai, Maharashtra, India

Saurabh Varshney
Professor and Head
Department of ENT
Himalayan Institute of Medical
Sciences, (HIHT University)
Jolly Grant; Doiwala
Dehradun, Uttarakhand, India

B K Venkatesha
Department of ENT
SS Institute of Medical Sciences and
Research Center
Davangere, Karnataka, India

Giovanni André Pires Viana MD
Cliniplast
Al. Jauaperi
São Paulo, SP, Brazil

Rohan R Walvekar MD
Associate Professor
Department of Otolaryngology
Head and Neck Surgery
Louisiana State University
Health Sciences Center
Bolivar Street
New Orleans, Louisiana, USA

Jeremy Warner MD
Division of Plastic Surgery
North Shore University Health
System, Central Street
Evanston, Illinois, USA

JJ Waterval
Department of Otorhinolaryngology
and Head and Neck Surgery
Maastricht University Medical Center
The Netherlands

Parag Watve
Resident
Department of ENT and
Head and Neck Surgery
TN Medical College and
BYL Nair Charitable Hospital
Mumbai Maharashtra
India

Stephen Wetmore MD
Professor and Chair
Department of Otolaryngology
West Virginia University
School of Medicine
Morgantown, West Virginia, USA

Jeremy B White
Plastic Surgeon
ARC Plastic Surgery
Stirling Road
Hollywood, Florida, USA

Adele P Williams
Department of Otolaryngology
Head and Neck Surgery
Louisiana State University
Health Sciences Center
Bolivar Street
New Orleans, Louisiana, USA

Eyal Winkler MD
Assistant Professor of Plastic Surgery
Director of the Division of Plastic
and Reconstructive Surgery
Sheba Medical Center
Tel-Aviv University
Ramat Gan
Israel

R Yadav MS (ENT) DORL FCPS
Assosiate Professor
Rajawadi Hospital
Mumbai, Maharashtra
India

Kazunari Yoshida
Associate Professor
Department of Neurosurgery
Keio University
School of Medicine, Japan

Ramzi Younis
Department of Otolaryngology
University of Miami School of Medicine, USA

Alper Yüksel
Fatih University, Faculty of Medicine
Department of Otorhinolaryngology
Head and Neck Surgery
Ankara, Turkey

Olaf Zagólski MD PhD
ENT
St John Grande's Hospital
Kraków, Poland

Diego Zanetti
Department of Otorhinolaryngology
San Gerardo Hospital
University of Milano Bicocca
Monza, Italy

Maria Zisiopoulou
Department of Otorhinolaryngology
The University of Mainz Hospitals and Clinics, Mainz, Germany

Foreword

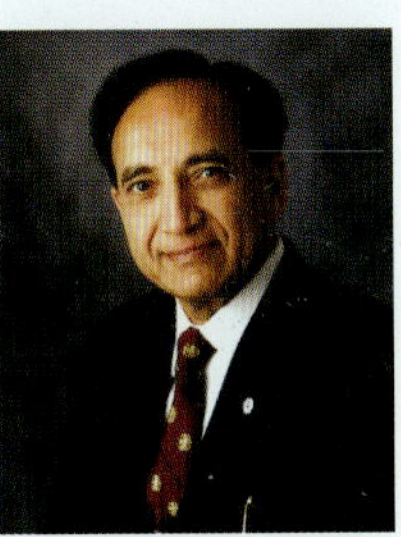

In spite of significant advances made in the multidisciplinary treatment of diseases and neoplasia in the head and neck region, surgery remains the mainstay amongst all therapeutic modalities currently available for these conditions. Surgical techniques have however, undergone significant evolution with major emphasis on preservation or restoration of form and function. This has resulted in the development of minimally invasive techniques. Technological advances in endoscopic instrumentation have ushered in the era of endoscopic surgery, replacing the well-established techniques of open surgery of the nasal cavity and paranasal sinuses. Major strides in imaging techniques over the past three decades, has facilitated accurate assessment of the extent of a neoplasm and has facilitated development of computer-assisted surgical techniques with intraoperative navigation and Robotic surgery. Thus, the surgical specialty of Otolaryngology and Head & Neck Surgery has dramatically changed over the years, and remains a challenging and continuously evolving field.

The editors of this magnificent work, Drs Bachi T Hathiram and Vicky S Khattar have done a splendid job in putting together a state-of-the art surgical atlas by recruiting specialists from all parts of the world who have contributed their specific areas of expertise in demonstrating surgical techniques. The atlas is lavishly illustrated with operative pictures, imaging studies, and superb artwork to accompany the procedural details and operative photographs. The rationale, indications, step-by-step details of the procedure, and postoperative management and complications, makes this a complete surgical treatise, equally useful to the trainee and the surgeon in practice.

This opus of operative surgery is presented in five volumes, covering a total of 195 operative procedures and their variations. The compilation covers nearly all the operative procedures from the 'Dura to Pleura', in the repertoire of the Otolaryngologist /Head and Neck Surgeon. This would be an essential textbook for a surgeon or surgeon in training, to familiarize oneself with an operative procedure, and go prepared to the operating room to carry out a safe and successful surgical procedure. The Editors and the Publishers of this excellent Atlas are to be commended for bringing about this excellent book, and offering it at an affordable price to surgeons of all generations. I am confident that this book will be an essential 'read', for Otolaryngologist / Head and Neck Surgeons, worldwide for years to come.

Jatin P Shah MD MS (Surg) FACS Hon FRCS (Edin)
Hon FDSRCS (London) Hon FRACS
Professor of Surgery
Elliot W Strong Chair in Head and Neck Oncology
Memorial Sloan Kettering Cancer Center
New York, USA

Foreword

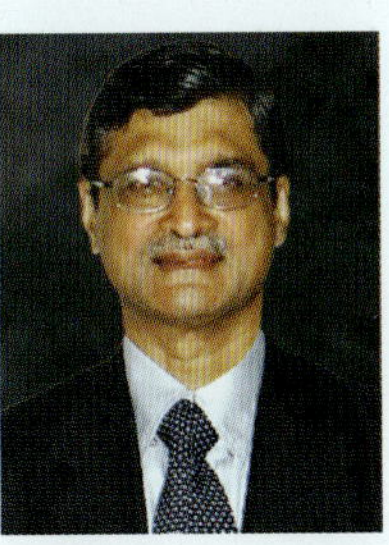

It is a pleasure to write the foreword for the *Atlas of Operative Otorhinolaryngology and Head & Neck Surgery*. Today, the field of Medicine and especially the field of Otorhinolaryngology and Head & Neck Surgery is advancing by leaps and bounds in expertise and technology. With evidence-based medicine being at the forefront of our practice, mastering the skills of the surgical technique and the rationale behind this is of equal importance to the surgeon. There are various centers of excellence all over the world specializing in particular aspects of our field and it is common practice for the trainee doctors as well as established surgeons to visit these from time to time to learn and to upgrade their skills.

This exhaustive compilation by the editors, Dr Bachi T Hathiram and Dr Vicky S Khattar is an attempt to bring together the best in the field of Otorhinolaryngology and Head & Neck Surgery under one title. With its five volumes on Otology and Lateral Skullbase Surgery, Rhinology and Anterior Skullbase Surgery, Facial Plastics, Cosmetics and Reconstructive Surgery, Voice and Laryngotracheal Surgery and Head & Neck Surgery, the editors have aimed to cover topics dealing with routine procedures as also, those that are at the cutting edge of technology.

The Atlas comprises of 195 Chapters with intraoperative images and clear line diagrams/figures making it easy to understand the surgical steps. There are contributors from all over the world, each a master in his/her own technique. More than 30 countries have participated in this mammoth and prestigious venture thus, making it unique in our field and one of a kind, lending to it a truly global perspective.

In addition to this pictoral step-by-step depiction of surgeries, there will follow a similarly exhaustive compilation of teaching DVDs which will further enhance the learning process.

I am sure this academic venture will go a long way in benefitting not only the trainees but also established specialists.

Milind V Kirtane

Professor Emeritus Seth GS Medical College
Hon Surgeon at KEM Hospital
Hon Consulting ENT Surgeon at PD Hinduja National Hospital
Hon ENT Consultant to his Excellency the Governor of Maharashtra
Hon ENT Consultant at Prince Aly Khan Hospital
Mumbai, Maharashtra, India

Preface

In today's age of rapid advances in science and technology, there is no dearth of learning material available to the avid learner. However, in the field of Otorhinolaryngology and Head & Neck Surgery, there seemed a lacuna between undergoing surgical training at various places and understanding the concepts/rationale behind the surgical technique. This book is a modest attempt by the editors to bridge this lacuna by going through each surgery in a simple step-wise manner using intraoperative images and illustrated figures, wherever required, to help understand the technique of surgery.

This is essentially an atlas and hence, the stress on learning through intraoperative images and illustrations, making it easy for the trainee as well as the ENT consultant to follow the surgery. The authors are masters in the field and this is a mammoth compilation from more than 30 countries from all over the world since knowledge cannot be bound by any barriers.

We feel that it is never too late to learn and especially as surgeons, it is imperative to keep in touch with the recent advances in our field and we hope to spread this message amongst our fraternity through this atlas. The Atlas discusses not only routinely performed surgeries, such as tonsillectomy, septoplasty, tympanoplasty, thyroidectomy and tracheostomy but also the latest advances in our field such as robotics, endoscopic skullbase surgery and sialoendoscopy. It is targeted to young trainee surgeons as well as specialists in the field who would like to learn the techniques of surgery from the masters.

Bachi T Hathiram

Vicky S Khattar

Acknowledgments

We would like to express our gratitude to our publishers, M/s Jaypee Brothers Medical Publishers (P) Ltd, New Delhi, India, especially Shri Jitendar P Vij for having the vision and faith in us, Ms Chetna Malhotra Vohra for her patience, perseverance and perfection, Ms Payal Bharti, Mr Arun Sharma and the entire team for their untiring efforts in completing this book on time. Also, we would like to thank all our students who have taught us in addition to learning from us; Reema Rai, Harshad Nikte, Parag Watve, Harshal Sonavane, Snigdha Devane, Anjoo Choudhary, Alok Nema, Supriya Rode, Balagopal Kurup, Hemant Sharma, Sunil Khot, Sanket Dani, Ankit Jain, Diptarka Bhattacharya, Sobhana Chandran and Lubna Sayed. They have all contributed to the making of this Atlas in significant ways. Most importantly, our teachers who have not only taught us surgery but, given us the drive to teach and impart knowledge.

Contents

Volume 3

3

Section

Facial Plastics, Cosmetics and Reconstructive Surgery

Chapters Outline

CHAPTER

89 Chemical Peels

Chitra Nayak

DEFINITION

Chemical peeling is defined as application of one or more chemoexfoliating agents to the skin resulting in destruction of portions of epidermis or/and dermis with resulting regeneration of new epidermal and dermal tissues.[1]

HISTORY

- *Egypt*:
  - First evidence of exfoliants use.
  - Sun-damaged skin was a sign of lower rank in society.
  - Sour milk containing lactic acid, an alpha-hydroxy acid (AHA), is commonly used today[1] (Fig. 1).
- *Turks*: Used fire to produce thermal exfoliation.

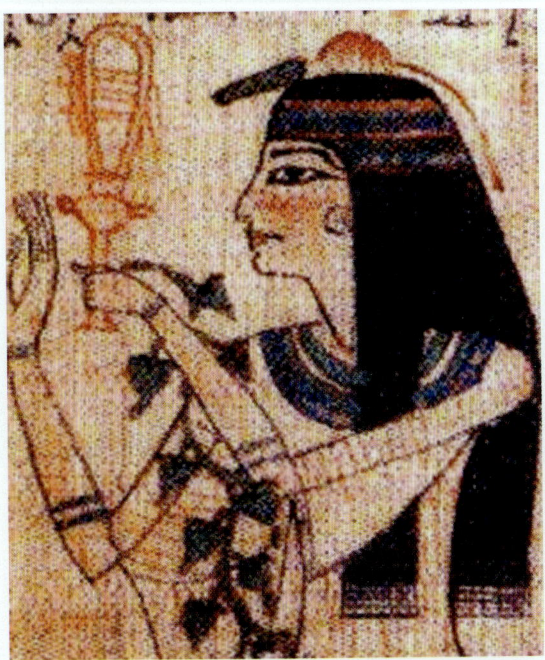

Fig. 1: An Egyption female using sour milk as a natural peel

Historical Timeline

- *1882*: PG Unna, German dermatologist described the use of resorcinol, salicylic acid (SA), phenol, trichloroacetic acid (TCA)
- *1903*: Mackee (Chairman of Dermatology at New York University) began using phenol for acne scarring.
- *1961*: Baker and Gordon presented a peel formula with one patient with a 3-month follow-up which became the standard formula.
- *1966*: Baker published results in 250 patients.

PRINCIPLE

Chemical peeling is used to create epidermal/dermal wounding enough to stimulate regeneration from the appendages and dermis via wound healing.[2]

HISTOLOGY

Actinic Changes[3]

Photochemical effects of solar radiation exposure:[3]

- Disorderly arrangement of epidermis
- Degeneration of the elastic network
- Mottled pigmentation
- Lymphocytic infiltration
- Decrease in collagen
- Flattening of the dermal-epidermal junction
- Epidermal cell atypia
- Increased melanocytes, but they were unevenly distributed and contained variable amounts of melanin.

Peel Skin Histology[4,5] (Figs 2 to 5)

- *At 2 weeks*:
  - New collagen formation begins and may continue up to 1 year
  - New bands of dermis 2–3 mm thick
  - Thin, compact and parallel collagen bundles arranged horizontally along the epidermal-dermal matrix.

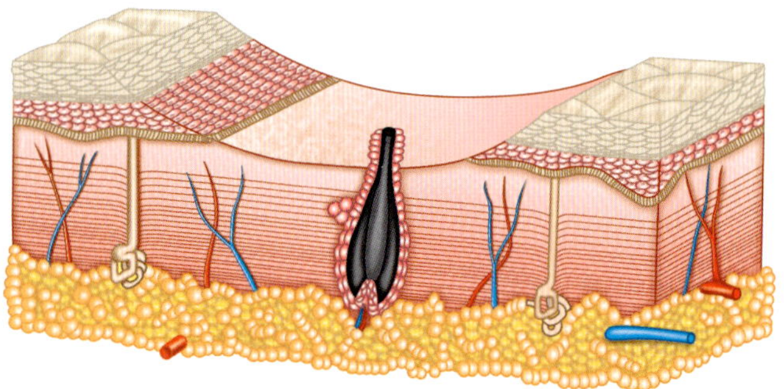

Fig. 2: Chemical burn of the epidermis and the outer dermis

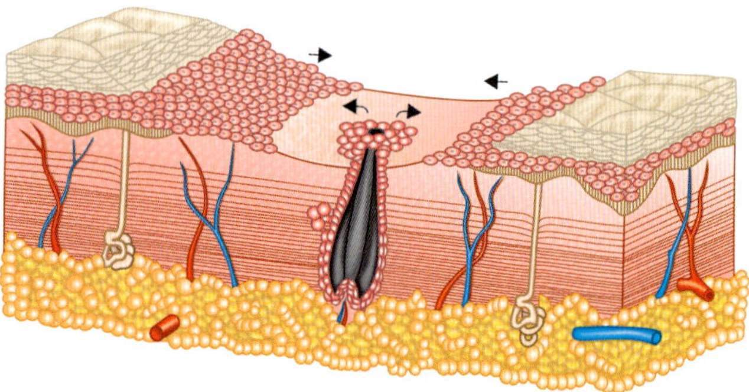

Fig. 3: First 2–5 days: Regeneration from follicular and eccrine duct epithelium

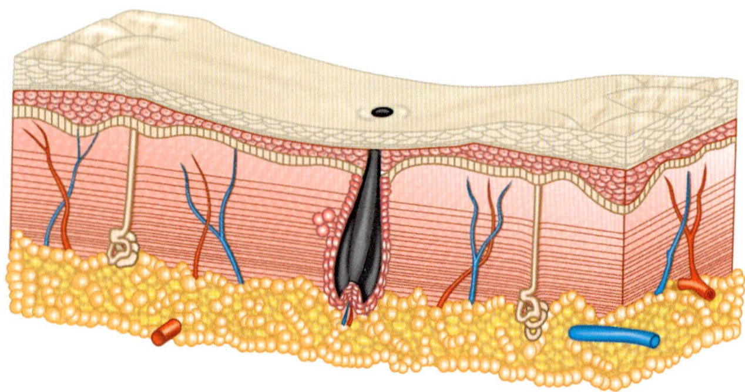

Fig. 4: Fresh, orderly and organized epidermis

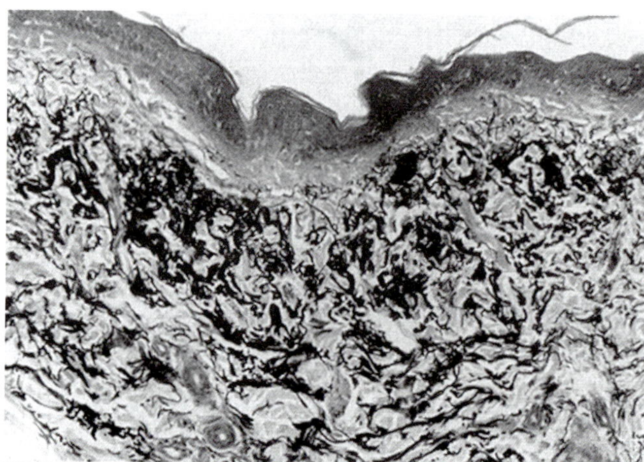

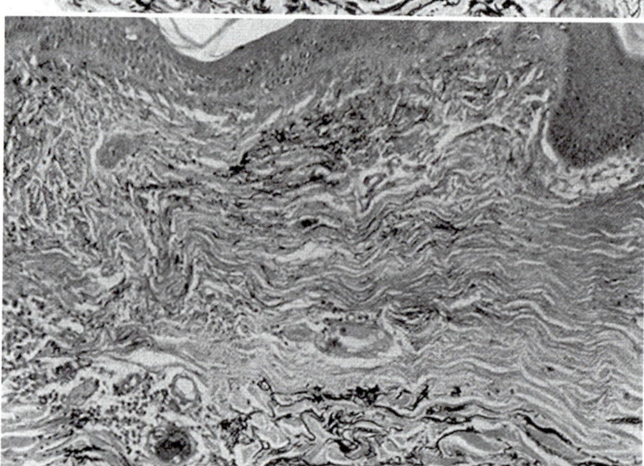

Fig. 5: Dermal collagen and extracellular matrix remodeling after deep peeling

Other Changes

- Melanocytes contain fine, evenly distributed melanin granules
- Impaired melanin synthesis with a generalized bleaching effect
- Decreased lymphocytic infiltration.

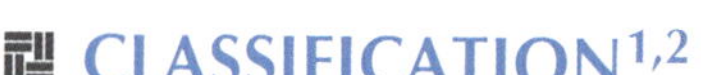

CLASSIFICATION[1,2]

- Brody's classification
- Mark Rubin's classification

Classification According to Depth of Peel

- Very superficial exfoliation
- Superficial (epidermal)
- Medium (papillary dermis)
- Deep (reticular dermis)

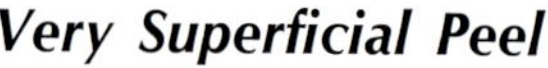

Very Superficial Peel

- Only stratum corneum is thinned out or removed without creating wound below stratum granulosum i.e. general epidermal wounding.
- It is suited for all skin types.
- It is also known as "freshening peel".
- *Solutions used*: Resorcinol, Jessner's solution, tretinoin, AHA [glycolic acid (GA), lactic acid], SA, TCA 10%, CO_2 slush, liquid nitrogen.

Superficial Peel

- Necrosis of part or all of epidermis from stratum granulosum to basal cell layer
- Solutions used
  - Trichloroacetic acid 15–20%
  - Glycolic acid 30–50%
  - Resorcinol
  - Jessner's solution.

Factors influencing depth of peel:

- Peeling agents and concentration
- Priming/degreasing done before
- *Mode of application*: Painting/rubbing
- *Current on-going medications*: Isotretinoin
- *Location*: Facial/non-facial peel
- *Skin condition*: Thin/thick, dry/oily.

Medium Depth Peel

- Peeling up to papillary dermis
- *Solutions used*:
  - Trichloroacetic acid 35%
  - CO_2 slush prior to TCA
  - Jessner's solution prior to TCA
  - Glycolic acid applied and washed off prior to TCA.

Medium-Deep Depth Peel

- *Solutions used*:
  - Trichloroacetic acid 50%
  - Combination of GA 50% + TCA 35%.

Deep Peel

- Peeling up to reticular dermal layer
- *Formula used*: Baker's/Gordon phenol formula.

MECHANISM OF ACTION[6]

- Creating wound/necrosis of epidermal cells leads to repair mechanism wherein damaged skin is replaced with normalized tissue thereby achieving better cosmic results.
- Removal of stratum corneum results in stimulation of epidermal growth.
- Inflammatory reaction in deep dermis activates mediators of inflammation resulting in angiogenesis and collagen remodeling; also increased production of glycosaminoglycans in dermis (Fig. 5).
- Epidermal regeneration within 2–7 days. Heals completely in 2 weeks.

INDICATIONS OF PEELS

- *Photoaging*: Actinic keratosis, solar elastosis, solar lentigines, pigmentary alterations, fine wrinkles.[7]
- *Pigmentary disturbances*: Melasma, postinflammatory hyperpigmentation, freckles, fixed drug eruption, lentigines.
- *Rhytids*: Actinic, dynamic, sleep
- *Others*
  - Rough, oily skin
  - Dilated pores
  - Superficial scarring
  - Radiation keratoses
  - Acne vulgaris and rosacea
  - Flat facial warts and milia
  - Pseudofolliculitis barbae
  - Xanthelasma and acanthosis nigricans

CONTRAINDICATIONS

- Keloidal tendencies
- *Active infection*: Herpes/bacterial
- Open wounds
- Unrealistic expectations
- Recent radiation treatment or surgery
- Warts

IMPROVEMENT IN PHOTOAGING (FIGS 6A AND B)

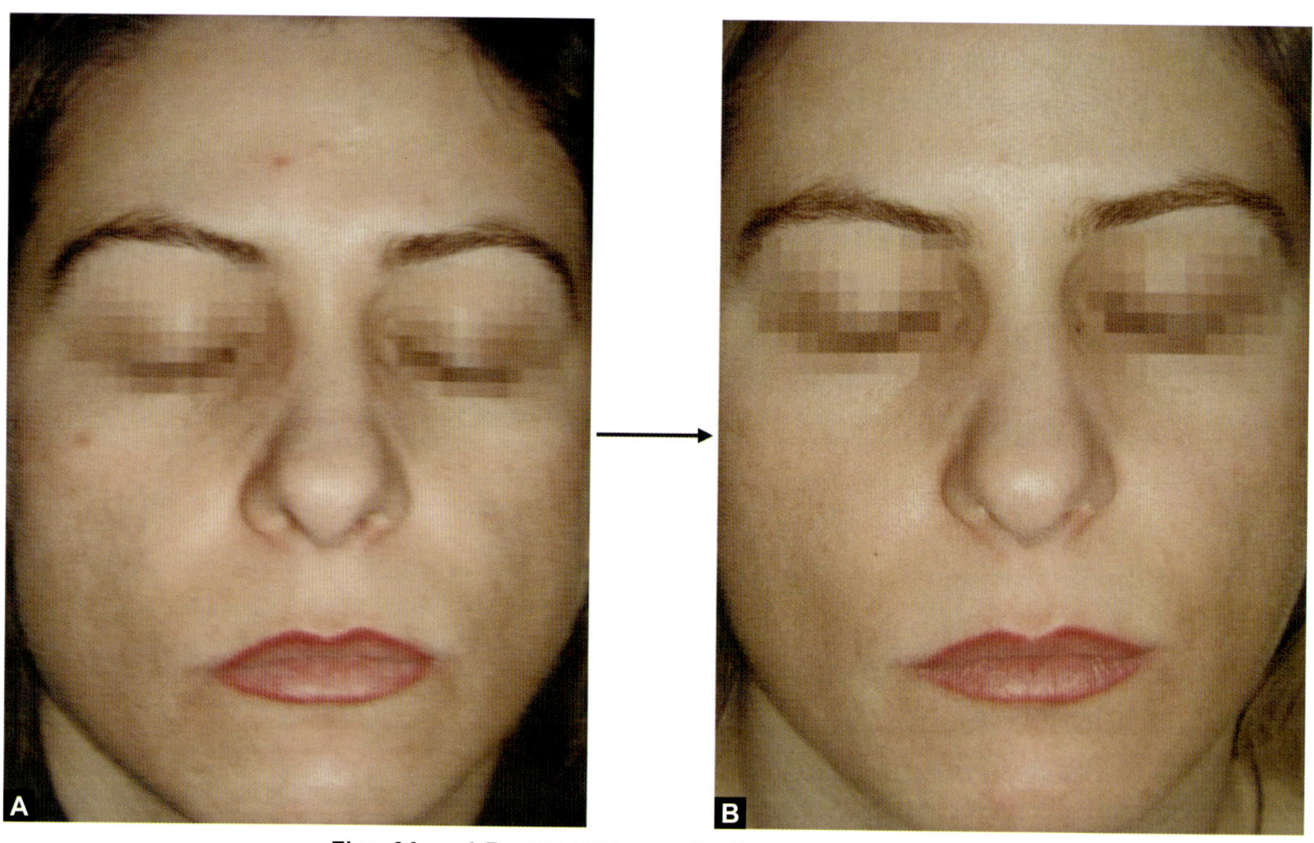

Figs 6A and B: 20% TCA-peel. (A) Pre-peel; (B) Post-peel

PATIENT SELECTION

- "The ideal patient is a thin-skinned female with fair complexion and fine rhytids."
- Skin type and the amount of photo damage present.
- Fitzpatrick classified the skin types on the basis of color and acute solar radiation response (Table 1).
- The Glogau classification is based on the degree of photoaging (Table 2).

History Taking

- History of recent facial surgery/peels and outcome
- Herpes simplex
- Current medications
- Immunocompromised states/susceptibility
- Recent facial X-ray therapy
- Recent isotretinoin
- Keloids/hypertrophic scarring
- Concurrent product/treatment used.

Fitzpatrick Classification (Table 1)

Table 1: Fitzpatrick classification

- Fitzpatrick skin type I and type II are good candidates
- *Type III and greater:* Increased risk pigment complications

Table 1: Fitzpatrick classification of skin types

Type	*Color*	*Tanning response*
I	White	Always burns, never tans
II	White	Usually burns, tans less than average
III	White	Sometimes burns mildly, tans about average
IV	Brown	Rarely burns, tans more than average and with ease
V	Dark brown	Very rarely burns, tans very easily
VI	Black	Never burns, tans very easily

Glogau Classification (Table 2)

Table 2: Glogau classification of photoaging

Group	*Classification*	*Skin characteristics*	*Peel*
I	Mild	Little wrinking or scarring and no keratoses	Superficial
II	Moderate	Early wrinkling, mid scarring, and sallow color with early actinic keratoses	Medium
III	Advanced	Persistent wrinkling, discoloration with telangiectasias and actinic keratoses	Medium
IV	Servere	Wrinkling—superficial to deep actinic keratoses ± skin cancer	Medium to deep

EXAMINATION PRIOR TO PEELS

- General cutaneous examination
- Fitzpatrick skin type to predict pigmentary response to peeling
- Degree of photoaging
- Degree of sebaceous secretions
- Laxity of skin
- Presence of keloid/hypertrophic scar
- Presence of active dermatitis/infection in areas to be peeled

ADVANTAGES OF PRIMING

- *Reduces wound healing time*: Speeds up re-epithelialization.
- More uniform penetration of peeling agent.
- Decreased risk of postinflammatory hyperpigmentation.
- Use of hydroquinone (HQ), kojic acid and azelaic acid enhance skin lightening with dispersion of melanin granules throughout epidermis.
- Enforces concept of maintenance regimen and helps to assess patient's skin tolerability.

PREPEEL PROCEDURES[8]

- Counseling
- *Test peel*: Postauricular
- Photodocumentation
- Written informed consent

Counseling

- Patient/physician expectations to avoid unrealistic expectations and disappointment
- Need for multiple office visits for staged peeling and improvement
- Enforce importance of post-peel care and treatment of complications.

Preparation of Skin

- *Keratotic lesions*: Seborrheic keratoses; warts to be removed 2 weeks prior to peeling
- *Priming*: Topical retinoic acid in acne vulgaris
- Alpha-hydroxy acid in acne and pigmentary alterations
- Hydroquinone and kojic acid in melasma and hyperpigmentation
- Broad-spectrum sunscreen
- Antiviral in patients with history of herpes simplex infection in areas to be treated.

Before Peel

- To wash face with soap and water to remove makeup and surface oils
- Wipe face dry
- Remove contact lenses if
- Hair should be secured off the face using clips/rubber band
- Place a fan 4 feet from patient's face to help keep the skin cool to reduce discomfort during procedure.

During Peel

- Patient should sit in reclining position with 45° head elevation to avoid the acid pooling around unwanted areas.
- *Degreasing of area*: To remove excess of sebum, dirt, debris and allow better, uniform penetration of peeling agent.
- *Commonly used agents*: Acetone, alcohol, chlorhexidine gluconate (Hibiclens®).
- Gentle wiping of area unidirectionally with gauze or cotton ball as scrabbing causes friction and damages the skin.

Precautions

- Position
- Label checking to confirm strength and substance.
- Avoid dripping of solution into non-peel areas
- Never pass on open container of acid over patient's face to avoid accidental spilling
- Water prefilled syringe to flush eyes in case of accidental spilling
- Stand in front of patient and watch for untoward reactions
- Give adequate post-peel care instructions
- Apply petrolatum to any cuts, abrasions, creases of mouth, nose and eyes.

TRICHLOROACETIC ACID PEEL[8]

- It is used to treat aging and premalignant skin conditions.
- It destroys epidermis and upper dermis; causes necrosed skin to exfoliate within 2–3 weeks.
- Sloughed epidermis is replaced by new epidermis within a week while regeneration of dermis takes 2–3 weeks and remodeling of collagen continue for up to 6 months.

Preparation of Solution

- 10 g of TCA United States Pharmacopoeia (USP) crystals w/v in 100 cc distilled water = 10% TCA
- *Brands*:
  - Easy TCA
  - Obagi Blue Peel®
  - Compositum Peel
  - AcuPeel

Depth and Concentration

- *Superficial peel (20%)*: Used for acne, photoaging, freckles, melasma, shallow complexion, vitiligo and seborrheic melanoses (Figs 6A and B).
- *Intermediate peel (35%)*: Used for lentigines, wrinkles and actinic keratoses.
- *Deep peel (50%)*: Used for xanthelasma, acne scars, severe photoaging and striae distensae (Fig. 7).

Advantages

- Safe and inexpensive
- Few medical contraindications
- No systemic toxicity and allergic reaction
- Depth of peel is achieved by adjusting TCA concentration
- No need to neutralize peel.

Trichloroacetic Acid in Combination

- Tape occlusion
- Trichloroacetic acid + Tretinoin cream preoperative and postoperative
- Trichloroacetic acid + 5-Fluorouracil (5-FU)
- Trichloroacetic acid + Microdermabrasion
- Trichloroacetic acid + Phenol
- Trichloroacetic acid + Solid CO_2
- Resorcinol/spot peel
- Lactic acid, GA, resorcinol and SA.

Application Protocol

- *Level 0*: No frost.
- *Level 1*: Irregular frosting giving skin a wispy appearance—superficial intraepidermal peel.
- *Level 2*: Skin shows white frost with pink red background colour—peel extends up to dermoepidermal junction.
- *Level 3*: Solid intense white frost with no pink/white background—peel up to papillary dermis.

Postpeel Events

- Area is pink for first 2–3 days when calamine lotion is applied to initiate exfoliation during next 2 days.
- Skin darkens by 5th day.
- Skin begins to peel and is complete in 10 days.

Postpeel Care

- Application of sunscreens or emollients immediately after peel
- Not to peel, pick, scratch or scrape the skin.
- Not to expose the skin to sun/sauna.
- Interval between two peels is 2–3 weeks and concentration can be increased 5–10% with each peel.

ALPHA-HYDROXY ACID PEEL[1,2]

- Most preferred
- They are group of nontoxic organic acids present in natural foods such as fruits, so known as fruit acid.
- *Natural sources*: Sugarcane (GA), sour milk (lactic acid), citrus fruit (citric acid), apple (malic acid), grapes (tartaric acid).

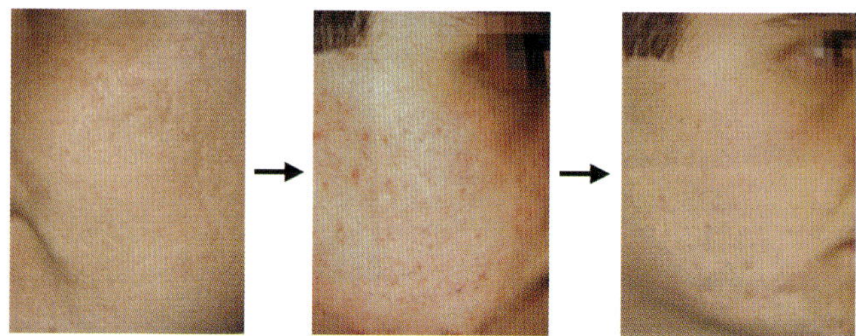

Fig. 7: Trichloroacetic acid (TCA) peel. 50% TCA in acne scars (three sittings)

Preparation and Formulation

- Solutions are made using water, alcohol and propylene glycol.
- In practice, solution is made by bubbling carbon monoxide through formaldehyde.
- *Glycolic acid formulations*: Partially neutralized, buffered, esterified, free GA.

Application Protocol

- Routine degreasing.
- Time bound peel so time to be noted at beginning of peeling using stopwatch.
- Application to be completed within 30 seconds to 1 minute.
- At end, sodium bicarbonate should be sprayed to neutralize action of acids. Bubbling and fizzing occurs on surface of skin. Continue the application till fizzing stops.

Postpeel Care

- Neutralization is exothermic reaction which produces heat making patient's face more erythematous and potentially inducing wounds, so immediately spray ice cold water.
- Dry with towel
- *Mild steroid cream*: Hydrocortisone or an emollient to apply
- Leave at least for 4 hours
- Emollient application: I------------I × 2–7 days to promote healing process
- Avoid products containing SA, AHA and retinoids until normal skin comes back
- Avoid makeup for 24 hours after peel
- Avoid sun exposure, scrubs, abrasive materials and artificial tanning devices

Postpeel Events

- Stinging, redness, burning and tightness, may be some mild swelling, superficial scabbing and peeling. These gradually disappear over period of week.
- Temporary darkening of skin.

Peels Timetable (Table 3)

Advantages

- *Biweekly serial peels*: Effective in treatment of atrophic acne scars
- Fifteen to sixteen peels effective in all types of acne including rapid improvement and appearance of normal skin
- Rapid improvement in comedogenic acne
- For papulopustular acne, average 6 applications.
- For nodulocystic acne, 8–10 applications.
- 50% GA peel/month for 3 months are sufficient for effective treatment in Indian women with melasma.
- No systemic toxicity and well tolerated.

SALICYLIC ACID PEEL[1] (FIG. 8)

- It is also known as beta-hydroxy acid (BHA).
- Popular and inexpensive.
- Superficial, facial and non-facial sites can be done.
- Salicylic acid is a keratolytic agent because of its lipophilic nature. It has strong comedolytic effect.
- It affects arachidonic cascade and thus acts as an anti-inflammatory.

Advantages

- Minimal downtime
- More efficacious when treating fine wrinkles, photoaging, keratoses, acne and depigmentation.

Formulations

- 20–30% on w/v basis in hydroethanolic solution
- 20% w/v: Treatment for facial skin
- 30% w/v: Non-facial sites
- *Brands*:
  - Beta-Lift
  - Bioglan pharmacy
  - Delasco

Procedure

- Application with cotton tip applicator or wedge sponge.

Table 3: Biweekly peel shedule for acne scars (GA peel)

CONC %	20	20	20	35	35	35	50	50
PEEL	1st	2nd	3rd	4th	5th	6th	7th	8th
TIME (MIN)	2-3	3-4	4-5	2-3	3-4	4-5	2-3	3-4

Fig. 8: 25% salicylic acid (SA) peel in melasma (three sittings)

- After 30 seconds, stinging and burning starts, which increases over next 2 minutes, reaches crescent at 3 minutes and then rapidly decreases to baseline over next minute.
- As hydroethanolic acid evaporates, it leaves behind a white precipitate of SA termed as SA frost.

Advantages

- Any area inadequately treated can be identified.
- Timing is not necessary.
- Risk of overpeeling is remote because once vehicle evaporate, little penetration of active agents takes place.
- Neutralization is unnecessary.
- Easier to apply on larger areas but risk of salicylism restricts their use.

Postpeel Events and Care

- Tightness, smoothness, immediate postpeel peeling begins 2 days post peel and extends up to 5–7 days.
- *Care*: Regular use of emollients and sunscreens
- Avoid sun exposure
- Avoid products containing AHA

Intervals

- Once in 2 weeks for 5–6 sessions for resurfacing photo-damaged facial skin moderately.
- Excellent improvement in rough and oily skin with skin type V and VI, enlarged pores
- To avoid in pregnant and breast-feeding mothers, and those allergic to aspirin
- Cautions in children, elderly and large body surfaces

PHYTIC ACID PEELS[6]

- Slow-release superficial peel for individuals who do not opt for visible desquamation.
- Molecule of inositol hexaphosphoric acid shows anti-oxidant, antityrosinase and iron chelating effects.

Indications

- Acne
- Photoaging
- Hyperpigmentation

Application

- 2 mL of product should be evenly applied with brush or cotton bud in two coats one after other without any rubbing. No frosting should occur. If accidental frosting occurs, neutralization with sodium bicarbonate is done.
- *Brand*: Easy phytic solution—mixture of phytic acid with glycolic, lactic or mandelic acid.

Postpeel Care

- Mild stinging persist up to 1 hour. The peel should be left on face 8–12 hours and then washed off.
- Three to four days later, skin sloughs off very little often not visible
- Sunscreens and moisturizers
- Interval: Once a week till results are obtained or once a month as maintenance treatment between TCA peels.

TRETINOIN PEELS[6]

- Retinoids are group of molecules consisting of vitamin A and their synthetic analogues.
- Topical application on daily basis causes keratinization.
- *Indications*
  - Melasma
  - Intrinsic and extrinsic skin aging.

Product and Procedure

- Solution containing 0.1 g of tretinoin solution solubilized by addition of 5 mL of ethanol and 5 mL of propylene glycol.
- Degreasing of skin followed by application—skin acquires yellowish discoloration—leave in contact for 6–8 hours then wash off.

Postpeel Care

- After 2 days, skin begins to peel mildly and complete in 7 days with no discomfort.
- One percent hydrocortisone along with sunscreens.
- *Advantages*: Safe and effective in improving skin texture and appearance.

Peels in Combination

Glycolic acid with TCA (medium depth peel) (Fig. 9): 70% GA was applied to the entire face and diluted with water after 2 minutes. Then, 35% TCA was applied over the same areas. It results in impressive improvement in pigmentary dyschromia and actinic damage.

Peel with Dermabrasion

- Fifty percent TCA application f/b dexamethasone acetate (DMA) with cryoanesthesia (CO_2 slush or liquid nitrogen).
- *Indications*:
  - Acne pitting
  - Acne scarring
  - Striae

Peel with LASER[9]

- First chemical peel followed by LASER resurfacing for eradication of wrinkles in perioral and periocular regions.

Peel with Manual Dermasanding

- First TCA application followed by local dermasanding using sandpapers and gauze roll dipped in normal saline until fine bleeding points are visualized.
- *Indication*: Fine and moderate rhytids.

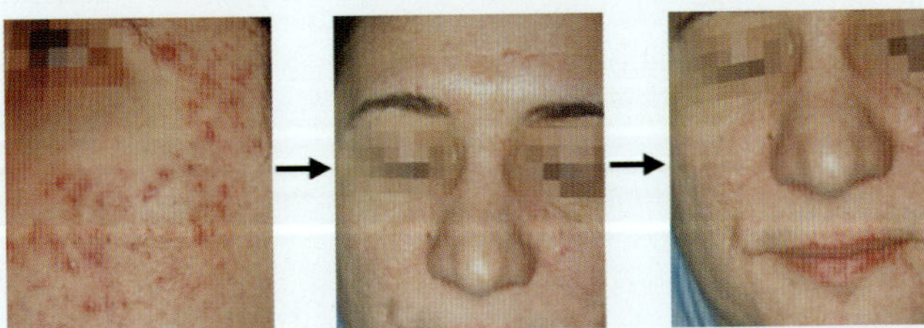

Fig. 9: 70% glycolic acid (GA) peel in active acne (three sittings)

Complications of Peels

- Pigmentary changes (Figs 10 and 11)
- Scarring
- Infections (e.g. Herpes simplex) (Fig. 12)
- Keratoacanthomas
- Textural changes
- Milia
- Acne

Toxicity

- Trichloroacetic acid or AHA have no systemic toxicity
- Urticaria with 30% TCA (cholinergic)
- Faint or lightheadedness (facial vasodilatation and tachycardia)
- Mottled hyperemia
- Allergic contact dermatitis (lactic acid)
- Non phenols (resorcinol and SA) can not be used in large area.

Resorcinol Toxicity[6]

- *Forty percent for 3–4 months*: Tremors, collapse and violet black urine, methemoglobinemia, hypothyroidism and syncope.
- *Guidelines to prevent toxicity*
  - Patch test
  - Perform resorcinol peeling with the patient lying down, and have them get up slowly after peel.

Salicylism

- Rapid breathing, tinnitus, decreased hearing, nausea, vomiting and abdominal pain.
- Rarely allergic reaction
- Guidelines to prevent toxicity
  - Do not peel large area
  - In kidney disease do small area
  - After peel drink lot of water.

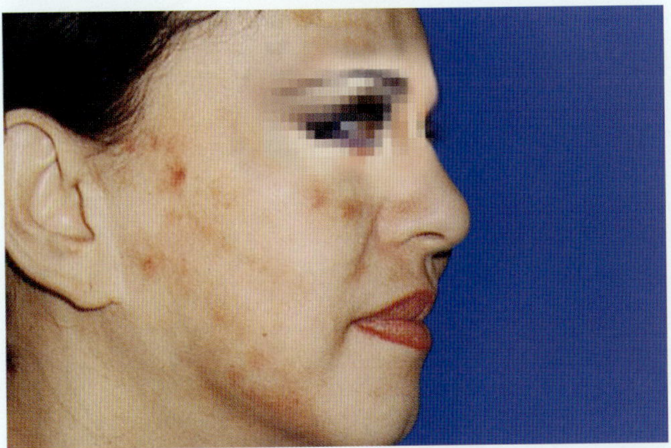

Fig. 10: Hyperpigmentation

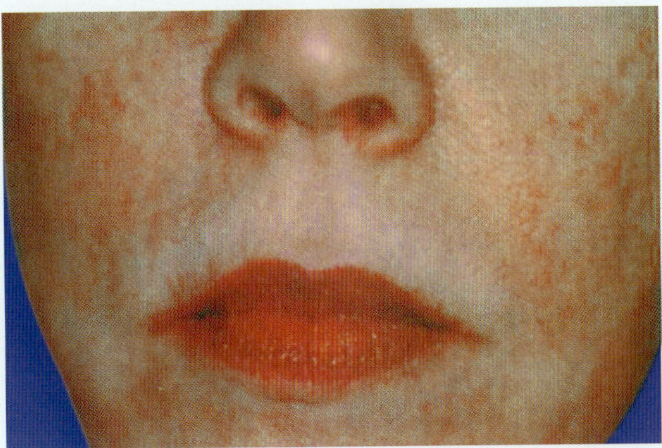

Fig. 11: Hypopigmentation

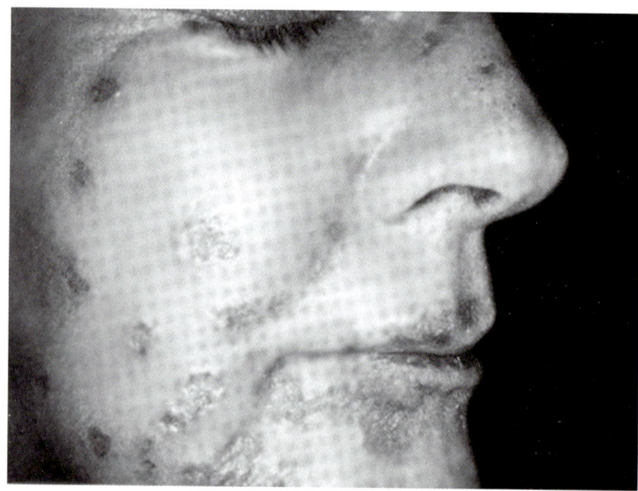

Fig. 12: Herpes outbreak

SEQUELAE

- Pigmentary changes
- Persistence of rhytids
- Prolonged erythema
- Hypertrophic subepidermal healing
- Milia
- Skin pore prominence
- Increased prominence of telangiectasias
- Darkening and growth of pre-existing nevi.

COMPLICATIONS

- Skin infection
- Herpes simplex virus
- Pseudomonas organisms
- *Staphylococcus/Streptococcus* organisms
- Candida organisms
- Ectropion
- Cardiac arrhythmias
- Renal failure
- Facial scarring

CONCLUSION

- Chemical peeling is a technique that removes superficial lesions and improves the texture of skin.
- Careful patient selection and education are crucial to both the patient's final result and his or her satisfaction.
- Learning the technique is a small part of the process; postoperative care and close patient follow-up are equally important.
- Clinical and histological changes are long-lasting (15–20 years) and may be permanent for some patients.
- A complication can also be permanent.

REFERENCES

1. Brody HJ. Chemical Peeling. St Louis, Mo: Mosby-Year Book; 1992. pp. 1-5.
2. Brody HJ. Chemical Peeling and Resurfacing. St. Louis: Mosby; 1997. pp. 109-10.
3. Tse Y, Ostad A, Lee HS, et al. A clinical and histologic evaluation of two medium-depth peels. Glycolic acid versus Jessner's trichloroacetic acid. Dermatol Surg. 1996;22(9): 781-6.
4. Kligman AM, Baker TJ, Gordon HL. Long-term histologic follow-up of phenol face peel. Plast Reconstr Surg. 1985;75(5):652-9.
5. Stegman SJ. A comparative histologic study of the effects of three peeling agents and dermabrasion on normal and sun-damaged skin. Aesthetic Plast Surg. 1982;6(3): 123-35.
6. Rubin M. Manual of Chemical Peels. Philadelphia: Lippincott; 1995. pp. 120-1.
7. Cummings C, Haughey B, Thomas R, et al. Management of aging skin. Otolaryngology: Head & Neck Surgery, 4th edition. Mosby; 2005.
8. Halaas YP. Medium depth peels. Facial Plast Surg Clin North Am. 2004;12(3):297-303.
9. Monheit GD, Zeitouni NC. Skin resurfacing for photoaging: laser resurfacing versus chemical peeling. Cosmet Dermatol. 1997;10:11-22.

CHAPTER

90 Head and Neck Tissue Expansion

Livnat Siman Tov, Alexander Margulis

INTRODUCTION AND BIOLOGY OF TISSUE EXPANSION

The expansion of skin was first reported in 1957 by Neumann,[1] who used a rubber balloon with an external port in reconstructing a traumatic ear defect. After almost 20 years, Radovan[2] presented his experience with breast reconstruction. In 1982, Austad and Rose[3] described a self-inflating expander.

Both animal and human studies have documented histological changes in soft tissue undergoing expansion. A mechanical force applied to skin influences numerous aspects of cellular architecture and function.[4-6]

Analysis of multiple sites of expanded flaps demonstrated an increase in epidermal thickness. A few weeks after the cessation of expansion and flap transposition epidermal thickness decreases, though not to pre-expansion thickness.[7] Hair follicles and skin appendages are compressed but do not degenerated. During the expansion, there is evidence of an increased melanocyte activity that returns to normal a few weeks after the transposition of the expanded flap.

Dermal thickness decreases dramatically during expansion and is most pronounced at the first weeks of the process.[8] On the other hand, collagen content in the dermis is increased with preservation of the relative proportion of type I and type III collagen.[9] A few week after the placement of the expander, a dense fibrous capsule is formed with gradual decrease in the number of cells within it. Mitotic activity of the capsule fibroblasts is maximal after 96 hours of pressure application by expansion and decreases gradually thereafter.[10]

Significant muscle atrophy is evident during the expansion period, regardless of the plane in which the expander is placed (above or below the muscle).[11] Histological examination shows ulceration, focal muscle fibers degeneration, mild fibrosis and disorganization of the myofibrils of the sarcomeres. Skeletal muscles regain normal architecture after the prosthesis is removed with normalization of muscle mass.[12]

Tissue expansion effect on underlying bone changes depending on the type of bone. Calvarial bone shows decreased thickness and volume at the area under the expander, and increased thickness at the periphery of the prosthesis.[13] Despite that, the process does not induce craniosynostosis. Observations by Colonna et al. showed that underlying bone reacts to the presence of an expander, but this reaction subsides within 9 months with moderate sequela in the general bony architecture.[14]

TYPES OF IMPLANTS

Tissue expanders are available in a variety of shapes, sizes, contours, and backing configurations and inflation ports. Jackson et al.[15] have described their experience with tissue expanders of the extremities and their successful use of external ports with only 6% of infection rate. Others, like the authors, are reluctant to the use of external ports due to fear of infection.[16]

INDICATIONS FOR THE SURGERY

The indications for tissue expanders are skin conditions that need to be excised for medical or cosmetic reasons, and in which primary closure or recruitment of local tissue flaps does not produce a pleasing esthetic result. These conditions include:

- Burn scars and scar contractures
- Congenital pigmented nevi
- Sebaceous nevus
- Cutis aplasia
- Hemangiomas and vascular malformations.

SPECIFIC PREOPERATIVE EVALUATION

During the preoperative evaluation of the patient, the amount of tissue needed to be excised and the amount and type of tissue needed for reconstruction is assessed. For skin lesions, that involve both hairy and non-hairy areas, two different tissue expanders should be used. The surgeon should decide on the type of reconstruction—using an expanded flap or expanded full-thickness skin graft. Further assessment should be made regarding the number of procedures needed for the final result. It is on this phase that the surgeon determines the volume of the tissue expander that would be used and where it would be inserted.

ANESTHETIC CONSIDERATIONS

The procedures are performed under general anesthesia and special attention should be made for tube placement in a way that would not distort the adjacent esthetic units. The tube should be firmly secured, sometimes, using silk sutures to the alveolus in order to avoid accidental extubation while maintaining the surgeon's ability to move the head relatively freely.

OPERATIVE TECHNIQUE

Reconstruction, using tissue expanders, involves at least two separate surgical procedures. The first procedure is the insertion of the expander (or expanders) and the second is removal of the expander, excision of lesion and reconstruction with expanded flaps, expanded full-thickness skin grafts, expanded free flaps, or expanded prefabricated flaps. The latter flaps are used less frequently. All procedures are performed under general anesthesia. Incisions for placement of the expanders are carefully planned, with the most important consideration being the visional design of the final flap.

SURGICAL STEPS

Insertion of Tissue Expanders

- The patient is intubated and the surgical field is washed with antiseptic solution
- Intravenous dose of cefazolin is given 1 hour preoperatively
- The skin is incised parallel and close to the lesion to be excised, and a subcutaneous pocket is prepared. The expander pocket should reflect the dimensions of the expander to be placed, being 1–2 cm larger in each dimension, so that the tissue expander will lie comfortably without sharp folds. Much care should be taken when dissecting the pocket to minimize trauma to the skin flap being elevated
- The authors use internal remote injection ports in all of their patients. The port should be low profile and placed in areas where there is no potential pressure on the overlying skin. Importantly, the port should be distanced from the expander to ensure that the expander is not punctured when accessing the port
- The authors routinely use drains, with one drain placed in each expander pocket. The drains are removed 4–5 days after the surgery
- After insertion of the expander, the pocket is closed with two layers of nylon sutures. The skin nylon suture is not removed throughout the entire process of expansion
- The authors continue antibiotic treatment until all drains are removed
- The wound is bandaged with xeroform, bacitracin and kerlix.

The inflation process is initiated a week after expander insertion and the injections are repeated on a weekly basis. The volume of expansion varies according to the size of the expander and the anatomical site in which it was implanted. Inspection of skin color, capillary refill and simple palpation are performed when administrating injections, and patient comfort is taken into consideration. Typically, 8–10 weeks are sufficient to fill the expanders. Expanders are typically overinflated beyond the manufacturer's recommended full capacity.[17,18]

Removal of Tissue Expanders

- The patient is under general anesthesia
- Intravenous dose of cefazolin is given 1 hour preoperatively
- The surgical field is prepared with antiseptic solution
- The tissue expander is removed and the expanded flap is transposed over the skin lesion. Flap borders are marked over the lesion. It is extremely important to avoid tension over the flap
- The skin lesion is excised according to markings. The skin lesion should not be resected until the extent of the transposition flap is determined
- Flap is transposed and sutured to place in layers
- Drains are left under the flap, and are removed when the secretions decrease
- The wound is bandaged with xeroform, bacitracin gauz and kerlix
- Antibiotic treatment is continued until the drains are removed.

Head and Neck Reconstruction

Scalp

Tissue expansion is a treatment modality of choice for reconstructing many scalp lesions.[19,20] As surgical experience increase and planning improves, larger defects can be reconstructed with fewer procedures and better restoration of normal hair patterns.[21-23] The expander is inserted in a subgaleal pocket, with the port placed at the preauricular area. The location of the future expanded flap is planned with consideration of axial arterial supply to the flap (based on the superficial temporal, postauricular, occipital and supraorbital). Treatment starts with patients as early as age 8 months, with some cranial molding expected by the time the expanders are removed. No long-term cranial deformity has been observed. Colonna et al.[8] showed that the underlying bone reacts to the presence of an expander, but this reaction subsides within 9 months with moderate sequela in the general bony architecture (Figs 1 to 3).

Face

Large and giant nevi of the face and extensive facial scars present some of the greatest challenges for the plastic surgeon. Facial reconstruction should be done with respect to facial esthetic units. Facial lesions are usually treated with expanded local flaps whenever possible, with the addition of expanded full-thickness skin grafts for the forehead, periorbital and eyelid areas and occasionally for the nasal dorsum.[24,25]

Planning the expansion and reconstruction of the forehead must be directed at minimizing any possibility of distorting the eyebrow and the normal distance from brow to hairline (Figs 4 to 8).

Nevi and extensive scars of the cheek are best reconstructed with expanded or non-expanded postauricular flaps. Use of advancement cervical flaps, distal to the cervicomental angle for reconstruction of cheek defects, is discouraged due to increased complication rate and increased possibility of secondary deformities as ectropion, lower lip drooping and oral incompetence (Figs 9 to 13).

Expanded full-thickness skin grafts have been used effectively for excision and reconstruction of nevi of the periorbital, eyelid and occasionally the nasal areas.[23] A single, large, expanded full-thickness graft from the supraclavicular area can cover eyelids, the canthus and the region between eyelid and brow, without the multiple "seams" that follow use of multiple smaller grafts (Figs 14 to 20).

Expanded full-thickness skin grafts or expanded forehead flaps can be used for nasal reconstruction as lining or for external coverage of nasal defects.

Neck

Posterior and posterolateral neck defects can be successfully reconstructed with expanded flaps from the upper back and the shoulders.[22] The flap is designed in such a

Fig. 1: A 5-month-old girl with congenital melanocytic nevus involving the left occipitoparietal scalp and posterior aspect of the left auricle

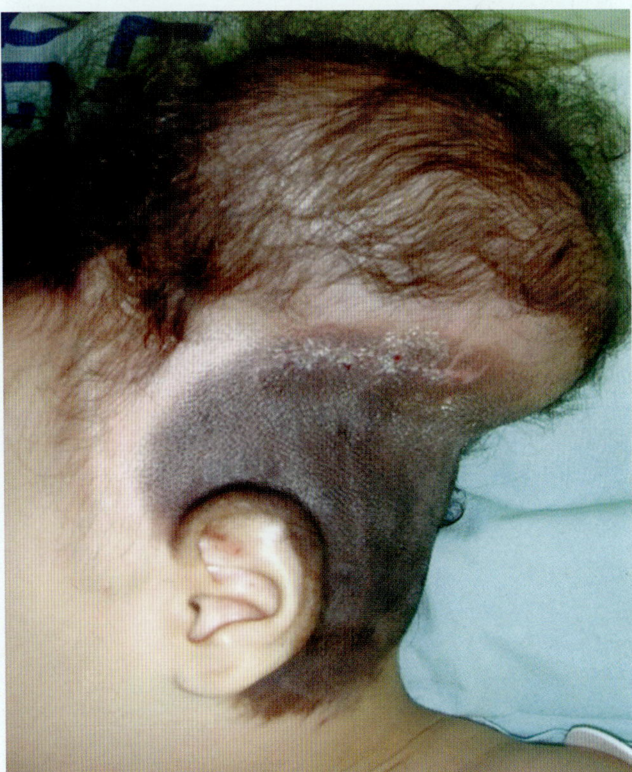

Fig. 2: Fully expanded tissue expander

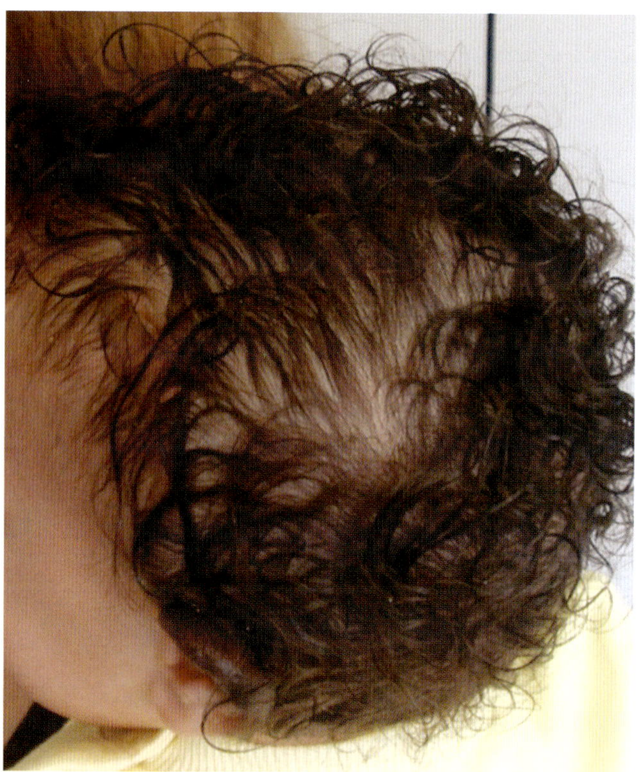

Fig. 3: Following removal of the tissue expander and left scalp reconstruction with expanded flap. Note residual nevus on auricle

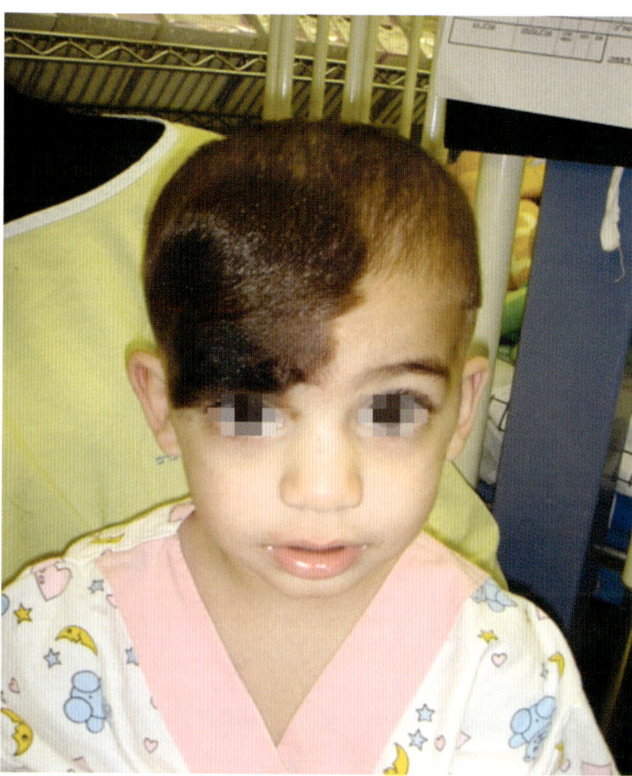

Fig. 4: A 3-year-old boy with congential melanocytic nevus involving the scalp, forehead, right eyebrow and upper eyelid

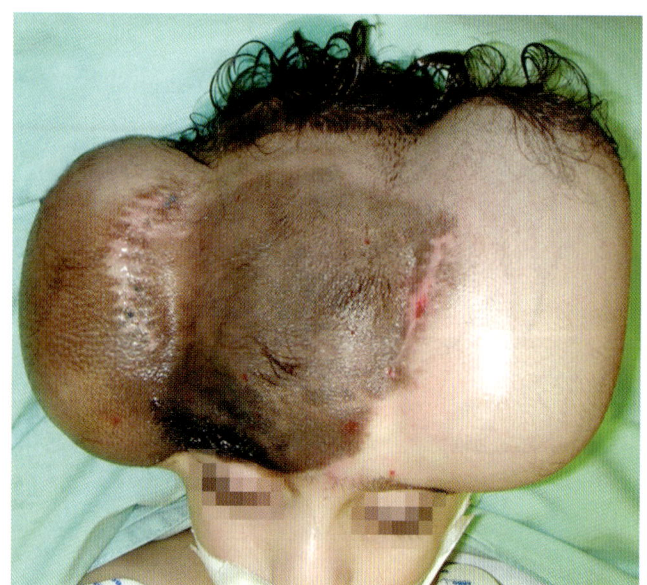

Fig. 5: Fully expanded scalp and forehead tissue expanders

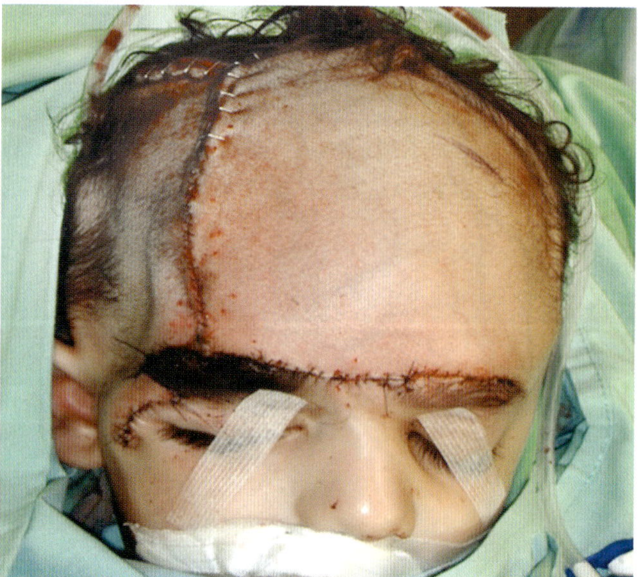

Fig. 6: The nevus was excised and forehead and scalp reconstructed with expanded flaps

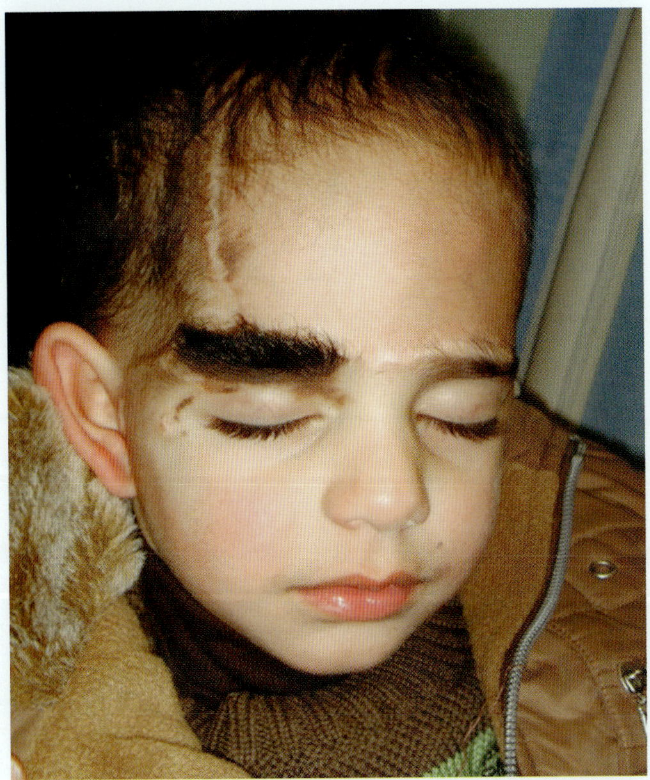

Fig. 7: Residual nevus at eyebrow and upper eyelid

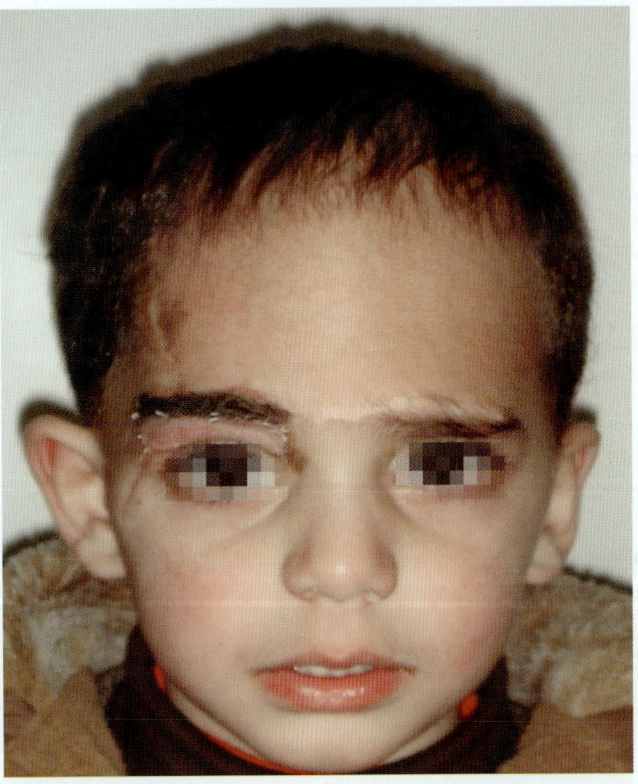

Fig. 8: Upper eyelid nevus was excised and lid reconstructed with full-thickness skin graft. The eyebrow was shaped, a part of the nevus was excised, and small part of the nevus was left to mimic the eyebrow

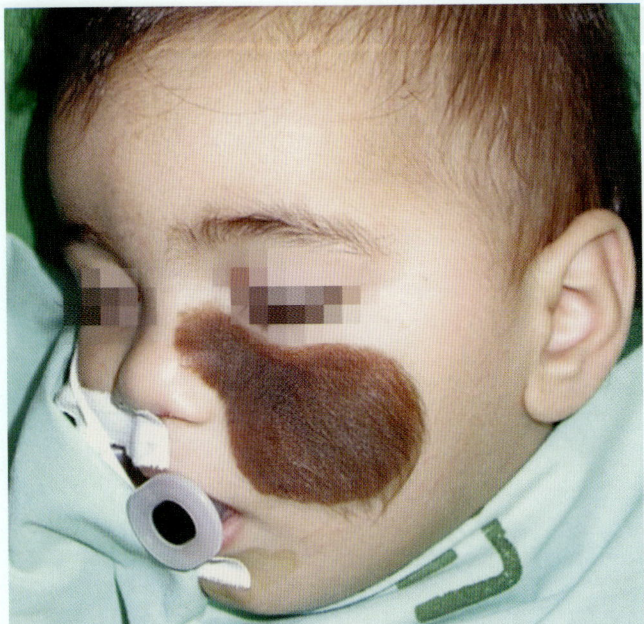

Fig. 9: A 6-month-old child with congenital melanocytic nevus involving the left cheek and lateral nasal sidewall

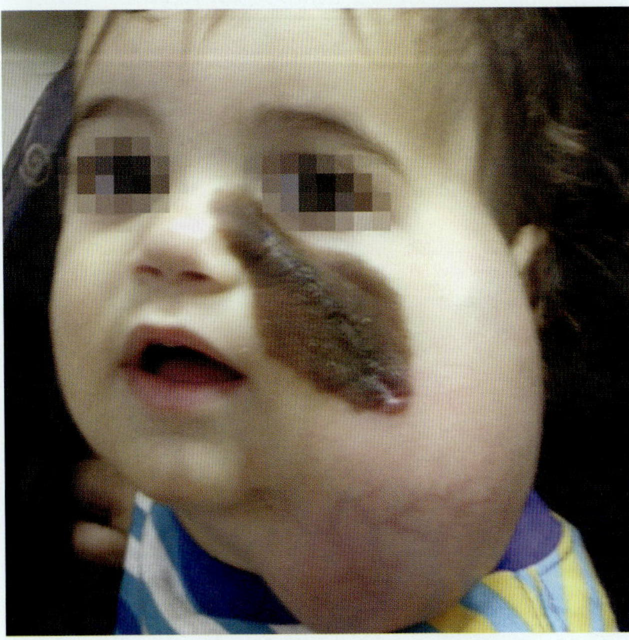

Fig. 10: Fully expanded tissue expander

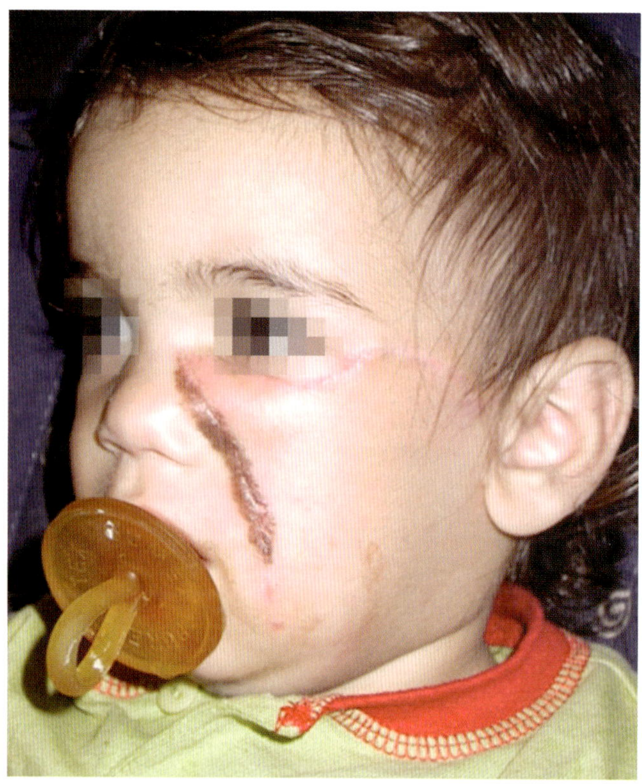

Fig. 11: The tissue expander was removed, cheek and part of nasal sidewall nevus were excised and reconstructed with expanded flap

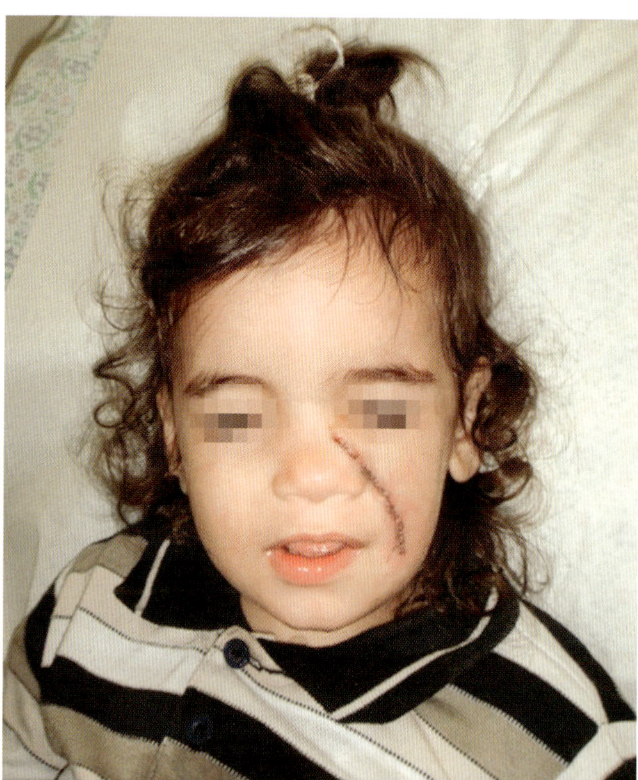

Fig. 12: Residual nasal sidewall nevus was excised and wound closed primarily

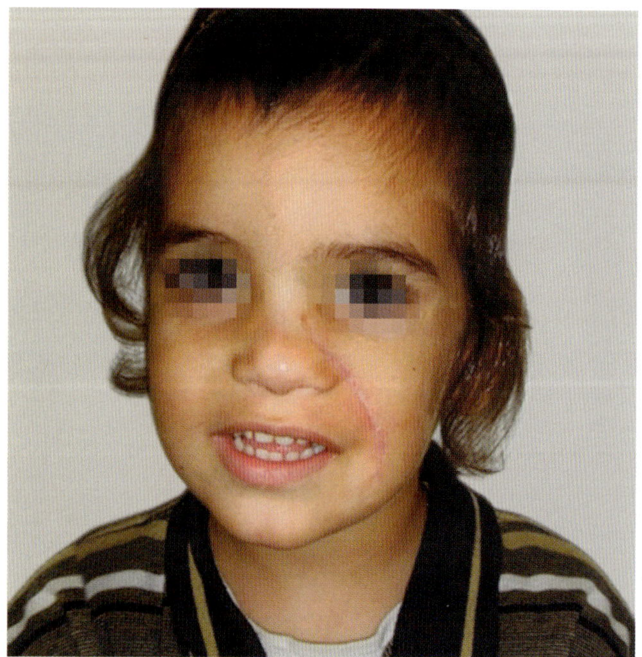

Fig. 13: Late result at 4 years of age

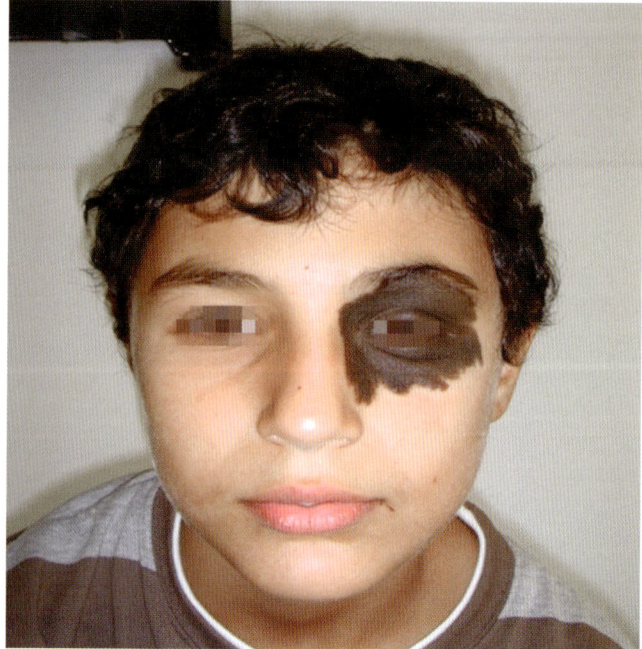

Fig. 14: A 12-year-old boy with congenital melanocytic nevus involving the left periorbital region—upper and lower eyelids and left nasal sidewall

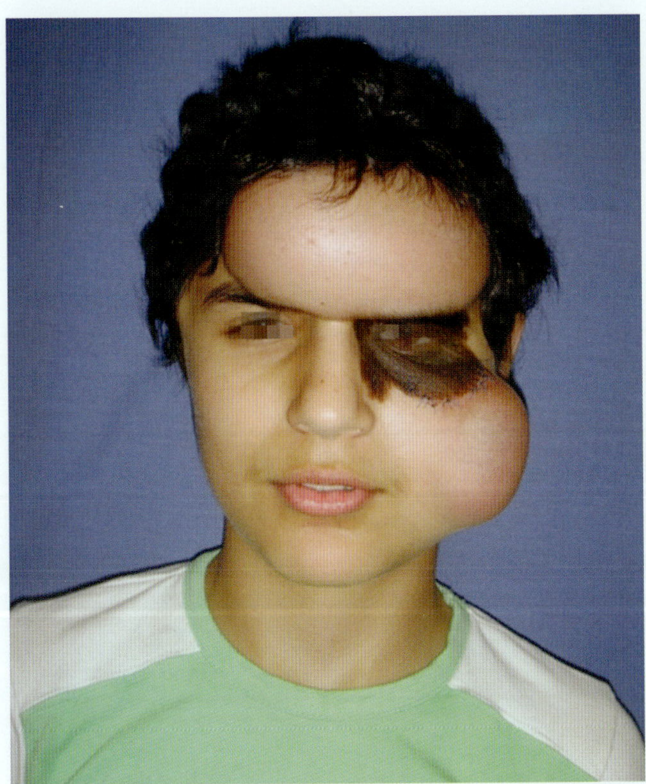

Fig. 15: Fully expanded forehead and scalp tissue expanders

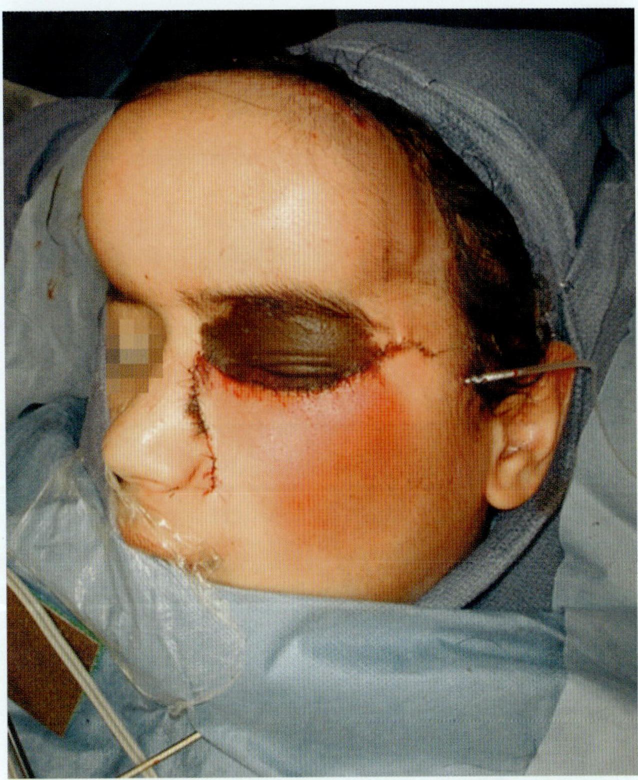

Fig. 16: The cheek expander was removed, lower eyelid and nasal sidewall nevus was excised and reconstructed with expanded flaps

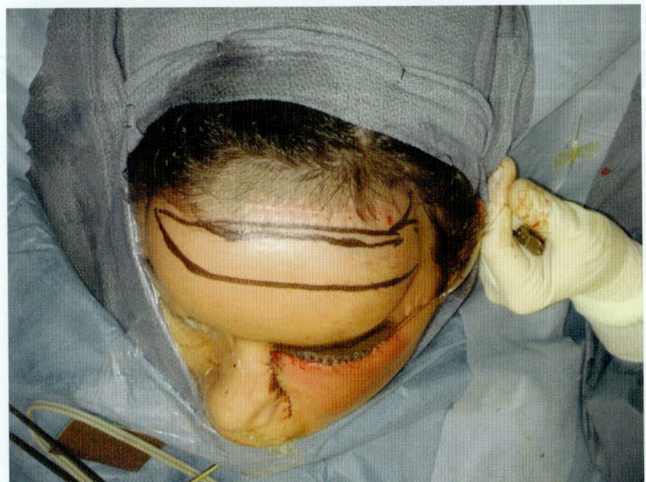

Fig. 17: Upper eyelid was reconstructed with pedicled tubed expanded flap

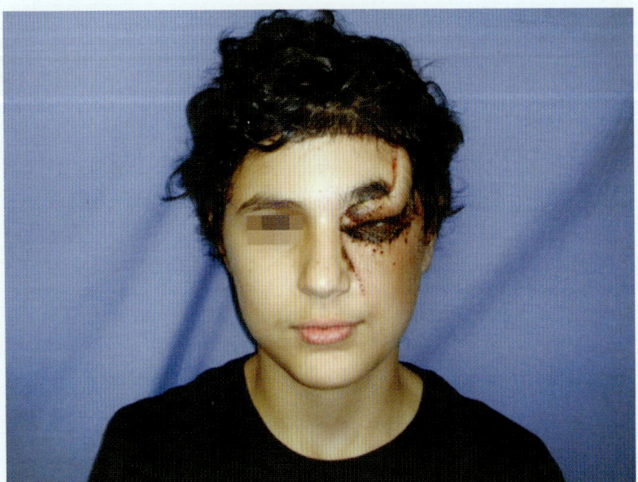

Fig. 18: The tubed flap is attached to its pedicle

way that it can be wrapped around the neck, eliminating the "webbing" created by pure upward advanced flaps. With this design, the reconstructed neck has a better contour and more favorable scar location. Care must be taken to avoid placement of the tissue expander under the platysma. Incorporation of this muscle in the expanded flap exposes the marginal mandibular nerve to trauma.

Tissue expansion is also very effective in treating anterior burn scar contractures of the neck. The expanders are placed in the unburned skin in the posterolateral neck or

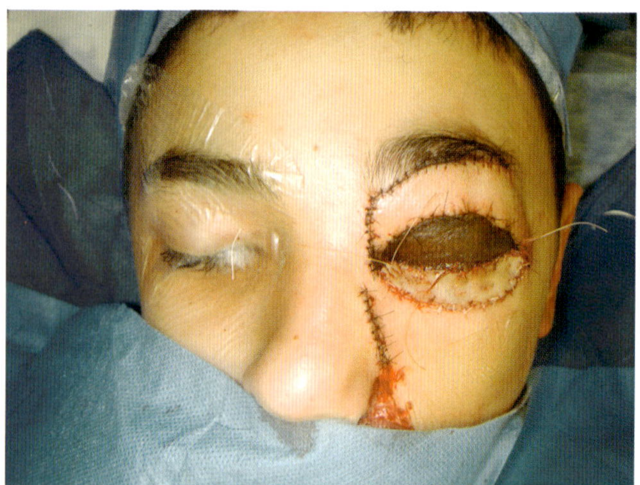

Fig. 19: The tubed flap was separated and upper eyelid reconstruction completed. Residual nevus at the nasal sidewall was excised. Lower eyelid nevus was excised, and eyelid reconstructed with full-thickness skin graft

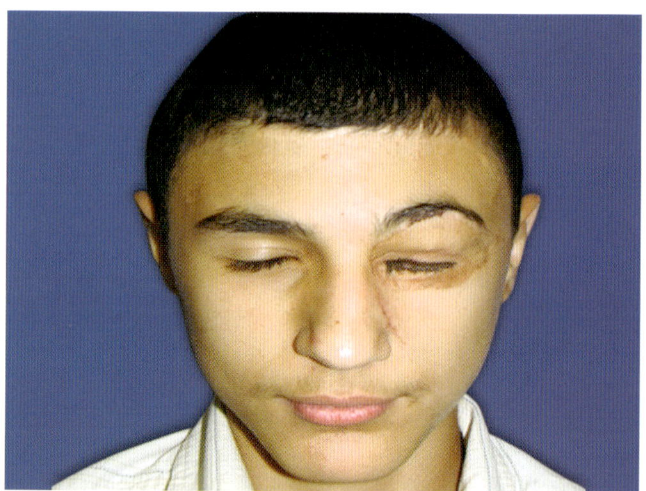

Fig. 20: Final result after fourth stage surgery in which the residual upper eyelid nevus was excised and reconstructed with full-thickness skin graft

the supraclavicular region. The flaps are designed as large transposition flaps, wrapped around the anterior neck to release these challenging mentosternal contractures. When no adjacent tissue is available for expansion, island or prefabricated expanded flaps from the supraclavicular areas can be transplanted into the anterior neck defect (Figs 21 to 26).

COMPLICATIONS

Tissue expansion has been associated with significant complications since its inception. The risks have been described in numerous studies and overall complication rates from 13% to up as high as 40% have been reported. Complication rates are higher among pediatric population. However, some of the minor complications will not delay the process of expansion and reconstruction, in contradistinction to major complications, such as infection or extrusion.

Infection

Careful patient selection and meticulous surgical technique are the two most important factors for avoiding complications.[6]

One has to envision the expanded flap for the final reconstruction during the expander's placement and plan the incisions and the pocket accordingly. In planning the design of the expanded flap, the authors found that there are significant advantages in using expanded transposition flaps over pure advancement. Restricting the expanded flap design to advancement alone, in order to minimize potential scarring, severely limits the reconstructive capabilities of the added tissue and distracts from the surgeon's ability to achieve the initial goal of reconstructive surgery. The cost of additional incisions is worthwhile in order to achieve a better final contour of the reconstructed part, a reduced risk of anatomic distortion, a better position of the scars and a reduced risk of scar contracture.

Implant Exposure

Implant exposure can occur early or late during the course of expander inflation. Early exposure is attributed to inadequate pocket dissection, inadequate wound closure or early inflation of the expander. Late exposure is usually attributed to overzealous inflation of the expander in a short period of time.

Once exposure occurs, the expander should be deflated; wound edges are debrided and sutured in layers. Antibiotic treatment is given for 5 days following the procedure. In case of late exposure, if there is sufficient amount of expanded flap, reconstruction can be carried out earlier than planned. If the expander was exposed for over 24 hours and there is high-risk for infection, the patient should be hospitalized, intravenous antibiotics should be administered, and one should consider removing the expander and reinserting it on a later date.

Expander Deflation

Deflation of an expander is usually caused by accidental puncture of the expander during its insertion or inflation. Rarely does it occur due to device failure. When deflation occurs, the expander should be removed and replaced by another.

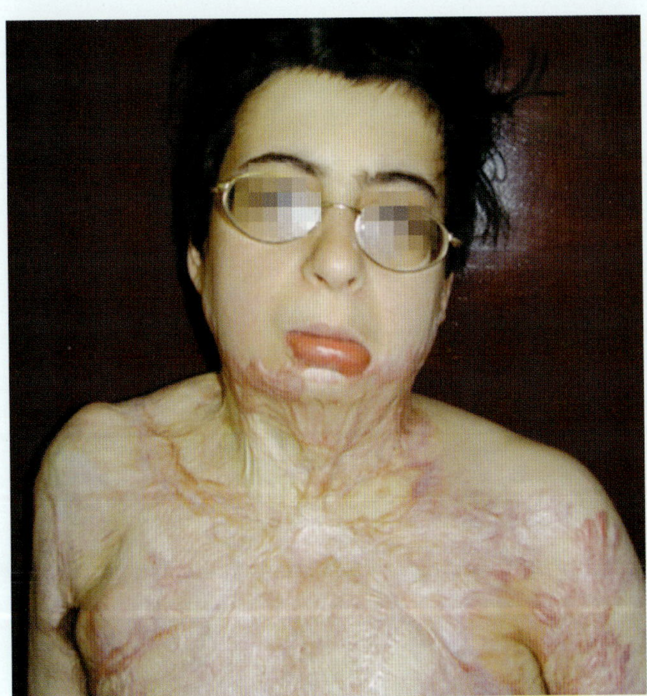

Fig. 21: A 26-year-old postburn patient with anterior neck scar contracture

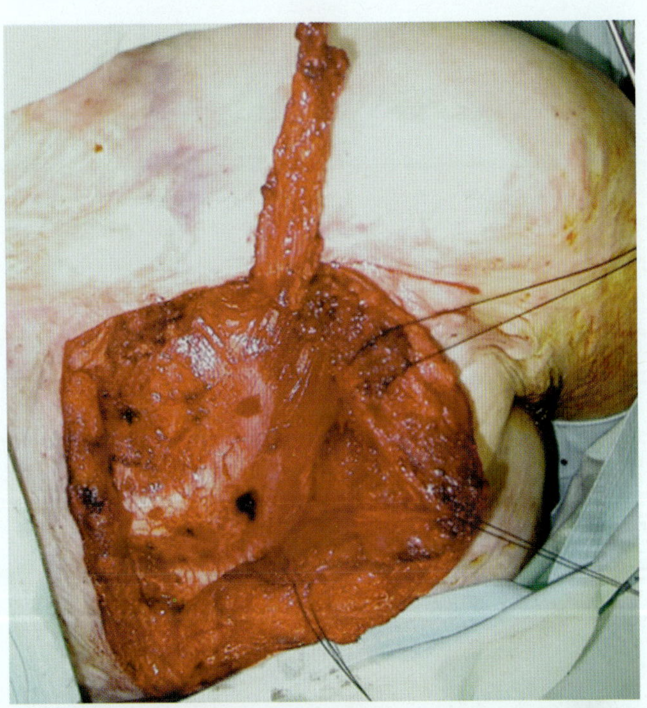

Fig. 22: Thoracoacromial vessels were separated and implanted under supraclavicular expanded skin

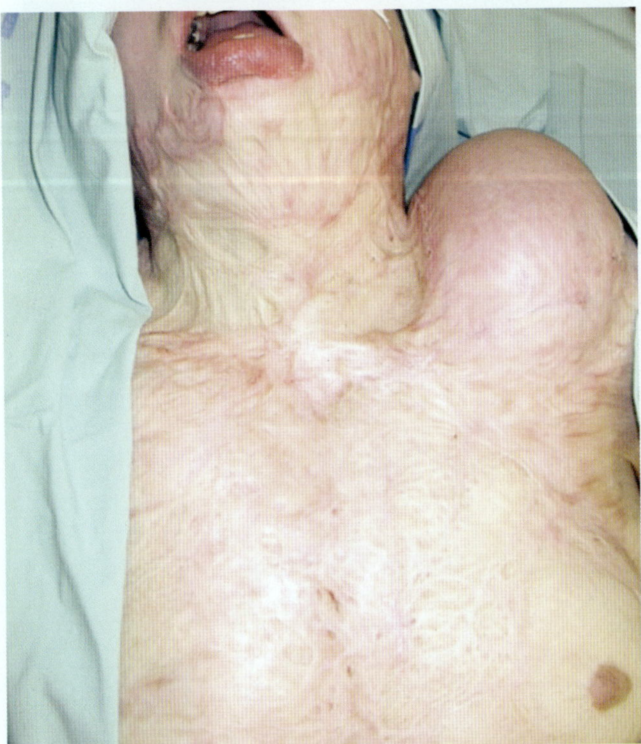

Fig. 23: Fully expanded left supraclavicular flap

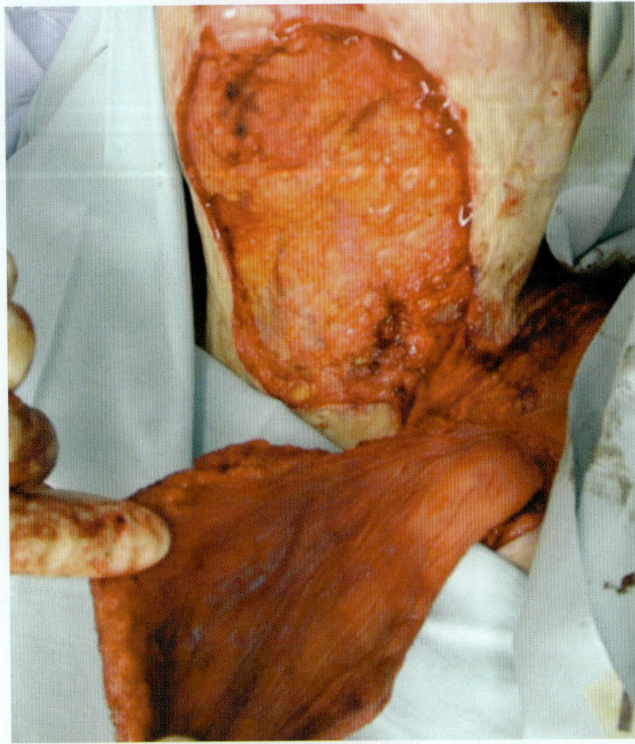

Fig. 24: Prefabricated flap elevation. Enriched blood vessels network is seen through capsule

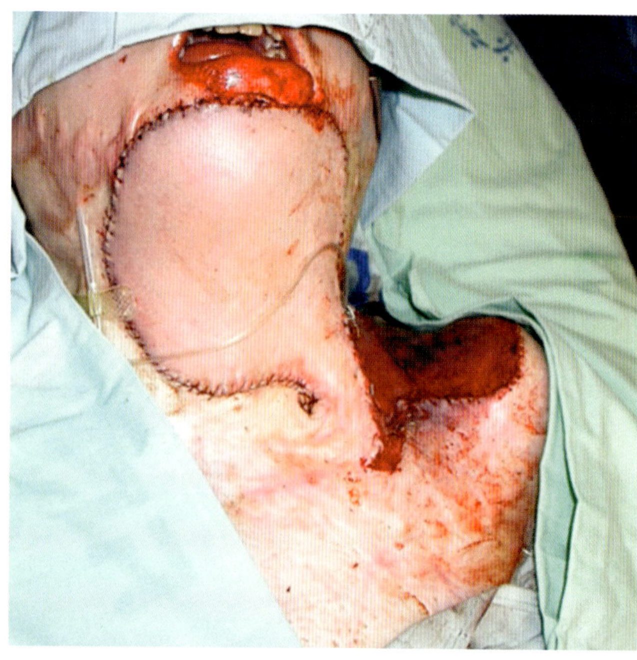

Fig. 25: Immediate result following anterior neck reconstruction with prefabricated expanded flap

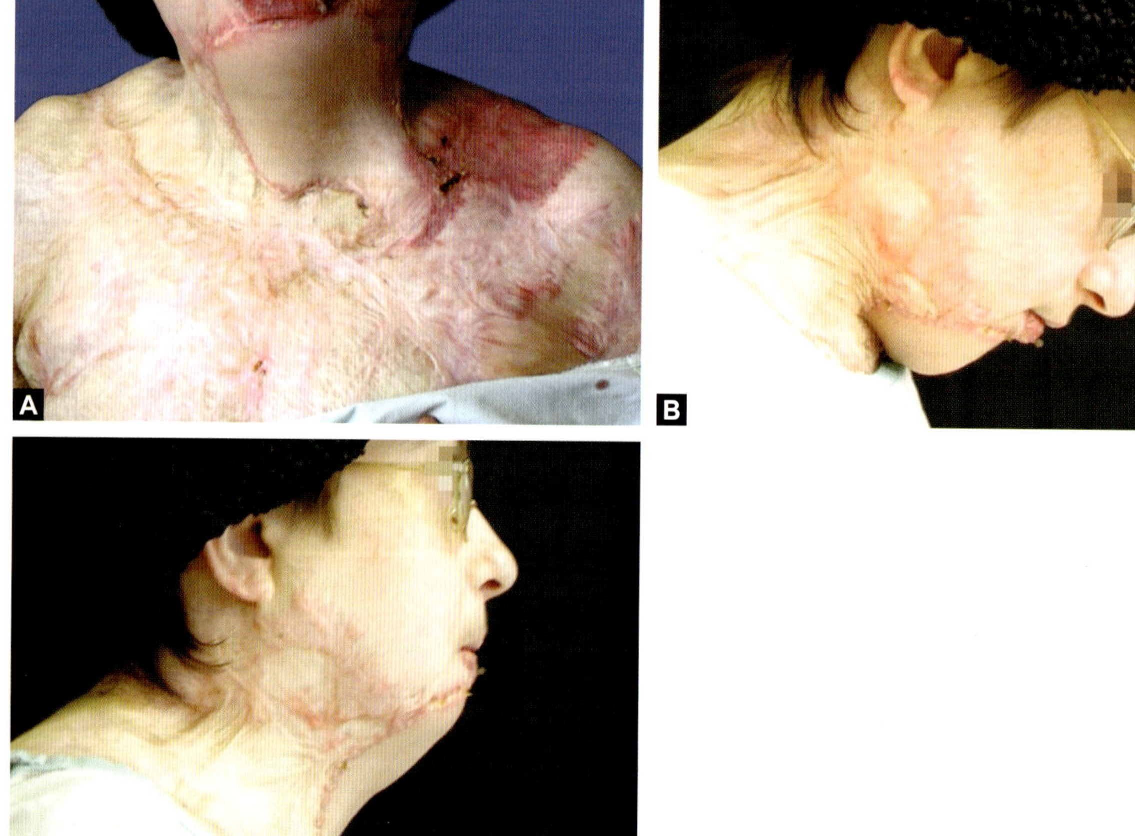

Figs 26A to C: Improved anterior neck esthetics and range of motion

REFERENCES

1. Neumann CG. The expansion of an area of skin by progressive distension of a subcutaneous balloon; use of the method for securing skin for subtotal reconstruction of the ear. Plast Reconstr Surg (1946). 1957;19(2):124-30.
2. Radovan C. Adjacent flap development using expandable silastic implant. Presented at the Annual Meeting of the American Society of Plastic and Reconstructive Surgeons. September 27-October 2, 1976, Boston, MA. 1976.
3. Austad ED, Rose GL. A self-inflating tissue expander. Plast Reconstr Surg. 1982;70(5):588-94.
4. Johnson TM, Lowe L, Brown MD, et al. Histology and physiology of tissue expansion. J Dermatol Surg Oncol. 1993;19(12):1074-8.
5. Takei T, Mills I, Arai K, et al. Molecular basis for tissue expansion: clinical implications for the surgeon. Plast Reconstr Surg. 1998;102(1):247-58.
6. Steenfos H, Tarnow P, Blomqvist G. Skin expansion. Long term follow up of complications and costs of care. Scand J Plast Reconstr Surg Hand Surg. 1993;27(2):137-41.
7. Simon PJ, Anderson LS, Manstein ME. Increased hair growth and density following controlled expansion of guinea pig skin and soft tissue. Ann Plast Surg. 1987;19(6):519-23.
8. Johnson PE, Kernahan DA, Bauer BS. Dermal and epidermal response to soft-tissue expansion in the pig. Plast Reconstr Surg. 1988;81(3):390-7.
9. Knight KR, McCann JJ, Vanderkolk CA, et al. The redistribution of collagen in expanded pig skin. Br J Plast Surg. 1990;43(5):565-70.
10. Lew D, Fuseler JW. The effect of stepwise expansion on the mitotic activity and vascularity of subdermal tissue and induced capsule in the rat. J Oral Maxillofac Surg. 1991;49(8):848-53.
11. Gur E, Hanna W, Anderighetti L, et al. Light and electron microscopic evaluation of the pectoralis major muscle following tissue expansion for breast reconstruction. Plast Reconstr Surg. 1998;102(4):1046-51.
12. Kim KH, Hong C, Futrell JW. Histomorphologic changes in expanded skeletal muscle in rats. Plast Reconstr Surg. 1993;92(4):710-6.
13. Moelleken BR, Mathes SJ, Cann CE, et al. Long-term effects of tissue expansion on cranial and skeletal bone developments in neonatal miniature swine: clinical findings and histomorphometric correlates. Plast Reconstr Surg. 1990;86(5);825-34.
14. Colonna M, Cavallini M, De Angelis A, et al. The effects of scalp expansion on the cranial bone: a clinical, histological, and instrumental study. Ann Plast Surg. 1996;36(3):255-60; discussion 260-2.
15. Meland NB, Loessin SJ, Thimsen D, et al. Tissue expansion in the extremities using external reservoirs. Ann Plast Surg. 1992;29(1):36-9; discussion 40.
16. Iconomou TG, Michelow BJ, Zuker RM. Tissue expansion in the pediatric patient. Ann Plast Surg. 1993;31(2):134-40.
17. Paletta C, Campbell E, Shehadi SI. Tissue expanders in children. J Pediatr Surg. 1991;26(1):22-5.
18. Neale HW, High RM, Billamire DA, et al. Complications of controlled tissue expansion in the pediatric burn patient. Plast Reconstr Surg. 1988;82(5):840-8.
19. Antonyshyn O, Gruss JS, Zuker R, et al. Tissue expansion in head and neck reconstruction. Plast Reconstr Surg. 1988;82(1):58-68.
20. Bauer BS, Vicari FA. An approach to excision of congenital giant pigmented nevi in infancy early childhood. 1988;82(6):1012-21.
21. Rivera R, LoGiudice J, Gosain AK. Tissue expansion in pediatric patients. Clin Plast Surg. 2005;32(1):35-44, viii.
22. Bauer BS, Margulis A. The expanded transposition flap: shifting paradigms based on experience gained from two decades of pediatric tissue expansion. Plast Reconstr Surg. 2004;114(1):98-106.
23. Bauer BS, Corcoran J. Treatment of large and giant nevi. Clin Plast Surg. 2005;32(1):11-8, vii.
24. Gur E, Zuker RM. Complex facial nevi: a surgical algorithm. Plast Reconstr Surg. 2000;106(1):25-35.
25. Bauer BS, Few JW, Chaven CD, et al. The role of tissue expansion in the management of large congenital pigmented nevi of the forehead in the pediatric patient. Plast Reconstr Surg. 2001;107(3):668-75.

CHAPTER

91 The Surgical Technique of LASER Skin Resurfacing

Zekayi Kutlubay, Murat Küçüktaş

The desire for cosmetic enhancement of facial skin with minimal risk and rapid recovery has inspired LASER mediated means of wrinkle and photodamage reduction. In the 1980s and early 1990s, continuous-wave carbon dioxide (CO_2) LASERS were used to resurface photodamaged skin in a procedure called "thermabrasion"; however, this ablative procedure was associated with an unacceptably high risk of scarring. The advent of short-pulsed, high-peak-power and rapidly scanned, focused beam CO_2 LASERS and normal mode erbium:yttrium-aluminum-garnet (Er:YAG) LASERS, which remove photodamaged skin layers in a precisely controlled manner, revolutionized skin rejuvenation and scar treatment.

The prolonged recovery time and complication risk of ablative LASER resurfacing prompted the development of nonablative and, more recently, fractional resurfacing in an effort to further minimize risk and recovery. Nonablative LASER resurfacing induces dermal-thermal injury to improve rhytides and photodamage without epidermal damage. Fractional resurfacing thermally ablates microscopic columns of epidermal and dermal tissue in a regularly spaced array comprising a fraction of the skin surface. This intermediate approach increases efficacy as compared to nonablative resurfacing and speeds recovery as compared to ablative resurfacing. Neither nonablative nor fractional resurfacing produces results comparable to ablative LASER skin resurfacing, but both have become much more popular than the latter because of minimal risks and acceptable improvement.[1]

INDICATIONS FOR LASER RESURFACING

LASER skin resurfacing has been employed to treat a large number of skin conditions, but the two most common indications are photoaging and scarring. A primary indication is photoaging, which includes rhytides, dyspigmentation (Figs 1 and 2), vascular changes, elastosis, actinic cheilitis, and actinic keratoses (Figs 3A to D) is highly responsive to LASER resurfacing.[2]

Perioral and periorbital rhytides, which are resistant to facelift procedures, are highly amenable to LASER resurfacing. Fine rhytides (particularly in the periorbital, perioral and cheek areas) may be completely eradicated with LASER resurfacing; deeper creases are also improved, probably secondary to a general tightening effect. Rhytides and creases that appear with active movement and facial expression, such as glabellar and nasolabial folds, tend to be more resistant to LASER resurfacing.[1]

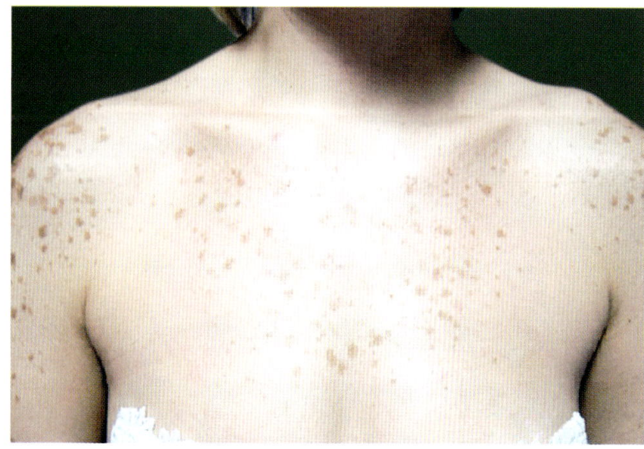

Fig. 1A: Solar lentigines before the operation

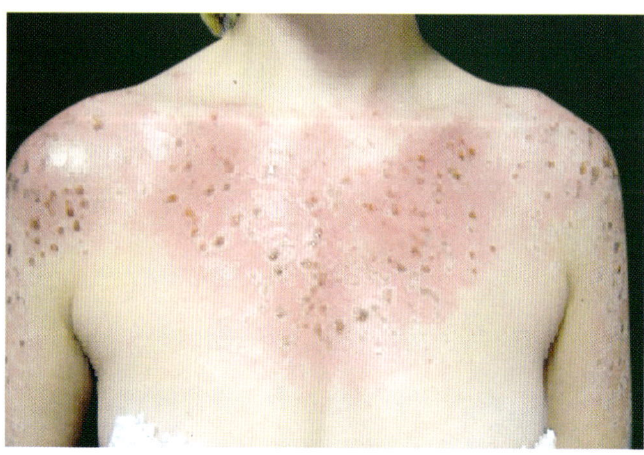

Fig. 1B: Immediately after operation

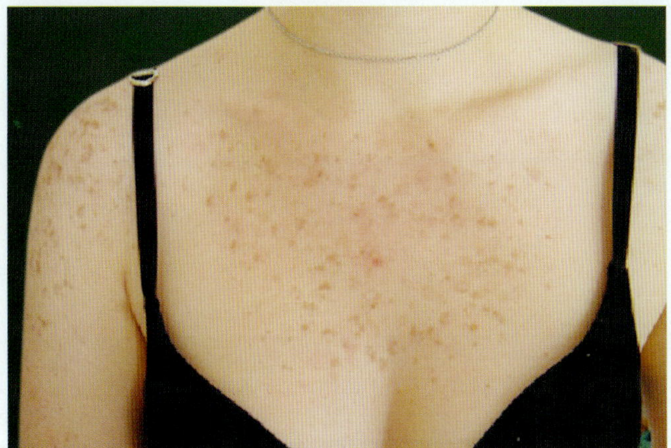

Fig. 1C: One month after LASER procedure

Ablative LASER resurfacing is effective for scars, including those caused by acne (Figs 4 to 6), trauma (Figs 7A to E) and surgery. It is most effective for elevated or deep, distensible acne scars (Figs 8A and B), in which the fibrotic tissue can be removed or the shoulders of the scars ablated, respectively. Ice-pick or bound-down scars are less responsive, requiring a combined approach of subcision and punch excision/grafting, followed by LASER resurfacing 6–8 weeks later. Varicella scars may be improved with spot LASER resurfacing, with fresh scars (6–10 weeks after varicella) responding more completely than older scars. Postsurgical and traumatic scars may achieve dramatic improvement, especially if resurfaced 6–10 weeks after the surgery or injury. Resurfacing well-vascularized wound edges immediately after surgery, prior to suture placement, may also improve cosmetic outcome.

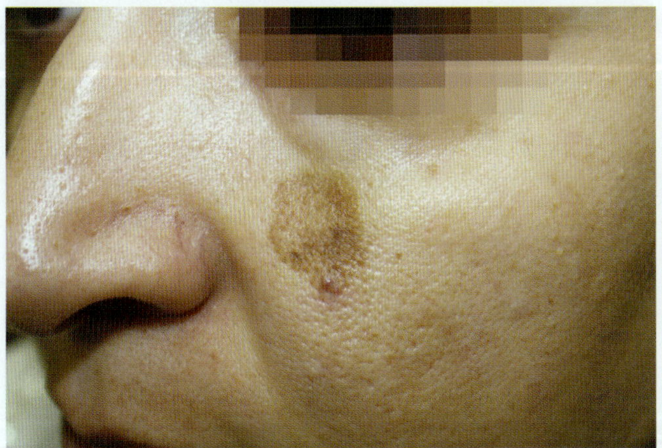

Fig. 2A: Solar lentigine before the operation

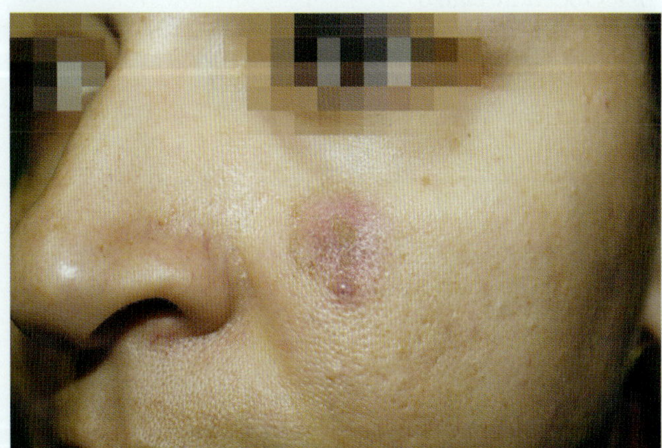

Fig. 2B: Seventh day post procedure

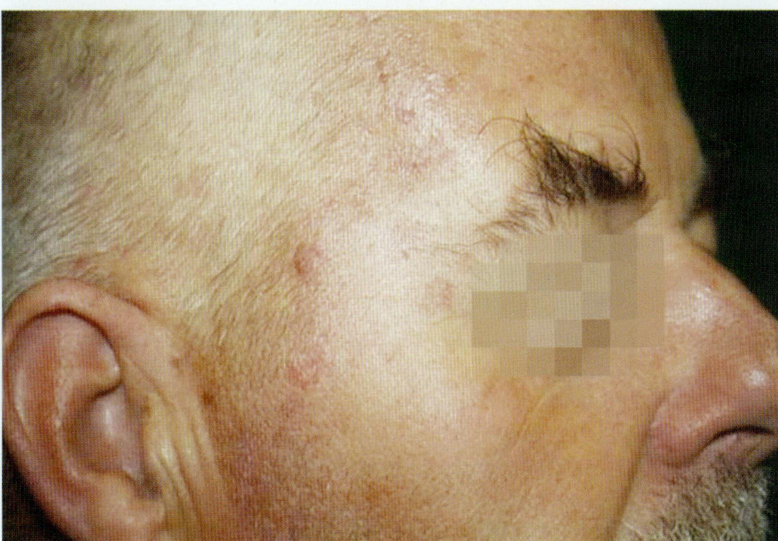

Fig. 3A: Ablative Er:YAG LASER resurfacing for actinic keratoses (before the operation)

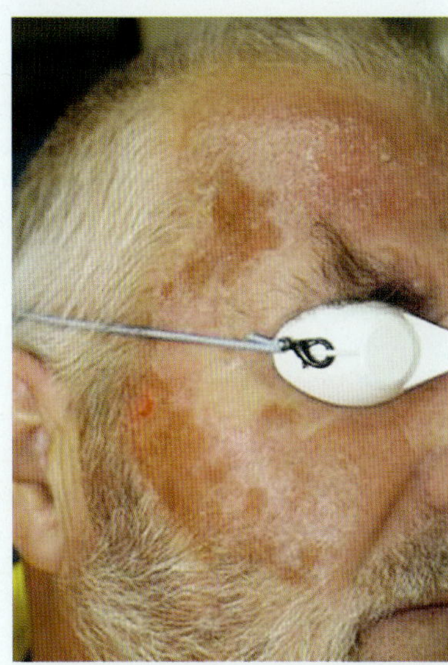

Fig. 3B: Immediately after LASER procedure

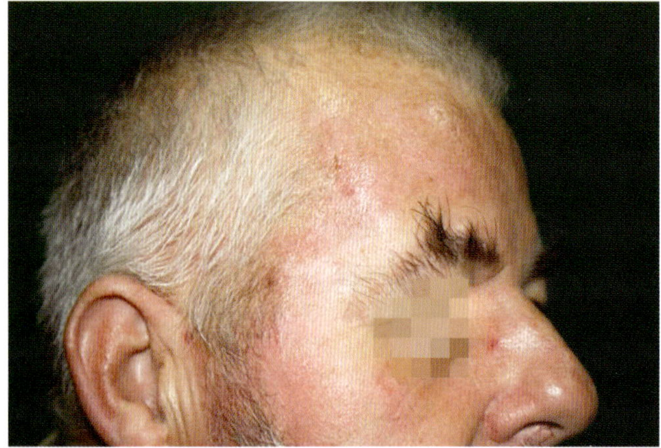

Fig. 3C: Seventh day after operation

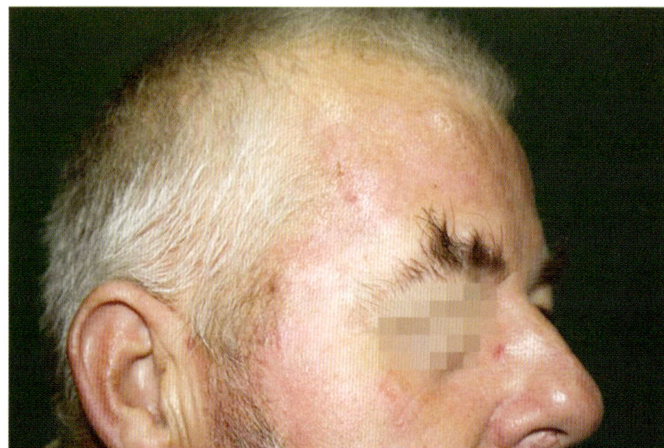

Fig. 3D: Twenty-eighth day after operation

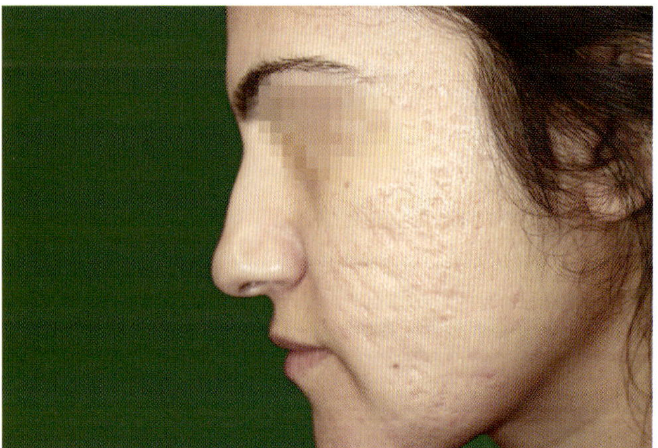

Fig. 4A: Acne scars treated by ablative mode of Er:YAG LASER (before the procedure)

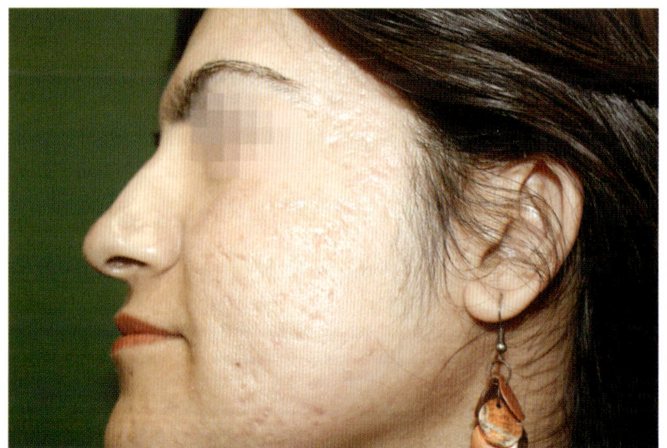

Fig. 4B: Seventh day after procedure

Other Indications

Since LASER resurfacing is relatively bloodless and allows for controlled tissue removal with a low risk of scarring, it has also been used to treat rhinophyma, diffuse actinic cheilitis, actinic keratoses, benign neoplasms/hamartomas (e.g. angiofibromas, appendageal tumors), verrucae, and eyelid laxity (Figs 9A to D).[1,2]

The ideal LASER resurfacing candidate is a healthy, lightly pigmented patient with realistic expectations. Patients with a history of keloids, radiation therapy to the area or scleroderma are not candidates. Diseases that exhibit Koebnerization, such as psoriasis and vitiligo, are relative contraindications.

Prior isotretinoin therapy has been associated with atypical scarring after dermabrasion or chemical peeling, even if the procedure were performed more than 1 year after isotretinoin treatment. Therefore, it is generally recommended that patients wait for at least 1–2 years before undergoing this procedure.

Resurfacing performed at the same time or soon after facelifting or blepharoplasty increases the risk of skin necrosis and scarring due to the altered blood circulation of the undermined skin following these procedures. Hence, LASER resurfacing of undermined skin should be deferred for at least 6 months after the original surgical procedure.

Ablative LASER skin resurfacing with either CO_2 or Er:YAG LASER systems is a well accepted treatment for facial rejuvenation.[3]

Carbon dioxide LASER resurfacing can achieve excellent results in patients with mild-to-moderate surface texture changes and fine superficial or moderate static wrinkles but not in those with deep furrows or severe dermatoheliosis.[4]

Acne scars can be classified into three basic types: (i) Shallow depressed scars, (ii) Wide-base atrophic scars, and (iii) Ice-pick scars. The first two types of acne scars generally are amenable to CO_2 LASER resurfacing; however, fibrotic or ice-pick scars often require punch excision, punch grafts, or punch elevation. Scar base lifting and injection of filling substances for atrophic acne scars (performed as a separate procedure at a different time) can also be combined with LASER resurfacing for optimal results.[5]

Carbon dioxide LASER resurfacing has proved to be a valuable method for facial rejuvenation of photodamaged skin with detectable improvement of fine lines and wrinkles, mottled dyspigmentation, rough-skin texture, and solar lentigines (Figs 10A and B). CO_2 LASER resurfacing can eradicate precancerous growths such as actinic keratosis, although prevention of future development of actinic keratosis has not been substantiated.

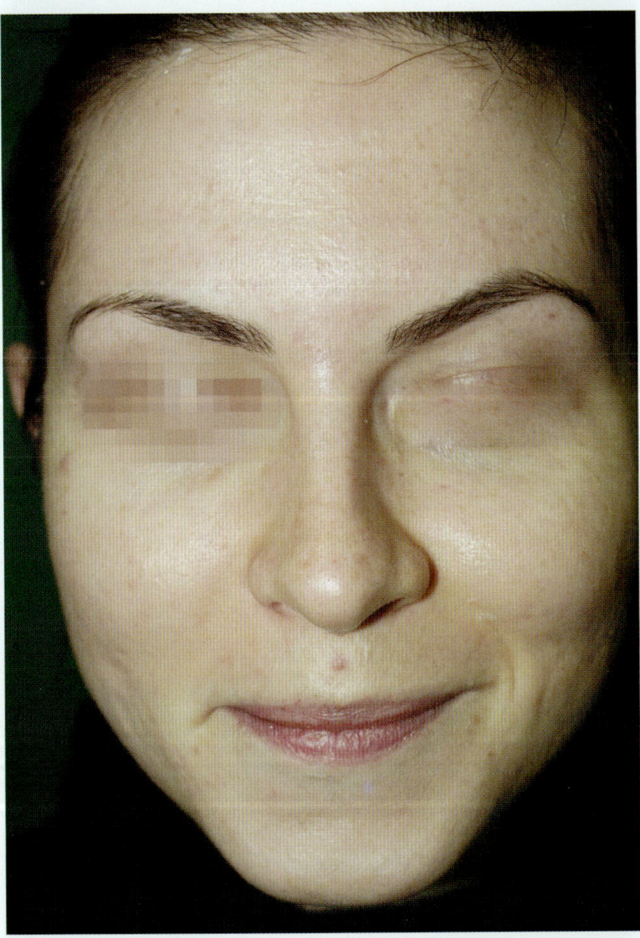

Fig. 5A: Preoperative photo of the patient with acne scars

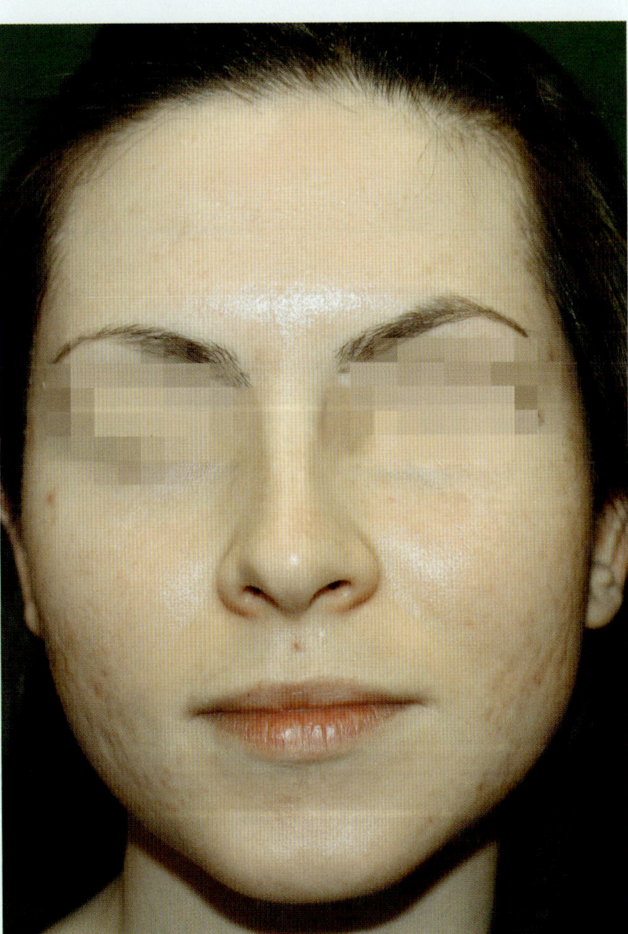

Fig. 5B: Seven days later after ablative Er:YAG

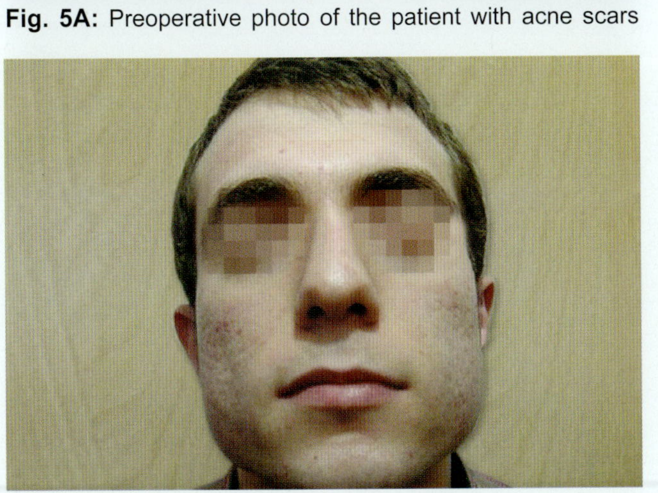

Fig. 6A: Before Er:YAG ablation

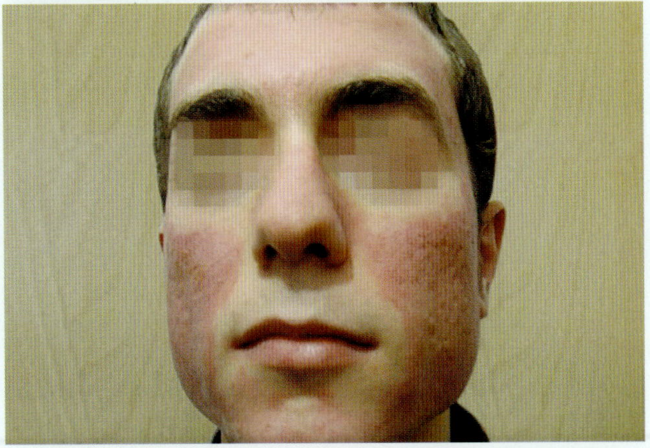

Fig. 6B: Immediately after the LASER procedure

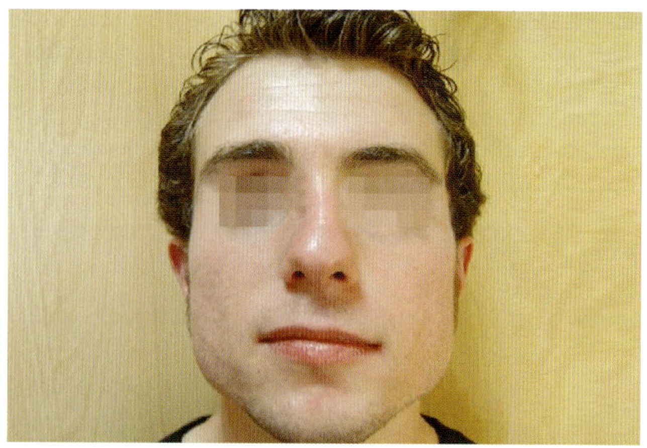

Fig. 6C: One month later from the ablation

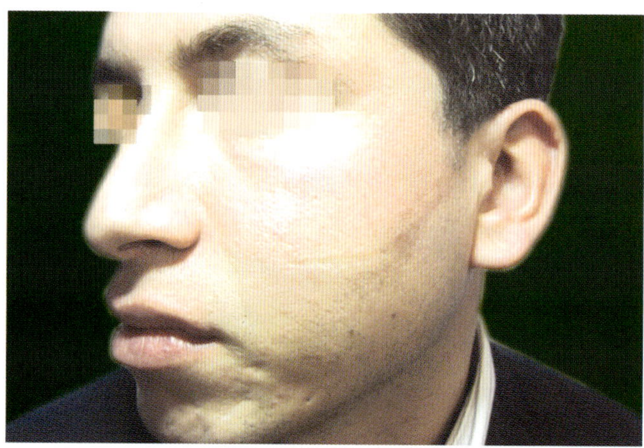

Fig. 7A: Blade cut trace, before fractional CO_2 LASER
Source: By the courtesy of Dr Şehriyar Nazari

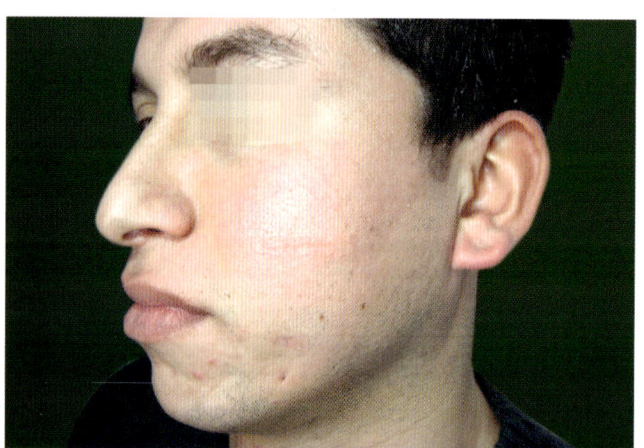

Fig. 7B: Blade cut trace, 7 days later

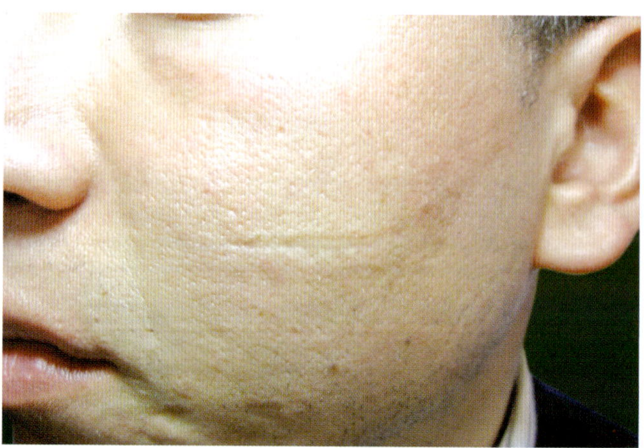

Fig. 7C: Blade cut trace, 15 days later

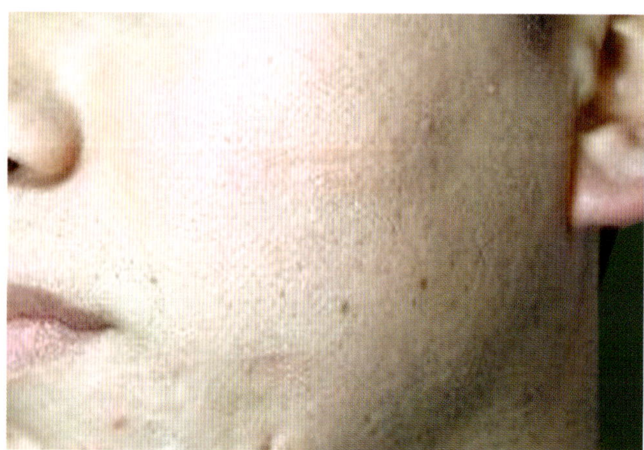

Fig. 7D: Blade cut trace, 20 days later from fractional CO_2 LASER

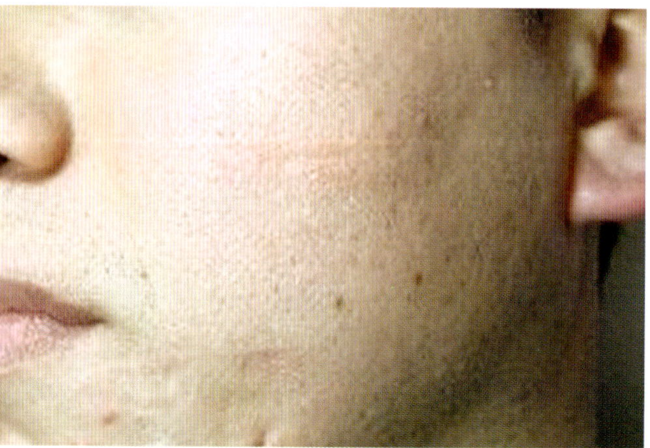

Fig. 7E: Blade cut trace, 30 days later from the fractional CO_2 LASER

The Er:YAG LASER is a powerful tool in the cosmetic surgeon's armamentarium that can have beneficial effects when used properly for the correct indication (Sample video). Mild-to-moderate photo-induced rhytides, superficial pigmentation, atrophic scars, and a variety of epidermal and dermal lesions can be treated successfully with the Er:YAG LASER (Figs 11A to E). Treatment with the short-pulsed Er:YAG LASER is particularly well suited for patients with darker skin phototypes. Several studies have documented a lower risk of pigmentary alterations as compared to CO_2 LASER resurfacing. Although studies suggest modulated Er:YAG LASERS are associated with a lower risk of pigmentary alterations than CO_2 LASER resurfacing, long-term data regarding the risks of delayed hypopigmentation are not yet available.

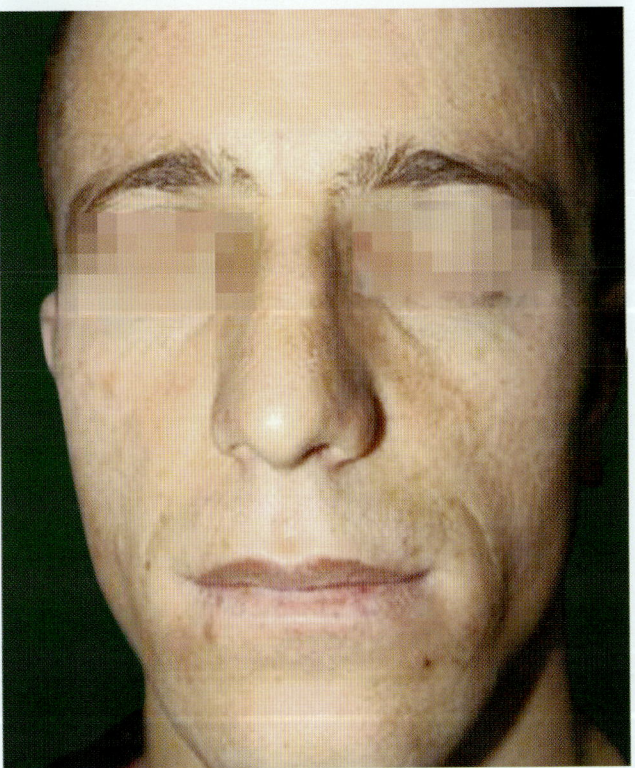

Fig. 8A: Acne scars, before the Er:YAG ablation

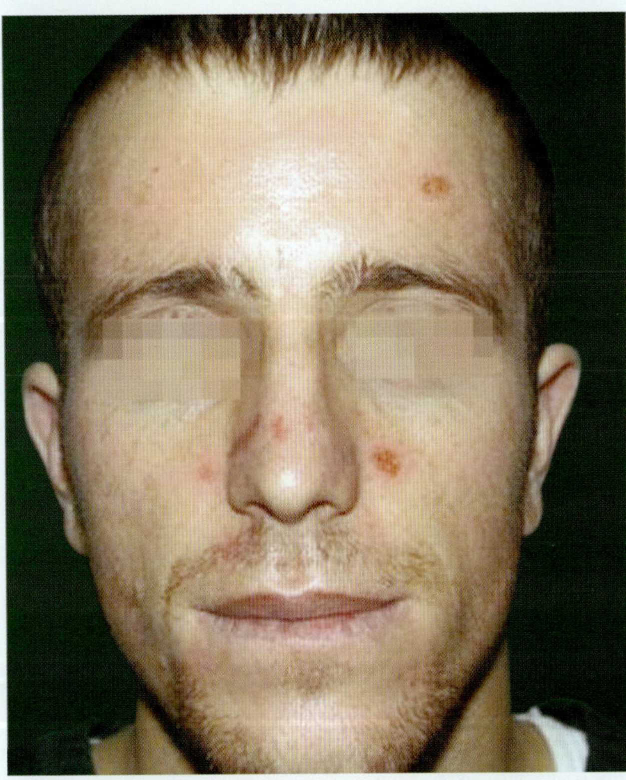

Fig. 8B: Seven days later (from the ablative procedure)

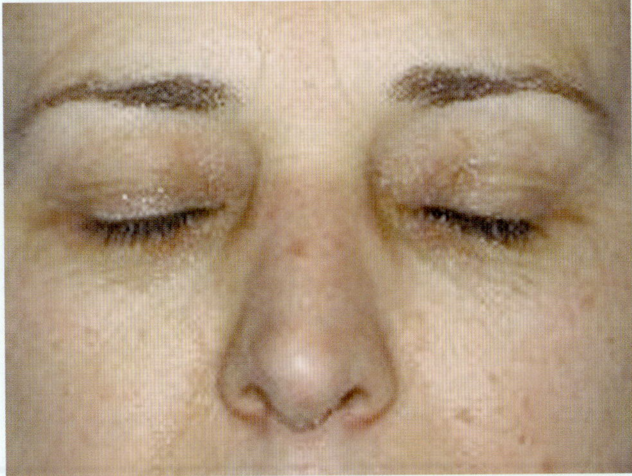

Fig. 9A: Eyelid laxity, before fractional CO_2 LASER treatment
Source: By the courtesy of Dr Şehriyar Nazari

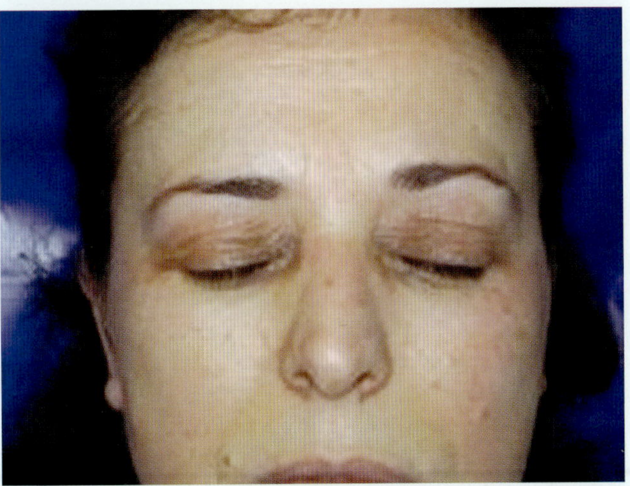

Fig. 9B: Eyelid laxity, 7 days later from fractional CO_2 LASER treatment

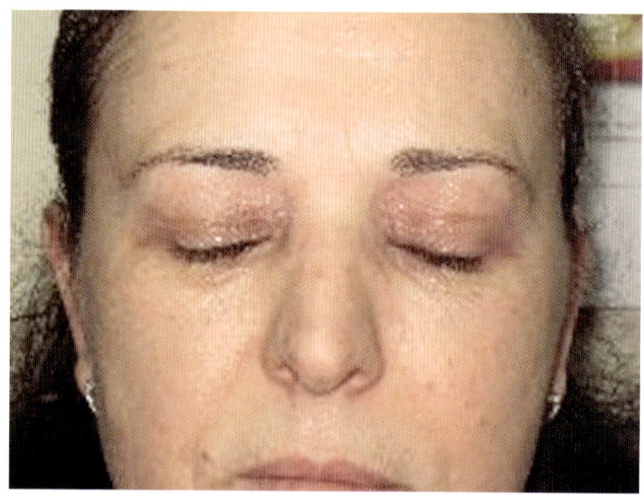

Fig. 9C: Eyelid laxity, 15 days later

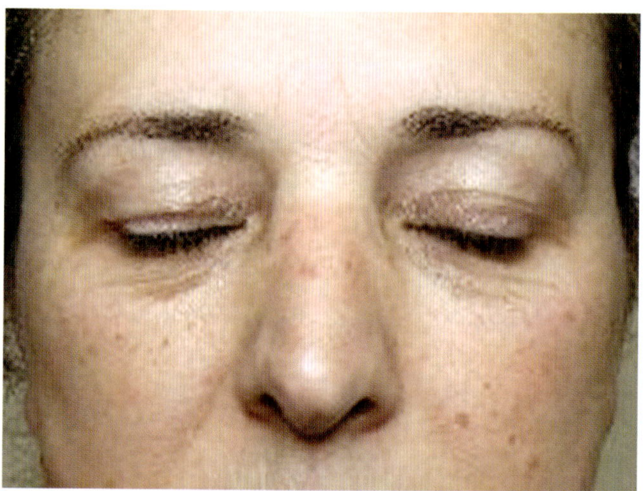

Fig. 9D: Eyelid laxity, 30 days later

Skin resurfacing with a short-pulsed Er:YAG LASER is most commonly used for the improvement of fine rhytides. For moderate photodamage and rhytides, modulated Er:YAG LASER skin resurfacing results in greater collagen contraction and improved clinical results as when compared to short-pulsed Er:YAG systems. Clinical improvement of severe rhytides treated with a modulated Er:YAG LASER can be impressive. However, the improvement seen is not equivalent to that of pulsed or scanned CO_2 resurfacing, even when equal depths of ablation are obtained. Newman et al.[6] compared a variable pulse Er:YAG LASER to traditional pulsed or scanned CO_2 resurfacing for the treatment of perioral rhytides. Although a reduced duration of re-epithelialization was noted with the modulated Er:YAG LASER (3.4 days vs 7.7 days with CO_2), the clinical results observed were less impressive than those following CO_2 LASER resurfacing.

Er:YAG LASER systems may greatly improve atrophic scars caused by acne, trauma, or surgery. In a series of 78 patients, Weinstein[7] reported 70–90% improvement of acne scarring in the majority of patients treated with a modulated Er:YAG LASER. Pitted acne scars may require ancillary procedures, such as subscision or punch excision, for optimal results. These procedures can be performed either prior to or concomitant with Er:YAG LASER resurfacing.

A variety of benign epidermal and dermal conditions respond favorably to Er:YAG LASER resurfacing, including sebaceous hyperplasia, eruptive hair cysts, adenoma sebaceum, angiofibroma, hidradenoma, xanthelasma, and syringomas.

LASER surgeons can combine Er:YAG LASER and CO_2 LASER to take advantage of the unique properties of each LASER. The addition of Er:YAG LASER following CO_2 LASER resurfacing may decrease the duration of postoperative crusting and edema, presumably by reducing the amount of thermal necrosis induced by the CO_2 LASER.

Nonablative procedures are ideal for the younger person who wishes to improve the quality, the tone, and the texture of his or her skin. It is a technique ideally suited for the individual with early photoaging, not for one with class III rhytides.

SPECIFIC PREOPERATIVE EVALUATION

Patient expectation, skin type and medical history should be thoroughly assessed before initiation. An ideal patient has reasonable expectations for cosmetic outcome. Patients should understand the side-effect profile, as discussed later, as well as being able to manage the necessary downtime following treatment.[1]

The ideal patient is of Fitzpatrick skin type I through IV, and has a primary concern cited or related to the indications described above. Because certain histories can directly, and negatively, influence outcome, a patient's medical history plays a critical role in patient selection. A patient with history of keloids should not undergo the procedure, as the procedure may trigger another keloidal response. Similarly, patients with dermatologic diseases that demonstrate Koebnerization, such as vitiligo, lichen planus, and psoriasis, should be cautioned and likely dissuaded from undergoing ablation.

Any suggestion of adnexal disease also serves as a contraindication to ablative LASER resurfacing. Ablative resurfacing relies on the repopulation of the epidermis from stem cells found in skin appendages. A deficiency of these appendages, as seen in morphea and scleroderma, for example, serve as contraindications because of their

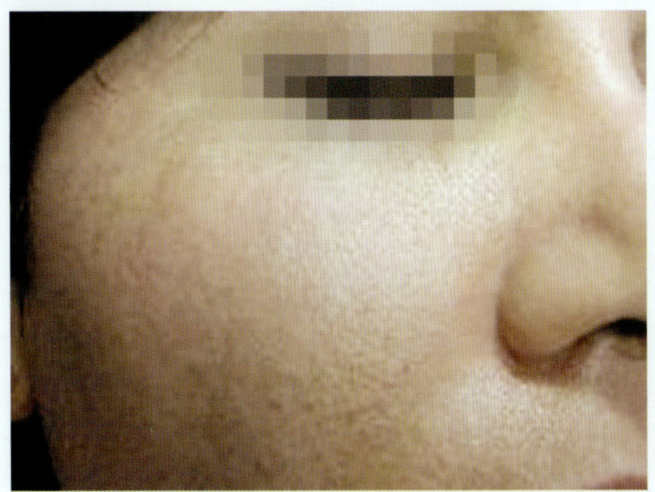

Fig. 10A: Before fractional CO_2 LASER treatment
Source: By the courtesy of Dr Şehriyar Nazari

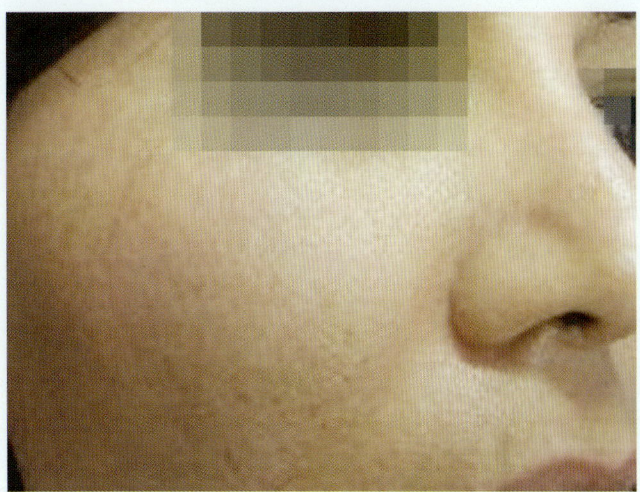

Fig. 10B: Fifteen days later from LASER treatment

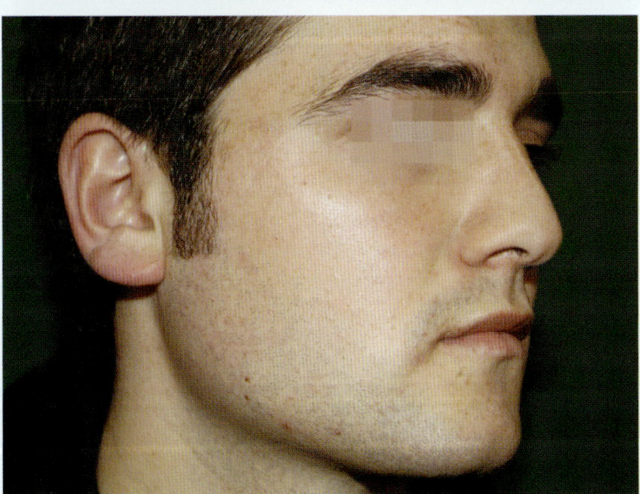

Fig. 11A: Before Er:YAG LASER ablation

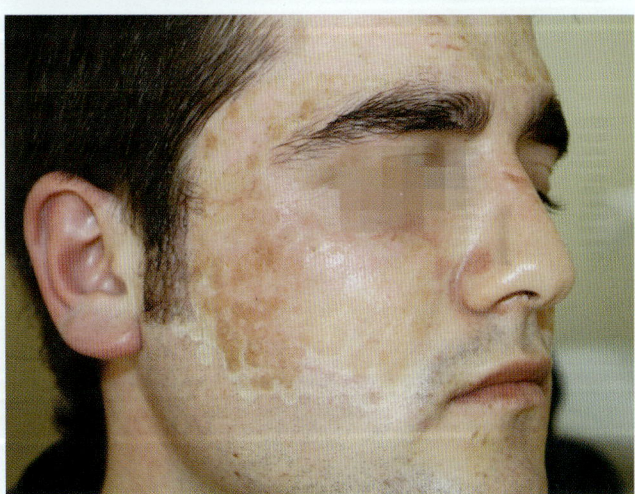

Fig. 11B: Immediately after operation

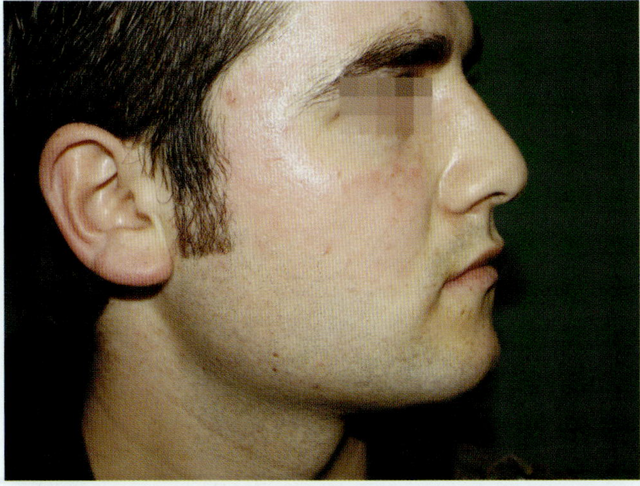

Fig. 11C: Seventh day

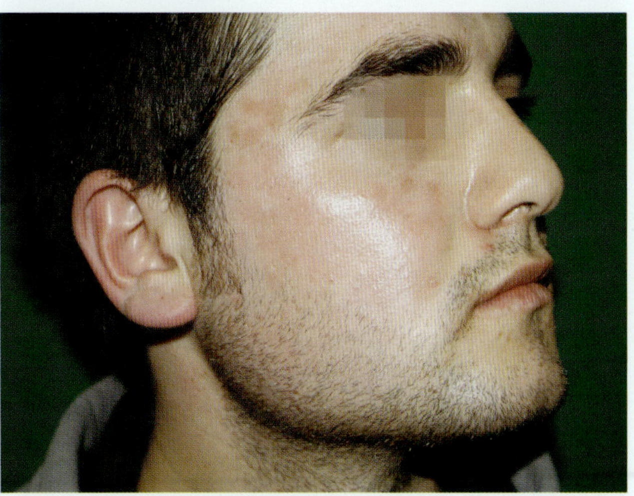

Fig. 11D: Twentieth day postoperatively

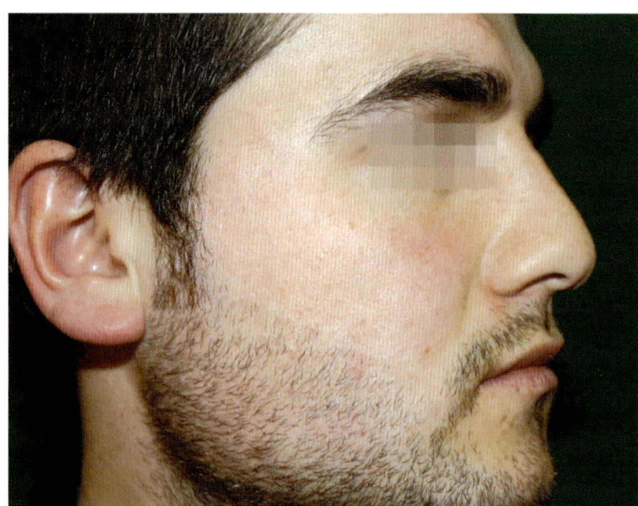

Fig. 11E: Four months after operation

diminished stem cell supply. Furthermore, while the number of sebaceous glands remains approximately the same throughout life, they tend to increase in size with age, and therefore younger patients may not be as suited to this form of treatment.

Several iatrogenic conditions can also serve as contraindications. Skin treated with radiation therapy should not undergo ablation for the same rationale just cited: namely, a relative absence of adnexal structures to repopulate the epidermis.

Recent treatment with isotretinoin also serves as a contraindication, since atypical scarring has been reported in dermabrasion and chemical peeling following its use. Though not evidence based, many consider a washout period of at least 1 year as adequate when treating patients who have been on isotretinoin. Ironically, despite the contraindication to ablative LASER resurfacing following systemic retinoid treatment, preoperative topical retinoids, often tretinoin, are often recommended. Tretinoin is thought to prime the skin for more rapid healing after ablation.

Finally, ablative resurfacing after extensive surgical procedures is also contraindicated.[2]

At the time of the consultation, patients are given prescriptions for an oral antibiotic, oral antiviral preparation.[8] Oral antiviral and antibacterial prophylaxis is generally recommended to prevent herpes and secondary bacterial eruptions.[2] Fluconazole administered postoperatively between days 3 and 8 significantly promotes re-epithelialization in patients undergoing full-face CO_2 LASER skin resurfacing. Fluconazole should be considered prophylactically in addition to antibiotic and antiviral medications in patients undergoing full-face CO_2 LASER resurfacing.[9]

ANESTHETIC CONSIDERATIONS

Prior to the procedure, the skin is cleansed with a mild cleanser to remove any makeup, sunscreen, creams, or lotions. Topical anesthetic cream is applied to the skin 60 minutes prior to treatment.

Options for anesthesia exist over a wide spectrum, from topical agents and local infiltration to nerve blocks and systemic agents.[1] A variety of topical anesthetics are available. Superficial LASER procedures are often managed with topical agents, such as lidocaine and prilocaine cream. However, with deeper and higher density treatments, topical anesthetic cream alone is not adequate to keep the patient comfortable during the treatment.[8] These can be combined with local infiltration of anesthetic, particularly when treating a specific cosmetic unit. When broadly treating the central forehead, median cheek, nose, upper lip, lower lip, and/or chin, a variety of blocks including supraorbital, supratrochlear, infraorbital, and mental nerve blocks may be employed as appropriate. Blocks may be achieved simply using lidocaine 1–2% with 1:100,000 or 1:200,000 epinephrine, but can be enhanced by bupivacaine 0.5%, 1:10 sodium bicarbonate ($NaHCO_3$) 8.4% to neutralize the pH and, subsequently, diminish pain.

Patients undergoing total face resurfacing and patients who are particularly sensitive may warrant the addition of systemic agents as well, including anxiolytics, narcotics, intramuscular sedation, or intravenous anesthesia.

If the edema is severe enough, oral corticosteroids may be prescribed over a short term. Cool compresses, head elevation, soaks in saline or water, and protection with a petrolatum ointment as well as bio-occlusive dressings are additional methods of caring for these patients postoperatively.

Additionally, patients must be strongly advised to use sunscreen and practice sun-protective behavior to reduce risks of postinflammatory hyperpigmentation.[2]

SURGICAL STEPS

Ablative LASER Resurfacing

Carbon Dioxide LASER

LASER resurfacing for rejuvenation was first widely offered in the 1980s using ablative CO_2 LASERS.[2] The CO_2 LASER emits a 10.600 nm wavelength which is strongly absorbed by tissue water (Table 1). The penetration depth is dependent upon the tissue water content, but not the melanin or hemoglobin content. With a pulse duration of less than 1 ms, CO_2 LASER light penetrates approximately 20–30 μm into the skin, and residual thermal damage can be confined to a 100–150 μm layer of tissue, although thermal coagulation up to 1 mm has been reported.[1]

Vaporization and removal of a surface layer of cells; coagulation necrosis of cells and denaturation of extracellular proteins in a subjacent residual layer; and nonfatal damage to cells in a deeper zone are all seen in CO_2 LASER resurfacing. The entire epidermis and varying thickness of the dermis are removed, and the patient's skin looks smoother and tighter during healing due to heat-induced shrinkage of collagen.[10]

The vaporization or boiling point of water at 1 atmosphere is 100°C. The fluence required to achieve pulsed-LASER ablation of skin tissue is 5 J/cm^2, with less energy producing diffuse tissue heating without vaporization. At these parameters, the skin temperature reaches approximately 120–200°C. The diameter of the beam plays a role, with small beams (100–300 μm in diameter) achieving high fluences and rapid tissue vaporization; however, the beam must be moved rapidly across the skin surface to avert desiccation, charring and heat diffusion. Beam diameters of greater than 2 mm induce nonvaporization heating and increase the risk of deep thermal damage due to the need to apply low fluences for longer periods of time in order for visible vaporization to occur. Based on these findings, the pulsed or scanned CO_2 LASERS were designed to combine high peak powers with short pulses and/or rapid movement across the skin surface.

Two basic CO_2 LASER systems have been utilized in cutaneous resurfacing. The first type is the high-powered pulsed CO_2 LASER system, which delivers energy in individual pulses of about 1 ms or less. This LASER produces up to 500 mJ of energy in each individual 600 μs to 1 ms pulse. Vaporization can be performed either with a 3-mm spot size or by a computer pattern generator, which can deliver various patterns of up to 80 pulses, each pulse measuring 2.25 mm in diameter.

The second type of CO_2 resurfacing LASER achieves well-controlled tissue ablation by rapidly scanning the focal spot of a focused continuous-wave CO_2 LASER over the skin. Computer-driven mechanical devices can scan a 0.2-mm spot in a spiral manner, ranging in diameter from 8–16 mm in several shapes at a constant velocity. No individual spot is irradiated more than once and the dwell time on any individual spot is less than 1 ms, while achieving fluences above the ablation threshold.[1]

Erbium: YAG LASER

The Er:YAG LASER was the next ablative LASER developed for skin resurfacing. It emits infrared (IR) LASER light with a wavelength of 2940 nm, which is close to the absorption peak of water and yields an absorption coefficient 16 times that of the CO_2 LASER (Table 1). Penetration depth of the Er:YAG LASER is limited to about 1–3 μm of tissue per J/cm^2 versus the 20–30 μm observed with the CO_2 LASER. This provides more precise ablation of skin with minimal thermal damage to the surrounding tissues; the residual thermal damage is estimated to be 10–40 μm. Operating the Er:YAG LASER at a fluence of 5 J/cm^2 vaporizes the epidermis in four passes, 8–12 J/cm^2 achieves this after two passes.

The Er:YAG LASER is almost totally absorbed by a very thin, superficial layer of skin and can be used for precise and superficial tissue ablation (Fig. 12). Additionally, the wavelength of the Er:YAG LASER is very close to an absorption maximum of collagen at 3030 nm. Therefore, skin containing 70–80% water has an absorption coefficient of approximately 8000–9000 cm^{-1} at 2940 nm.[11]

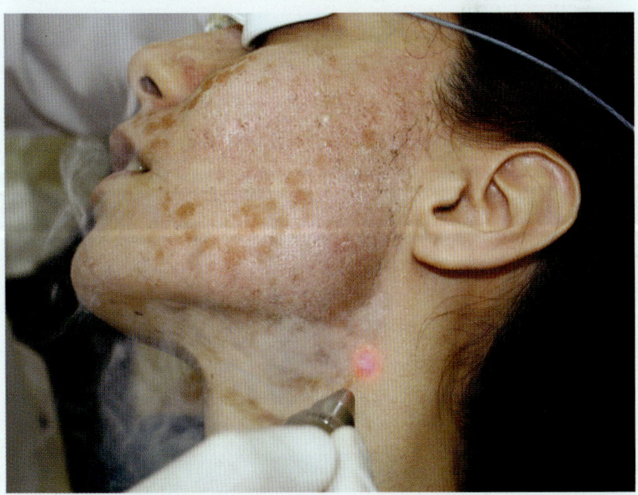

Fig. 12: Er:YAG LASER skin resurfacing

Table 1: Ablative LASER devices for rejuvenation and resurfacing

LASER/Device	*Target*	*Advantages*	*Disadvantages*
Carbon dioxide (10.600 nm) LASER	Water	Excellent efficacy for rhytides and photoaging	3-week recovery time, higher risk profile
Erbium:YAG (2.940 nm) LASER	Water	Excellent efficacy for rhytides and photoaging	3-week recovery time, higher risk profile
Nitrogen plasma	Cell membranes	Moderate to excellent efficacy for rhytides and photoaging	3-day to 3-week recovery time

Overall efficacy of the Er:YAG is rather similar to the CO_2 LASER, although the CO_2 LASER has been found to be superior in most comparative studies. Er:YAG LASER ablation is more superficial and wounds heal more quickly, but efficacy is less when fluences per pulse and number of passes similar to those of the CO_2 LASER are used. Er:YAG LASER treatment also produces less dermal collagen remodeling than the CO_2 LASER.[10] The variable-pulsed Er:YAG LASER (pulse durations of 10–50 ms) demonstrates immediate tissue contraction and a healing rate that is intermediate between the short-pulsed Er:YAG (pulse durations of 250–350 μs) and CO_2 LASERS. In comparative studies, the variable-pulsed Er:YAG LASER was very effective in the removal of rhytides, although the CO_2 LASER was still found to be slightly more efficacious.

The Er:YAG LASER results in less severe side effects of discomfort, erythema and edema, and overall healing times are faster than with the CO_2 LASER. When compared according to the depth of ablation performed, healing times for the two LASERS have been similar. In contrast to the bloodless nature of CO_2 LASER treatment (due to photocoagulation of blood vessels less than 0.5 mm in diameter), bleeding increases with successive passes with the Er:YAG LASER.[1]

Plasma Skin Resurfacing

Plasma skin resurfacing (PSR) is a relatively new nonablative and fully ablative strategy.[1] This novel device for ablative resurfacing works by passing radiofrequency (RF) energy into nitrogen gas. The "nitrogen plasma" causes rapid heating of the skin with limited tissue ablation and minimal collateral thermal damage (Table 1). Preliminary reports indicate improvement in facial rhytides and scars following treatment. However, PSR offers improvement of moderately photodamaged skin of the neck, chest, and dorsal hands with limited side effects.[12] Epidermal regeneration occurs by 7 days postoperatively, with neocollagenesis visible on histologic analysis at 90 days.[1]

This technology is based on delivery of high-energy RF into nitrogen gas, which generates nitrogen plasma targeted at the treatment area. Heat is transferred to the skin, driving the collagen denaturation and subsequent neocollagenesis. Although promising, this technology has not yet been fully evaluated in comparison to the CO_2 and Er:YAG LASERS.[2]

A pulse of ultrahigh-energy RF from the device generator converts nitrogen gas into plasma within the handpiece. The plasma emerges from the distal end of the device handpiece and is directed onto the skin area to be treated. Rapid heating of the skin occurs as the excited gas transfers heat to the skin. Fibroblast activity is increased during dermal regeneration, with the retained necrotic epidermis serving as a biologic dressing for the formation of a new stratum corneum and epidermis.

Ablative LASERS offer maximum clinical benefit with increased prevalence of dermal wounds and morbidity while nonablative LASERS offer minimal clinical benefit and minimal morbidity. This novel PSR system offers a compromise between the two treatments, providing patients with ablative like clinical results as well as the minimal morbidity associated with nonablative techniques.[12]

Nonablative Resurfacing

Nonablative LASER and light systems can be classified into three main groups: (i) Vascular LASERS such as the pulsed dye LASER (PDL) and pulsed potassium titanyl phosphate (KTP) LASER; (ii) Mid-IR LASERS targeting the dermis; and (iii) Intensed pulsed light (IPL) (Table 2). Initially, the Q-switched Nd:YAG LASER (1064 nm) was shown to induce dermal remodelling. Subsequently, vascular LASERS such as the PDL and pulsed 532 nm LASERS were employed but with minimal efficacy. Longer-wavelength IR LASERS, which more effectively target the mid dermis, have since become the most prominent nonablative LASERS, resulting in more consistent mild improvement in rhytides. IPL improves dyspigmentation and vascularity while at the same time emitting near-IR wavelengths that target the dermis, thereby resulting in global improvement in photodamage. More recently, RF systems have been developed, delivering electrical energy (with or without concomitant LASER or light) that results in more pronounced reduction of skin laxity and rhytides. The mechanisms for nonablative rejuvenation involve photothermal and other effects resulting in collagen contracture and neocollagenesis.[1]

The greatest advantage to nonablative LASERS over their ablative and fractional ablative counterparts is their more attractive side-effect profile. However, efficacy of a single treatment may be considered less than ideal. It is the responsibility of the physician to be certain that the patient has reasonable expectations and may require a series of treatments to achieve desired outcome.[2]

Nonablative LASER procedures selectively injure the dermis but protect the epidermis by cooling during treatment. Like ablative LASERS, nonablative LASERS emit coherent light at wavelengths absorbed by water.[1]

Fractional Resurfacing

In 2004, the concept of fractional photothermolysis (FP) was introduced. In photothermolysis, only a specific fraction of the epidermal and dermal architecture is treated.[13] The theory of fractional photothermolysis, pioneered by Anderson and colleagues, along with the technology of

Table 2: Nonablative LASER devices for rejuvenation and resurfacing

LASER/Device	*Target*	*Advantages*	*Disadvantages*
Vascular LASERS (532 nm pulsed KTP, 585 and 595 nm pulsed dye)	Dermal vasculature	Excellent safety, no recovery time, improvement in telangiectasias	Minimal efficacy, multiple treatments necessary
Near-infrared LASERS (1310 nm diode, 1320 nm long-pulsed Nd:YAG, 1450 nm diode, 1540 nm Er:glass) and light devices (1100–1800 nm)	Dermal collagen and water	Excellent safety, no recovery time, greater efficacy for rhytides	Modest efficacy, multiple treatments necessary
Intensed pulsed light source	Dermal vasculature, pigment, collagen and water	Moderate safety, no recovery time, improvement in telangiectasias and dyspigmentation	Minimal to modest efficacy, multiple treatments necessary
Radiofrequency energy source	Dermal collagen; dermal and subcutaneous charged particles and water	Excellent safety, no recovery time, greater efficacy for rhytides and laxity	Modest efficacy, multiple treatments necessary

traditional ablative LASERS, has spawned the rise of the field of fractional ablative therapy (Table 3).[2]

Fractional photothermolysis is based upon the scientific concept of creating microscopic thermal wounds deep to the surface of the skin, which allow for tissue contraction, stimulation of collagen, and rapid wound healing. Fractionated LASERS drill microscopic holes into the dermis in a grid pattern. FP has been likened to aerating a lawn. The "lawn plugs," termed microscopic epidermal necrotic debris, are expelled via a transepidermal elimination process over 7–10 days. The consequences are twofold: (i) Dermal conditions that have been approached indirectly in the past via epidermal wounding are now directly wounded as portions of the normal dermis are removed; and (ii) The remaining adjacent intact dermis and epidermis allow for rapid healing without relying on the presence of adnexal structures to regenerate the epidermis.[8]

Fractionated 1.410-nm erbium-doped fiber, 2.940-nm erbium: YAG and 10.600-nm CO_2 LASERS have also been developed.[1] The first LASERS employing this concept were the nonablative fractional technologies, such as the 1.550-nm erbium-doped fiber LASER.[2] A 1.550-nm erbium-doped fiber LASER causes cylindrical areas of thermal damage to the epidermis and upper dermis, which are spaced at a density of approximately 1.000–3.000 microscopic treatment zones of photothermolysis per cm^2. Each column or 'microthermal zone' is approximately 70–150 µm in width with a vertical thermal injury depth of 400–700 µm into the dermis. Approximately 15–25% of the skin surface area is ablated per treatment session.[1]

Histologic studies examining fractional ablative devices have demonstrated that typical microthermal zones consist of a tapered ablative zone, surrounded by eschar and a thermal coagulation zone, with maximum lesion depths ranging from 300 µm to over 1 mm and lesion widths of 140 µm to almost 300 µm. More recently, it has been reported that fractional ablative LASERS can achieve a depth of over 1.5 mm into the dermis at higher energy levels (70 mJ). Furthermore, re-epithelialization was shown to be complete in a matter of 2 days, with extrusion of the coagulated tissue, or microepidermal necrotic debris.[14]

Following full-face resurfacing with ablative fractional photothermolysis (AFP), complete re-epithelialization is generally seen in 3–6 days. This is in contrast to the 2–3 weeks of recovery following full-face resurfacing with traditional CO_2 LASER systems. Rapid re-epithelialization after AFP treatment results in very few infections, which are further reduced with the use of prophylactic antiviral and antibiotic therapy. Faster re-epithelialization also results in patients requiring fewer days of occlusive ointment application. This greatly reduces the rate of acneiform eruptions, which are seen in up to 83% of patients treated with traditional CO_2 LASERS. The rapid recovery times seen with fractionated CO_2 LASER marks a significant improvement over traditional CO_2 and Er:YAG LASER resurfacing.[8]

Practical Tips for Treatment of LASER Resurfacing

Prior to treating patients with any of the available ablative LASER systems, it is important for the practitioner to have

Table 3: Indications and parameters for fractional LASER resurfacing

Indication	*Energy/MTZ (mJ)*	*Density (MTZ/cm²)*	*Number of passes*	*Total treatment density (MTZ/cm²)*
Melasma				
Skin types I–II	6	250	12	3,000
Skin types III–VI	6	250	8	2,000
Rhytides				
Mild	12	125	12	1,500
Moderate	15	125	8	1,000
Severe	20	125	8	1,000
Acne scarring				
Skin types I–II	15–20	125	8–12	1,500–1,000
Skin types III–VI	15	125	8	1,000
Photoaging				
Skin types I–II	10	250	8	2,000
Skin types III–VI	8	250	8	2,000

an understanding of the extent of tissue injury produced by the device at various settings and consider the thickness of the skin and the depth required to ablate the skin abnormality, in order to choose safe and effective treatment settings.

Published histologic studies on the thickness of the skin, and the depth and number of adnexal structures at various anatomic sites, and histologic studies showing the depth and width of tissue injury with varying LASER parameters are helpful in guiding the clinician in the choice of appropriate LASER settings.

When using AFP devices with small spot sizes, increasing energy results in deeper tissue injury. Increasing energy with both of these devices also increased the width of the zones of ablation and coagulation of tissue. Treatments utilizing higher energies increase the time required for resolution of edema and erythema following treatment. In addition, deeper treatments result in more pinpoint bleeding during and following treatment. It is important to use lower energies when treating areas with thinner skin, such as the eyelids and neck.[1,2,8]

Spot sizes less than 200 μm allow for deeper penetration into tissue, whereas spot sizes greater than 300 μm result in a shallower depth of penetration at the same energies. When superficial treatment is the goal, as in treatment of dyschromia, the practitioner may choose a larger spot size, whereas for treatment of skin conditions, such as scars and rhytids, a small spot size will result in deeper tissue injury required to achieve a clinical result.

Density determines the distance between microthermal zones (MTZs). Increasing the density decreases the distance between MTZs, resulting in treatment of a larger percentage of the skin surface. Treatments at higher densities increase the duration of edema and erythema following treatment. It is prudent to use lower densities in areas with lower density of hair follicles, such as the neck and lower eyelid. Higher densities are necessary and can be used safely to treat deep rhytides in the perioral region.

In general, shorter pulse durations are desirable. Longer pulse durations result in more collateral heating of the tissue. When using LASERS that have pulse durations greater than 2 milliseconds, the authors recommend compensating for the increase in collateral tissue heating by using lower densities.[8]

COMPLICATIONS OF LASER SKIN RESURFACING

- Prolonged erythema
- Acne and milia
- Contact dermatitis
- Recall phenomenon
- Infection
- Pigmentary alteration
- Eruptive keratoacanthomas
- Hypertrophic scarring
- Ectropion formation
- Delayed purpura
- Superficial erosions
- Anesthesia toxicity[11,15-17]

Prolonged Erythema

Immediate post-treatment erythema (Figs 13A and B) is an expected consequence of fractionated LASER skin resurfacing that usually resolves within 3–4 days. Prolonged erythema is defined as post-treatment

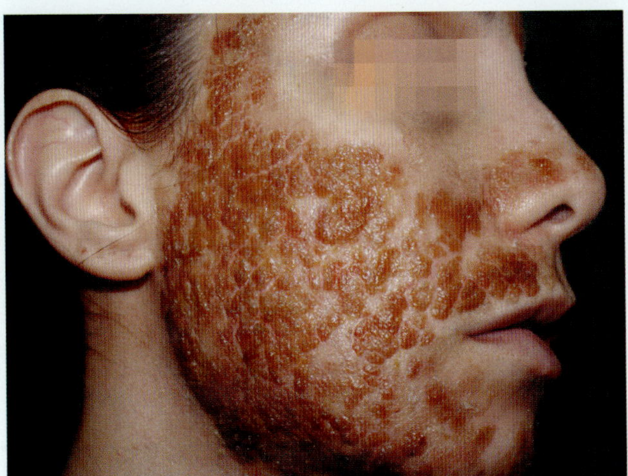

Fig. 13A: Post-treatment crusting. Five days later Er:YAG ablation

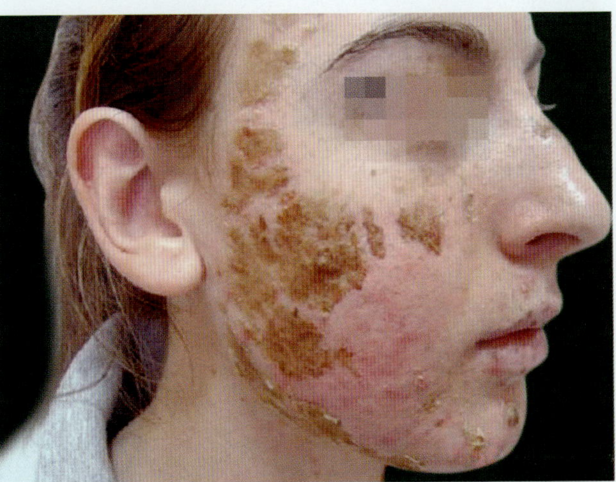

Fig. 13B: Post-treatment erythema and crusting. Four days later Er:YAG ablation

erythema that persists longer than 4 days with nonablative resurfacing and beyond 3–4 months with ablative treatment.[8,15] Flushing within the treated site upon physical exertion or emotional stress may occur for up to 1 year after resurfacing.[1]

Photomodulation with a 590-nm-wavelength LED array can decrease the intensity and duration of postfractional LASER treatment erythema.[18] In addition, given its anti-inflammatory properties, topical ascorbic acid should be considered because a previous study reported less severe and shorter postablative LASER resurfacing erythema with its use.[15]

Infection

Given that viral, bacterial, and fungal infections usually present during the first postoperative week, proper identification and treatment are essential to avoid further complications, including delayed wound healing, scarring, co-infection with other pathogens, and systemic dissemination.

Infection rate ranging from 6–8% for all patients is treated with ablative resurfacing devices.[19] The rate of Herpes simplex virus (HSV) infection, the most common type of infection after fractional LASER skin resurfacing, has been reported in 0.3–2% of cases. In contrast, infection rates with traditional (nonfractionated) LASER treatment are higher, with 2–7% of cases developing HSV reactivation. Patients may not present with classic herpetiform vesicopustules but instead may demonstrate only superficial erosions that develop during the first week after treatment. To minimize the risk of HSV reactivation with fractional resurfacing, antiviral prophylaxis should be administered when a prior history of facial HSV is documented or if full-face ablative LASER procedures are performed. In these patients, oral antiviral agents should be initiated concomitant with or 1 day before treatment and continued for 5–7 days.[11,15] The agent of choice for HSV prophylaxis remains acyclovir 400 mg orally twice a day,[19] or famciclovir 250 mg or 500 mg twice day.[20] Antiherpetic prophylaxis is recommended for all patients undergoing full-face or perioral LASER resurfacing regardless of past HSV history.[20] Furthermore, fractional skin resurfacing should not be performed on patients with active HSV infection, given the risk of HSV exacerbation.[15]

The rate of bacterial infection with traditional LASER vaporization tends to be low (0.5–4.5% of cases).[15] Prophylactic systemic antibiotics and appropriate topical care are used to minimize the risk of bacterial infection.[1] Excessive wound occlusion during the early postoperative period can enhance the likelihood of pathogen overgrowth, primarily *Staphylococcus aureus* and *Pseudomonas aeruginosa*.[13] The increased prevalence of methicillin-resistant *Staphylococcus aureus* in the community (with carrier rates as high as 40% in some regions) warrants the use of topical mupirocin three times a day.[19]

Disseminated infection, the causative agents and appropriate treatment are essential, especially in light of possible methicillin resistant *Staphylococcus aureus*. Notwithstanding, controversy remains with regard to the use of prophylactic systemic antibiotics in all patients but should be standard practice in patients at high risk, especially those who are immunosuppressed or have documented mitral valve prolapse with regurgitation or other valvular heart disease.[15]

Acne and Milia

Transient acneiform eruptions and milia are relatively common after traditional nonfractionated LASER resurfacing, with up to 80% of cases developing the former and more than 14% developing the latter. Although the rates of acneiform eruptions are significantly lower (2–10%) with fractional skin resurfacing, the incidence of milia development has been reported in as many as 19% of treated patients.

Given that occlusive moisturizers and dressings can exacerbate such eruptions, most authors recommend their avoidance or a change to noncomedogenic equivalents. Disruption of follicular units during treatment and aberrant follicular epithelialization during healing may further contribute to acne exacerbation.

In moderate to severe acne flares, short courses of oral tetracycline-based antibiotics have been advocated. Antibiotics can also be prescribed during subsequent treatments to prevent future outbreaks.[11,15]

Dermatitis

Irritant contact dermatitis may be observed following application of topical anesthetics; it does not correlate with patch test findings but resolves with appropriate treatment (e.g., topical corticosteroids). This occurrence increases the likelihood of postoperative erythema and hyperpigmentation. Irritant or allergic contact dermatitis due to other etiologies (e.g. wound dressings, topical antibiotics) may also develop during the first 4 weeks after treatment and also responds to mid to high-potency topical corticosteroids. Perioral dermatitis is infrequently observed 1–3 months after resurfacing of the perioral region, and responds to oral doxycycline.[1]

Pigmentary Alteration

Postinflammatory hyperpigmentation (PIH) is much less frequent with fractional LASER skin resurfacing than with other ablative procedures but is observed in 1–32% of patients, depending on the system used, parameters applied, and skin phototypes treated. Patients with darker skin phototypes (Fitzpatrick III–VI) have a higher likelihood of developing PIH.[15] Both the density and energy of the treatment determines the risk of PIH in dark-skinned patients.[21]

In general, fractional resurfacing of darker skin should use higher fluencies, lower density settings, and longer treatment intervals. To further minimize the risk of PIH, patients should avoid sun exposure at least 2 weeks before and after fractional skin resurfacing. In contrast to traditional nonfractionated LASER resurfacing, PIH is typically less intense and of shorter duration.

Hypopigmentation is an extremely uncommon complication of fractional LASER skin resurfacing. One reported case involved transient hypopigmentation 15 days after treatment that was attributed to the prophylactic use of topical tretinoin and hydroquinone.[15]

Scarring

Hypertrophic scarring is a known and rare complication of ablative skin resurfacing using CO_2 and Er:YAG LASERS.[15] Focal areas of erythema and induration 2–4 weeks after treatment are the first signs of potential scar formation. Nine of ten published cases involved fractional ablative skin resurfacing of the neck, resulting in multiple vertical and horizontal hypertrophic scars.

Scarring after LASER therapy may be due to overly aggressive treatments of insensitive areas (including excessive energy, density, or both), lack of technical finesse, associated infection, or idiopathic. Care should be taken when treating sensitive areas such as the eyelids, upper neck, and especially the lower neck and chest by using lower energy and density. Postoperative infections may lead to scarring and may be prevented by careful taking of history, vigilant postoperative monitoring and/or prophylactic antibiotics.[22]

The neck is also a well-recognized site that is especially susceptible to the development of scarring because of the small number of pilosebaceous units and poor vasculature in this region, which are essential for wound healing. In addition, the thin skin of the neck renders it more susceptible to thermal injury.[15,23]

Other scar-prone anatomic locations that also require more conservative treatment protocols include the periorbital and mandibular regions.[15]

Ectropion Formation

Cicatricial ectropion is a rare and serious complication that has recently been reported after fractional CO_2 LASER treatment. The lower eyelid is typically involved. Careful intraoperative detection of excessive collagen contraction and use of lower energy density settings help to minimize ectropion formation.[15]

Eruptive Keratoacanthomas

Keratoacanthomas are low-grade malignant skin tumors that are known to arise over sites of trauma. Although previously described in association with ablative LASER treatment of the face,[24] the development of multiple eruptive keratoacanthomas after fractional resurfacing has more recently been reported on the legs of two patients.[25]

Recall Phenomenon

Heat-induced recall phenomenon has been observed after skin resurfacing with a combination (1.320/1.440 nm) fractional LASER. After resolution of transient post-treatment wheal-like erythema, some patients experience reappearance of erythematous patches after a hot shower or prolonged exposure to direct sunlight, resulting in a "recall" phenomenon. The exact mechanism has not been fully elucidated, but it appears that there is activation of neurogenic or histamine or mast cell-dependent mechanisms responsible for high levels of molecules that produce erythema in the skin.[15]

The wavelengths or deep heating component of this combination device might be responsible for the phenomenon through the activation of pathways or increased levels of molecules that produce erythema in the skin: histamine, 5-hydroxytryptamine, phospholipase A_2, cyclooxygenase, interleukin-1, and tumor necrosis factor. However, in contrast to this line of thinking, a previous study assessing the wheal and flare reaction following treatment of human forearm skin with an argon LASER demonstrated that the reaction could not be blocked by pretreatment with acetylsalicylic acid or antihistamines, suggesting a neurogenic rather than a histamine or mast cell-dependent mechanism.[26]

REFERENCES

1. Armenakas MRA, Dover JS, Arndt KA. Laser therapy. In: Bolognia JL, Jorizzo JL, Rapini Rp (Eds). Bolognia Dermatology, 2nd edition. Spain: Mosby Elsevier; 2008. pp. 2099-120.
2. Brightman LA, Brauer JA, Anolik R, et al. Ablative and fractional ablative lasers. Dermatol Clin. 2009;27(4):479-89; vi-vii.
3. Tanzi EL, Wanitphakdeedecha R, Alster TS. Fraxel laser indications and long-term follow-up. Aesthet Surg J. 2008; 28(6);675-8.
4. Sandel HD 4th, Perkins SW. CO_2 laser resurfacing: still a good treatment. Aesthet Surg J. 2008;28(4):456-62.
5. Avram MM, Tope WD, Yu T, et al. Hypertrophic scarring of the neck following ablative fractional carbon dioxide laser resurfacing. Lasers Surg Med. 2009;41(3):185-8.
6. Newman JB, Lord JL, Ash K, et al. Variable pulse erbium:YAG laser skin resurfacing of perioral rhytides and side-by-side comparison with carbon dioxide laser. Lasers Surg Med. 2000;26(2):208-14.
7. Weinstein C, Scheflan M. Simultaneously combined ER:YAG and carbon dioxide laser (derma K) for skin resurfacing. Clin Plast Surg. 2000;27(2):273-85.
8. Tierney EP, Eisen RF, Hanke CW. Fractionated CO_2 laser skin rejuvenation. Dermatol Ther. 2011;24(1):41-53.
9. Conn H, Nanda VS. Prophylactic fluconazole promotes reepithelialization in full-face carbon dioxide laser skin resurfacing. Lasers Surg Med. 2000;26(2):201-7.
10. Geronemus RG. Fractional photothermolysis: current and future applications. Lasers Surg Med. 2006;38(3):169-76.
11. Kutlubay Z, Gokdemir G. Treatment of atrophic facial acne scars with the Er:YAG laser: a Turkish experience. J Cosmet Laser Ther. 2010;12(2):65-72.
12. Alster TS, Konda S. Plasma skin resurfacing for regeneration of neck, chest, and hands: investigation of a novel device. Dermatol Surg. 2007;33(11):1315-21.
13. Manstein D, Herron GS, Sink RK, et al. Fractional photothermolysis: a new concept for cutaneous remodeling using microscopic patterns of thermal injury. Lasers Surg Med. 2004;345):426-38.
14. Hantash BM, Bedi VP, Kapadia B, et al. In vivo histological evaluation of a novel ablative fractional resurfacing device. Lasers Surg Med. 2007;39(2):96-107.
15. Metelitsa AI, Alster TS. Fractionated laser skin resurfacing treatment complications: a review. Dermatol Surg. 2010; 36(3):299-306.
16. Fisher GH, Geronemus RG. Short-term side effects of fractional photothermolysis. Dermatol Surg. 2005;31(9 Pt 2): 1245-9.
17. Graber EM, Tanzi EL, Alster TS. Side effects and complications of fractional laser photothermolysis: experience with 961 treatments. Dermatol Surg. 2008;34(3):301-7.
18. Alster TS, Wanıtphakdeedecha R. Improvement of postfractional laser erythema with light-emitting diode photomodulation. Dermatol Surg. 2009;35(5):813-5.
19. Setyadi HG, Jacobs AA, Markus RF. Infectious complications after nonablative fractional resurfacing treatment. Dermatol Surg. 2008;34(11):1595-8.
20. Alster TS, Nanni CA. Famciclovir prophylaxis of herpes simplex virus reactivation after laser skin resurfacing. Dermatol Surg. 1999;25(3):242-6.
21. Chan HH, Manstein D, Yu CS, et al. The prevalence and risk factors of post-inflammatory hyperpigmentation after fractional resurfacing in Asians. Lasers Surg Med. 2007; 39(5):381-5.
22. Fife DJ, Fitzpatrick RE, Zachary CB. Complications of fractional CO_2 laser resurfacing: four cases. Lasers Surg Med. 2009;41(3):179-84.
23. Avram MM, Tope WD, Yu T, et al. Hypertrophic scarring of the neck following ablative fractional carbon dioxide laser resurfacing. Lasers Surg Med. 2009;41(3):185-8.
24. Gewirtzman A, Meirson DH, Rabinovitz H. Eruptive keratoacanthomas following carbon dioxide laser resurfacing. Dermatol Surg. 1999;25(8):666-8.
25. Mamelak AJ, Goldberg LH, Marquez D, et al. Eruptive keratoacanthomas on the legs after fractional photothermolysis: report of two cases. Dermatol Surg. 2009;35(3):513-8.
26. Foster KW, Fincher EF, Moy RL. Heat-induced "recall" of treatment zone erythema following fractional resurfacing with a combination laser. Arch Dermatol. 2008;144(10): 1398-9.

CHAPTER 92

Hair Transplantation

Jumroon Tungkeeratichai

INDICATIONS

Primary Alopecia

- Genetic hair loss (85% are men)[1]

Secondary or Traumatic Alopecia

- After trauma or surgery procedures such as endoscopic forehead facelifts, forehead facelift or facelifts
- Previous hair transplantation to improve hairline and unnatural large plug grafts[2,3]

The hair follicles begin to develop between 9 weeks and 12 weeks of gestational age from ectodermal and mesodermal cells. The ectoderm gives rise to the hair matrix cells and the melanocytes responsible for the pigmentation of hair. Two buds form off of this layer, one gives rise to the sebaceous gland. Hair production can typically be seen by 16–20 weeks of gestation[4] (Fig. 1).

Fig. 1: Hair follicle

The scalp contains approximately 100,000–125,000 terminal hairs.[5] Transverse or horizontal sections of the scalp show that hair follicles are organized into follicular units. Each unit contains one to four terminal hairs, one or two vellus hairs, nine sebaceous glands and arrector pili muscle insertions and a perifollicular vascular plexus, neural net and connective tissue (Fig. 2).

The scalp consists of five layers—SCALP; the outer layer is the skin. The subcutaneous layer contains fat, connective tissue, vessels, lymphatics and nerves. The galea aponeurotica combines with the frontalis muscle anteriorly and the occipitalis muscle posteriorly. Loose connective tissue lies between the galea and periosteum of the skull. The arterial supply to the scalp is provided by five pairs of arteries: the supraorbital and supratrochlear arteries in front, the superficial temporal and retroauricular arteries laterally and the occipital arteries posteriorly[4] (Fig. 3).

Hair growth can be divided into three phases. Anagen is the active (growth phase), about 90% of hair follicles are in the anagen phase and its duration is between 2 years and 8 years. The catagen is the active loss (regression

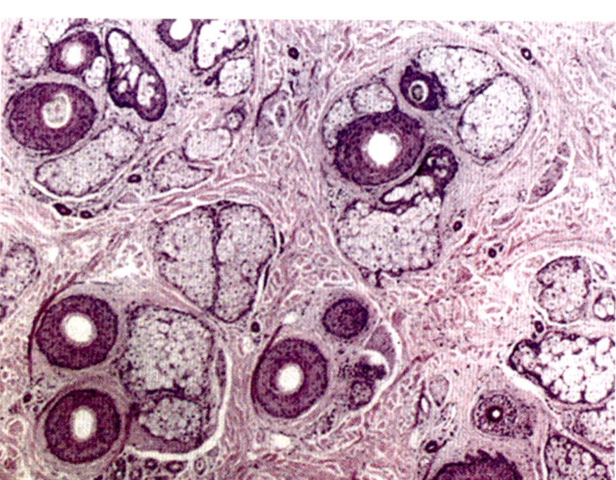

Fig. 2: Follicular units

phase), shortest of three phases and its duration between 2 weeks and 4 weeks, is characterized by separation of the hair shaft from the dermal papilla and migration toward the epidermis. The telogen follicles are in active and hair growth stop (resting phase) or resting phase, about 10% hair follicles are in this phase, which lasts 2–4 months, hair shaft detaches from the dermal root resulting in the hair falling out. Scalp hair growth occurs at a rate of approximately 37–44 mm/day and normal scalp hair loss is 50–100 hairs/day[6-8] (Figs 4A and B).

ANDROGENETIC ALOPECIA

The term androgenetic alopecia (AGA), both androgens and genetic factors work together to produce hair loss pattern. The most common form of hair loss is androgenetic alopecia or male-pattern balding (MPB). Typically, it affects the bitemporal and frontal hairline first, followed by diffuse thinning of hair over the vertex. The dermal papilla is most likely the target for these androgen-induced changes. As the follicle becomes smaller, hair becomes finer and less pigmented. Also, the time of each cycle spent in anagen becomes shorter while the telogen phase becomes longer. The ratio of time spent in anagen compared to telogen reduces from 12:1 to 5:1[9] (Fig. 5).

Both men and women are affected by AGA. It is transmitted in an autosomal dominant pattern. Approximately 33% of people with a positive family history of AGA will be affected. In most patients, 30–50% of hair losses occur before it becomes apparent. Thirty percent of white men have AGA by age 30 years, 50% are affected by age 50 years and 40% of women are affected by age 70 years.

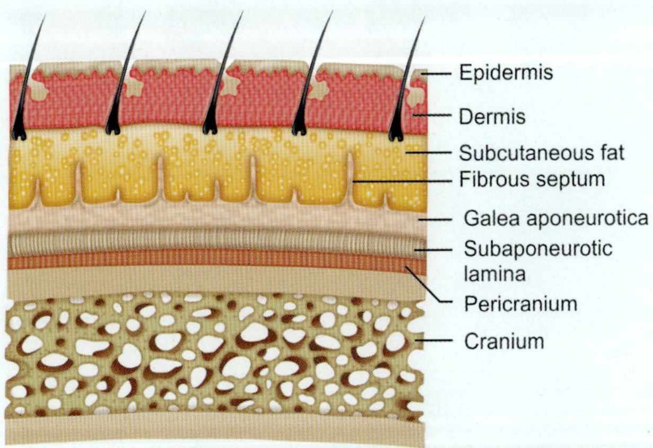

Fig. 3: Outer layer of the skin

CLASSIFICATION

Many classification systems of hair loss in androgenetic alopecia have been devised. Hamilton, in 1951,[10] was the first to publish such a schematic but his system was later revised by Norwood in 1973. Today, the Norwood system is most commonly used to classify MPB. Female androgenetic alopecia follows the Ludwig classification system that was introduced in 1977[7] (Figs 6 and 7).

PATIENT EVALUATION FOR SURGERY

Age is not a contraindication for hair replacement surgery.[11] It is important to emphasize that the hair replacement techniques available today do not result in new hair growth, but instead involve redistribution of

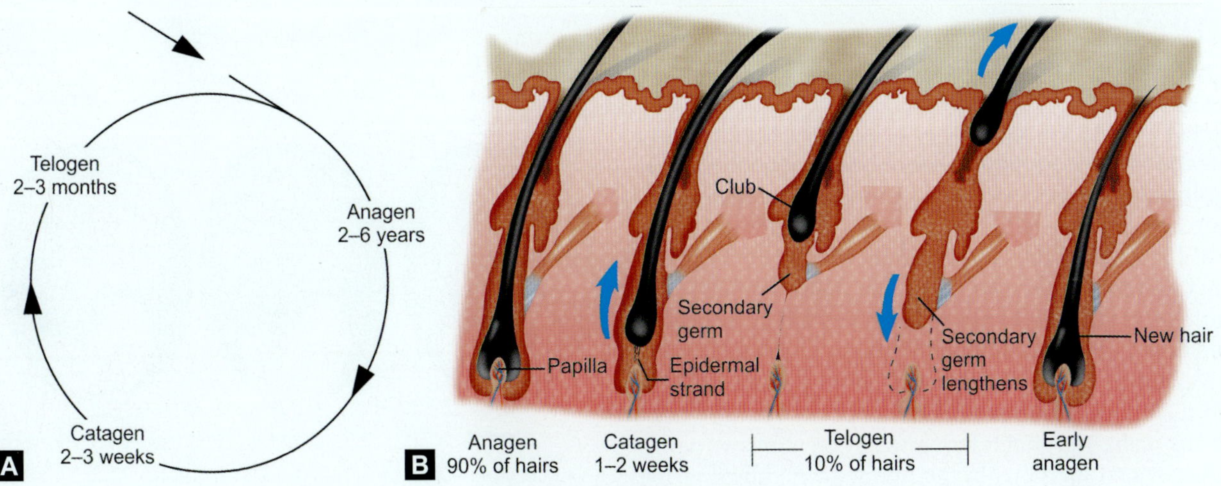

Figs 4A and B: Hair cycle

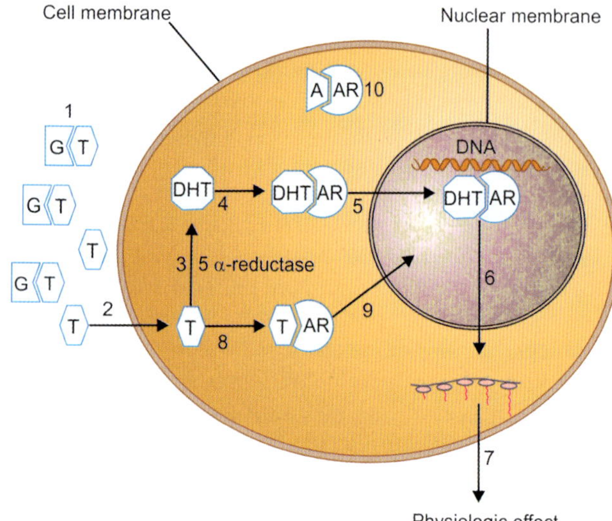

Fig. 5: Androgen pathway

1. Testosterone (T) bound to circulating binding globulin (G)
2. T enters target cell.
3. Conversation of T to dihydrotestosterone (DHT) 5 alpha-reductase.
4. DHT binds to cytosol androgen receptor (AR).
5. DHT-AR complex enters cell nucleus.
6. DHT-AR complex binds to DNA, producing cell-spacific mRNA.
7. Protein synthesis produces physiologic effect.
8. Direct binding of T to alternate cytosol AR.
9. T-AR complex enters cell nucleus.
10. Antiandrogen (A) binds to cytosol AR.

remaining hair. Therefore, in order to be a candidate for these procedures, a patient must have adequate donor hair at occipital and parietal scalps.

FOLLICULAR UNIT HAIR TRANSPLANTATION

In 1939 Okura, a Japanese dermatologist, was the first to describe to using small full-thickness autografts of hair-bearing skin to correct alopecia. In 1959 Orentreich, a New York dermatologist, discovered the principle of donor dominance. He harvested via 4 mm round punch grafts from the occipital scalp.[5]

This provides grafts that typically contain 10–20 hairs/punch depending on hair density of the donor site. Hair distribution can be visualized and the remaining spaces filled in with new grafts.[12,13]

Vallis was the first to describe strip grafting in 1964. This technique involves a free composite graft of hair-bearing scalp. The graft is harvested by creating two parallel, horizontal incisions in the donor scalp, down to the

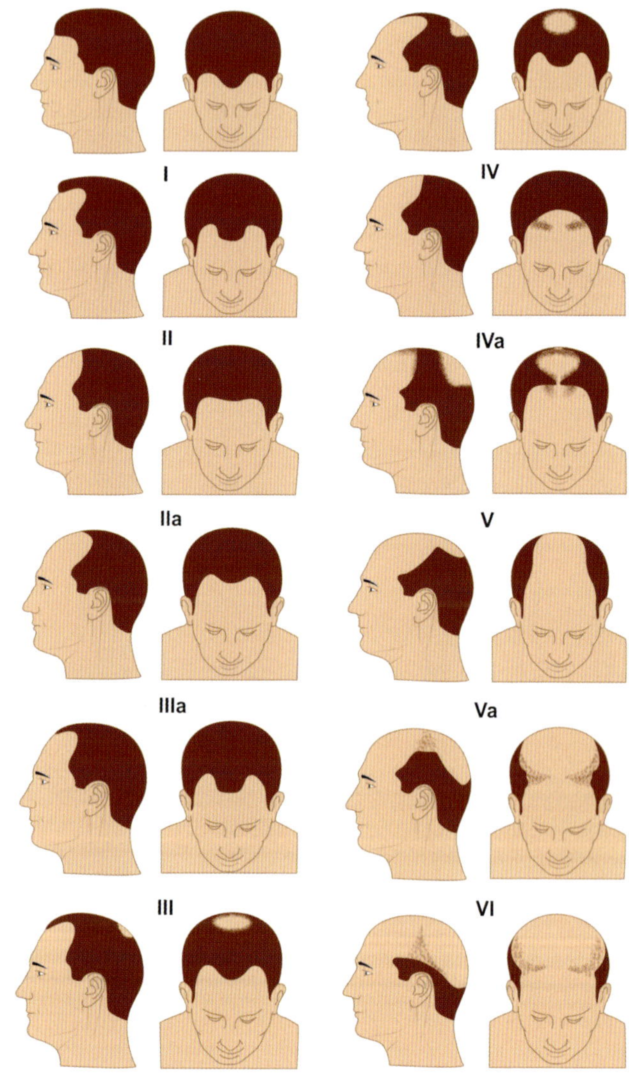

Fig. 6: Norwood classification

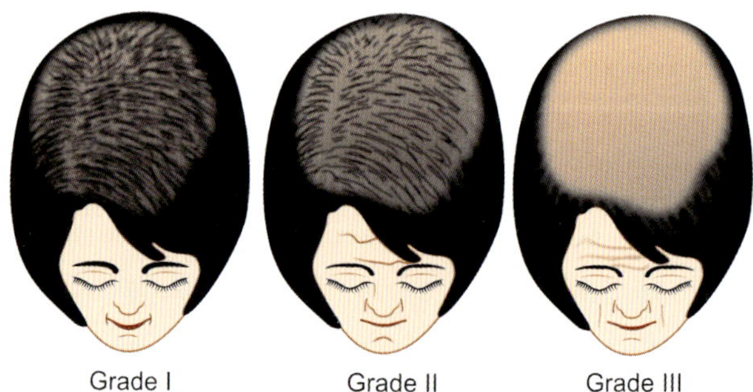

Fig. 7: Ludwig classification

level of the galea. It is elevated in this plane and the donor site closed.[14]

In 1980, Bobby Limmer began to transplant grafts that were dissected along these natural cleavage planes. Thus was born Total Follicular Unit Transfer.[5]

Follicular-unit transplantation is probably the most widely used hair grafting method today. In this technique, large numbers of minigrafts (3–4 hairs/graft) and micrografts (1–2 hairs/graft) are utilized to cover significant areas of balding scalp. Several different methods of follicular-unit transfer are described by various authors; herein is the technique as outlined by Barrera. Donor hair is harvested from the occipital scalp in one large ellipse, the size of which is determined by hair density, scalp elasticity and the area of alopecia to be covered. Graft dissection proceeds on a separate table under bright lighting and magnification. The donor tissue is first cut into 2 mm segments, aligning all incisions in the direction of follicle growth. Then, a #10 blade is used to further dissect the segments into micrografts and minigrafts, taking care to preserve natural groupings of hair follicles. The grafts are kept moist and cool while the recipient area is prepared. The direction of grafted hair growth can be controlled by changing the angle of the scalpel when creating the slits. This is particularly important along the frontal hairline where the direction of growth should be angled 45–60 degrees anteriorly. If there are residual native hairs in the region being grafted, the slits should be placed parallel to the existing hairs. Barrera advocates placement of a moist, light pressure dressing that is removed after 48 hours. Patients are then instructed to shampoo daily and begin applying minoxidil 2% topical spray twice daily.[7]

Six Steps for Hair Transplantation

1. Patient Preparation
2. Anesthesia
3. Donor Strip Harvest
4. Donor Strip Dissection
5. Recipient Sites
6. Postoperative Care

1. Patient Preparation

Hairline design: The midpoint of the forehead is normally 8 cm from the glabella. Then, estimate the number of hair for transplantation after design of frontal hairline (Fig. 8)

- Average non-balding scalp has 100 follicular units per square centimeter
- 50% of hair may be lost before noticeable thinning
- Aim density at approximate 30–40 units per square centimeter

How many grafts must be harvested are based on donor hair density; typically donor density in mid-occiput contained 70–100 follicular units per square centimeter. If surgeon needs 1,000 grafts, the projected numbers reflect 10 cm long by 1 cm wide strip of donor hair.[15] Measurement of scalp laxity is done to estimate the maximal donor strip width that can be safely removed during hair transplantation. Trim donor area to 2 mm with electric clippers from occipital protuberance medially to over ears laterally and then the donor area has been planned out and marked (Figs 9A and B).

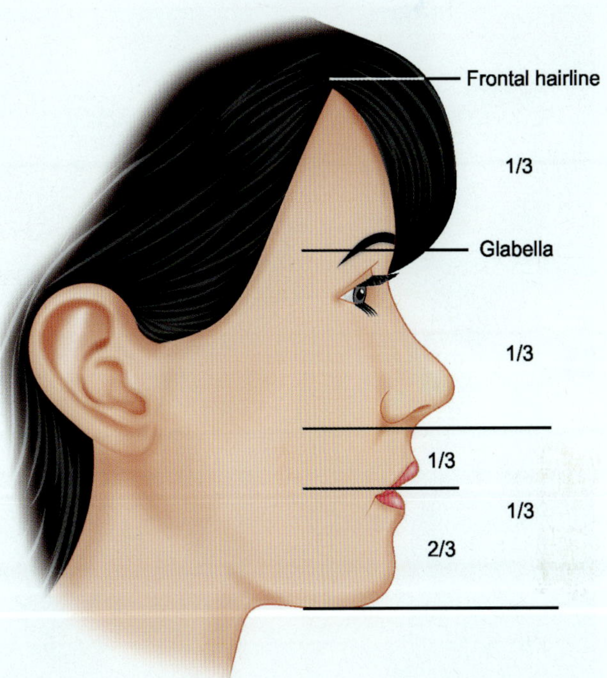

Fig. 8: Horizontal role of third

2. Anesthesia (Figs 10A and B)

- Oral sedation with Dormicum 15 mg; 1 tablet 20 minute before surgery
- Local anesthesia for donor and recipient sites
  - 1% Lidocaine with Epinephrine 1:100,000 (20 mL)
  - +0.9% NSS (20 mL) + 0.5% bupivacaine (20 mL)
  - +7.5% sodium bicarbonate (3 mL)
    - Lidocaine for quick onset
    - Bupivacaine for increased duration
    - Epinephrine for hemostasis and increased duration
    - Sodium bicarbonate to decrease stinging
- Donor-recipient tumescent solution after injection of local anesthesia (Fig. 11)
  - 1% Lidocaine (10 mL) + 0.9% NSS (100 mL) + epinephrine (0.3 mL)
  - Purpose of injection tumescent solution is to :

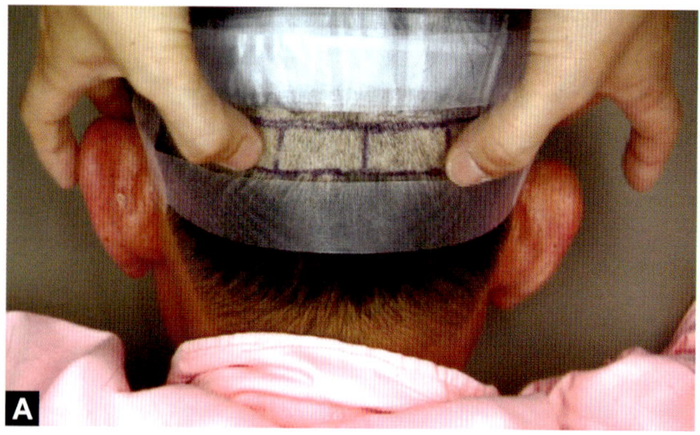

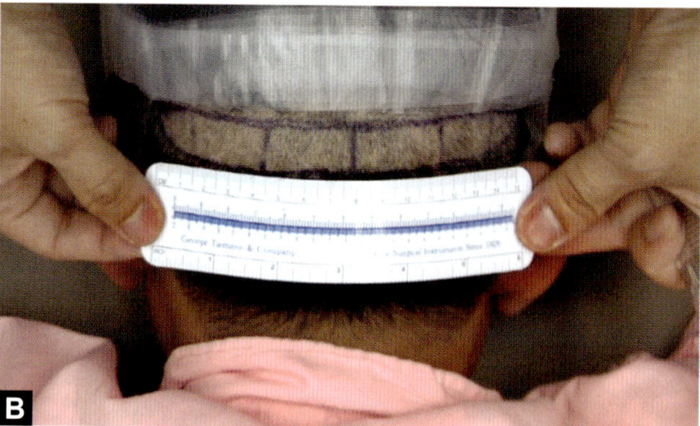

Figs 9A and B: Scalp laxity

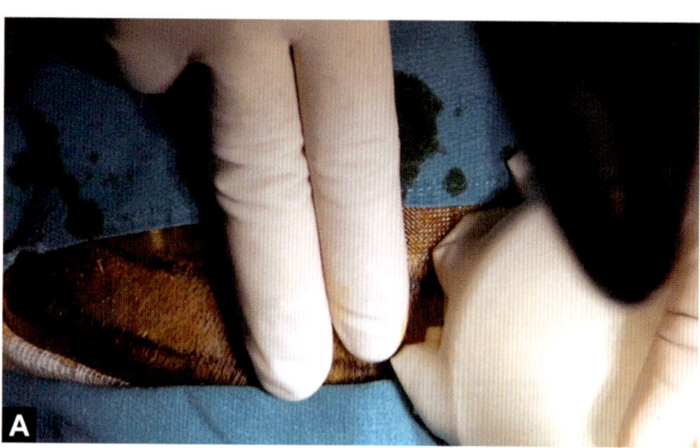

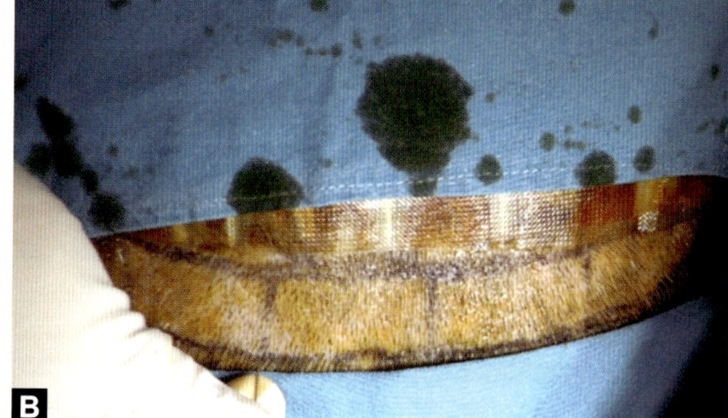

Figs 10A and B: Local anesthesia

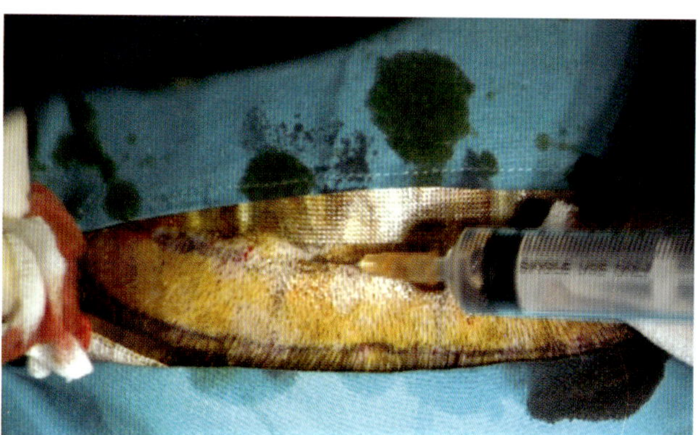

Fig. 11: Donor-recipient tumescent

  - Increase follicular distance from blood vessels and nerves
  - Increase rigidity of donor area
  - Decrease bleeding
  - Reduce total amount of anesthesia required
- The procedure starts with the patient sitting up or in prone position for ring-block anesthesia and donor harvest

3. Donor Strip Harvest

Donor area preparation: The donor area is shaved and the ellipse is marked. The hair-bearing ellipse is cut with an oblique angle parallel the hair axis angle to avoid damaging the hair follicles. Just deep from hair follicle not deeper than vessel The midline of the donor area is determined by the landmark of the bony occipital protuberance. The lateral limit of hair transplant is defined by the auricle about two finger breadths or approximately 2 cm above the top of the ear. If width of donor strip more than 1.5–2 cm subcutaneous suture with 3-0 vicryl suture is necessary for prevent scar. Before suture skin superior edge of epithelium 1 mm is removed for trichophytic wound closure,[16-18] then suture skin with 4-0 nylon suture continuous locking fashion (Figs 12A to F).

4. Donor Strip Dissection

To avoid follicular transection all graft dissections are under binocular stereo microscopic 10-power magnification.[19,20] Right now all graft dissections are under LED monitor that has more power magnification than binocular stereomicroscopic. Preparing the follicular units: the

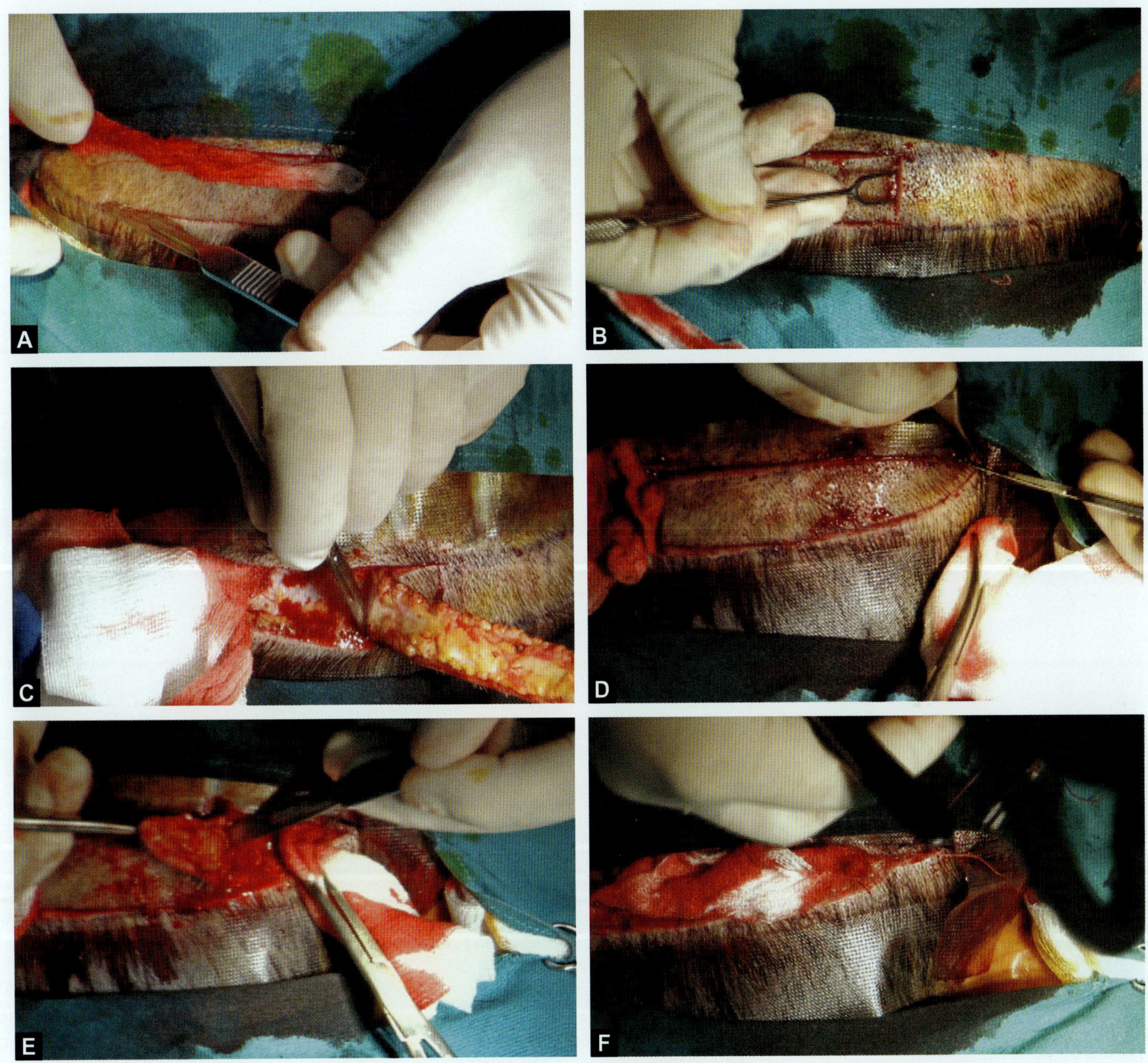

Figs 12A to F: Donor strip harvest

hair-bearing ellipse is placed on a hard wooden and cut into several slices. The grafts are divided into two groups: micrografts consisting of one or two hair follicles and minigrafts consisting of three or four hair follicles.[21] After the grafts have already been divided, they are soaked in 0.9% normal saline and kept under control temperature at 4° C (Figs 13A to F).

5. Recipient Site (Figs14A to E)

- Average non-balding scalp has 100 follicular units per square centimeter
- 50% of hair may be lost before noticeable thinning
- Aim density approximately 20–40 units per square centimeter
- Keep recipient sites small, but large enough so that grafts do not need to be forced in place
- Visible scars are not produced by needles 18 gauge or less
- Recipient sites

Instrument size guide equivalents

20 gauge = 1-hair unit

19 gauge = 2-hair and thin 3-hair units

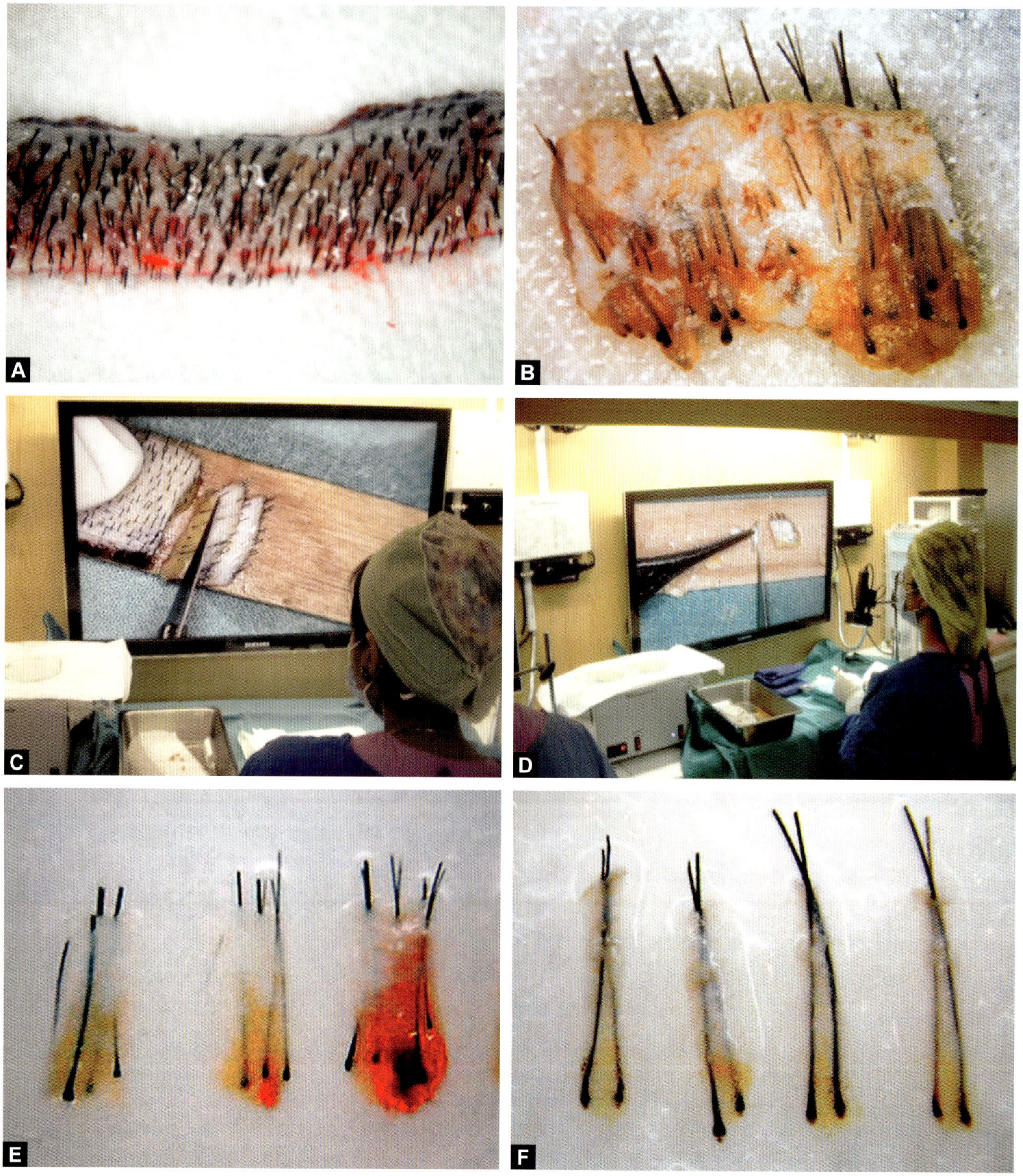

Figs 13A to F: Donor strip dissection. (A to D) Minigraft Unit; (E and F) Micrograft Unit

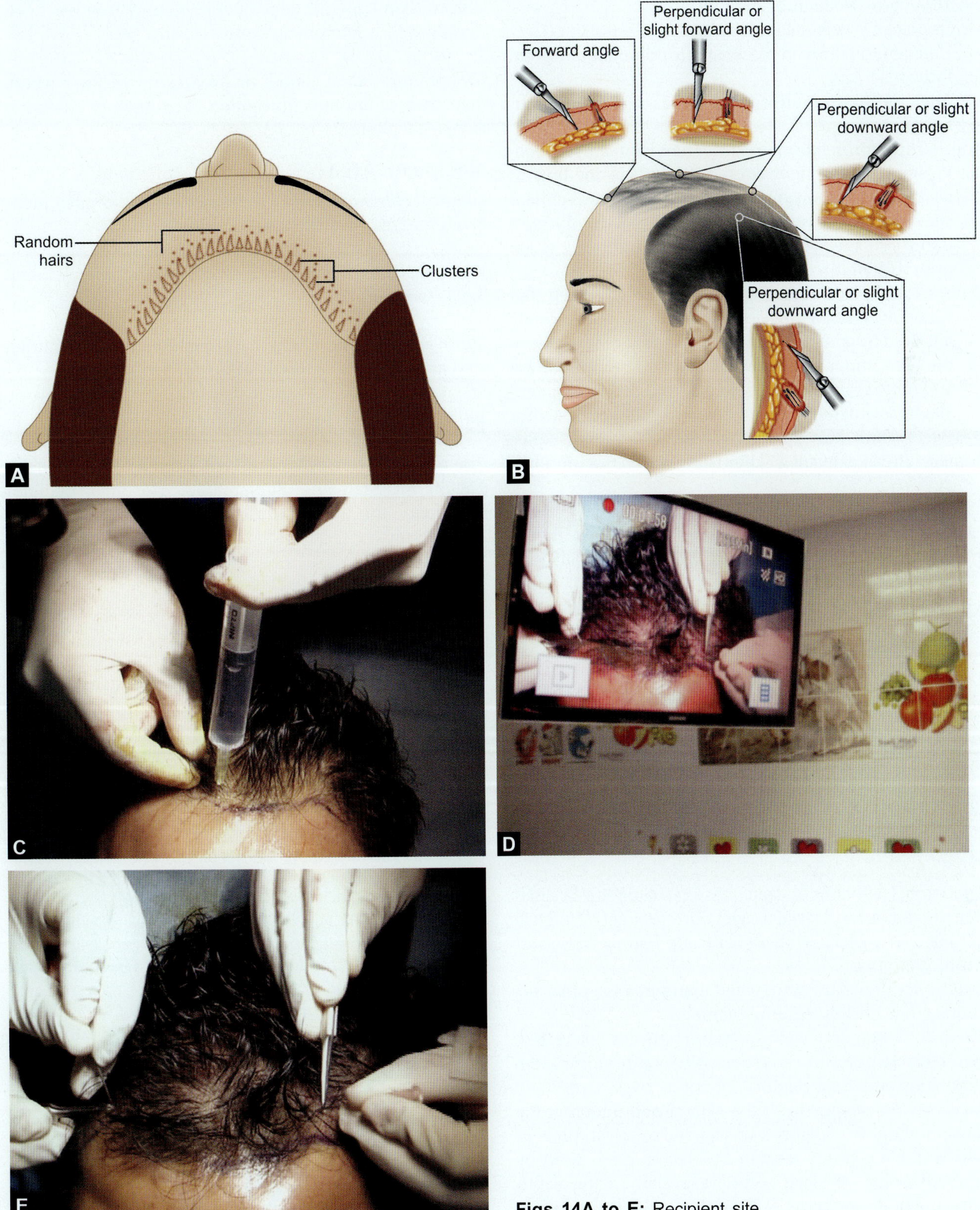

Figs 14A to E: Recipient site

18 gauge = 3-hair and 4-hair units

Grafts placed at original growing angle

- Hair anterior to vertex transition point should point forward
- Angle becomes more acute as it reaches the anterior hairline

There are two principle methods for recipient-site creation:

1. Pre-making recipient sites describe the method in which the surgeon makes almost all of the recipient sites after which the surgical assistant[16] places the graft into these sites at the end of procedure (sites made prior to graft insertion).[5,22]
2. Stick-and-place describes a method in which the surgeon makes a single site (stick) and immediately followed by graft insertion (place). Right now we place the graft under LED monitor to so that more precise and more graft can be inserted per square centimeter.

The transplanted hairs usually fall out within 3–6 weeks and hair growth will begin 3 months after surgery. The final result will be visible within 6–8 months.

6. *Postoperative Care*

Wash scalp with sterile water

- Apply antibiotic ointment and pressure headband dressing to donor
- Patient to have hair washed on postoperative day 3 to remove crusts
- Pain medication and antibiotic for 1 week
- No strenuous activity for 1 week
- Return to clinic in day 2 to remove dressing and day 10 for stitch off donor site
- Wait for at least 6–8 months between sessions

COMPLICATION[5,23,24]

Donor Area

Effluvium: Hair in the anagen phase can suddenly be shed due to a temporary lack of oxygen during surgery. Hair will fall out 2–3 weeks postoperatively and regrow will occur within 3 months.

Dehiscence: It occurs more when epidermis to epidermis contact than dermis to dermis contact.

Necrosis: When too wide, a donor strip is harvested, extremely tight closure cause a massive compromise of the circulation and tissue death.

Excessive donor scarring: If the skin closed under strong tension, there is a high risk of scar widening. To prevent scar widening, severe tension free technique is used by sunbcutneous 3-0 vicryl suture, especially if the width applying of donor strips is more than 1.5-2.0 cm. Before suture, skin superior edge of epithelium 1 mm has been removed for trichophytic wound closure.

Donor harvesting: Blood vessel and nerve transection, hair transection and Prevention the tumescent solution subgaleal plane.[18]

Recipient Area

Surgical effluvium: Hair will fall out 2–3 weeks postoperatively and regrow will occur in 3 months.

Cysts, pustules: Burying of grafts by making the recipient holes too deep.

Pitting and tenting: Grafts are placed too deeply in pitting and are placed too superficially in tenting.

ACKNOWLEDGMENTS

The authors are thankful to Prof Amnuay Thithapangha Faculty of Medicine Ramathibodi Hospital, Mahidol University for advice during the preparation of this manuscript.

REFERENCES

1. Fisher J. Management of alopecia. In: Guyuron B, Elof Eriksson, Murray JE, et al. (Eds). Plastic Surgery: Indication and Practice, volume 2. Philadelphia: Saunders; 2009. pp. 1391-1408.
2. Vogel JE. Correction of the cornrow hair transplant and other common problems in surgical hair restoration. Plast Reconstr Surg. 2000;105(4);1528-36.
3. Epstein JS. Revision surgical hair restoration: repair of undesirable results. Plast Reconstr Surg. 1999;104(1); 222-32.
4. Nordstrom RE. Scalp, hair, baldness, and surgery. Facial Plast Surg. 1985;2(3);173-7.
5. Hair Transplant Preoperative 360. In: Lam SM (Ed). Hair Transplant 360: For Physicians, volume 1. New Delhi: Jaypee Brothers Medical Publishers (P) Ltd.; 2011. pp. 1-45.
6. Nigman AM. The human hair cycles. J Invest Dermatol. 1959;33:307.
7. Barrera A. Hair Transplantation: The Art of Micrografting and Minigrafting. St. Louis: Quality Medical Publishing Inc.; 2002.
8. Abell E. Embryology and anatomy of the hair follicle. In: Olsen EA (Ed). Disorders of Hair Growth, Diagnosis and Treatment. New York: McGraw-Hill Inc.; 1994.
9. Sinclair R. Male pattern androgenetic alopecia. BMJ. 1998;317;865-9.
10. Norwood OT. A classification of male pattern baldness. South Med J. 1975;68:1359.

11. Nordstrom RE. The initial interview. Facial Plast Surg. 1985;2(3):179-87.
12. Unger WP. Construction of the hairline in punch transplanting. Facial Plast Surg. 1985;2(3):221-30.
13. Vallis CP. Treatment of male pattern baldness by punches, strips, and flaps. In: Courtiss EH (Ed). Male Aesthetic Surgery, 2nd edition. St. Louis: Mosby; 1991.
14. Vallis CP. The strip graft. Facial Plast Surg. 1985;2(3); 245-52.
15. Hair transplant preoperative 360. In: Lam SM (Ed). Hair Transplant: For Physicians, volume 1. New Delhi: Jaypee Brothers Medical Publishers (P) Ltd.; 2011. pp. 47-126.
16. Frechet P. Donor harvesting with invisible scars. Hair Transplant Forum Int. 2005;15:119-20.
17. Marzola M. Trichophytic closure of the donor area. Hair Transplant Forum Int. 2005;15:113-16.
18. Marzola M. Single-scar harvesting technique. In: Haber RS, Stough DB (Eds). Hair Transplantation. Philadelphia: Elsevier Saunders; 2006. p. 83.
19. Limmer BL. The history of follicular unit micrografting technique: A personal view. In: Unger W, Shapiro R (Eds). Hair Transplantation. New York: Marcel Dekker Publishers; 2004. pp. 383-8.
20. Limmer BL. Donor strip slivering and microscopic dissection. In: Haber RS, Stough DB, (Eds). Hair Transplantation. Philadelphia: Elsevier Saunders; 2006. pp. 87-9.
21. Pathomvanich D. Donor harvesting: a new approach to minimize transection of hair follicles. Dermatol Surg. 2000;26:345-8.
22. Pathomvanich D. Hair Transplantation in Asians. In: Haber RS, Stough DB (Eds). Hair transplantation. Philadelphia: Elsevier Saunders; 2006. pp. 149-56.
23. Cooley JE. Complication of hair transplant. In: Unger W, Shapiro R (Eds). Hair Transplantation. 4th edition. New York: Marcel Dekker Publishers; 2004. pp. 568-73.
24. Marzola M, Vogel JE. Complication: Haber RS, Stough DB, (Eds). Hair Transplantation. Philadelphia: Elsevier Saunders; 2006. pp. 173-85.

CHAPTER

93

Surgery for Alopecia

Arunesh Gupta, Dipesh J Malviya, Akshay P Deshpande

INTRODUCTION

The surgical treatment of alopecia includes:

- Synthetic hair grafting
- Hair transplant
- Scalp reduction surgery
- Scalp flaps
- Expanded scalp flaps

SYNTHETIC HAIR GRAFTINGS

In this technique, synthetic hairs made up of polyethylene terephthalate (PET) are inserted percutaneously into the scalp.

Requirements for Synthetic Hair

The synthetic hair should have the following properties.

- It must not dissolve after placement
- It must be completely removable without fragmentation
- It must have low potential for infection
- It must have no residual toxicity or mutagenicity after sterilization
- It must have long-term durability
- It must be heat stable
- It must have appearance of natural hair.

Advantages

- Supply is infinite
- Simple procedure
- Variety of hair styles can be achieved.

Disadvantages

- Chances of infection exist
- Not all grafted hair are permanently fixed, thus requires follow-up sittings
- Facial swelling
- Loss of natural hair
- Foreign body reaction
- Fiber breakage
- Risk of carcinogenesis from deeply embedded bits of fibers
- Pruritus.

HAIR TRANSPLANT

It is the redistribution/rearrangement of the existing hair follicles in a particular pattern by various techniques so as to cover the bald areas of alopecia and give a good cosmetic camouflage. In this, a horizontal strip of scalp is harvested from occipital area; its hair units with follicle are separated under magnification and implanted over the area of baldness under local anesthesia.

Indications for Hair Transplant

- Male pattern alopecia
- Female androgenic alopecia
- Cicatricial alopecia
- Reconstruction of eyebrows, eyelashes and side burns.

Contraindications

- Large bald area
- Small donor area
- Low hair density
- Progressive microscopic polyangiitis (MPA) in young patient with strong family history
- Bleeding disorders
- Keloidal tendency
- Systemic debilitating disease
- Patient with unrealistic expectation.

Preoperative Evaluation

- Whether or not the donor site has adequate hair
- To design a hair pattern that is appropriate not only as patient ages but also on the basis of progressive hair loss
- Patient's family history specially from maternal side
- *Classification of hair loss*: Norwood classification (Fig. 1)

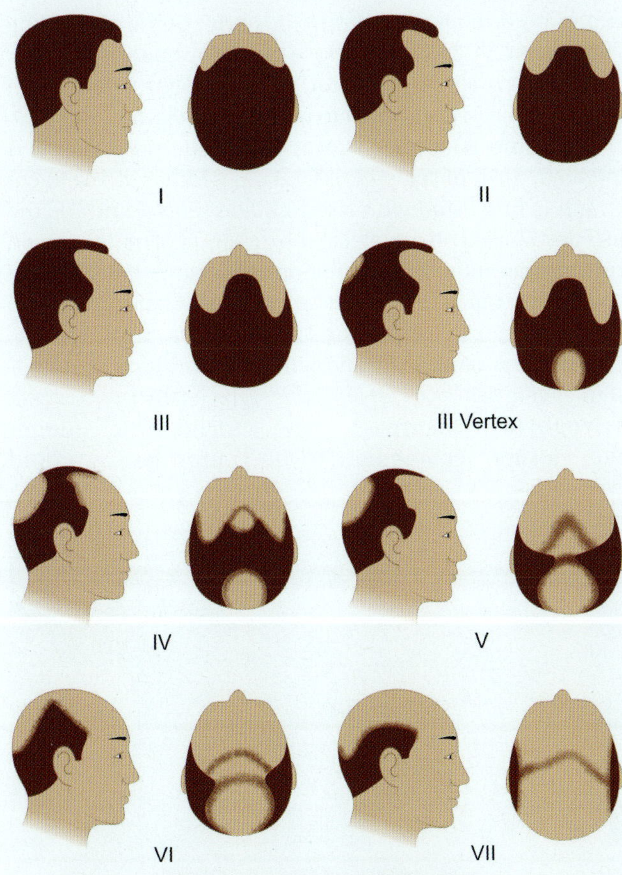

Fig. 1: Norwood classification

The recommended number of follicular unit grafts for hair transplantation is indicated in Table 1.

- *Type of hair*: Color, texture, density, curling, straightness
- Assessment of frontotemporal angle (Fig. 2)
- Medical history
- *Drug history*: Aspirin, anticoagulants, etc. should be discontinued 2 weeks prior
- Alcohol, caffeine, smoking should be avoided
- Number of sittings required
- Previous procedures like scalp reduction, etc.
- Informed consent
- Premedications
  - Minoxidil lotion/foam Local Application at bedtime (should be stopped 1 week before surgery)
  - Tab. Finasteride 1 mg OD
  - Multivitamin tab. I OD.
- Shampooing
- Trimming
- Preoperative photographs.

Assessment of density of hair and dimension of strip to be harvested—photo of 1 × 1cm square from donor site is taken and hairs are counted. This gives density of hairs. According to the requirement of grafts based on Norwood classification, strip of scalp is excised with width of around 1–1.5 cm.

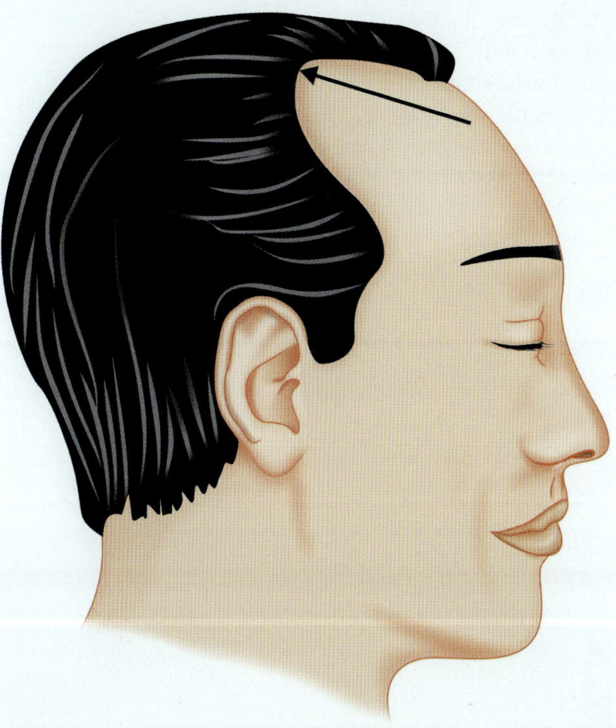

Fig. 2: Frontotemporal angle

Table 1: Requirement of follicles

Norwood class	*Follicular units*
III	800–1,000+
III Vertex	800–1,000+
IIIA	1,300–1,600+
IV	1,100–1,400+
IVA	1,700–2,100+
V	1,500–1,800+
VA	2,200–3,000+
VI	2,000–3,200+
VII	2,000–3,500+

Anesthesia

Procedure is done under local anesthesia. (for average 70 kg adult). Tumescent solution is prepared by mixing:
20 mL 2% xylocaine
10 mL sensorcaine
2 mL adrenaline

70 mL ringer lactate.
102 mL- total
Infiltration - Occipital region for strip harvest - 20 mL
Frontal hairline - 20 mL
Supratrochlear and supraorbital block - 2 mL + 2 mL
50 mL of remaining solution + 50 mL ringer lactate for tumescent infiltration over recipient area.
Some patients require light sedation.

Steps of Surgery

Preparation of Donor Site and Harvesting of Strip

Donor site is approximately marked as follows. Lateral border at a line perpendicular to external auditory canal, superior border is according to posterior border of balding zone generally 11–12 cm above posterior hairline, inferior border 4 cm above posterior hairline. Light trimming of hairs is done over the area to be excised (Fig. 3).

Betadine is applied. Local anesthetic preparation is injected. Strip of scalp of 0.5–1.5 cm width and 10–20 cm length is harvested with No. 10 blade (Figs 4 and 5). The incision should be parallel to the direction of hairs to avoid cutting the bulb. The strip is raised in supragaleal plane just below the hair follicles and fat. The harvested strip with intact hair follicles and shaft is shown in Figure 8. Donor site is closed with prolene 4-0 continuous sutures/ staples (Fig. 6).

Tricophytic closure—A new "trichophytic" donor site closure technique ("tricho") provides improved

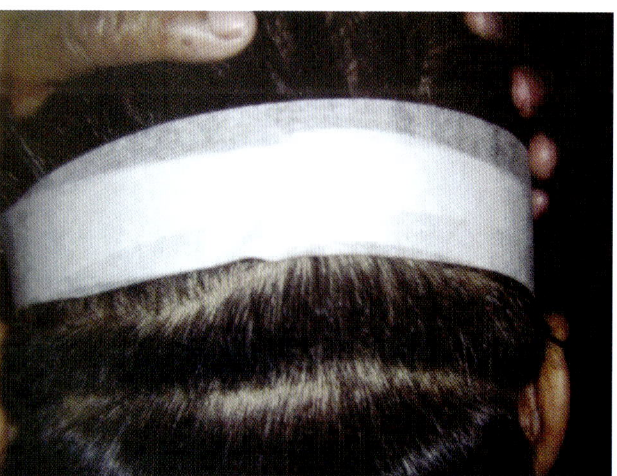

Fig. 3: Donor site preparation

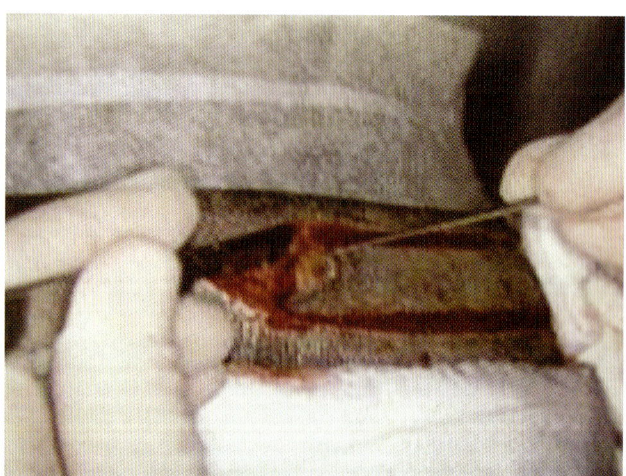

Fig. 4: Donor strip harvesting

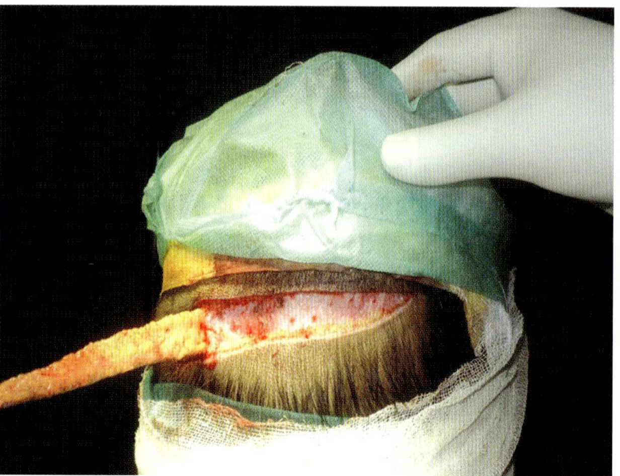

Fig. 5: Donor strip harvesting completed

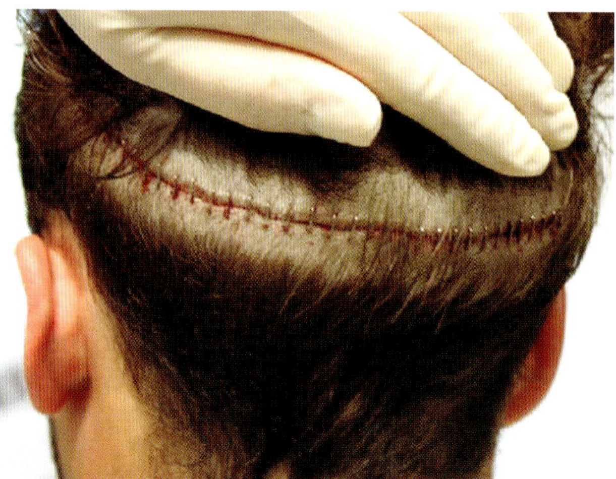

Fig. 6: Donor site closure completed

camouflage of a linear donor scar in Follicular Unit Transplantation. Normally, in FUT, the surrounding hair easily covers the scar. For some patients with very short hairstyles, the resulting donor scar may be visible. With the trichophytic closure technique, one of the wound edges (upper or lower) is de epithelised , allowing the edges to overlap each other and the hair to grow directly through the donor scar. This can significantly improve the appearance of the donor area in patients who wear their hair very short and who had previous transplant surgery.

Graft Preparation

Slices containing 1 to 3 follicular units(FUs) are separated from harvested strip under magnifying glass or loupes (Fig. 10). This process is called "slivering" (Fig. 9). The grafts and strip are always kept in cold saline in petri dish to prevent desiccation (Figs 7 and 11).

Recipient Site Preparation

Recipient area is anesthetized with prepared solution by supratrochlear and supraorbital blocks and tumescent infiltration .Marking is done as discussed with patient (Fig. 12).

Incisions are made 0.5-2 mm apart, more closely over frontal and central scalp, either by 18 G/19 G needle or miniblades. In needle and stick technique, after puncturing the scalp, about 5 mm deep or till the beveled edge of needle just disappears, needle is slightly withdrawn, the hair graft inserted in the incision with follicle down and simultaneously needle is withdrawn. Grafts should be placed from front to back and should snugly fit in the incision (Fig. 13).

Direction of grafts — frontal region- forward
Parietal region — downward and forward
Vertex — radiating and spiral manner
Occipital region — downward

No dressing is applied, antibacterial ointment is applied. Follicular Unit transplant has been completed (Fig. 14). Patient is kept under observation for 2 hours and discharged with antibiotics, analgesics. Finasteride and minoxidil are continued postoperatively.

Complications

Donor site

- Hypertrophic scar and keloid
- Infection
- Wound dehiscence
- Hematoma, neuroma
- Cyst formation.

Recipient site

- Poor graft survival
- Chronic folliculitis
- Elevated or depressed grafts
- Changes in hair texture.

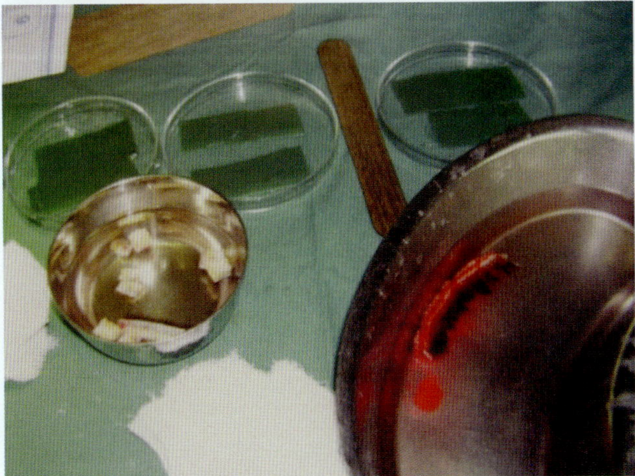

Fig. 7: Scalp strip kept in cold saline

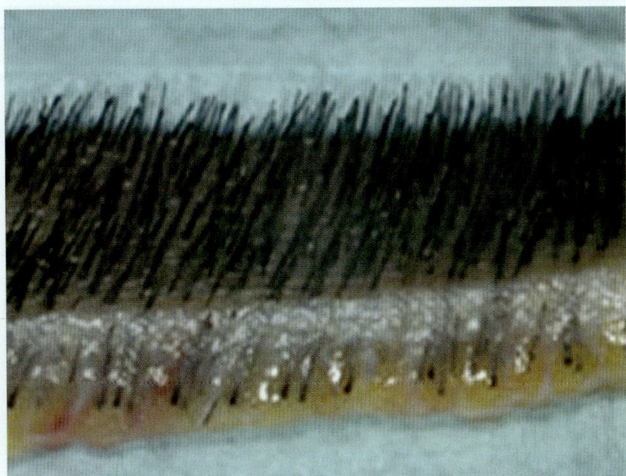

Fig. 8: Close up view of strip with visible hair shafts and follicles

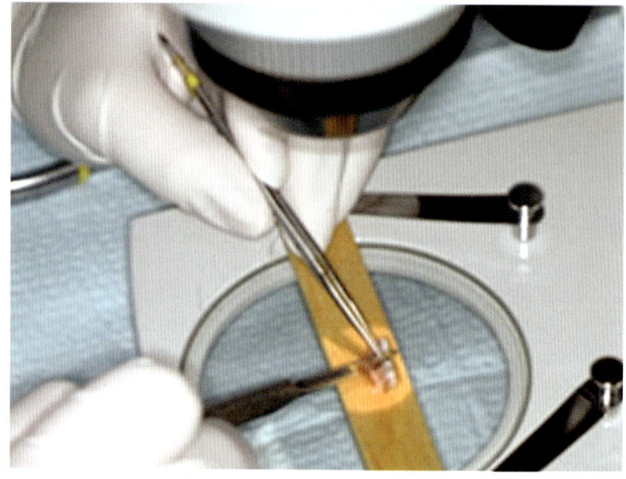

Fig. 9: Slivering of strip

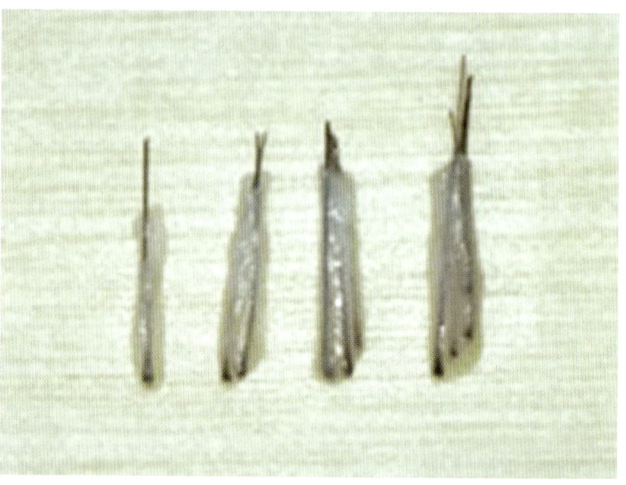

Fig. 10: Follicular units (FUs) with 1, 2 and 3 FU grafts

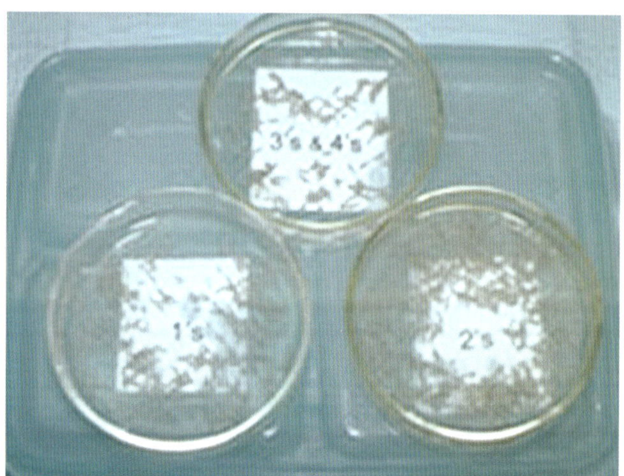

Fig. 11: Follicular unit (FU) grafts kept in cold saline in petri dish till grafting is done

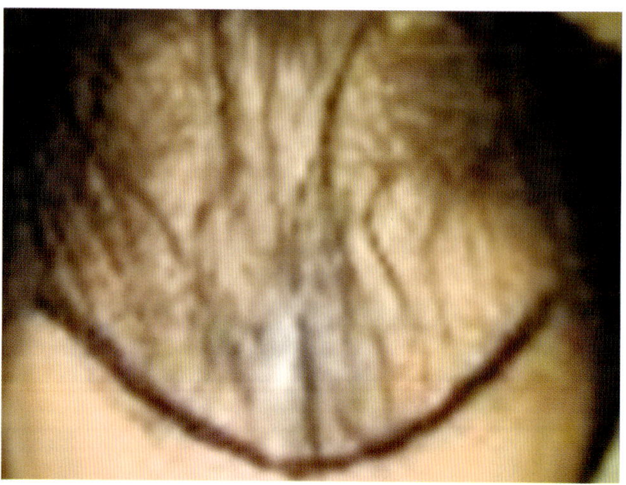

Fig. 12: Marking on recipient site

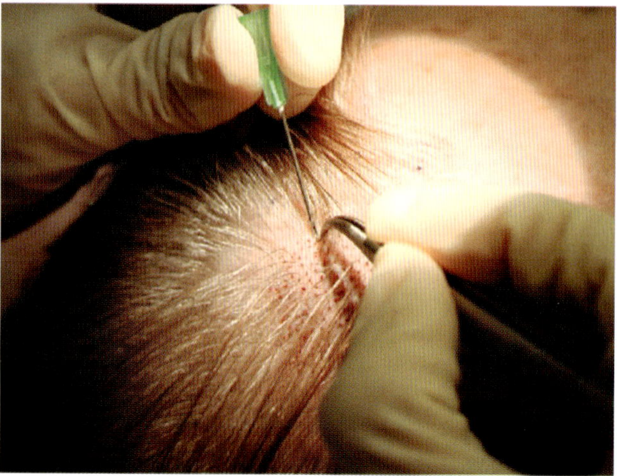

Fig. 13: Simultaneous incision with needle and grafting

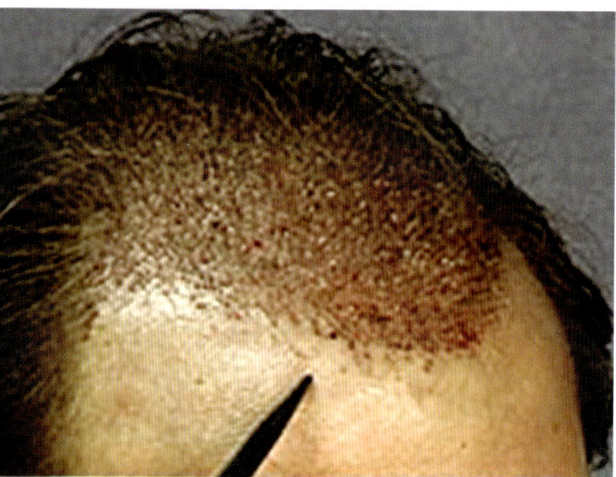

Fig. 14: FU transplant completed

Special Instruments

The following special instruments, used in surgery for alopecia, are given in Figures 15 to 19.

SCALP REDUCTION SURGERY

It is defined as the surgical excision of redundant tissue from one or more areas of scalp alopecia. There are different types of scalp reduction techniques that can be performed (Figs 20A to H).

Indications

- Extensive baldness with limited donor site
- Patient with large circular bald spots over crown or at the back of scalp.

Advantage

- Immediate results in limited alopecia.

Disadvantages

- Stretch back phenomenon
- Widening of scars
- Secondary procedures required
- Exposure of scars.

SCALP FLAPS

In this technique, scalp tissue having hairs is transposed and redistributed to bald area.

Types

1. Temporo-parieto-occipital flap
2. Temporo-occipital flap

The design of triple advancement transposition flap is given in Figure 21.

Advantages

- Immediate results with dense frontal hairline
- Useful for treatment of vertex.

Disadvantages

- Unnatural appearance of frontal hairline
- Inadequate coverage
- Incorrect hair direction
- Scarring
- Necrosis.

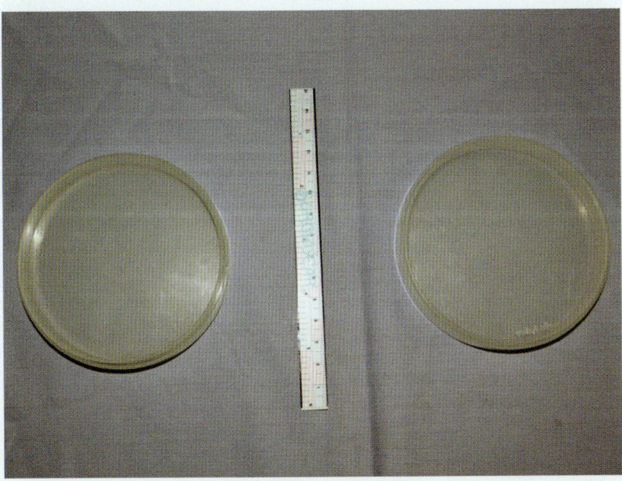

Fig. 15: Petri dish

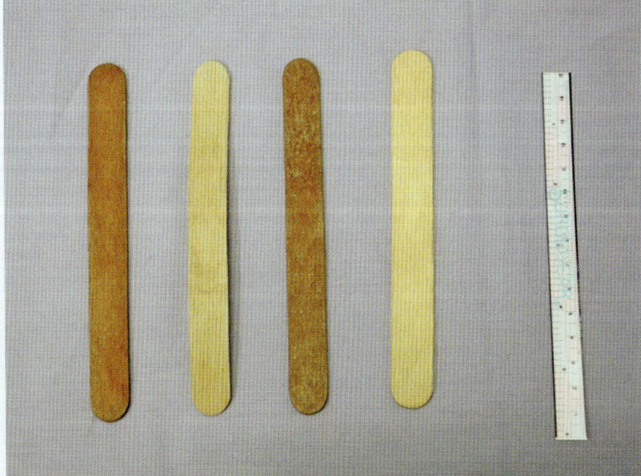

Fig. 16: Wooden sticks

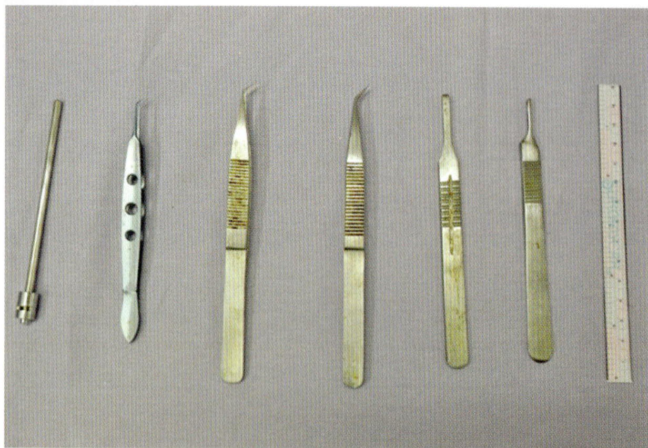

Fig. 17: Curved microforceps, scalpel

Fig. 18: Magnifying glass with light

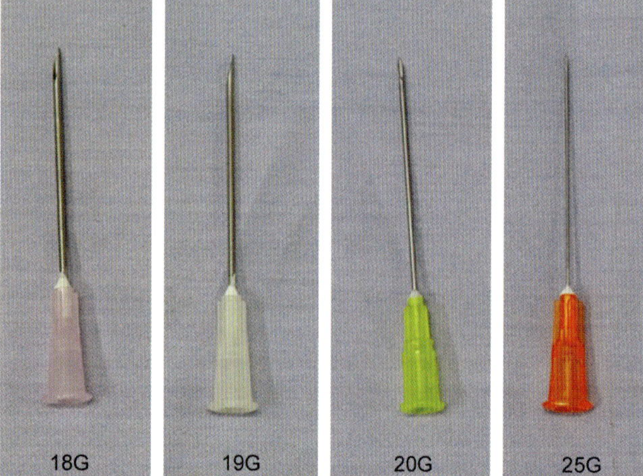

Fig. 19: Needles—smaller caliber needles are used in the front of the area to be grafted and preferably FU containing single hair are grafted. As we go posteriorly, FU containing 2 or 3 hairs are grafted to increase density and larger caliber needles are used

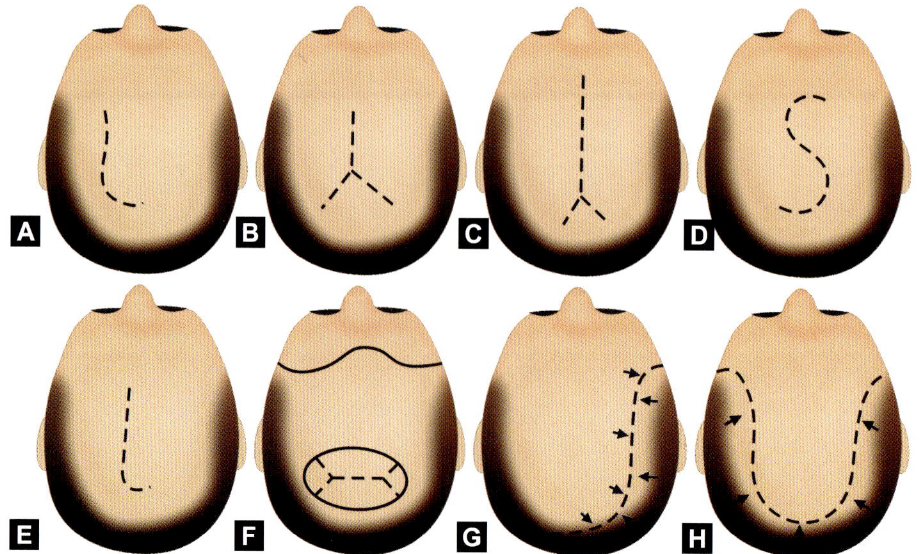

Figs 20A to H: Different types of scalp reduction techniques. (A) L pattern; (B) Mercedes Benz pattern; (C) Y-shaped pattern; (D) S-shaped pattern; (E) J-shaped pattern; (F) Midline reduction pattern; (G) Lateral pattern; (H) U-shaped pattern

EXPANDED HAIR BEARING FLAPS

It is a staged procedure. A patient with post burn alopecia over scalp reconstructed by this method is shown in Figure 22.

Stage 1 – Appropriate size and shape of tissue expander (for e.g. crescentric shaped tissue expander shown in Figure 25) is inserted into the surrounding hair bearing area of scalp in subgaleal plane.

Stage 2 - Serial expansion is done till adequate size of flap is achieved: approximately 1.5 to 2 times the capacity of expander (Fig. 23)

Stage 3 - Expander removal and advancement of scalp flap. (Figs 24 A and B)

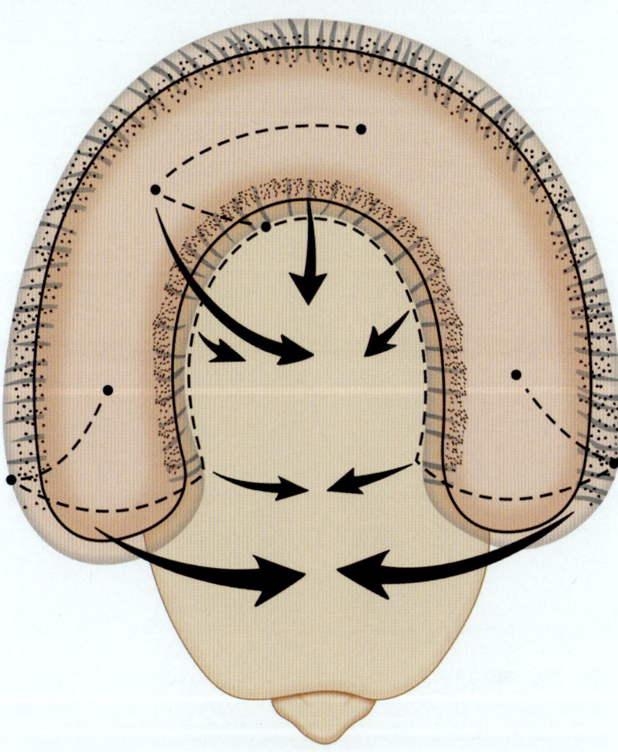

Fig. 21: Design of triple advancement transposition flap

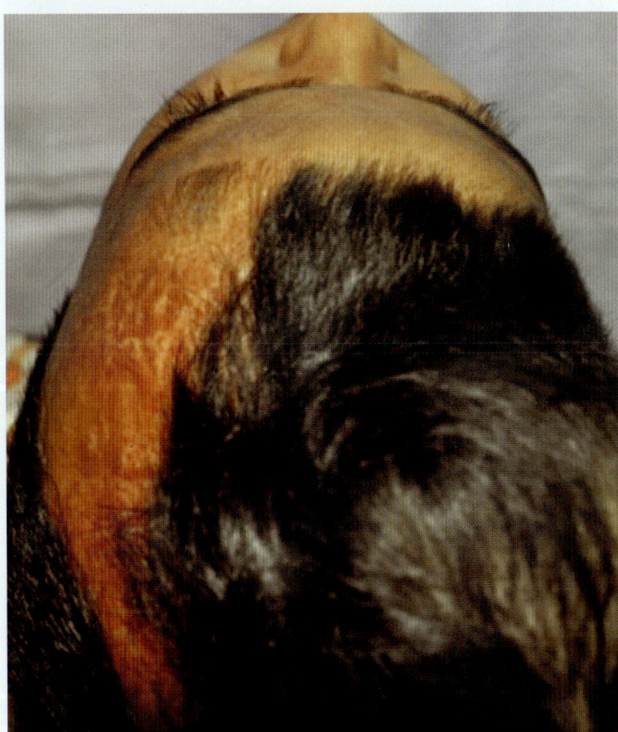

Fig. 22: Patient with post-burn scalp alopecia over left parietal region

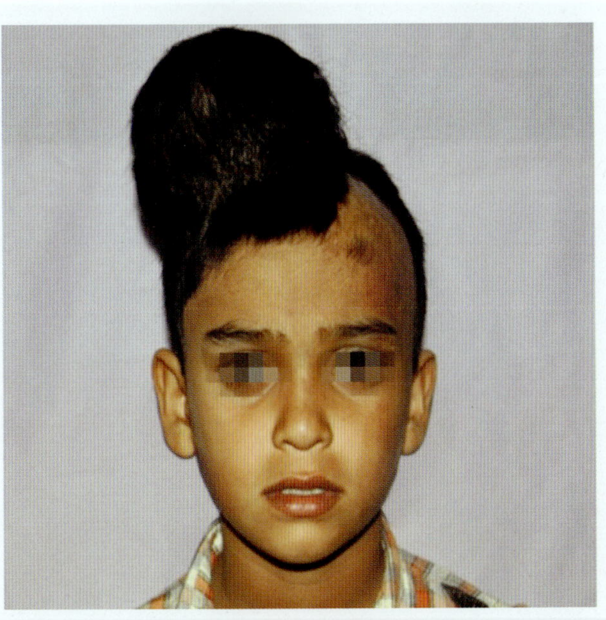

Fig. 23: Tissue expander inserted below the hair bearing scalp in subgaleal plane and serial expansion done

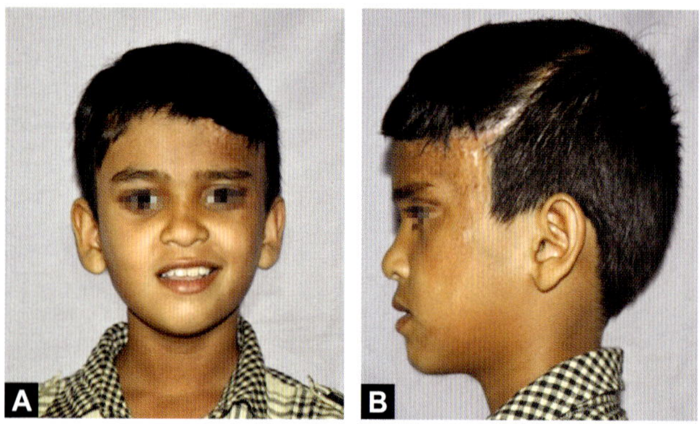

Figs 24A and B: Postoperative results of patient after excision of alopecia segment with coverage using expanded scalp flap

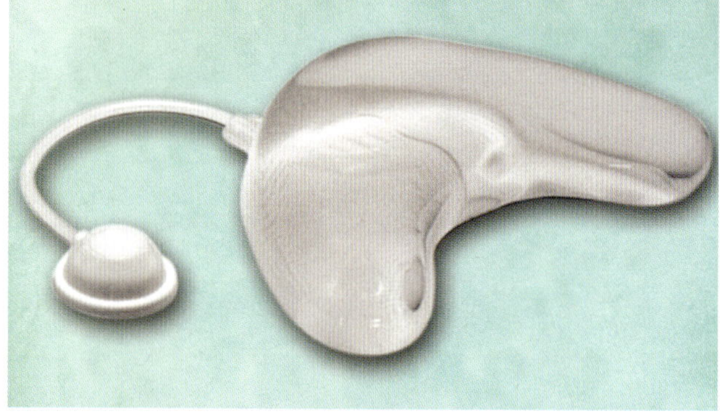

Fig. 25: Crescentric shaped tissue expander

Few words about female alopecia—Hair loss in females is often of diffuse nature which frequently results in lack of donor area. However a subgroup of females show male pattern which has familial predisposition. These are candidates of hair transplant. Unlike male pattern, they maintain low frontal hairline. In female candidates of hair transplant Finasteride is not used.

CHAPTER

94 Upper and Lower Lid Blepharoplasty

Giovanni André Pires Viana

HISTORICAL PERSPECTIVE

The history of periorbital surgery has been traced as far back as the 18th century BC, when Hammurabi's code detailed the contract between a surgeon and patient undergoing the lancing of an infected lacrimal sac.[1] The medical therapy of eye disease was documented throughout ancient Egyptian times between 1550 BC and 3000 BC.[1] It is in the Edwin Smith papyrus that the earliest known description of stitching the eyebrow is found.[1]

The eyelid surgery was described in an Indian document, the Susruta, more than 2000 years ago.[2] The recorded history of blepharoplasty dates back to the first century when the Roman Aulus Cornelius Celsus described excision of skin for "relaxed upper eyelids" in his compendium De Re Medicina (25–35 AD).[1,3] As early as the 10th century, Avicenna devised ways to excise skin folds in the upper eyelid that impaired vision.[1-3] Ambroise Paré described the functional correction of excess eyelid skin in the 16th century.[2]

The term blepharoplasty itself is derived from Greek term "blepharon", meaning "eyelid," and "plastos," meaning "formed", and was initially used by Carl Ferdinand von Graefe in the early 19th century when reporting a reconstructive technique for defects caused by resection of cancer in the eyelids.[1-3] Jules Sichel, in 1844, provided the first accurate description of herniated orbital fat in association with skin excess, to which he attributed decreased movement of the lid and overhanging of the eyelid margin.[1-3] Ernst Fuchs observed that the excess skin fold was caused by weakening of the fascial attachments of the skin and the tendon of the levator muscle.[1]

In 1907, Charles Conrad Miller wrote the first book on cosmetic surgery and also published the first photography depicting a marking of upper and lower eyelid surgery that was similar to those used today.[1,3] Frederick Kolle was the first to stress the importance of preoperative measurements and markings of excess skin.[1] Julian Bourguet reported separate fat compartments in the eyelids and was the first to describe a transconjunctival approach to the resection of herniated periorbital fat in 1924. One year later, he published before and after photographs of his procedure.[1,2] Madame Noël, a French female surgeon, was the first to stress the importance of before and after photographs in cosmetic surgery.[1]

The modern concept of blepharoplasty and detailed anatomy of the orbital fat compartments were described by Castanãres in 1951.[4] In the years between 1951 and 1967, Castanãres described seven treatable cosmetic eyelid deformities and their treatments: (i) Blepharochalasis, (ii) Dermatochalasis, (iii) Hypertrophy of the orbicularis muscle, (iv) Protusion of intraorbital fat, (v) Combination of these conditions, (vi) Hooding of upper eyelid skin due to brow ptosis, and (vii) Lid cheek bags.[1-3]

Over the past 40 years, surgeons have generally moved away from traditional techniques of the subtractive approaches, described by Castanãres, to a more conservative approach.

In upper blepharoplasty, the "anchor blepharoplasty" described by Flowers in the 1970's represented the esthetic ideal, but this approach has fallen into disfavor with many surgeons and recently, a more conservative, reconstructive surgery with attention to the repair of anatomic defects from levator aponeurosis to replacement of lost fat volume in the lateral brow has become popular.[5,6]

In lower eyelid surgery, Raul Loeb was one of the first surgeons to preserve adipose tissue during the lower lid blepharoplasty, but since de la Plaza and Arroyo described their approach for lower lid hernia repair, there has been a great deal of interest in fat-preservation techniques in lower lid blepharoplasty.[7-9]

SPECIFIC PREOPERATIVE EVALUATION

Preoperative Assessment

Preoperative patient evaluation for blepharoplasty should include lifestyle history (smoking, exercise tolerance, and alcohol use), history of chronic illness, hypertension, diabetes, cardiac disease, bleeding and/or clotting disorders, thyroid disturbances, or previous operations.

Medications, including aspirin and other anticoagulants, should be listed and withheld for at least 2 weeks preoperatively. Dietary supplements should be listed as they may affect clotting; for instance, Dong Quai (anticoagulants effects), omega 3-fatty acids in fish oil, ajoene in garlic, ginger, Ginkgo, and vitamin E (antiplatelet properties), Fucus (heparin-like activity), Danshen (antithrombin III-like activity and anticoagulant bioavailability), and St. John's Wort and American Ginseng (interference with drug metabolism).[2,3,10]

Ophthalmologic history should be obtained, including vision, correction lenses, trauma, glaucoma, allergic reactions, excess tearing, and dry eyes. Specific history pertaining to LASER-assisted in situ keratomileusis (LASIK) and other refractive surgery should be documented, as they predispose the patient to postblepharoplasty dry eye exposure and visual changes. No cosmetic surgery of the periorbital region should be performed for a minimum of 6 months following corneal refractory surgery and when in doubt, clearance from the refractive surgeon should be obtained. Schimmer's test should be considered if there is a history of dry eyes.[2,3,10-13]

Physical Examination

Evaluation of the patient for blepharoplasty should include a general physical examination, including blood pressure, height, and weight of the patient. Visual acuity should be registered. Pupillary response and extraocular muscles including evaluation for amblyopia and an intact Bell's phenomenon should be documented. The evaluation of the periorbital area should take into account skin quality and quantity, underlying soft-tissue positioning, and skeletal support.[2,3,10-13]

Dermatochalasis is the loss of elasticity and support in the skin. In the upper eyelid, this can create a fold of excess skin, which can impair the function of the eye, specifically, by superior and lateral visual field obstruction. Lower eyelid should be assessed for skin excess secondary to dermatochalasis. Age-associated changes in the orbicularis oculi muscle are attributable to increased muscle relaxation and ligamentous attenuation. This can cause lower lid malposition and, in association with malar ptosis, can result in inferior muscle border prominence, creating a festoon or malar crescent. Fat herniation can accentuate lower eyelid fullness. This may be attributed to weakening of the lower eyelid septum and can be localized to one or all three fat pads (medial, central, lateral).[2,3,10,11,13]

Blepharochalasis is a recurrent, intermittent, inflammatory condition of the eyelids resulting in edema, erythema, and thin skin excess eyelid secondary to histamine response and related to increased immunoglobulin E. In contrast to dermatochalasis, blepharochalasis is difficult to correct and likely to recur.[2,3,10,11,13]

Upper eyelid ptosis should be evaluated by the relation of the eyelid margin to the superior limbus in neutral gaze, since it can be corrected simultaneously. The normal position of the upper lid margin covers 2–3 mm of the superior limbus but does not cover any aspect of the pupil. Pseudoptosis, the excess lateral skin and hooding of the upper lid, can be differentiated from true ptosis by elevating the lateral brow.[14]

Evaluation of the upper eyelid must include an evaluation of the eyebrow.[2,3,10,11,13,15] In the male patient, the brow should be at the superior orbital rim, whereas the female brow should be above the rim with the arch apex inline with lateral limbus.[16,17] Brow ptosis should be corrected to achieve repositioning of heavy eyebrow skin, which may be compensated by frontalis contraction to keep the eyebrows above the orbital rim. Once the visual obstruction has been removed by eyelid skin resection, the brows may look even heavier since elevation is no longer needed for the visual field. This results in a more aged appearance.[2,3,10-13,15-17] This should be performed before upper blepharoplasty so that correct brow position is ensured before upper lid skin excision. Asymmetry in upper and lower eyelids and brow position is common and should be appreciated individually. Correction to attain exact symmetry is unreasonable.

The pathogenesis of aging within the lower eyelid is multifactorial, and varies among patients. Periorbital age-related changes include crow's feet and lower eyelid rythides, scleral show, infraorbital hollowing, herniated fat pads, excess or laxity of lower lid skin, festoons, and eyelid hooding. Common complaints include eyelid bags, circles under the eye, wrinkles around the eye or a tired look. Lower eyelid fat becomes more prominent in upgaze and less prominent in downgaze.[4,7-11] In addition, attenuation of the lateral canthal tendons results in loss of the youthful architecture of the eye secondary to a decrease of the esthetically pleasing upward tilt. The change in the lateral canthal complex position is functionally important, as its changes contribute to lower eyelid laxity, which may result in rounding of the lateral commissure and narrowing of the palpebral fissure.[9-11,18]

Lower eyelid displacement with anterior traction (distraction test) can precisely determine the degree of laxity and guide lower eyelid canthal repositioning; greater than 6 mm of anterior distraction from the globe indicates significant lid laxity, which may require lateral canthal repositioning. The anatomical relationship of the orbital region should also be evaluated secondary to the direct effect of lower blepharoplasty. The posterior displacement of the orbital rim in relation to the anterior cornea and lower lid margin, a negative vector, should be appreciated preoperatively. Proeminent or deep-set eyes should be documented. A more detailed analysis can be performed using exophthalmometry with Hertel or Lued exophthalmometer (Fig. 1), which measures the position of the globe relative to the lateral orbital rim (normal range: 16–18 mm). Malar anatomy should be evaluated for tear trough deformities or prominent nasojugal folds, which may guide lower eyelid operative plans.[9-11,18]

Photography Documentation

All patients should be submitted to a preoperative photo evaluation. Standardized digital photographs should be taken as following, one frontal (eyes opened, neutral-gaze), one frontal (eyes closed), one frontal (upgaze), one frontal (downgaze), and lateral views (neutral-gaze).

ANESTHETIC CONSIDERATIONS

The surgeon must consider the risk factors associated with each blepharoplasty procedure when deciding whether such procedures should be performed in a hospital or an office-based setting. The postblepharoplasty patient may have temporary decreased visual acuity and limited visual fields. This may be secondary to temporary tarsorrhaphy sutures, edema, and chemosis, which may require hourly care. Patient assistance in postoperative period should be part of the preoperative plan and may dictate the location of the operation and postoperative care.

Blepharoplasty may be performed under different anesthesia modalities, depending upon the surgical plan, patient and surgeon preference, and need for concomitant operations.

A simple upper or lower eyelid blepharoplasty, where only skin or fat is excised, can be performed under local anesthesia with small volume of 2% lidocaine with epinephrine, and may be combined with intravenous sedation. Other more invasive procedures, such as lower blepharoplasty combined with fat repositioning, mid-face lifting or endoscopic browlift, may need intravenous sedation with local anesthetic infiltration or general anesthesia. The modality of anesthesia should be discussed preoperatively with patient, surgeon and anesthesia provider.

Complications during anesthesia should be diagnosed and treated promptly. Changes in vital signs or end-tidal carbon dioxide may be early warning signs of impending complications. Events, such as laryngospasm, hypotension, or hypertension, may occur at anytime during the perioperative period. Close monitoring of the patient should persist during the postoperative period, as cardiac arrhythmias, cardiac standstill, fluid overload, and pulmonary edema may manifest hours after surgical procedure is complete.[10]

SURGICAL STEPS

Upper Eyelid Blepharoplasty

Preoperative Marking

Preoperative marking should be made with the patient sitting upright in neutral gaze with the brow properly positioned. The eyelid crease is situated above ciliary margin approximately 8–9 mm in women and 7–8 mm in men (Fig. 2).[11] The lower limit of excision should be along the eyelid crease, and lateral extent of the marking should be limited by an imaginary line joining the lateral end of

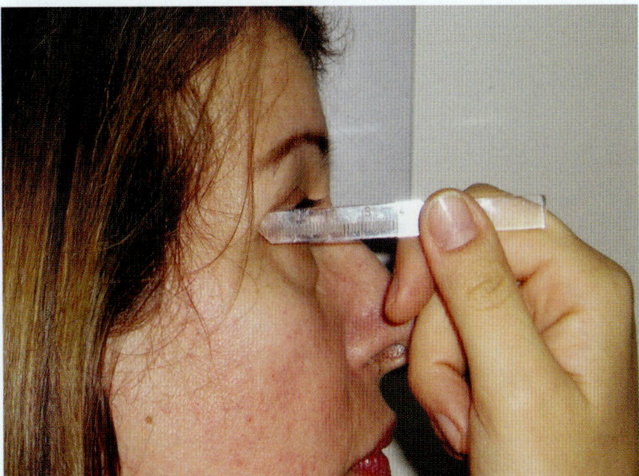

Fig. 1: Exophthalmometry with Lued exophthalmometer

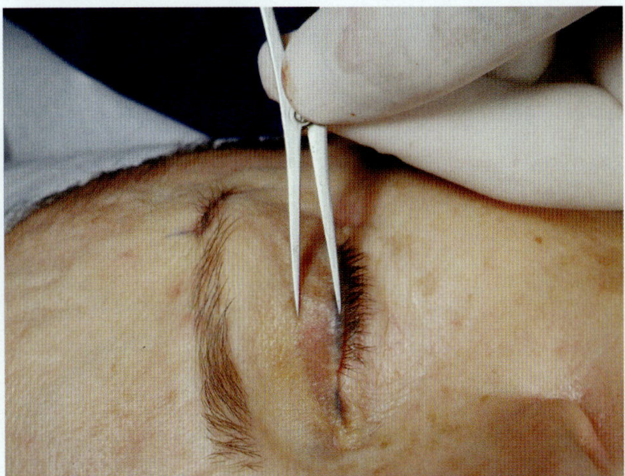

Fig. 2: Measuring the eyelid crease with caliper

the brow to the lateral canthus, because a poorly planned incision in this location can be noticeable, especially in male patients and patients with thick skin. Similarly, the medial markings should not be extended medial to medial canthus for larger resections because extensions onto the nasal sidewall result in webbing. The extent of the excision should be at least 10 mm from the inferior border of the brow, so as to not include any brow skin, making a pattern of skin excision as shown in Figure 3. The pattern of skin excision should be lenticular in the younger patient and more trapezoid-shaped laterally in the older patient (Fig. 4). Using the midpupil line as the reference point, more skin is excised laterally and less medially. A skin pinch test can confirm the preoperative markings (Fig. 5). A minimum of 20 mm of vertical lid height should be preserved for normal eye closure (Figs 6A and B). The location of fat should be determined and marked preoperatively, with the patient in upgaze, downgaze, and medial and lateral ranges of motion, with photographic documentation.

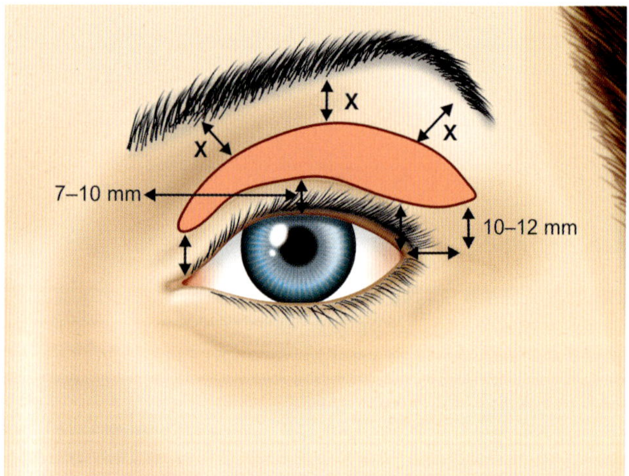

Fig. 3: A careful evaluation and particular attention to precise incision planning can lead to a more accurate and youthful result

Source: Adapted from Fagien S. Advanced rejuvenative upper blepharoplasty: enhancing aesthetics of the upper periorbita. Plast Reconstr Surg. 2002;110(1):278-91

Surgical Technique

The upper lids should be injected superficially to avoid any subcutaneous or intraorbicularis hematoma formation, with 2% lidocaine with epinephrine using a 30-gauge needle (Fig. 7). Incisions are made superficially with a fresh No. 15 blade through the epidermis only, and the premarked strip of skin is resected with fine curved scissors, scalpel or a needle-point Bovie (Fig. 8). If definition of the supratarsal fold is desired, some surgeons recommend that a small strip of orbicularis be resected, as described by Baker et al.[19] Hemostasis is obtained using pinpoint cautery (Fig. 9). Conservative fat excision can be performed as part of upper lid blepharoplasty. There are two fat compartments—medial or nasal (white fat) and central (yellow fat)—that can be accessed through small incisions in the septum, teased out, and resected using pinpoint cautery (Figs 10A to D). Of the medial and central fat, only the fat that comes easily into the wound is excised. It is important not to aggressively pull fat from the orbit to avoid injury to neurovascular structures or extraocular muscles and lead to a "hollowed-out" appearance.

Retro-orbicularis oculi fat can be accessed beneath the lateral orbicularis oculi muscle overlying the superior orbital rim.[20] Resection has been described to help decrease heaviness of the upper lid and lateral brow.

Supratarsal fixation at the conclusion of an upper lid blepharoplasty can secure the pretarsal orbicularis oculi muscle or dermis to the levator mechanism to reconstitute and define the supratarsal fold.[21]

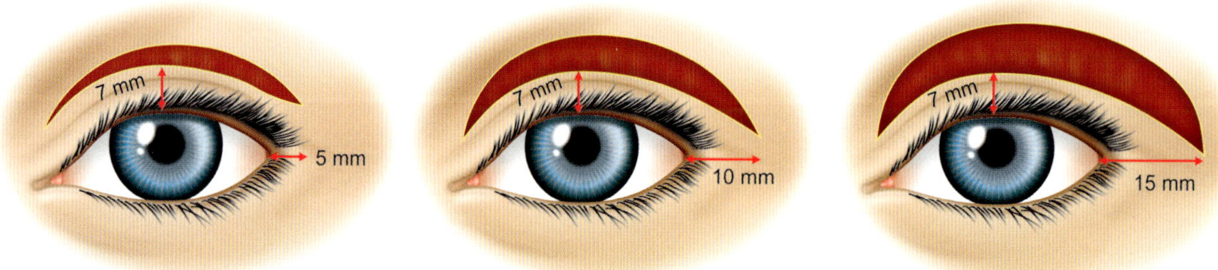

Fig. 4: Upper eyelid skin resection increases in size both vertically and laterally as the periorbital area ages: young (left), middle age (center), and old (right)

Source: Adapted from Fagien S. Advanced rejuvenative upper blepharoplasty: enhancing aesthetics of the upper periorbita. Plast Reconstr Surg. 2002;110(1):278-91

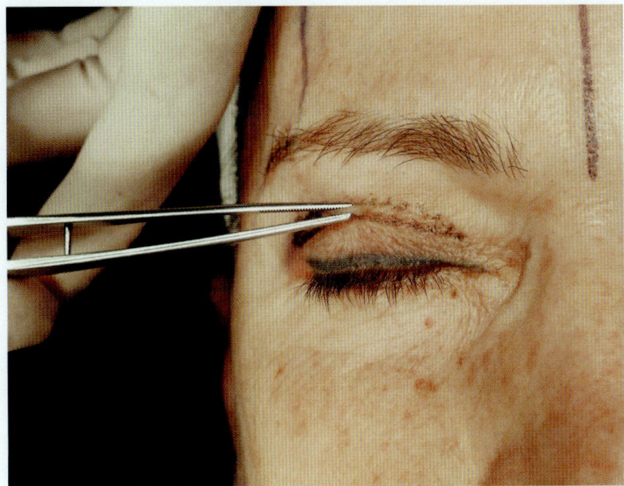

Fig. 5: Skin pinch test

The skin incision can be closed using running subcutaneous 6-0 nylon suture or interrupted sutures with 6-0 nylon sutures to achieve an esthetic outcome (Fig. 11). Bandage strips are applied at the end of bilateral procedure (Fig. 12).

In male blepharoplasty, a more natural look is preferred, and the "operate look" will not be tolerated well by most male patients. Men will typically not be wearing cosmetics, so all scars must be carefully concealed. The lateral incision should only infrequently be extended beyond the later orbital rim. In men with heavy brows, resection of upper eyelid skin will only result in profoundly ptotic brows. Therefore, one should counsel combined brow surgery with upper blepharoplasty. Often, conservative eyelid resection is all that is required.

In Asian patients, blepharoplasty represents a unique set of challenges. The eyelid anatomy, esthetic goals

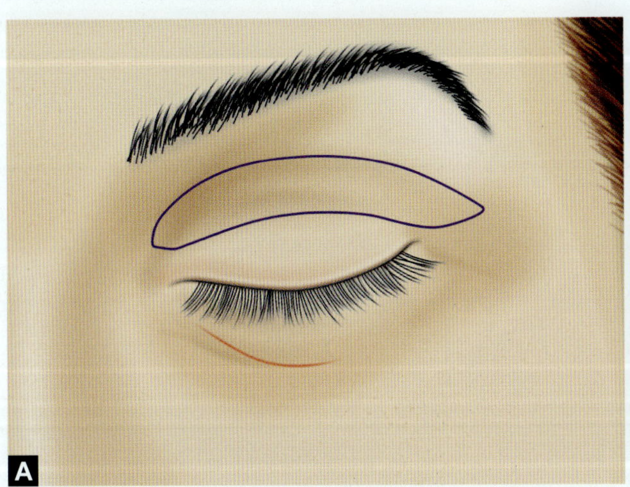

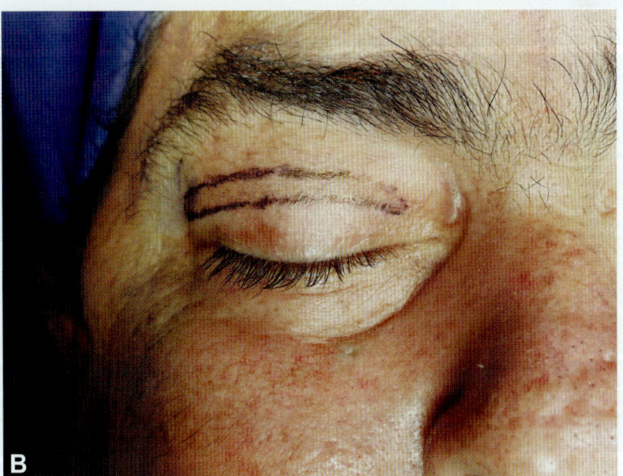

Figs 6A and B: Final marking. (A) Schematic figure; (B) Real patient

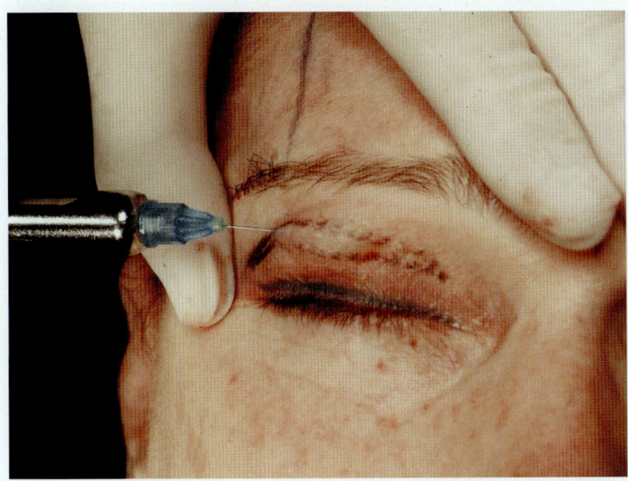

Fig. 7: Local anesthetic infiltration

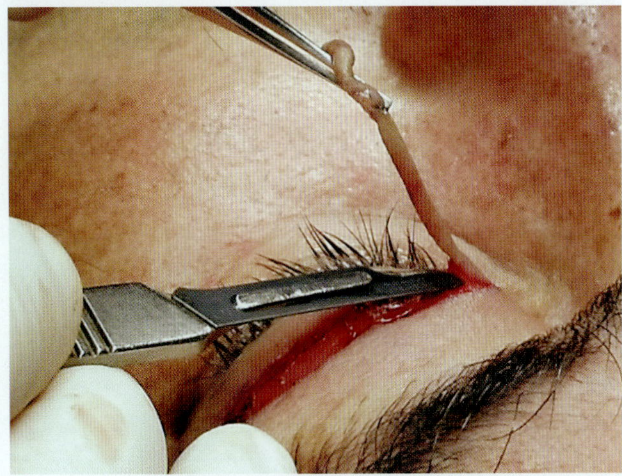

Fig. 8: Skin resection with scalpel

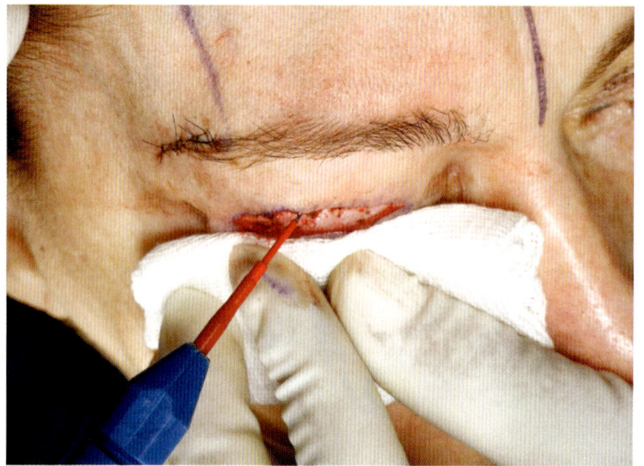

Fig. 9: Hemostasis

and surgical techniques are vastly different from that of Caucasian patients. Approximately 50% of Asians have an upper lid crease, which can be complete, partial or intermittent. Many patients requesting blepharoplasty desire the formation of a crease or a double eyelid. A common misconception is that the endpoint of Asian blepharoplasty is the creation of a more "Westernized" appearance. In Asians, the primary goal is to create an eyelid crease to enhance their natural Asian features.

Postoperative Care

Methylcellulose eye drops are recommended while the patient is awake, and lubricating ointment for night-use for several days postoperatively. The patient's head should remain elevated to reduce edema and ophthalmic pressure. Patients are advised to avoid strenuous lifting,

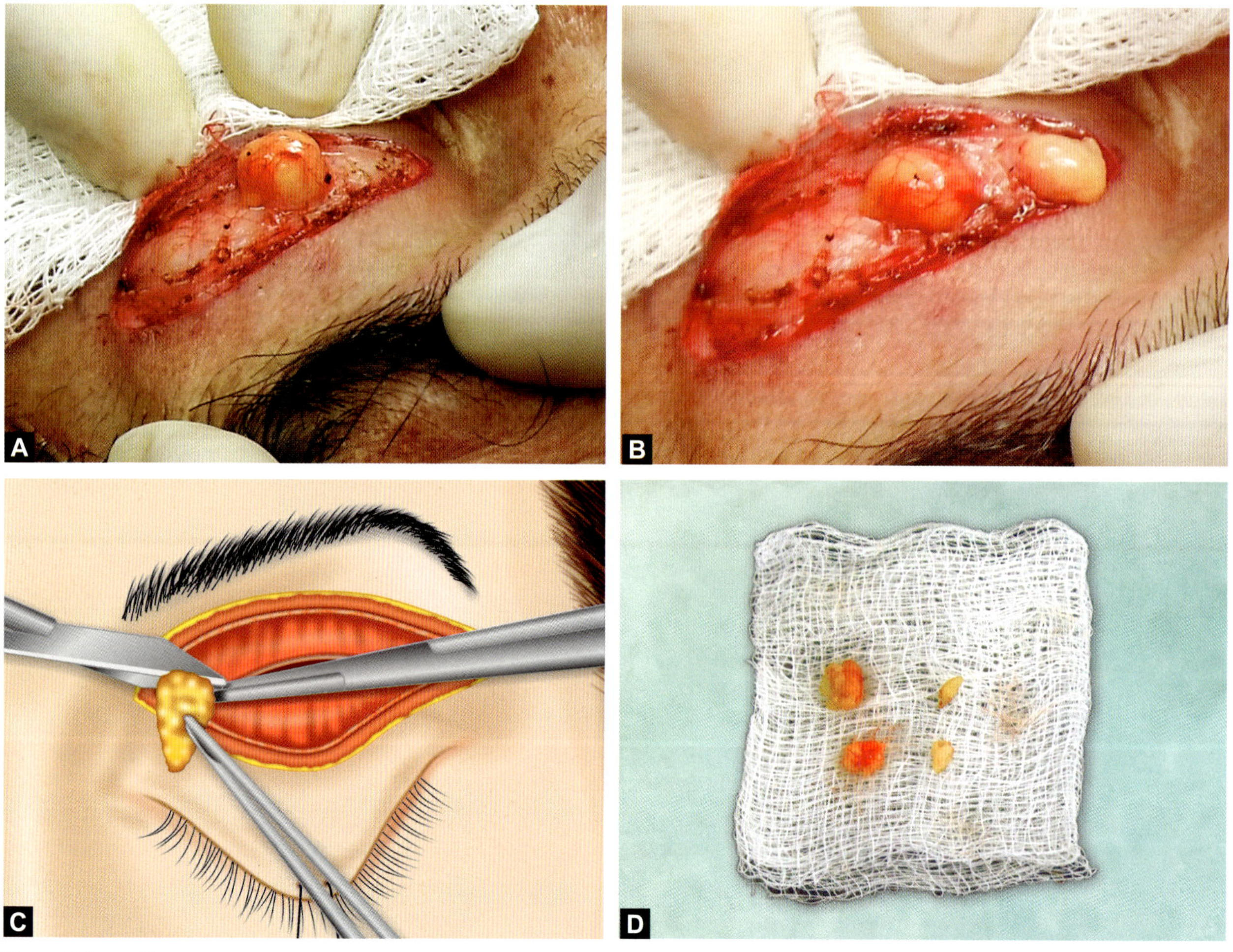

Figs 10A to D: Both fat compartments and respectively fat pads exposed through small incisions. (A) Central fat pad; (B) Central and medial fat pads; (C) Schematic figure showing the fat being placed in the tips of the clamp, the fat being removed with either scissors, knife or pinpoint cautery. Then, the stump is coagulated with bipolar cautery to obtain hemostasis and, after hemostasis is obtained, the instruments are withdrawn; (D) After excision (both eyelids)

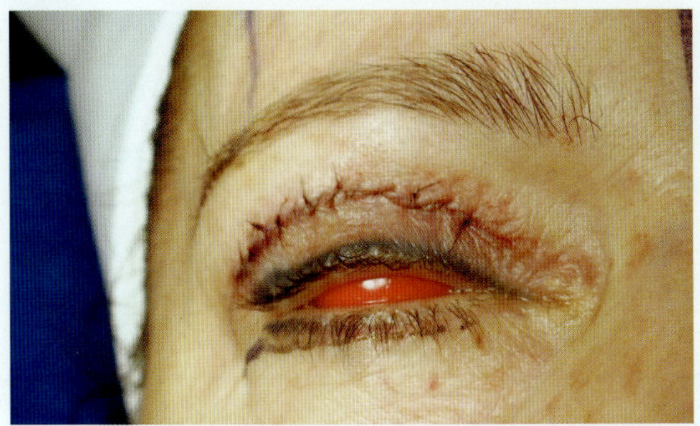

Fig. 11: Final upper blepharoplasty closure

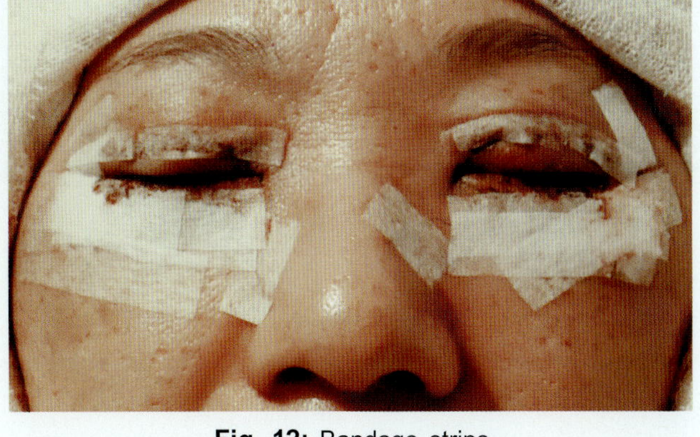

Fig. 12: Bandage strips

bending, and vigorous activities for 2 weeks following the procedure. Lagophthalmos is usually secondary to periorbital edema and resolves in 1–2 weeks. The patient is advised to return to full activities 2 weeks following upper blepharoplasty. Suture removal is performed 5 days postoperatively, and bandage strips may be removed on the first postsurgery visit, which is usually 1–3 days following surgery.

Complications

Thorough preoperative planning and meticulous surgical technique will avoid or decrease the risk of serious complications in upper blepharoplasty. The surgeon should focus intraoperatively on executing the surgical plan, emphasizing conservative skin excision maintaining symmetry of the lid crease and managing any intraoperative findings, such as levator dehiscence. The most common complication of cosmetic surgery is failure to meet the patient's expectations.

Post surgery mild pain, ecchymosis, eyelid edema, lagophthalmos, blepharoptosis, subconjunctival hemorrhage, and diminished sensitivity of the eyelids should resolve within the early postoperative period. Other complications, such as persistent fat, skin or textural irregularities may require minor secondary procedures.

The major complications of blepharoplasty are blindness, hematoma, and globe injury. Visual loss due to retrobulbar hematoma is the most feared complication; fortunately, the occurrence is rare.[10,22] Acute retrobulbar hematoma may compress neurovascular structures, leading to ischemia of the retina, central artery, and optic nerve. Symptoms include severe pain, visual changes, including hemianopia or amaurosis fugax, and scintillating scotomas. Examination will often reveal a tense and protuberant periorbital area with diminished or absent extraocular movements. Once the diagnosis is made, treatment should be implemented immediately because 90–120 minutes of ischemia leads to irreversible blindness.[2] All dressings should be removed and sutures need to be released. An ophthalmologic consultation should be obtained immediately. The patient should be given mannitol 20% 1.5 g/kg to 2 g/kg intravenously (with the first 12.5 g over a 3-minute period and the remainder over a 30-minute period), 95% oxygen/5% carbon dioxide to dilate intraocular vessels, methylprednisolone 100 mg intravenously (Solu-Medrol®), Betaxolol Hydrochloride Ophthalmic Suspension (Betoptic®) one drop immediately, then twice daily. These actions should be taken as the patient is being taken back to the operating room for re-exploration and evacuation of hematoma, as well as possible lateral canthotomy and release of the arcus marginalis.[2,3,10,23,24]

Visual changes, including diplopia, are generally temporary and can be attributed to wound reaction, edema, and hematoma. Damage to extraocular muscles and nerves may cause permanent strabismus. The most common structures damaged in blepharoplasty are the inferior oblique muscle and superior oblique muscle. Conservative management is recommended, though refractory cases should be referred to an ophthalmologist. Vision loss can also result from globe perforation during infiltration with local anesthetic.[10,25] This is extremely rare and along with corneal abrasion, can be prevented with corneal protectors.

Lower Eyelid Blepharoplasty

Lower eyelid rejuvenation is more complex and has several treatment options, such as blepharoplasty, fillers and skin resurfacing. Most surgeons have developed a customized approach to eyelid surgery in which the specific anatomic problems are identified and the operation is individualized to address these problems.

The approach to the lower eyelid remains a controversial issue within plastic and oculoplastic surgeons.

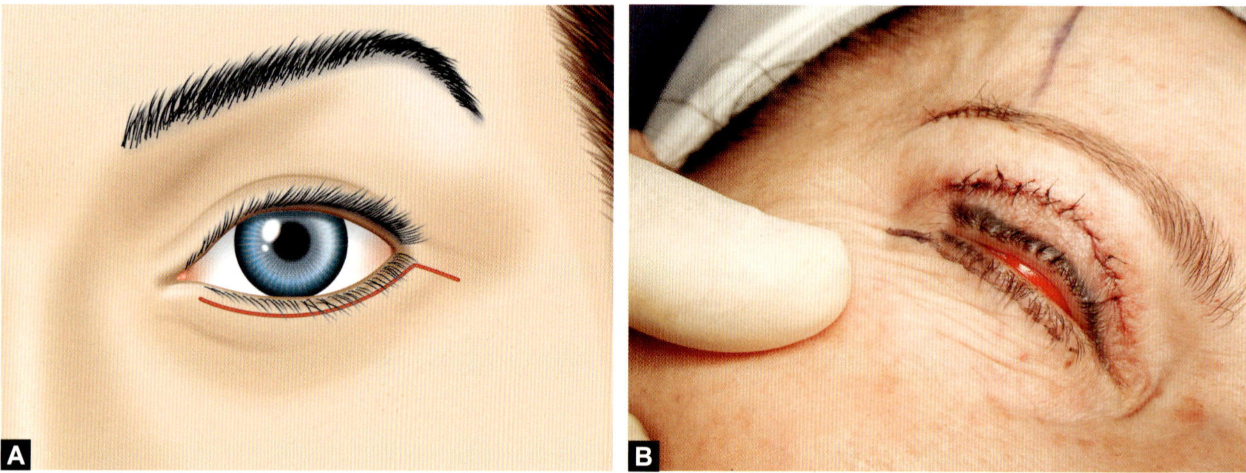

Figs 13A and B: Subciliary incision. (A) Schematic figure; (B) Real patient

The evolution of lower eyelid blepharoplasty has resulted in divergent concepts; some authors favor the maintenance of the fat bags, others are against touching the orbicularis oculi muscle and still, others recommend muscle cutaneous flaps and ample undermining of the orbicularis oculi muscle.[9]

Transcutaneous Lower Eyelid Surgery

Traditional transcutaneous lower blepharoplasty corrects multidimensional aspects of periorbital aging through tightening of the lower eyelid skin and muscle and manipulation of orbital fat.

Preoperative Marking

The incision should be marked with the patient in the supine position. The scar in the lower eyelid will become less visible when placed just beneath the lashes and restricted to the lateral canthus, and certainly extending no further than the orbital rim (Figs 13A and B). The amount of skin and fat in excess should be noted previously.

Anesthesia

No matter which kind of approach may be performed in the lower lid, different anesthesia modalities would be done and in all cases, lower eyelid is anesthetized with 2% lidocaine (Fig. 14).

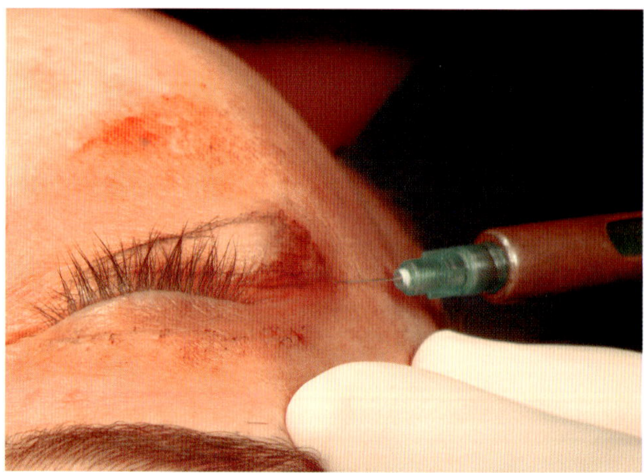

Fig. 14: Local anesthetic infiltration

Operative Technique

The skin flap method of lower blepharoplasty has the advantage of maintaining the integrity of the orbicularis (Figs 15A and B). It is ideal for skin laxity alone with no fat prolapse. The amount of skin to be resected can be estimated with a skin pinch between forceps and usually represents 3 mm of tissue. The technique is approached through a subciliary incision with the skin elevated off the orbicularis to the level of the infraorbital rim. Redundant skin can be removed conservatively and redraped without disturbing the underlying orbicularis oculi muscle.[10,11]

The more aggressive skin-muscle flap method is again approached through a subciliary incision with dissection through skin and orbicularis oculi muscle. The pretarsal orbicularis fibers should remain intact and the skin and preseptal orbicularis are elevated as one flap (Figs 16A to C). Dissection can be continued along the orbital septum to the level of the orbital rim. Periorbital fat is approached through small incisions in the septum. Orbicularis oculi muscle fibers and skin can be excised at closure; however, damage to the muscle may lead to lower eyelid malposition and muscle denervation (Figs 17A and B).[9-11]

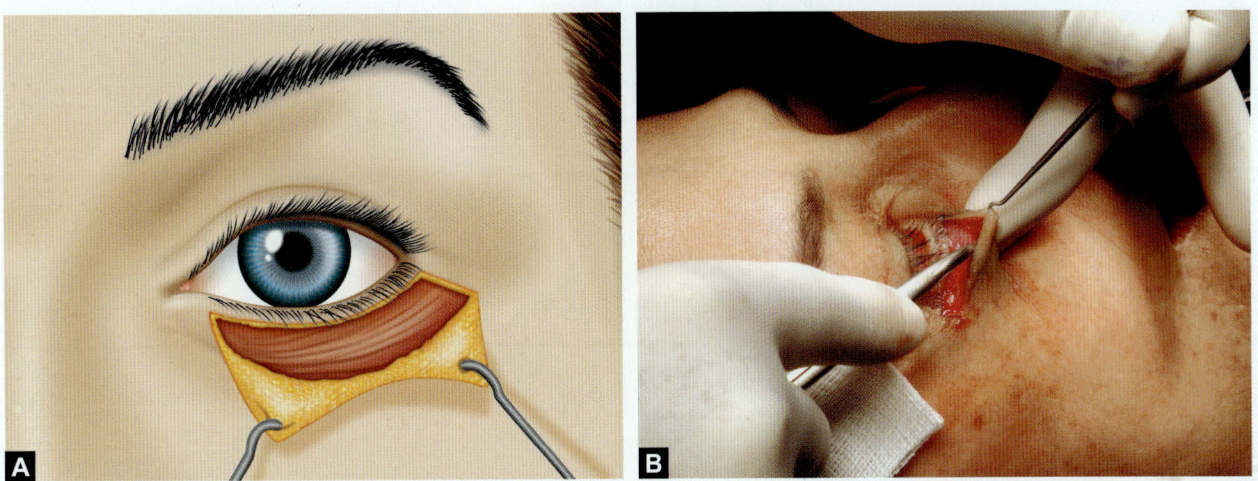

Figs 15A and B: Skin flap figure. (A) Schematic figure; (B) Undermining with curved scissors

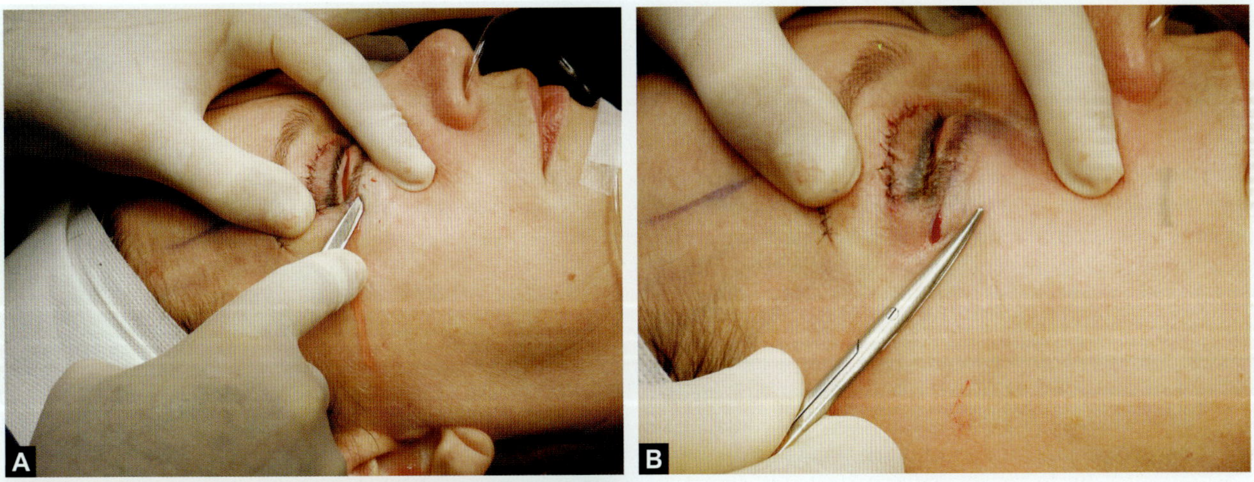

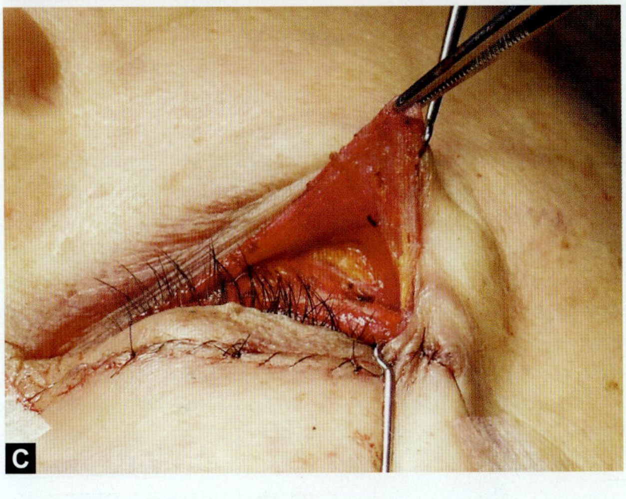

Figs 16A to C: Skin-muscle flap. (A) Dissection through skin and orbicularis oculi muscle with curved scissors; (B) The curved scissors used; (C) After complete dissection of the skin-muscle flap

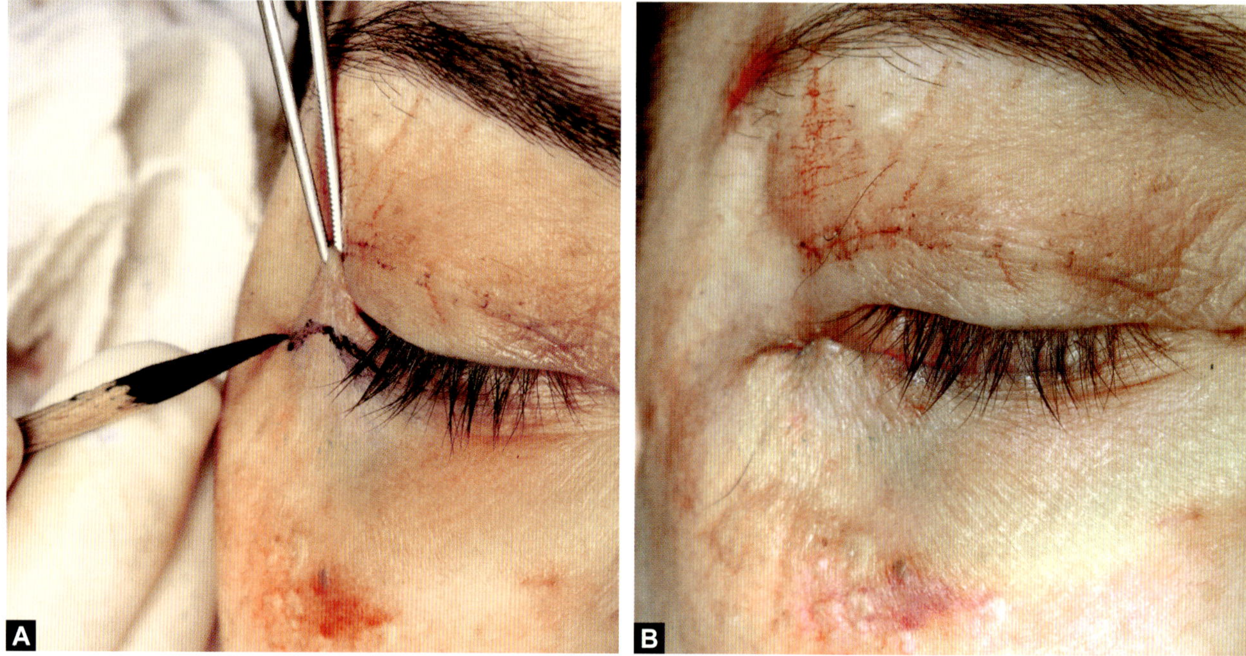

Figs 17A and B: Skin excision. (A) Marking the amount to be excised; (B) After skin excision

Separate skin and muscle flaps are developed to maximally preserve the pretarsal orbicularis oculi fibers on the tarsal plate. This leaves the orbicularis-tarsus relationship intact and possibly preserves innervation to the muscle. Periorbital fat, muscle and skin can be addressed separately.[9-11,26]

It is important to remember that three fat compartments are associated with the lower eyelid. The medial and central fat pads are separated by the inferior oblique muscle. However, an isthmus of fat generally lies anterior to the muscle belly. Its course makes it susceptible to injury during surgical dissection of the surrounding fat pads. The medial and lateral fat pads are separated by the arcuate expansion, a fascial band extending from the capsulopalpebral fascia to the inferolateral orbital rim. Notably, the inferolateral orbital septum inserts 2 mm outside the orbital rim, creating the recess of Eisler, allowing the lateral fat pad to just spill over the orbital rim.[20] If necessary, fat pads can be accessed through small incisions in the septum, teased out, and resected using pinpoint cautery (Fig. 18). Only the fat that comes easily into the wound is excised. It is important not to aggressively pull fat from the orbit to avoid injury to neurovascular structures or extraocular muscles and lead to a "sunken eyes" appearance.

The skin incision can be closed using running subcutaneous 6-0 nylon suture or interrupted sutures with 6-0 nylon sutures to achieve an esthetic outcome (Fig. 19). Bandage strips are applied at the end of bilateral procedure (Fig. 12).

Transconjunctival Lower Eyelid Blepharoplasty

Surgery is performed through an incision made several millimeters below the tarsal plate through conjunctiva and lower eyelid retractors (Fig. 20). This incision would be continuous or discontinuous. This can be done by sharp dissection with scissors, radiofrequency monopolar cautery or LASER. Gentle pressure on the eyeball prolapses the fat compartments and aids in identification of the medial, central and lateral fat pads. Conservative fat removal is achieved using radiofrequency monopolar or bipolar cautery (Fig. 21). Care is taken not to damage the inferior oblique muscle that separates the medial from central fat pocket. The end point for excision is reached when gentle pressure on the globe results in the anterior aspect of the orbital fat being flush with the orbital rim. The transconjunctival incision is left unclosed, but the inferior and superior edges of the conjunctival epithelium are well apposed to avoid overlap. The incision usually heals within a week.[10,11,26,27]

The advantage of the transconjunctival approach is not violating the middle lamella. Lower eyelid skin can be addressed with a conservative "pinch" excision or through skin resurfacing with chemical or LASER peels.

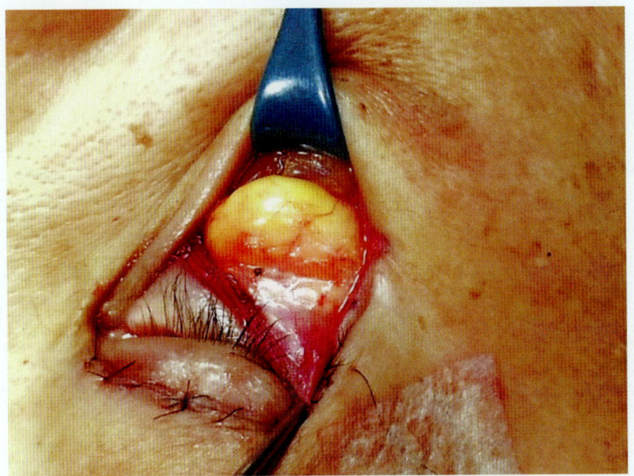

Fig. 18: Inferior fat pads

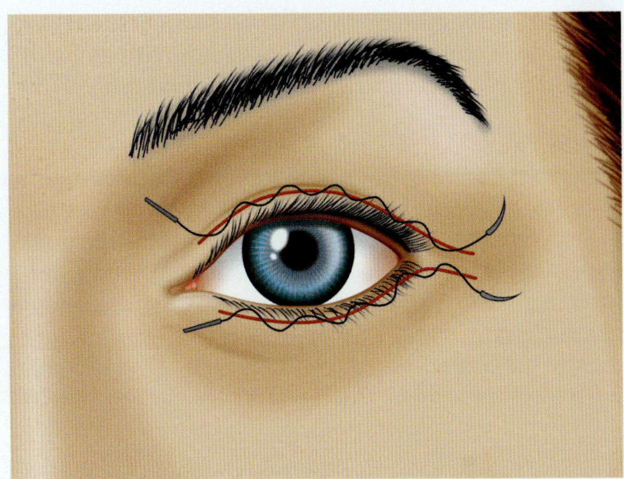

Fig. 19: Final upper and lower lid closure

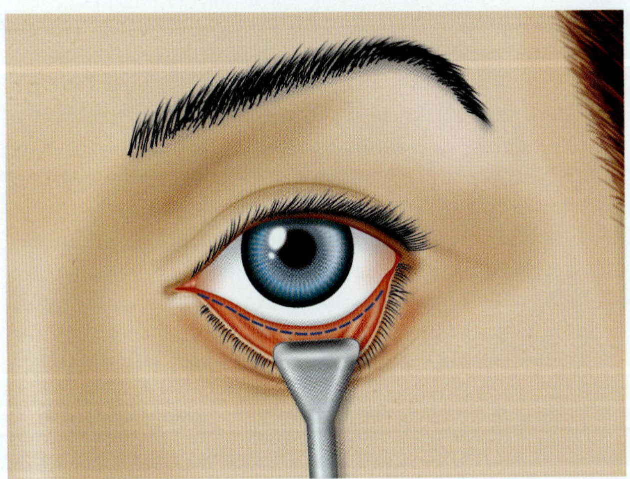

Fig. 20: Transconjunctival incision at the inferior edge of the tarsus

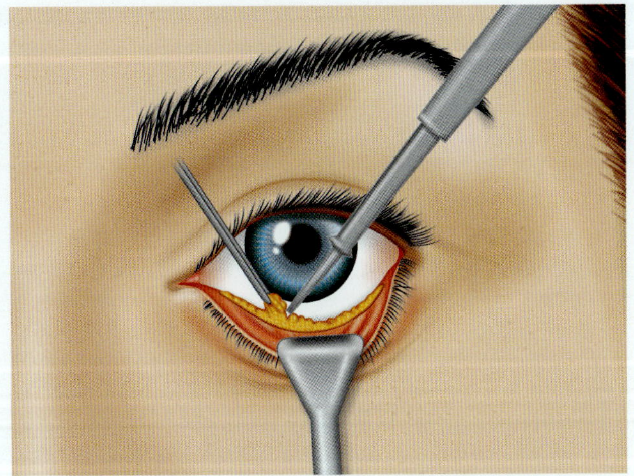

Fig. 21: Fat pads compartments through transconjunctival approach

The disadvantage of this approach is a limited exposure, leading to inadequate fat removal and possible injury to lower extraocular muscles.[10,26,27]

Lower Eyelid Fat Repositioning

Transposition of periorbital fat from the retroseptal position to redrape over the arcus marginalis can be used to fill out the nasojugal deficiencies and soften lower eyelid depressions.[7,9,28,29] Advantages to this technique include the ability to use a pedicle, vascularized fat graft to precisely fill out a depression, though in reality, the periorbital fat is delicate and difficult to reliably secure in position.

Fat repositioning surgery includes release of the arcus marginalis and advancement of the orbital fat beyond the infraorbital rim underneath the orbicularis oculi muscle with the help of temporary exteriorized sutures. The fat can be placed either in the subperiosteal or supraperiosteal plane, with no apparent effect on esthetic results. This technique camouflages the lower orbital rim anatomy and provides more youthful rejuvenation of the midface.[7,9,28,29] This procedure is difficult secondary to the limited exposure and delicate septal tissues. It should be performed only by an experienced surgeon prepared for the frequent complications of ectropion and lower lid malposition.

Other methods suggested to correct tear through deformity include orbital fat removal, fat injections or grafts and temporary soft-tissue fillers, such as hyaluronic acid.[7,28,30]

Postoperative Care

Methylcellulose eye drops are recommended while the patient is awake, and lubricating ointment for night use for several days postoperatively. The patient's head should remain elevated to reduce edema and ophthalmic pressure. Patients are advised to avoid strenuous lifting, bending, and vigorous activities for 2 weeks following the procedure. Suture removal is performed 5 days postoperatively, and bandage strips may be removed on the second postsurgery visit, which is usually 5–7 days following surgery.

Complications

Historically, the most common complication following lower lid blepharoplasty is lower eyelid malposition, with published complication rates ranging from 5% to 90%.[9,10,24,31] Causes include excessive skin, fat or muscle removal, scar contracture, intramuscular hematoma, orbicularis oculi muscle paralysis, adhesions in the middle lamella, uncorrected lower lid laxity, and proptosis (Fig. 22A). The most prevalent etiological factor in post-blepharoplasty lid malposition is vertical deficiency of the anterior or posterior lamella in the setting of tarsoligamentous laxity.[9,10,24,31] To avoid the typical deformity seen after this procedure, canthopexy and canthoplasty have been adopted into cosmetic surgery, as the presumed rationale for correction of (or prophylaxis of) lower lid malposition in an attempt to optimize vertical eyelid position by tightening or shortening the lower eyelid horizontally.[9,24,31-34] In general, all methods of canthopexy/canthoplasty correct tarsoligamentous laxity, thereby counteracting the downward forces of healing.[9,24,31-34] Its treatment can include simple massage exercises as advocated by Carraway, lateral canthal repositioning, vertical skin recruitment and spacer grafts.[9,10,31-36]

Severe complications, such as visual loss from orbital hemorrhage, orbital injection or posterior optic nerve infarction are extremely rare, but have been described.[23,24,26,37] Other possible complications are lagophthalmos, corneal exposure and acquired strabismus (Fig. 22B). Among the potential risks with lower eyelid fat repositioning are temporary skin irregularities from fat and edema, fat granulomas, restricted ocular motility or new-onset diplopia.[23,24,26,37,38]

GENERAL COMPLICATIONS

Early Complications

Dry eye syndrome is a clinical diagnosis. Symptoms include itching, foreign body sensation, burning, mucoid secretions, frequent blinking, and conjunctival infection. Pre-existing dry eyes may be aggravated by perioperative lagophthalmos. Abnormal preoperative ocular history, such as documented dry eyes, history of dry eyes, LASIK surgery and/or history of frequent eye drop use, and abnormal orbital and periorbital anatomy, such as lower eyelid laxity and a negative vector, are all predictors of postoperative dry eye complications.[10,11,24,26] Ocular protection with patches, temporary tarsorrhaphy, and/or lateral canthopexy/canthoplasty should be combined with aggressive corneal lubrification, warm compresses and edema control.

Infection is a rare complication of blepharoplasty. Dry eye syndrome may predispose the cornea to superinfection. It can be treated with topical and/or systemic antibiotics. A fluid collection, if present, should be drained.

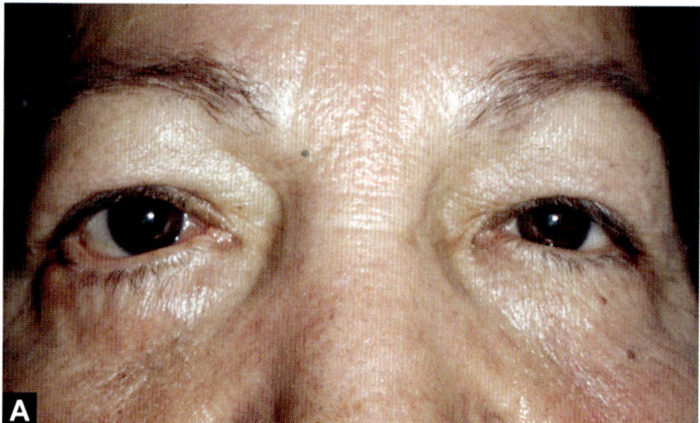

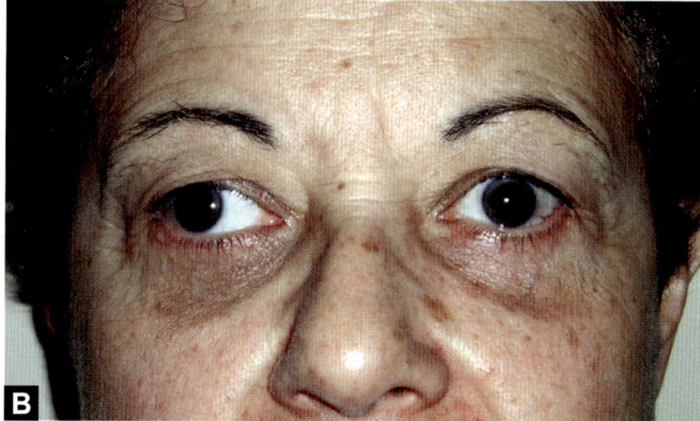

Figs 22A and B: Complications. (A) Lower eyelid malpositioning (ectropion—OD) after blepharoplasty. The surgery was performed at another hospital by another surgeon; (B) Acquired strabismus after lower blepharoplasty (40 days). However, the etiology of this case was Lambert-Eaton syndrome

Chemosis is a common complaint after blepharoplasty that is caused by lymphatic disruption of the eyelid, with development of milky conjunctival and corneal edema. Corneal injury and infection should be ruled out. It can be limited by atraumatic dissection, protective tarsorrhaphy, and edema-limiting maneuvers, such as cold compresses, elevation, massage, and corneal lubrification. It is usually self-limiting and resolves spontaneously, though prolonged chemosis can be treated with topical steroids.

Asymmetry is a common complication that can be addressed with revision procedures once edema and inflammation resolve completely.

Iatrogenic ptosis can result from injury to the levator aponeurosis during the inferior skin muscle excision upper lid blepharoplasty. Other causes include local anesthetic, edema, intramuscular hematoma, and traumatic operative technique. If levator injury is recognized intraoperatively or postoperatively, it should be repaired. Mild cases may resolve spontaneously.

Late Complications

Lagophthalmos can be caused by upper eyelid edema, iatrogenic orbital septal elevation or excessive skin resection. It usually resolves spontaneously, as edema resolves and muscles relax. Treatment is conservative with patient reassurance, light massage, taping and proper nocturnal lubrification. If conservative treatment fails, surgical treatment includes upper lid scar release with full-thickness interposition skin grafting.

Undercorrection of upper lid skin can be treated with secondary excision if necessary or, if pseudoptosis is the cause, lateral brow elevation.

Excess fat removal can result in hollowing of the socket. Fat transposition or soft-tissue fillers along the orbital rim may help mask this complication.

Inadequate fat resection, usually medial fat compartments, may be amenable to secondary transconjunctival resection. Residual lower lid rhytides can be treated with resurfacing modalities such as, chemical peels and ablative LASER resurfacing and/or soft-tissue fillers.

REOPERATIONS

Secondary blepharoplasty is a challenging and demanding procedure. It should not be performed until more than 3 months after the previous operation. Patients, who are to undergo secondary surgery to correct eyelid irregularities, should be evaluated carefully and counseled to ascertain a concurrent goal for surgery.

CONCLUSION

This chapter briefly describes the techniques of standard upper and lower blepharoplasty. Blepharoplasty is most of all about anatomy, and once the surgeon understands the surface anatomy of the eyelid complex and its deep underpinnings, the surgeon is prepared to assess the individual patient and formulate an individual surgical plan.

Practically, rejuvenation of this complex anatomical area requires a combination of therapies including fat excision, repositioning or transfer, simultaneous brow or midface lift, and adjunctive treatment for skin resurfacing and periorbital hollows.

Physicians should be receptive to patient feedback and continually evaluate their results to ensure patient satisfaction and safety. Refinements can be based on constructive criticism and can be incorporated into the entire blepharoplasty process.

REFERENCES

1. Espinoza GM, Holds JB. Evolution of eyelid surgery. Facial Plast Surg Clin North Am. 2005;13(4):505-10.
2. Rohrich RJ, Coberly DM, Fagien S, et al. Current concepts in aesthetic upper blepharoplasty. Plast Reconstr Surg. 2004;113(3):32e-42e.
3. Gentile RD. Upper lid blepharoplasty. Facial Plast Surg Clin North Am. 2005;13(4):511-24.
4. Castanãres S. Blepharoplasty for herniated intraorbital fat; anatomical basis for a new approach. Plast Reconstr Surg 1951;8(1):46-58.
5. Flowers RS. Upper blepharoplasty by eyelid invagination. Anchor blepharoplasty. Clin Plast Surg. 1993;20(2):193-207.
6. Fagien S. The role of the orbicularis oculi muscle and the eyelid crease in optimizing results in aesthetic upper blepharoplasty: a new look at the surgical treatment of mild upper eyelid fissure and fold asymmetries. Plast Reconstr Surg. 2010;125(2):653-66.
7. Loeb R. Fat pad sliding and fat grafting for leveling lid depressions. Clin Plast Surg. 1981;8(4):757-76.
8. de la Plaza R, Arroyo JM. A new technique for the treatment of palpebral bags. Plast Reconstr Surg. 1988;81(5):677-87.
9. Viana GA, Osaki MH, Nishi M. Comparison between two surgical techniques for lower eyelid rejuvenation: safety analysis and outcomes. Graefes Arch Clin Exp Ophthalmol. 2010;248(4):555-63.
10. Trussler AP, Rohrich RJ. MOC-PSSM CME article: Blepharoplasty. Plast Reconstr Surg. 2008;121(1 Suppl):1-10.

11. Naik MN, Honavar SG, Das S, et al. Blepharoplasty: an overview. J Cutan Aesthet Surg. 2009;2(1):6-11.
12. Lima CGMG, Siqueira GB, Cardoso IH, Sant'Anna AEB, Osaki MH. Avaliação do olho seco no pré e pós-operatório da blefaroplastia (Evaluation of dry eye in before and after blepharoplasty). Arq. Bras. Oftalmol. 2006; 69:227-32.
13. Brazzo BG, Nesi FA. Evaluation of the cosmetic patient. In: Nesi FA, Lisman RD, Levine MR (Eds). Smith's Ophthalmic Plastic and Reconstructive Surgery. Mosby, St Louis. 1998; 411-5.
14. Beard C. Examination and evaluation of the ptosis patient. In: Nesi FA, Lisman RD, Levine MR (Eds). Smith's Ophthalmic Plastic and Reconstructive Surgery. Mosby, St Louis. 1998; 339-44.
15. Viana GP, Viana GAP. Approach to eyebrow ptosis through the modified technique of Castanãres. Indian J Plast Surg. 2009; 42:58-62.
16. Feser DF, Gründl M, Eisenmann-Klein M, Prantl L. Attractiveness of eyebrow position and shape in females depends on the age of the beholder. Aesth Plast Surg 2007; 31:154-60.
17. Knize DM. Anatomic concepts for brow lift procedures. Plast Reconstr Surg. 2009; 124:2118-26.
18. Jelks GW, Jelks EB. The influence of orbital anatomy and eyelid anatomy on the palpebral aperture. Clin Plast Surg. 1991; 18:183-95.
19. Baker TJ, Gordon HL, Mosienko P. Upper lid blepharoplasty. Plast Reconstr Surg. 1977;60(5):692-8.
20. Zide BM, Jelks GW. Surgical anatomy of the orbit. New York: Raven; 1985.
21. Sheen JH. A change in the technique of supratarsal fixation in upper blepharoplasty. Plast Reconstr Surg. 1977;59(6):831-4.
22. Callahan MA. Prevention of blindness after blepharoplasty. Ophthalmology. 1983;90(9):1047-51.
23. Wolfort FG, Vaughan TE, Wolfort SF, et al. Retrobulbar hematoma and blepharoplasty. Plast Reconstr Surg. 1999;104(7):2154-62.
24. Lowry JC, Bartley GB. Complications of blepharoplasty. Surv Ophthalmol. 1994;38(4):327-50.
25. Schechter RJ. Management of inadvertent intraocular injections. Ann Ophthalmol. 1985;17(12):771-5.
26. Goldberg RA, Charonis GC, Baylis HI, et al.Upper and lower eyelid blepharoplasty. In: Nesi FA, Lisman RD, Levine MR (Eds). Smith's Ophthalmic Plastic and Reconstructive Surgery. St Louis: Mosby; 1998. pp. 416-35.
27. Baylis HI, Long JA, Groth MJ. Transconjunctival lower eyelid blepharoplasty. Technique and complications. Ophthalmology. 1989;96(7):1027-32.
28. Goldberg RA. The three periorbital hollows: a paradigm for periorbital rejuvenation. Plast Reconstr Surg. 2005;116(6):1796-804.
29. Hamra ST. The role of the septal reset in creating a youthful eyelid-cheek complex in facial rejuvenation. Plast Reconstr Surg. 2004;113(7):2124-41.
30. Viana GA, Osaki MH, Cariello AJ, et al. Treatment of the tear trough deformity with hyaluronic acid gel filler. Arg Bras Oftalmol. 2011;74(1):44-7.
31. Codner MA, Wolfi JN, Anzarut A. Primary transcutaneous lower blepharoplasty with routine lateral canthal support: a comprehensive 10-year review. Plast Reconstr Surg. 2008;121(1):241-50.
32. Flowers RS. Canthopexy as a routine blepharoplasty component. Clin Plast Surg. 1993;20(2):351-65.
33. Jelks GW, Glat PM, Jelks EB, et al. The inferior retinacular lateral canthoplasty: a new technique. Plast Reconst Surg. 1997;100(5):1262-70.
34. Lessa S, Sebastiá R, Flores E. Uma cantopexia simples. Rev Bras Oftal. 1999;58:779-86.
35. McCord CD Jr. The correction of lower lid malposition following lower lid blepharoplasty. Plast Reconstr Surg. 1999;103(3):1036-9.
36. Carraway JH, Mellow CG. The prevention and treatment of lower lid ectropion following blepharoplasty. Plast Reconstr Surg. 1990;85(6):971-81.
37. Trelles MA. Sight lost after lower lid laser blepharoplasty. Ann Plast Surg. 2000;45(6):678-9.
38. Goldberg RA, Yuen VH. Restricted ocular movements following lower eyelid fat repositioning. Plast Reconstr Surg. 2002;110(1):302-5.

CHAPTER

95 SMAS Rhytidectomy: Preoperative Evaluation, Surgical Techniques and Pitfalls

Jeremy B White, Mark Domanski, Steven B Hopping

INDICATIONS FOR THE SURGERY

Subcutaneous dissection with Superficial Muscular Aponeurotic System (SMAS) rhytidectomy is indicated for patients who have developed jowls and cervical skin laxity and wish to restore a more youthful appearance. The midface is not fully resuspended with this procedure so alternative approaches or adjunct procedures should be considered if this result is desired. Treatment of the midface can be accomplished by a combination of methods, including, but not limited to filler or fat injections to the midface, malar implants, and extended supra-SMAS, midface, deep plane or subperiosteal rhytidectomies.

The ideal candidate is one who is in the early forties to late fifties, has minimal sun damage to the skin, mild-to-moderate skin laxity and mild-to-moderate jowls. The thickness of the skin and soft tissues is important since those who have thicker, heavier tissues may experience decreased longevity to the lift due to the gravitational effect over time. A strong bony structure is also crucial as this will provide the platform upon which skin redraping will occur and the most pleasing results are usually obtained when mandibular and malar angularity can be restored. Some patients may require implants to achieve this effect. Along the same line, a patient with a low lying hyoid bone and microgenia is not ideal since tightening the SMAS alone may not restore a sharp cervicomental angle. This anatomic problem can be aided, to some effect, by submental liposuction and chin augmentation, if necessary. If the patient has platysma bands, it is often necessary to make a separate submental incision to remove excess platysma and reapproximate the edges in the midline.

SPECIFIC PREOPERATIVE EVALUATION

Patients often present for facial rejuvenation consultations because they desire to recapture their youth. During the preoperative assessment, it is important to gain a thorough understanding of the patient's motivations for surgery. If the patient is relying on this surgery to get a new job, find a new spouse and completely change his or her life, one must be cautious. Any dissatisfaction with these additional expectations postoperatively may be associated with surgeon failure in the patient's mind. It is therefore of utmost importance to establish a bond of trust and understanding between the physician and patient at this first encounter.

A second preoperative consultation is often necessary to solidify this relationship, to answer any questions, and to make sure that the patient's and surgeon's expectations are similar. Risks of the surgery should be reviewed thoroughly at this time to enhance the patient's understanding of the surgical complexity and to minimize patient resentment towards the surgeon if complications do occur. One should proceed with particular caution if the patient has had multiple cosmetic surgeries and still is not satisfied with the results. This may mean that the previous surgeries were poorly executed, expectations were not shared by both the surgeon and patient preoperatively, the patient has some impediment to optimal healing, or that the patient has a psychiatric disorder, such as body dysmorphia. In these situations, one should strongly consider obtaining an official psychiatric evaluation. If the patient has such a disorder, he or she will likely continue to be dissatisfied with any further procedures that are conducted, as will the surgeon.

In addition to the psychological evaluation, the physician should take a complete medical history. This should include a list of any dermatologic diseases, such as uncontrolled lupus or propensity to develop keloids that the patient may have. These problems will have negative effects on the patient's healing process. Moreover, if the patient has significant medical problems, such as diabetes or peripheral vascular disease, which can impact wound healing and skin flap survival significantly, the surgeon should consider performing a less extensive procedure and limiting the adjunct procedures.

A full list of medications should be obtained, but particular attention should be paid to patients who are taking anticoagulants, long-term steroids, which can cause wound healing complications and any alternative medicines that the patient might not have remembered to mention. Retinoids should not be used perioperatively as isotretinoin has been demonstrated to delay healing and the wound contraction response in animal models.[1,2] Certain herbal medicines and vitamins, such as vitamin E, feverfew, ginkgo, ginseng, ginger, garlic and green tea can cause an increase in intraoperative and postoperative bleeding either directly or via interactions with other medications. These medicines should be discontinued two weeks before surgery. Any history of propensity to bleed should prompt obtaining a CBC and coagulation profile.

Most importantly, the patient should not smoke tobacco for at least two to four weeks before and after surgery. Rhytidectomy skin flap necrosis has been shown to occur anywhere between four and 12.5 times more frequently in smokers than in nonsmokers.[3,4] Urine anabasine, which does not test positive with nicotine replacement product use and serum or urine cotinine measurements can be obtained to confirm the patient's smoking status. Given the added risk to this elective procedure, if the patient continues to smoke despite having received extensive counseling, one should consider either limiting the extent of flap undermining or canceling the surgery altogether.

The consultation should then continue with the physical examination. The surgeon should begin with a careful assessment of the facial skin for color, thickness, evidence of solar damage, scars and any lesions that are concerning for neoplasia. Rhytids, jowls, deepened nasolabial folds, platysma bands and areas of particular laxity should be identified with the patient in front of a mirror to enable a shared understanding of the most problematic regions to target. Moreover, the surgeon should discuss areas of hollowing where the malar fat pads have begun to atrophy and displace inferiorly. Midface descent can be treated with a lift, but is often in need of volume restoration as well. Autologous fat injection and other fillers can be extremely useful to accomplish this task. In the lower third of the face and neck, the cervicomental angle should be examined with respect to the hyoid bone. It may be more difficult to restore a youthful neck profile and a well-defined jaw in a patient with a low hyoid and an obtuse cervicomental angle. Adjunctive procedures, such as conservative midline cervical skin excision and submental liposuction may be necessary to achieve the best outcome in these cases. Incision lines should be drawn on the patient to communicate where scars will be placed and hidden. In planning these incisions, the surgeon must pay heed to the temporal hair line position as this may influence the optimal location of the incision.

Even after extensive discussion and patient evaluation, the preoperative dialogue is not complete without taking patient photographs. This should be performed against a light blue background in the Frankfort horizontal plane, which is parallel to a line that extends from the supratragal notch to the infraorbital rim. Frontal and bilateral lateral and oblique views should be obtained, however, additional photos should be taken if there are plans to perform other adjunctive surgery. Examination of these photographs with the patient gives the opportunity to address any further concerns from the patient and to finalize preoperative documentation.

Categories of Subcutaneous SMAS Facelifting

Anterior scar, short flap (S-Lift): Patients who are in their 30s or 40s and have early jowl and neck laxity.

Anterior scar, long flap (S-PlusLift): Patients who are in their 40s to 60s and have moderate jowl, neck and midface laxity.

Posterior scar (Neck Lift): Patients who are in their 30s to 60s, often men with moderate-severe neck laxity.

Platysmaplasty: Patients are of any age, but demonstrate platysma bands at rest.

ANESTHETIC CONSIDERATIONS

Excellent anesthesia management is essential since it sets the tone for the entire surgical experience. Patients often view cosmetic surgery as a venture without risks and it is therefore most important to educate the patient regarding these real risks without contributing excessively to his or her anxiety. Once this has been done, the anesthesiologist or CRNA must make certain key assessments to give the highest probability for a safe surgery. First, the surgeon and anesthesia provider must decide on the appropriate setting in which the surgery should be performed, whether in the office, at an outpatient ambulatory facility, or on a 23-hour observation status at a hospital. If the patient has sleep apnea or is obese, strong consideration should be given to admit the patient postoperatively. Patients with sleep apnea, which is often undiagnosed, can be more difficult to intubate if the necessity arises and are more sensitive to narcotics than patients without sleep apnea. The latter factor is crucial since narcotics can depress their respiratory drive postoperatively so these patients may require continuous pulse oxygen monitoring overnight.

If the patient is over 50 years old, an electrocardiogram should be performed. Preoperative medical clearance should be obtained from the appropriate physician if the patient has any significant medical problems. Anticoagulants, such as aspirin and coumadin should be stopped one to two weeks prior to surgery. A urine pregnancy test is conducted on the day of surgery for all premenopausal women as general anesthesia can have significant consequences for a fetus. Patients are asked not to eat or drink after midnight the night before surgery. If patients do not adhere to this and surgery proceeds with some level of sedation, the patient is at risk for aspiration pneumonia.

Patients who will receive general anesthesia or IV sedation are also at risk for deep vein thrombosis, particularly if the procedure is long and combined with other surgeries, such as abdominoplasty. There is additional cause for concern in patients who smoke, take oral contraceptive hormones, or have hypercoagulability disorders. Sequential compression devices are placed on the patient's lower extremities to minimize this risk of DVT and pulmonary embolus. Considering the precision that is required to perform this operation well, every attempt should be made to maintain a blood-free surgical field. This can be aided by giving the patient 0.2 mg of clonidine fifteen minutes prior to surgery, unless preoperative blood pressure is quite low. Intraoperative blood pressure should be maintained at the low range of normal for that patient while allowing for occasional raises in pressure due to stimulation or pain.

In the senior author's practice (SBH), patients are given IV sedation anesthesia intraoperatively with combinations of versed, diprivan, fentanyl and ketamine. Some patients prefer only oral-versed sedation. The patient's head is elevated just above the heart. A helpful method to optimize the surgical field is to instill tumescent local anesthesia solution subcutaneously over the SMAS ten minute prior to dissection. This will not only aid in hemostasis, but also increase the ease of operation with hydrodissection of the surgical plane. To avoid postoperative bucking, which can lead to bleeding and hematoma, dexamethasone and ondansetron are provided intraoperatively. Lastly, there should be good communication between the surgeon and anesthesia provider towards the end of the case. This will help to ensure that the sedation agent is titrated off at the appropriate time, leading to a smooth wakeup.

SURGICAL STEPS

Contemporary facelifting involves reversing the aging effects of atrophy and gravity by lifting the skin and SMAS of the face in a superior and posterior direction. Incisions are hidden anterior and posterior to the ears and in the hairline. Facelifts involve subcutaneous dissection, SMAS plication or imbrication, and sometimes deep plane (beneath SMAS) or subperiosteal dissection. The following will discuss the senior author's (SBH) technique for superficial plane SMAS rhytidectomy.

SPECIAL INSTRUMENTS USED FOR THE SURGERY

Instrumentation for rhytidectomies can vary widely from surgeon to surgeon.

A basic facelift set would include:

- Blunt facelift scissor
- Curved, sharp scissor
- Suture scissor
- Skin hook, two prong
- Deaver retractor
- Scalpel
- Adson forceps with teeth
- Needle holder
- Hemostats
- Bipolar or unipolar cautery Unit

Additional Instruments:

- Flap demarcator
- Facial liposuction cannulas
- Lighted facelift retractor

Operative Technique

Modified tumescent anesthesia (1000 cc saline, 100 cc 1% lidocaine plain, 2 cc epinephrine 1:1000) is infiltrated into the subcutaneous-supra SMAS tissue planes utilizing a 20 gauge spinal needle. Approximately 200 mL is infused into the neck and 100 mL into the anterior face. The face is then prepped with betadine and a light massage of the facial tissues is performed for 5 minutes to diffuse the tumescent solution evenly into the tissues.

Five stab incisions are made with a No. 15 blade: one submental, two supra-auricular and two infra-auricular. Criss-cross liposuction is performed with 1 or 2 mm blunt cannulas with the openings down, away from the skin. Criss-crossing tunnels helps to maximize skin tightening (Fig. 1).

Starting on the patient's right, incisions are made with a No. 15 blade from the infra-auricular ear to the supra-auricular area, with extensions horizontally into the temporal hairline, designed to preserve pretemporal hair. A preauricular strip for improved exposure is optional (Fig. 2). The incision is retrotragal in women and pretragal in men, if there is a history of nicotine use, however, a pretragal incision is favored because of concerns about distal flap viability. The incision is beveled towards the SMAS keeping the distal flap as full thickness as possible. Next, a two-pronged skin hook provides counter traction as the flap is extended anteriorly 2–3 centimeters using the beveled No. 15 blade. Face-lift scissors are now utilized to extend the flap widely inferiorly and anteriorly. As the dissection extends anteriorly beyond the parotid gland, be sure to remain in the subcutaneous plane to avoid injury to deeper facial nerve branches (Fig. 3).

In patients with fatty or heavy necks, open liposuction with a 3 mm spatula cannula is now performed.

Next, purse-string SMAS plication sutures are placed starting at the fixed fascial tissues overlying the zygomatic arch extending inferiorly to the platysma SMAS tissues at the angle of the mandible ("U suture"). A firm bite in this ESP (extended SMAS platysma) tissue allows dramatic tightening of the neck when the purse-string suture is tightened. A second purse-string suture ("O suture") is placed if lifting of the jowl is desired. A 2-0 Ethibond suture is used for the purse string SMAS plication and the knot is buried using a horizontal mattress suture of 3-0 Vicryl (Figs 4A and B). Any redundant tissue bunching that is created by the purse-string sutures is trimmed flat with the scissors. The skin flap is pulled superolaterally and held in position with a temporary surgical clip in the pre-auricular area. Other plication sutures can be placed to lift the jowl or midface as indicated. While the senior author has experienced excellent results using the purse string suture technique, there are many ways of plicating the SMAS, some of which have been evaluated in biomechanics studies.[5]

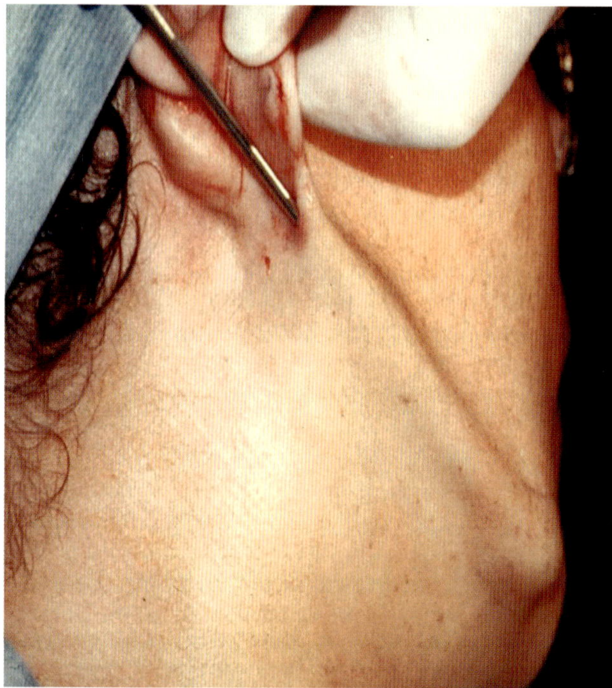

Fig. 1: Liposuction of neck, jowl and face. A 1 mm cannula is used for pretunneling and liposuction after tumescent anesthesia infusion

The same maneuvers are now performed on the patients left side.

Once the left side plication is completed, return to the right side and irrigate the flap with jets of saline from a 10 cc syringe. Complete hemostasis is obtained with bipolar forceps.

Superior rotation of the facelift flap skin is then performed. Measuring with a flap demarcator, the maximum tension of the closure is placed at the supra-auricular point of the anterior incision using a 3-0 vicryl, horizontal mattress suture to secure the flap to the fixed SMAS tissues below (Fig. 5).

At this point, tissue redundancy is created by the superior flap rotation. The horizontal, temporal hair preserving incision is extended utilizing sharp scissors. If excessive redundancy is present, the incision is curved sharply

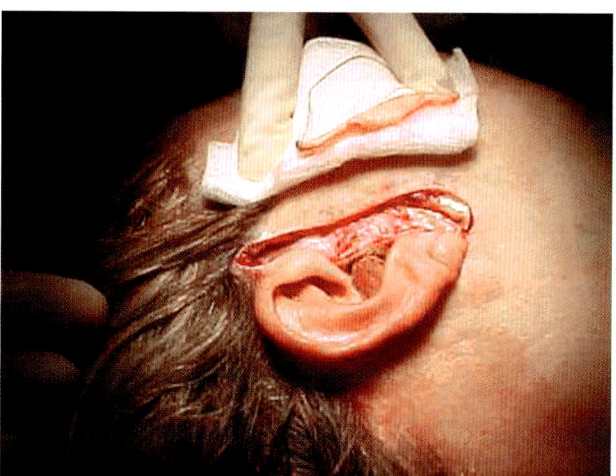

Fig. 2: Anterior facelift incision. Pre-excision strip can be performed for improved exposure prior to flap elevation

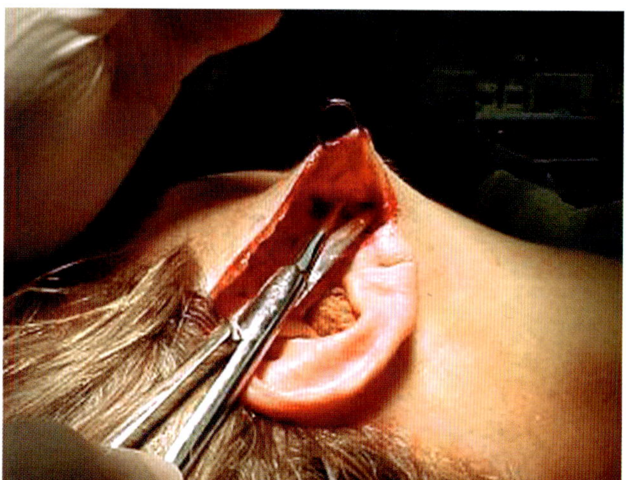

Fig. 3: Scissor elevation of facelift flap is best performed under direct vision

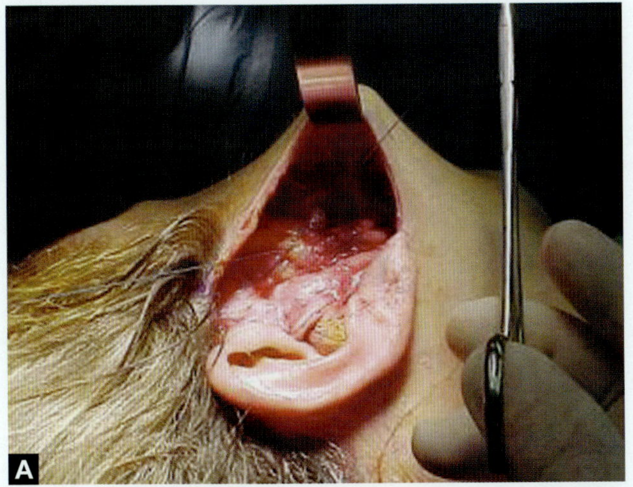

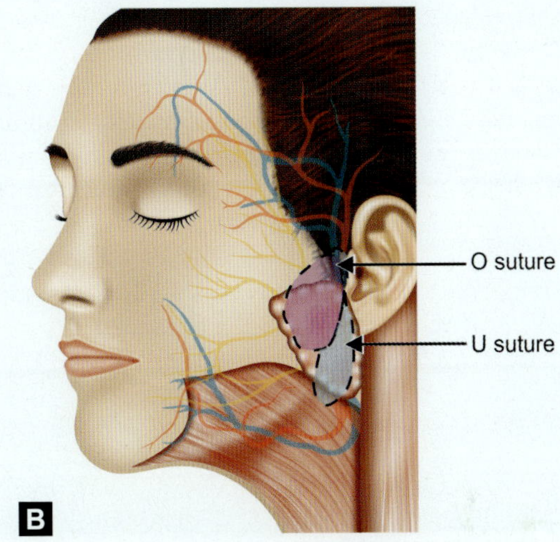

Figs 4A and B: SMAS plication sutures secured to fixed fascial tissues above the zygomatic arch

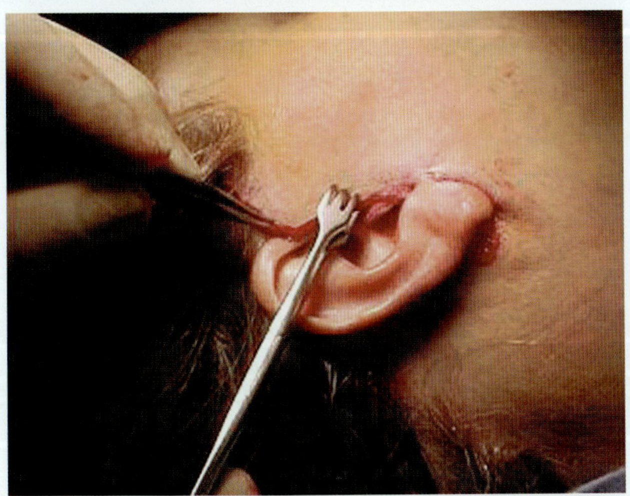

Fig. 5: Flap demarcator assists in calculating extent of skin excision. The point of maximum tension is just above the ear

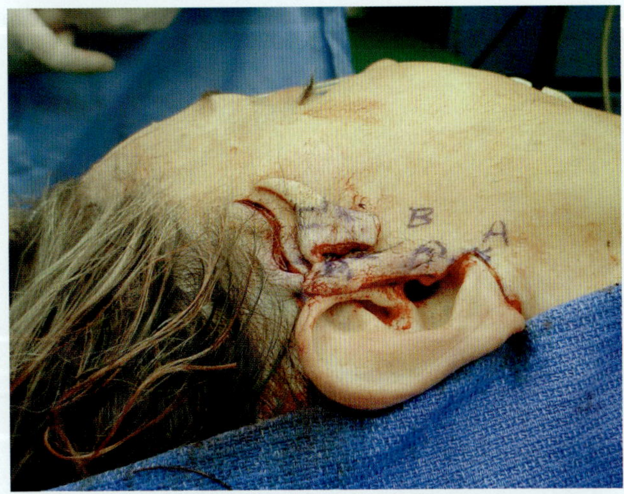

Fig. 6: The vector of pull is superolaterally as depicted. Note the excess skin superior to the ear

superiorly into the temporal hair. Redundant tissue (scalp) is removed and the superior "dog-ear" is corrected with a cut back into the temporal hair (Fig. 6).

Having resolved the superior redundancy issue, the flap demarcator assesses the amount of preauricular skin to be excised. No tension should be present in this anterior-inferior portion of the closure. Correct any infra-auricular redundancy or dog-ear as necessary. Generally, the extreme superior rotation of the flap minimizes redundancy in the infra-auricular area.

Closure of the subcutaneous tissues is accomplished with 3-0 vicryl interrupted sutures. This includes a tight adhesion of the infra-auricular flap to the conchal cartilage perichondrium of the ear to prevent inferior migration of the scar and a "pixie ear" deformity. The anterior skin incision is closed with subcuticular 5-0 monocryl (Fig. 7). Surgical clips are used to close all scalp incisions. Any postauricular incisions are closed loosely with interrupted 4-0 chromic suture. This allows easy egress of fluid or blood from beneath the flaps.

A light compressive dressing is applied for 24 hours. The patient is seen the next day and the dressing is replaced with a velcro head band, which is worn intermittently throughout the day and during sleep for one week. The surgical clips in the temporal and occipital hairline are removed on postoperation day 9 or 10.

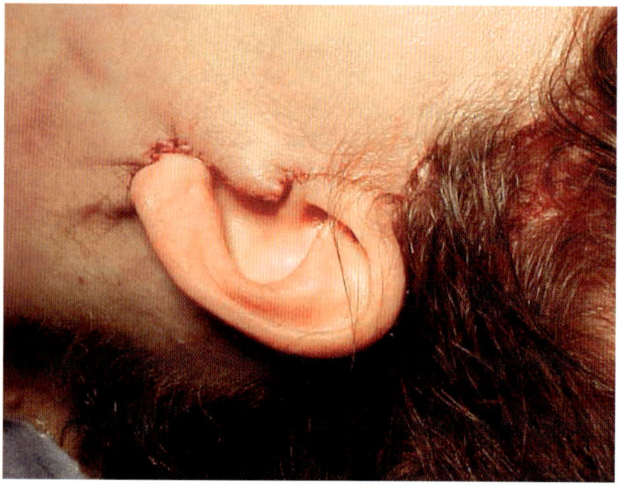

Fig. 7: Incision closed anterior to ear without tension. Note redundant skin left over the tragus to prevent postoperative tragal retraction

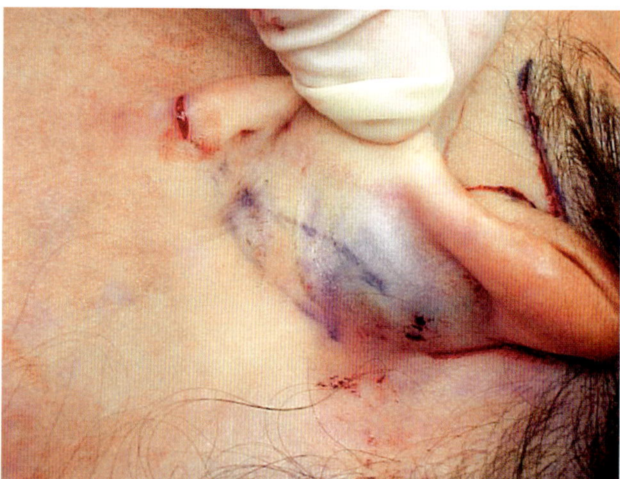

Fig. 8: Postauricular M-plasty to handle postauricular skin excess

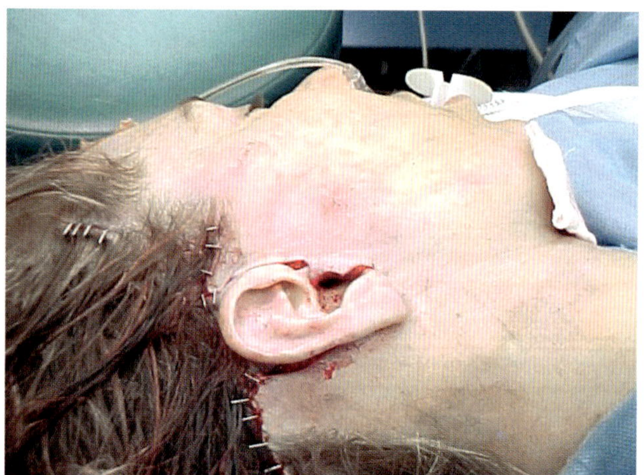

Fig. 9: Closure with extended postauricular and scalp skin excision, often needed for cases of excess neck laxity

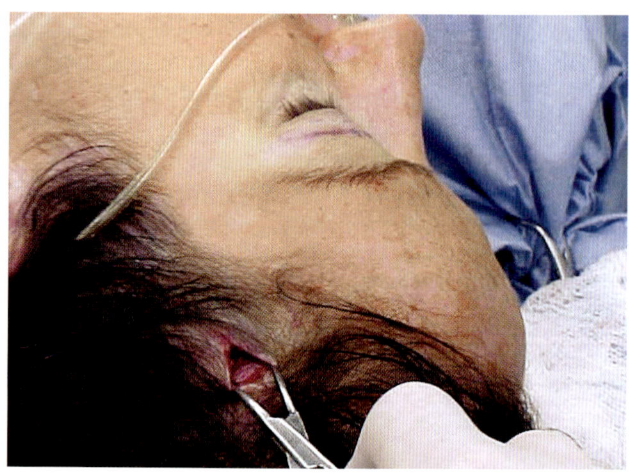

Fig. 10: Temple lift incision for superior temple scalp advancement

Special Considerations

If excessive skin redundancy exists postauricularly after superior rotation of the anterior flap, the incision should be extended into the postauricular sulcus and posterior hair as necessary. A postauricular M-plasty is useful for small skin redundancies (Fig. 8). For more excessive skin excess as in cases with advanced neck laxity, the incision must be extended into the postauricular sulcus and posterior scalp (Fig. 9).

If excessive redundancy exists in the temple area after flap rotation, perform a temple lift by widely undermining in the sub-SMAS plane between the temporoparietal fascia and the superficial layer of the temporalis fascia. This provides a safe plane away from the facial nerve branches, which lie within the temporoparietal fascia. Advance the temple tissues superiorly by attaching the temporoparietal fascia to a more superior level on the temporalis fascia using a 3-0 Vicryl horizontal mattress suture (Fig. 10).

If excessive or redundant SMAS tissues exist, perform SMASectomies to debulk excess SMAS before closure with purse-string sutures (Figs 11 and 12).

If excessive midface laxity exists, extend the midface dissection to the level of the infraorbital neurovascular bundle and plicate up the mobile malar soft tissues to the fixed orbicularis muscle fascia 1 cm below the lateral canthus. Use two or three 3-0 vicryl interrupted sutures with the knots buried (Figs 13 and 14).

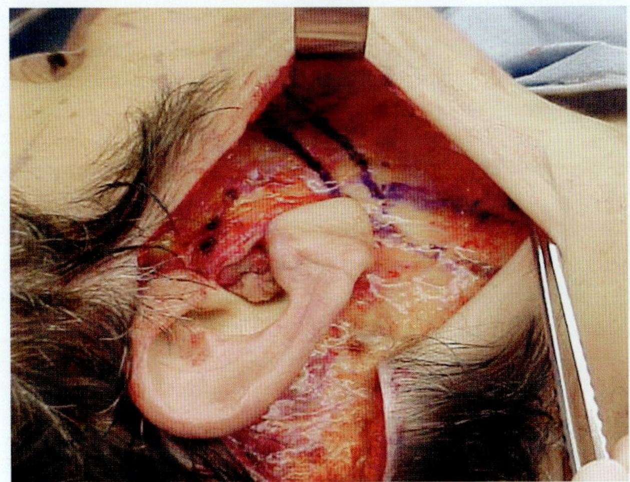

Fig. 11: Intraoperative photo showing planned SMASectomies

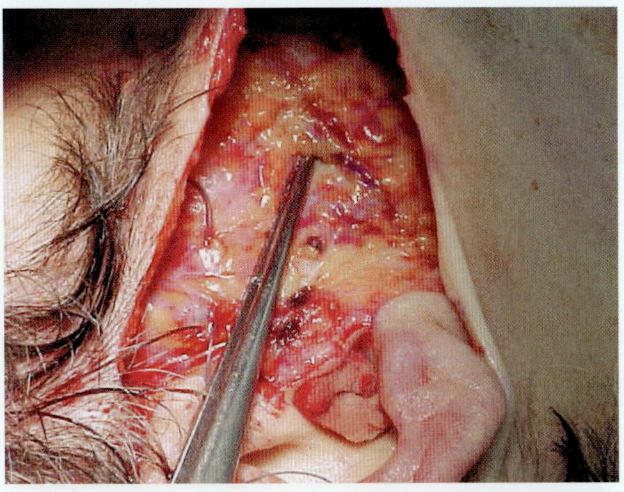

Fig. 12: SMASectomy defect closure. Note superior movement of the distal midface tissues

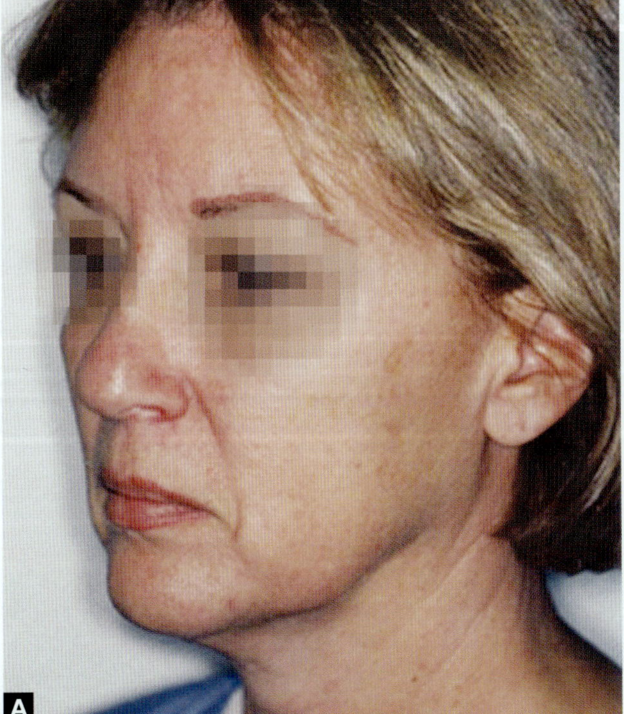

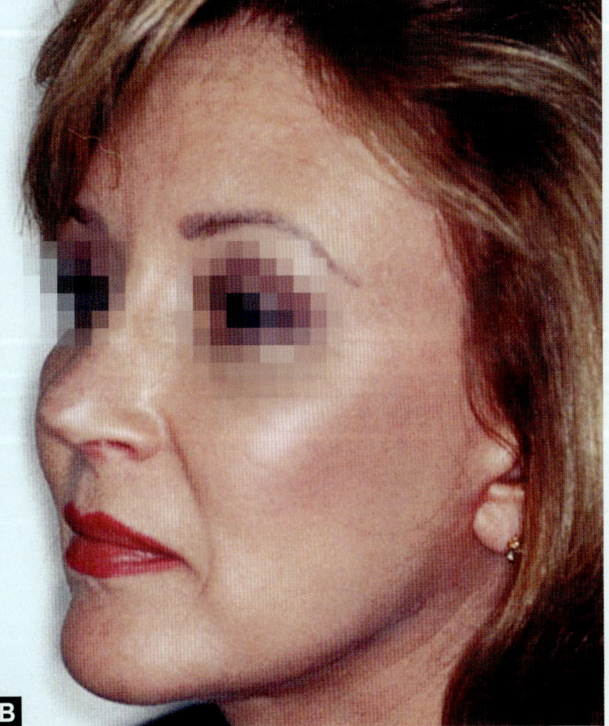

Figs 13A and B: Preoperative (A) oblique view of the face demonstrating the presence of jowls and a slightly obtuse cervicomental angle. She underwent SMAS rhytidectomy with autologous fat grafting to the midface; (B) and had significant improvement in these areas

If excessive submental fullness exists after lateral flap tightening or if there are platysma bands at rest, the neck should be opened by extending the horizontal submental incision to 3 cm and remove the soft tissue excess in the midline with scissors. Liposuction any excessive subplatysmal fat. Perform backcuts on the platysma muscles at the level of the hyoid bone. Approximate the cut edges of the platysma with interrupted 3-0 vicryl sutures with knots buried completing the platysmaplasty. Wide undermining of the skin of the neck is necessary to prevent postoperative irregularities.

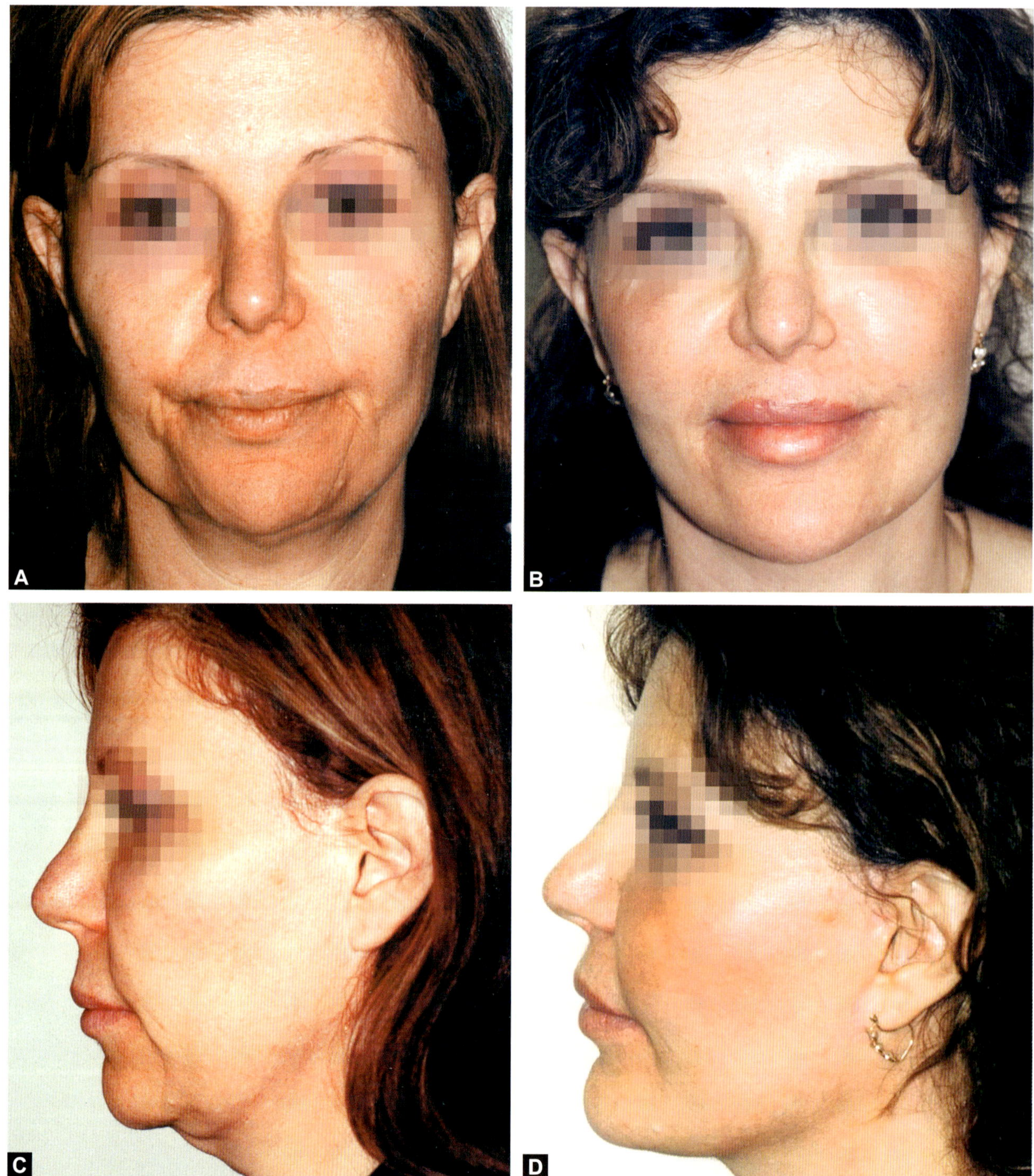

Figs 14A to D: Preoperative (A and C) and postoperative (B and D) anterior and lateral views of a patient who underwent SMAS rhytidectomy with autologous fat grafting to the midface

COMPLICATIONS

As with any surgical procedure, rhytidectomy has its own complications. If a complication occurs, early recognition and proper treatment is paramount to salvage a successful outcome. Moreover, if an adverse event occurs and the patient becomes upset, it is essential to see this patient more often, rather than distance oneself. This will help to maintain good rapport between the surgeon and patient.

Hematoma

The most common complication of rhytidectomy is hematoma, which is reported to occur in 0.3–8.1% of cases.[6] Avoidance of hematoma begins in the preoperative setting by discontinuing anticoagulants and avoiding herbal supplements that can contribute to bleeding, as mentioned previously. If a patient has a medical condition that requires a blood thinner, the patient's internist should evaluate the risks of discontinuing the medication prior to surgery.

Intraoperative avoidance of hematoma requires meticulous technique. Common practice involves preoperative injection of lidocaine with epinephrine into the planned incision sites. While this allows for better intraoperative hemostasis, this may mask blood vessels that may bleed postoperatively. Intraoperative dissection in the appropriate surgical planes will minimize bleeding. Bipolar coagulation of bleeding vessels is performed. Bipolar cautery is more focused and precise than monopolar cautery and thus carries less risk to nearby structures, such as nerves. Cauterization of the skin flap should be performed only where necessary as to minimize the risk of flap necrosis.

Prevention of hematoma continues postoperatively. Gentle emergence from anesthesia is paramount to prevent patient bucking and associated rises in blood pressure. A gentle pressure dressing in the form of a head wrap is placed on the wound site at the end of the procedure. Appropriate postoperative pain management helps to control blood pressure and potentially reduces the risk of hematoma. For this reason, the patient should have their postoperative prescriptions filled prior to the date of surgery to avoid any medication access problems.

If they occur, hematomas usually present within the first 24 hours postoperatively. Symptoms can include pain that is greater than expected, swelling or increased drain output. It should be emphasized that drains prevent seromas not hematomas. Evacuation of the hematoma is important to ensure skin flap survival. The wound site should be irrigated with saline to attempt to locate the source of bleeding. Unfortunately, the bleeding vessel often will remain elusive. Small hematomas may only present after facial edema has decreased and, at times, may be treated by repeat needle aspiration.

Infection

Infection is a risk in any surgery. Patients at increased risk for infection include those that are at risk for poor wound healing, such as diabetics and smokers.

Prevention of infection is focused on the minimization of bacterial load. The patients should be instructed to shower and shampoo the morning of surgery. Some centers recommend that patients bathe with hexachlorophene (Phisohex) before elective surgery. The theory is that this decreases bodily bacterial load and thus decreases wound infections. Phisohex should not be used around the eyes.

The role of preoperative antibiotics continues to evolve. Preoperative parenteral antibiotics given within one hour of skin incision has been shown in the general surgery literature to decrease wound infections. Common antibiotics include cefazolin or clindamycin.

Routine use of postoperative oral antibiotics after facial plastic surgery is common, but varies considerably between practitioners. Many practitioners like to apply bacitracin or mupirocin ointment to wound edges after closure. This theoretically decreases bacterial exposure to the wound while maintaining tissue moisture. However, such ointment may actually prevent adequate cleansing of the wound edge by trapping sloughed skin and debris next to the wound. Therefore, some practitioners recommend daily removal of clots from the wound with q-tips and hydrogen peroxide. Regardless of the method recommended, much about postoperative wound care is more empiric than evidence based.

If postoperative infection is suspected, antibiotics should be started. The antibiotic coverage should be broadened if the patient is already on antibiotics. If purulence is expressed from the wound edge, the wound should be opened, cultured and irrigated. Treatment should be tailored to the extent of the patient's infection.

Skin Slough/Flap Loss

Skin slough or flap loss occurs when the blood supply is inadequate to support live tissue. This has been reported to occur in 1–3% of rhytidectomies. Blood supply can become compromised if the skin flap is too thin or the flap is placed on excessive tension. If hair follicles are visible on the undersurface of the skin flap, the flap is too thin. Hematoma can cause increased tissue pressure and thus lead to reduced blood flow and flap loss. Similarly, infection compromises capillary blood flow. Smokers and diabetics have impaired microcirculation and are at increased risk of flap loss. Smokers should cease smoking at least two weeks prior to the surgery. Since nicotine also causes vasoconstriction, nicotine gum and other cigarette substitutes should be avoided as well.

Initial treatment of partial thickness loss involves dressing changes and observation. Many partial thickness losses will re-epithelialize with little noticeable cosmetic impairment. Skin flap re-advancement can be considered for more noticeable losses. The surgeon should be aware that blood supply is compromised each time tissue is advanced. Therefore, readvancement of the skin flap should be performed only once the wound is stable and the vasculature of the skin flap has accommodated to having been advanced previously.

Great Auricular Nerve Injury

Impairment to the sensation of the ear can be very significant to females, especially those that wear earrings. Sensation to the earlobe and helix is provided by a branch of the great auricular nerve. This nerve arises from the second and third cervical spinal rootlets and travels posterior to the sternocleidomastoid muscle. It then wraps around the posterior edge of the sternocleidomastoid muscle at Erb's point to course anteriorly and superiorly along the superficial aspect of the muscle. This portion is typically encountered approximately 6.5 cm below the external auditory meatus. The great auricular nerve then gives off several branches, one of which courses superiorly toward the earlobe.

One can prevent greater auricular nerve injury by avoiding deep dissection at the level of the sternocleidomastoid muscle. Some surgeons prefer to identify the nerve during dissection and then preserve it. Either way, most rhytidectomy patients experience some postoperative anesthesia to the earlobe and helix that is usually transient. Patients must be counseled to this fact.

Facial Nerve Injury

Facial nerve injury is the most devastating complication of rhytidectomy. An understanding of facial nerve anatomy is critical to avoid such a complication. The facial nerve exits the temporal bone at the stylomastoid foramen. The main nerve trunk can be found one centimeter deep, anterior and inferior to the tragal pointer. There is no need to be this deep in a face-lift and thus injuries to the main branch of the facial nerve are rare.

The facial nerve travels through the parotid gland, which is divided by this into a superficial and deep lobe. This division is somewhat arbitrary as there is no fascial plane dividing the parotid into lobes. The facial nerve divides within the parotid gland at the pes anserinus ("goose's foot") into a superior and inferior division and then into smaller branches. The branches of the facial nerve exit the parotid gland anteriorly and travel along the parotidomasseteric fascia. The facial nerve lies deep to the superficial musculoaponeurotic system and innervates the muscles of facial expression from the deep surface except for the buccinator, levator anguli ori and mentalis muscles, which receive their innervation on their superficial surfaces. The concept here is that the facial nerve lies deep in the lateral face but becomes more superficial toward the midline.

The most commonly injured branch of the facial nerve is the buccal branch. The buccal branch runs in close proximity to Stensen's duct (the parotid duct). Due to significant cross innervations of the buccal branch, injuries are often not disfiguring. The marginal and temporal branches of the facial nerve have few cross-innervating arcades and injury to these branches is more obvious postoperatively. There is controversy in the medical literature as to which of these two branches is injured most often. The temporal branch of the facial nerve is particularly vulnerable to injury because of its superficial location as it crosses the midportion of the zygomatic arch.

If a facial nerve branch is transected during surgery, it should be repaired immediately using a small suture, such as 9-0 nylon. A microscope or high powered loupes will be required. If there is a weakness from a traction injury, high dose steroids, such as dexamethasone (10 mg IV) followed by an oral taper may reduce inflammation and thus reduce neuropraxia.

Pixie Ear Deformity

Reattachment of the facial cheek skin to the ear can result in an elongated earlobe, which obliterates the definition of the lobule. This is often referred to as a pixie ear or satyr earlobe deformity.

Prevention of this deformity centers around minimizing skin tension at the lower earlobe upon closure. A generous amount of perilobular skin flap should be left around the earlobe. Closure of the infra-auricular flap to the conchal cartilage perichondrium or mastoid fascia reduces skin tension. The pull on the SMAS in this region should also help to redistribute the forces from the skin.

Pixie ear deformities may not manifest for some time after surgery. If present, it can be repaired with a V to Y advancement flap. The drawback of this procedure is a small scar that presents anterior to the earlobe. Another option is to perform a platysmaplasty or neck lift to resuspend the SMAS and thus remove tension from the skin. If this is a revision platsymaplasty, little skin needs to be excised other than the original incision since the problem is tension forces and not redundant skin.

Unhappy Patient

In order to succeed, one must first identify the problem, conceive an achievable goal, and then design and execute a tenable plan. Failure anywhere along this pathway will preclude success and result in an unhappy patient.

Patients have various motivations for rejuvenating procedures. This motivation may not have to do with any objective physical deformity and therefore, addressing physical appearance will not lead to patient satisfaction. If a patient seeks facial rejuvenation because they are distraught over their recent divorce, rhytidectomy will not change the divorce. The desire to create an external appearance commensurate with the patient's internal vigor is reasonable.

Rhytidectomy cannot make someone look like they did twenty years ago, but it can reduce the stigmata of aging and create a more youthful appearance. This difference is subtle, but extremely important. In the end, the problem of the unhappy patient is best managed preoperatively by making sure to establish a trusting bond with the patient and establishing realistic expectations with goals that can be accomplished.

OTHER TREATMENT OPTIONS AVAILABLE FOR THE SAME CONDITION

"It is tempting, if the only tool you have is a hammer, to treat everything as if it were a nail." In this regard the facial plastic surgeon should think beyond surgical rhytidectomy as the sole solution for facial rejuvenation. Patients sometimes may not be emotionally or fiscally ready to undergo extensive cosmetic surgery. Other times, they simply cannot spare the time off from work that is required for recovery. There are multiple rejuvenation therapies that can be offered to these patients, many of which can be used as adjuncts to rhytidectomy.

Chemical Peels

Chemical peels are commonly used to treat rhytids of various depths. This technique can be used at the same time as the rhytidectomy, but one must be careful to consider the possibility of an increased risk in flap necrosis.[7] Nonetheless, superficial peels can be a safe adjunct to surgery as long as the flap is not made extensively thin.[8] Pretreatment with tretinoin can accelerate the healing process and increase the peel penetration depth.[9-11] For fine wrinkles, superficial peeling agents, such as lactic acid, glycolic acid and 10–20% TCA formulas can be used. Jessner's solution is another popular agent that can be used alone for a superficial peel or prior to TCA application to increase penetration depth. These treatments are repeatable with minimal risk of scar or pigmentation problems. TCA concentrations higher than 20% can provide deeper peels, but there is more concern for scar formation and pain with more concentrated formulas over 35%. Phenol-based solutions, which typically contain croton oil, can produce deep chemical peels. These should be used with caution as they cannot only lead to hypopigmentation and scar, but can cause cardiac arrhythmias, particularly, if the treatment is not distributed slowly over an hour. It is because of this last concern that cardiac monitoring should be employed during phenol peels.

Dermabrasion

Dermabrasion is a useful adjunct to rhytidectomy to smooth fine rhytids, particularly around the mouth. This should not be performed on cervical skin since there is an increased risk of hypertrophic scar and hypopigmentation due to thin dermis. Use of a powered dermabrader has the disadvantage of causing a hazardous splatter. Sandpaper can be used instead to avoid this exposure while accomplishing this result, but it can occasionally cause adverse healing and scarring. Potential complications include hypopigmentation, scar, milia, acne flare-ups, infection, photosensitivity and erythema.

LASER Resurfacing

LASER resurfacing with CO_2 or Er:YAG LASER is indicated for fine and moderate rhytids. Discoloration from previous scars, acne, trauma or surgery can also be improved.

Facial resurfacing uses LASERS with wavelength ranges that allow absorption by water. The Er:YAG LASER is considered more conservative and fosters faster recovery, while the CO_2 LASER can produce greater smoothing and tightening of the skin. LASER resurfacing works by creation of a zone of reversible thermal damage that allows for collagen contraction and remodeling. The facial skin is rich with skin appendages that are thought to be responsible for a low incidence of scarring. In contrast, the neck, with a lower concentration of skin appendages, is at higher risk of poor healing and scaring.

Contraindications to LASER resurfacing include isotretinoin (Accutane) use within 12 months of the procedure. Isotretinoin increases the risk of hypertrophic scarring. Radiation therapy or collagen disorders, such as Ehlers-Danlos are also contradictions to resurfacing. A history of prior resurfacing procedures (LASER, chemical peel or dermabrasion) may predispose the patient to prolonged healing and possible scarring. Previous

Table 1: Injectable fillers and their effects

Injectable Brand Name	*Composition*	*Effect*
Artefill	Polymethylmethacrylate	Permanent
Evolence	Porcine collagen	Temporary
Juvéderm	Hyaluronic acid	Temporary
Radiesse	Calcium hydroxylapatite	Temporary
Restylane	Hyaluronic acid	Temporary
Sculptra	Poly-L-lactic acid	Temporary

blepharoplasy will predispose the patient to eyelid malpositioning. Previous facial herpetic infections and smoking are not absolute contraindications but should be noted and, in the former situation, should be treated prophylactically with valacyclovir.

The ideal candidate for LASER facial resurfacing has fine to moderate rhytids. Those with facial soft tissue ptosis or laxity will benefit more from surgical rhytidectomy, which addresses larger wrinkles. Previous LASER resurfacing does not preclude surgical rhytidectomy. Some surgeons caution that LASER resurfacing may increase the risk of wound complications when done concurrently with surgical rhytidectomy.[12] This has been shown not to be the case in a more recent study and meta-analysis with the right balance between LASER settings and amount of flap undermining.[13] Despite this controversy, most surgeons agree that LASER facial resurfacing can safely be used as a touch up procedure after all the healing from surgical rhytidectomy has occurred.

Fillers

Injectable fillers may be useful to augment the lips and to reduce prominent creases, such as nasolabial folds or forehead lines. The patient incurs minimal to no bruising and social recovery time. In the context of surgical face lifting, the most important concept is that most injectables are temporary and thus their behavior in the context of a surgical rhytidectomy is unpredictable. If a patient received an injectable a month prior to undergoing surgical rhytidectomy, the facial plastic surgeon will not be able to account for how the face will look after the injectable has been reabsorbed. Therefore, it may be advantageous to wait until the injectable has worn off before proceeding with a permanent surgical procedure. Autologous fat is used very commonly in the senior author's practice to rejuvenate the face in a 3D manner at the time of rhytidectomy. This can be a permanent filler, but only approximately 50% of the fat survives after each injection, thereby necessitating overinjection and repeated treatments. Some of the injectable fillers are given in Table 1.

REFERENCES

1. Arboleda B, Cruz NI. The effect of systemic isotretinoin on wound contraction in guinea pigs. Plast Reconstr Surg. 1989; 83(1):118-21.
2. Zachariae H. Delayed wound healing and keloid formation following argon laser treatment or dermabrasion during isotretinoin treatment. Br J Dermatol. 1988;118(5):703-6.
3. Riefkohl R, Wolfe JA, Cox EB, et al. Association between cutaneous occlusive vascular disease, cigarette smoking, and skin slough after rhytidectomy. Plast Reconstr Surg. 1986;77(4):592-5.
4. Rees TD, Liverett DM, Guy CL. The effect of cigarette smoking on skin-flap survival in the face lift patient. Plast Reconstr Surg. 1984;73(6):911-5.
5. White JB, Barraja M, Mengesha T, et al. Avoiding early revision rhytidectomy: a biomechanical comparison of tissue plication suture techniques. Laryngoscope. 2008; 118(12):2107-10.
6. Baker DC. Complications of cervicofacial rhytidectomy. Clin Plast Surg. 1983;10(3):543-62.
7. Hayes DK, Stambaugh KI. Viability of skin flaps subjected to simultaneous chemical peel with occlusive taping. Laryngoscope. 1989;99(10 Pt 1):1016-9.
8. Dingman DL, Hartog J, Siemionow M. Simultaneous deep-plane face lift and trichloroacetic acid peel. Plast Reconstr Surg. 1994;93(1):86-93.
9. Hevia O, Nemeth AJ, Taylor JR. Tretinoin accelerates healing after trichloroacetic acid chemical peel. Ach Dermatol. 1991;127(5):678-82.
10. Vagotis FL, Brundage SR. Histologic study of dermabrasion and chemical peel in an animal model after pretreatment with Retin-A. Aesthetic Plast Surg. 1995;19(3):243-6.
11. Kim IH, Kim HK, Kye YC. Effects of tretinoin pretreatment on TCA chemical peel in guinea pig skin. J Korean Med Sci. 1996;11(4):335-41.
12. Spira M, Gerow FJ, Hardy SB. Complications of chemical face peeling. Plast Reconstr Surg. 1974;54(4):397-403.
13. Koch BB, Perkins SW. Simultaneous rhytidectomy and full-face carbon dioxide laser resurfacing: a case series and meta-analysis. Arch Facial Plast Surg. 2002;4(4):227-33.

CHAPTER

96 Planning and Facial Analysis before Rhinoplasty

Fabrizio Moscatiello, Javier Herrero Jover

The nose is the most prominent feature of the human face and is significantly involved with the perception of beauty. Although the canons of beauty can vary according to the fashions, attractive faces follow having precise proportions and relations. Leonardo da Vinci studied in detail the relationships of beauty.

INDICATIONS FOR THE SURGERY

Facial Analysis

In the frontal view, the face can be divided in five equal parts by the aid of four vertical lines that intersect the medial and lateral canthus. The medial intercantal distance has to be equal in length to the eye width (Fig. 1).

In the same frontal view, the face can be divided in three equal thirds with segments between four horizontal lines that run through the chin, the base of the columella, the glabellar area and the hair line (Fig. 2).

The width of the alar base is evaluated with the aid of two vertical lines from the two medial canthus. Alar edges have to be situated 1–2 mm within these lines. A widened nasal base could require a partial resection of the nostrils (Fig. 3).

In the frontal view, the nasal dorsum is made of two parallel or concave lines, starting from the eyebrow and ending in the nasal tip. The width of the nasal dorsum is similar to the distance between the two lateral tip defining points. A surgeon has to evaluate the symmetry and the width of the dorsum. If the dorsal width is approximately 80% in length (or more) of the alar base, nasal pyramid has to be narrowed.

It is very important to study the tip defining points according to the thickness of the skin and the presence of sebaceous glands. A very thick skin could be not adequate coverage and could require fat removal, cartilage grafts or other corrective procedures. With thin skin, the nasal tip will show three defining points that correspond to the alar doms in the upper part and the junction of the medial with inferior crura in the lower part.

In the lower part of the nasal tip, a small portion of the columella has to be visible. An increased or decreased projection of the columella has to be corrected.

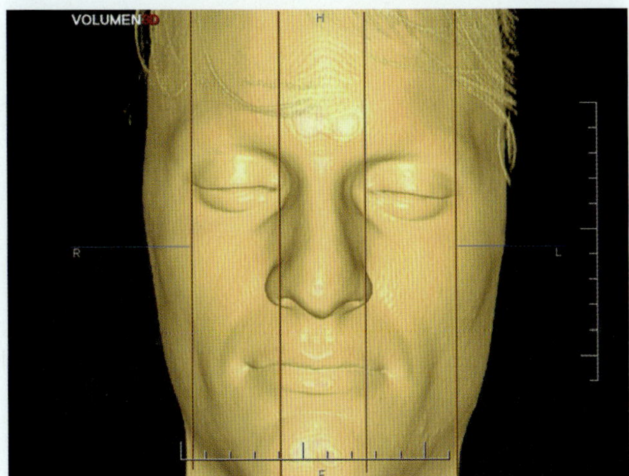

Fig. 1: Anthropometric measures in frontal view
Courtesy: Image has been produced by the aid of the software Alma IT Systems (Barcelona, Spain)

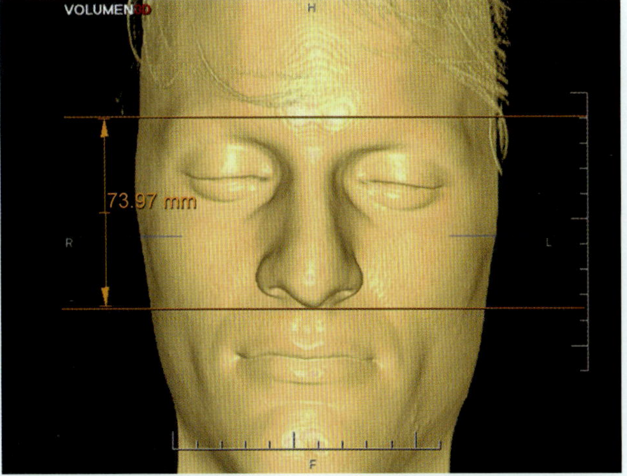

Fig. 2: Anthropometric measures in frontal view
Courtesy: Image has been produced by the aid of the software Alma IT Systems (Barcelona, Spain)

In the lateral view, with the head in a vertical position, a horizontal line is marked from the upper part of the tragus until to the inferior orbital rim. This line corresponds to the Frankfort horizontal plane.

To evaluate the facial convexity, a vertical line from the glabellar area is traced. In a well-proportioned face, this vertical line intersects the upper lip at the base of columella. With the aid of this vertical line, the authors are able to measure the nasolabial angle, that can vary in a woman between 90° and 110°, in a man between 80° and 90° (Fig. 4).

In the lateral view, the columella has to be 4 mm approximately lower than the alar edge. It is very important for the columello-alar relationship. As suggested by Gunter, the larger axis of the nasal orifice has to divide, in equal parts, the distance from the nostrils until to the columellar edge. Alterations in these relationships can correspond to an excessive or retracted columella, to an excessive or retracted ala, or to a combination of both defects. Each problem can require different surgical techniques.

In the lateral view, frontonasal angle is also examined. This 4-6 mm depression (named nasion) is between the superior edge of the tarsus and the upper lid rim (Fig. 5).

If a straight line is marked between the nasion and the nasal tip, nasal dorsum has to be 2 mm approximately behind this line. Nasal length corresponds to the distance from the nasion and the nasal tip. Nasal projection is the length between nasal tip and alar groove in the cheek. An adequate ratio between nasal length and projection is 1:0.6 (Fig. 6).

In the basal view, the nose has to appear as an equilateral triangle that can be divided in three equal thirds. Two thirds correspond to the length of the nasal orifice or the columella, the remaining third is the length of the nasal lobule (from the superior margin of the nasal orifice until to the end of the nasal tip) (Fig. 7).

In the basal view, the length and the width of the columella are recorded. The inferior third of the columella has to be wider than the upper thirds. If its width is excessive, the internal crura will be reduced, sutured and defatted.

SPECIFIC PREOPERATIVE EVALUATION

Clinical Evaluation

It is essential that the surgeon and the patient communicate thoroughly and realistically concerning the aesthetic goals before entering the operating room. Communication is the basis of preoperative analysis and planning for rhinoplasty.

From the patient's point of view, a surgeon's communication skills are nearly as important as his or her surgical skills. In addition to carefully analyzing a patient's anatomy and basic physiological profile, it is paramount that the physician understands the patient's emotional goals and motivation.

During the first visit, there are a lot of characteristics that the surgeon has to explore in detail: facial proportions; nasolabial and nasofrontal angles; height, width and length of the nasal dorsum; the width and the projections of the nasal tip; the tip defining points; thickness and texture of the skin.

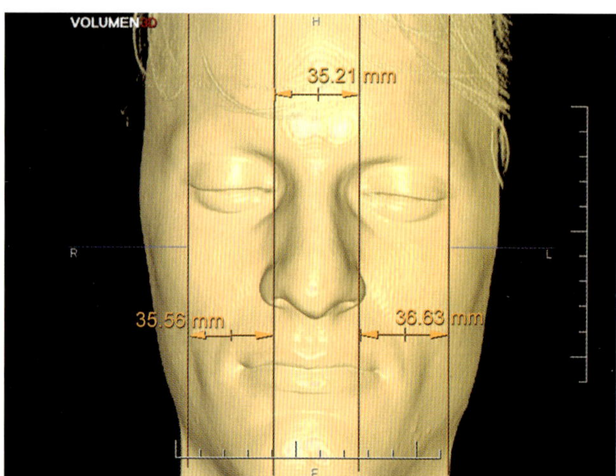

Fig. 3: In the frontal view, alar base width is evaluated
Courtesy: Image has been produced by the aid of the software Alma IT Systems (Barcelona, Spain)

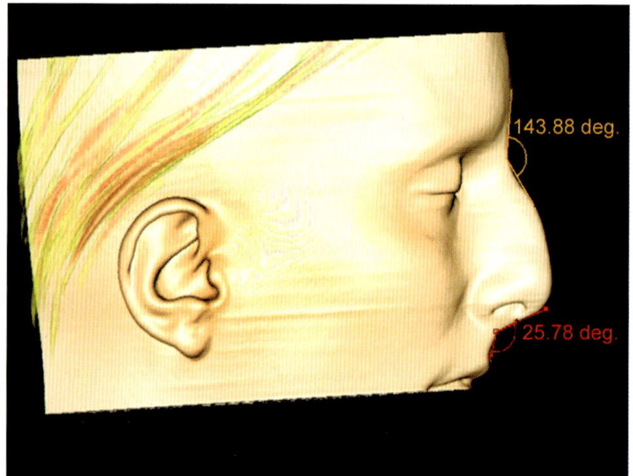

Fig. 4: Nasolabial and nasofrontal angles
Courtesy: Image has been produced by the aid of the software Alma IT Systems (Barcelona, Spain)

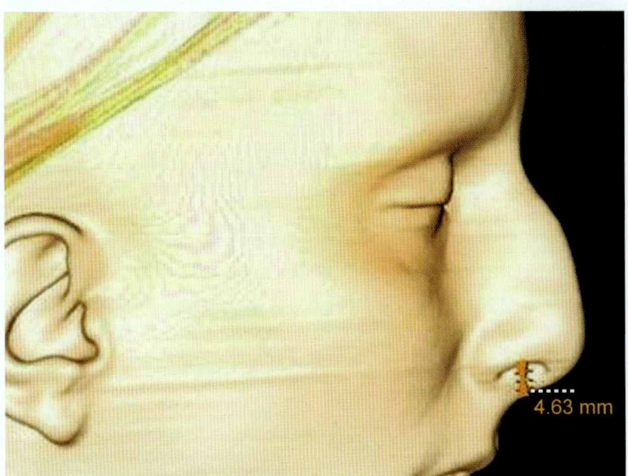

Fig. 5: Relationship between columella and nasal ala
Courtesy: Image has been produced by the aid of the software Alma IT Systems (Barcelona, Spain)

Fig. 6: Nasal length/tip projection ratio
Courtesy: Image has been produced by the aid of the software Alma IT Systems (Barcelona, Spain)

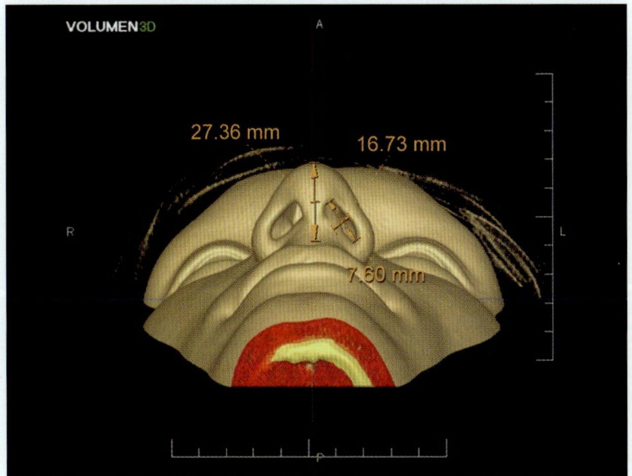

Fig. 7: Anthropometric measures in the basal view
Courtesy: Image has been produced by the aid of the software Alma IT Systems (Barcelona, Spain)

With the aid of a nasal speculum, alterations in the nasal anatomy, that could affect the vestibule, the nasal valve, the septum and the turbinates, have to be evaluated.

The patient should be informed about the possible outcome and the risks of the suggested treatment and it is very important to use every instrument that helps to improve communication with patients.

Photographic Study

Photographic documentation is indispensable in the planning of rhinoplasty and in the postoperative period to value the results of the authors' work. Usually, six static photos (frontal, left oblique, right oblique, left profile, right profile, basal) and two dynamic photos (frontal and profile) with the patient smiling are taken.

Patient photos are required also in the surgical theatre during the operation. They have to be of adequate size and in each profile (frontal, lateral and basal), it can be useful to write the desired modification both with the surgical planning.

In a lot of cases, the lateral profile image is the most important. In this profile, the authors advocate considering in detail: nasal length/projection ratio, nasofrontal angle, supratip region, nasolabial angle, columelloapical angle, relationship between the columella and the nasal orifice.

Complementary Exams

The development of the surgical technique in rhinoplasty is, these days, accompanied by the progress in more and more sophisticated diagnostic methods. Modern rhinoplasty has to achieve a natural aesthetic result without affecting the respiratory physiology. All preoperative diagnostic tests, that can clearly demonstrate the inner anatomy of the nose and avoid, intraoperatively, unexpected anatomic alterations, can be a useful tool for the positive outcome of the operation.

A complementary important method of preoperative evaluation is the nasosinusal fibroendoscopy. This method allows directly viewing the nasal fossas, posterior septal deviation, rhinopharynx alterations, rhinosinusitis and other sinus pathologies.

These days, although rhinomanometry can be used in the preoperative period, it is not useful in studying the internal nasal valve. Rhinomanometry can register flow and resistance alterations but cannot allow identifying the anatomic defect. To solve this problem, arose the acoustic rhinomanometry that allow understanding the anatomic region of the nasal cavity where flow and resistance are altered.

Multidetector CT scan is a very useful method to preoperatively study a patient that will undergo an aesthetic or functional rhinoplasty. CT scan allows valuing, in detail, the nasal and paranasal anatomy, identifying all the possible alterations that have to be corrected during the operation (Fig. 8).

Through static and dynamic details, it establishes a correlation between the different planes: superficial (skin), intermediate (subcutaneous and cartilages) and deep (bones) (Fig. 9).

CT scan can be considered the main test in detecting inflammatory rhino and sinusopathies, nasofacial traumas, planning primary, secondary or tertiary rhinoplasty (aesthetic, functional and posttraumatic) (Fig. 10).

The authors ask for a preoperative CT scan also in patients that do not complain respiratory difficulty.

CT Scans

Nowadays, there are different types of tomography: conventional, helicoidal and multislice. The use of different windows in tomography allows the study of the bones, discerning between cortical and medullar bone, and of the soft tissues, discriminating between skin, subcutaneous tissue and cartilages. Multislice CT scan, also known as multidetector CT scan, is the imaging diagnostic method that uses between 2–256 detector channels where thin sections of anatomic regions are generated through volumetric and sequential acquisitions. This allows a safer and more precise evaluation than conventional and helicoidal scan, with a final better quality (Fig. 11).

Computer Imaging

Personal computer is a very useful instrument when adequately used. In the XXI century, it is not allowed that a surgeon does not use this resource in his or her daily activity. Patients prefer the aid of computer imaging during the preoperative consultations rather than simple photos

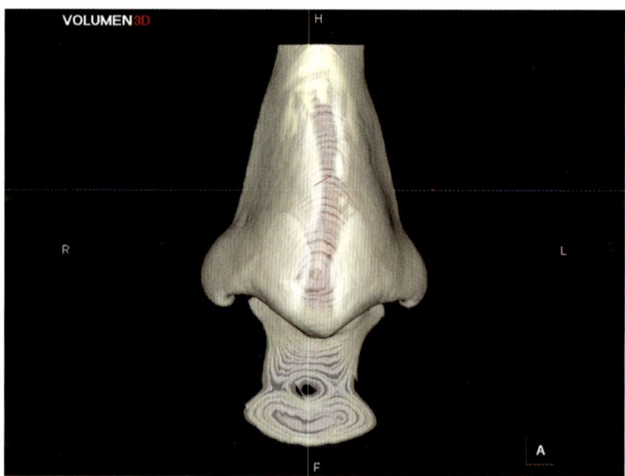

Fig. 9: Close-up view of cartilaginous structures
Courtesy: Image has been produced by the aid of the software Alma IT Systems (Barcelona, Spain)

Fig. 8: This patient has a complete cleft of the superior maxillary bone. An osteal graft could be considered during rhinoplasty
Courtesy: Image has been produced by the aid of the software Alma IT Systems (Barcelona, Spain)

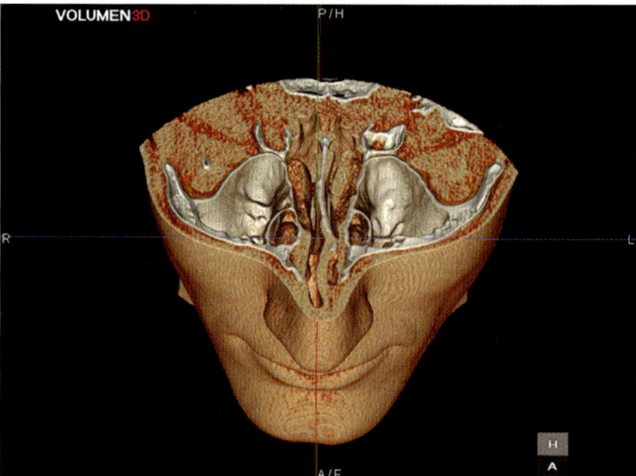

Fig. 10: 3D facial reconstruction
Courtesy: Image has been produced by the aid of the software Alma IT Systems (Barcelona, Spain)

and schemes. They had become aware of computer imaging and frequently asked for it when making an appointment by telephone.

Although the simulation (morphing) of a possible postoperative result by common imaging software can be very effective during the preoperative period in impressing patients and convincing them to undergo surgery, it is not an advisable procedure. In the postoperative period, patients cannot be satisfied with the final outcome due to unclear expected result.

Informatic items, dedicated to rhinoplasty, can help in the following: record pre, post, intraoperative images; comparative study of results; improving patient-surgeon relationship; recording files for medicolegal purposes; and technical planning of rhinoplasty.

3D Radiologic Viewer in the Office

A 3D radiologic viewer, in the authors' hands, has proved to be a sophisticated instrument for communicating with the patient during consultation. Imaging in front of the patients, that offers them the possibility of accurately studying their own anatomy and planning their own surgical procedure, is very impressive and helpful. With this imaging, patients better understand the anatomy, the procedures, and the possible results. The authors think that the 3D radiologic viewer increases the patients' trust in their operations (Fig. 12).

The 3D viewer allows for preoperatively studying the following clearly:

- The nasal dorsum (including any deviation, characteristics of the nasal bones, relative height of the nasal bridge, width of the dorsum and bony base, and transition into the nasal tip) (Fig. 13).
- The nasal tip (including tip shape, definition or lack of definition of the tip, presence of surface defects, relationship of the columella to the alar rims, and nasal base width) (Fig. 14).
- Profile characteristics (including position of the radix, slope of the dorsum, dorsal irregularities, presence or absence and location of a supratip break, amount of tip projection, nasal length, columellar/labial angle, columellar/lobular angle, nostril height and shape, prominence of the columella, length and relative position of crura, and nasal spine) (Fig. 15).
- Basal characteristics (including nostril size, symmetry, nasal width, columellar width, alar position and symmetry, and tip definition) (Fig. 16).
- Inner characteristics (including nasal valve morphology, septal deviations, cornet malformations, and sinus pathologies) (Fig. 17).
- Close-up of anatomic elements (Fig. 18).

In addition, full facial views, to determine the relative size of the nose and its relationship with other facial features, are possible. By determining preoperatively which structures need modification, stress can be reduced for the surgeon who can now go directly, with confidence, to change an already "known" nasal subunit, both functionally and aesthetically, without wasting time. Furthermore, it has become a marketing tool that should not be underestimated (Fig. 19).

SURGICAL STEPS

Surgical Planning

Surgical planning starts when patient and surgeon agree about the aesthetic modifications of the nose and when

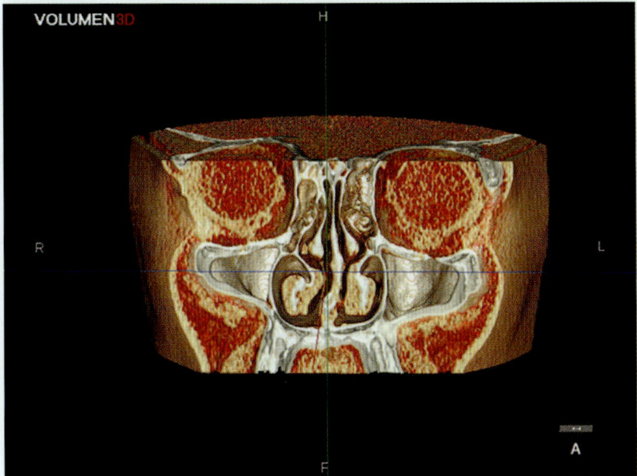

Fig. 11: Detail of septum, turbinates and maxillary sinus
Courtesy: Image has been produced by the aid of the software Alma IT Systems (Barcelona, Spain)

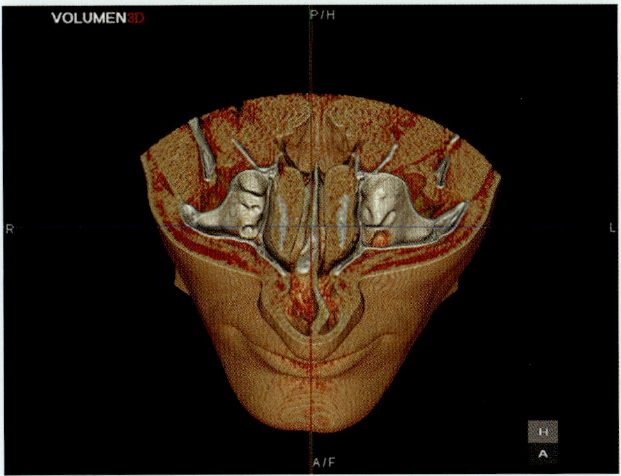

Fig. 12: 3D facial reconstruction
Courtesy: Image has been produced by the aid of the software Alma IT Systems (Barcelona, Spain)

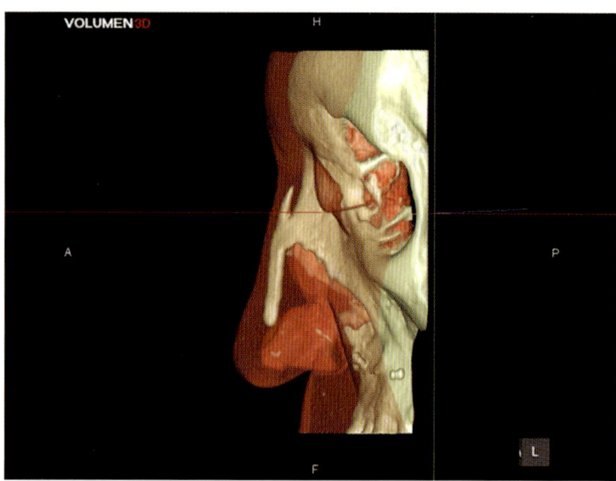

Fig. 13: A dorsal bone graft of several years of evolution
Courtesy: Image has been produced by the aid of the software Alma IT Systems (Barcelona, Spain)

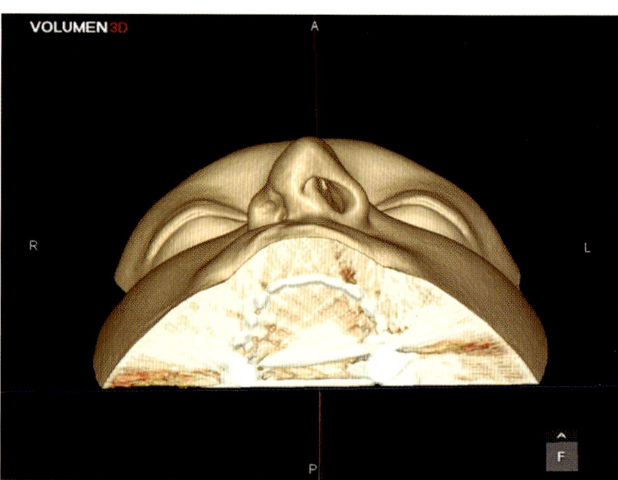

Fig. 14: The same patient of Figure 8 with a scar retraction of the whole nasal tip and a complete occlusion of right nostril
Courtesy: Image has been produced by the aid of the software Alma IT Systems (Barcelona, Spain)

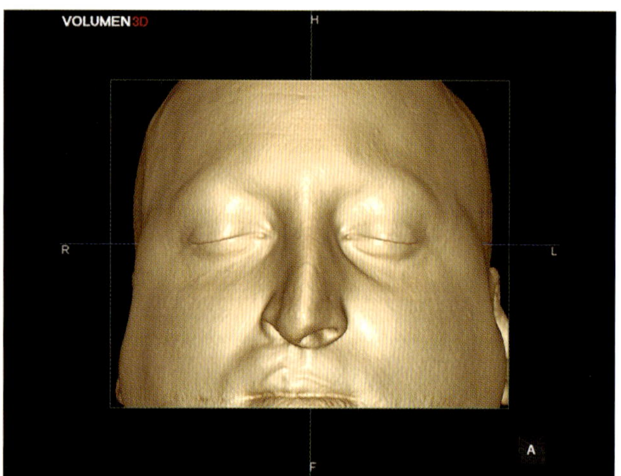

Fig. 15: Nasal tip right deviation
Courtesy: Image has been produced by the aid of the software Alma IT Systems (Barcelona, Spain)

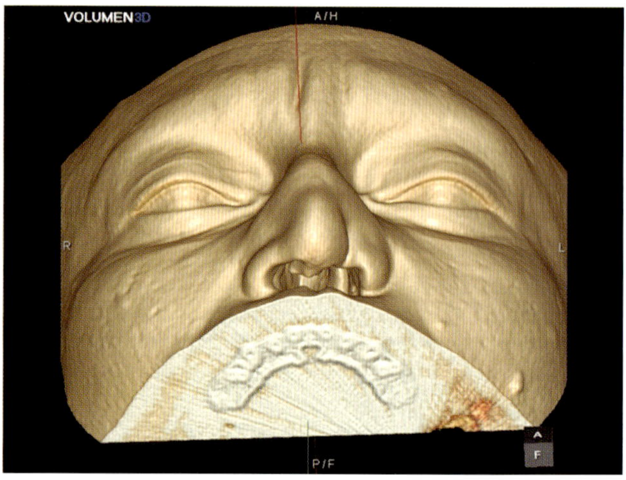

Fig. 16: A cocaine nose with left ala retraction and necrosis of columella and anterior septum
Courtesy: Image has been produced by the aid of the software Alma IT Systems (Barcelona, Spain)

the patient understands the surgical process. This first evaluation with the patient is very important because the basic surgical principles about patient's demand and surgical options will be established.

With the aid of the surgical model (SM), the authors are able to quantify, objectify, estimate and customize the habitual workflow of the rhinoplasty to each patient. The SM, obtained from patient radiological images, allows the authors to make a surgical planning more precise and structured, clarifying possible doubts both of the patient and the surgeon (Fig. 20).

The process starts with a dynamic vision of the 3D model that can be rotated 360° in each plane. Anteroposterior, caudal, lateral and intermediate views can be studied whenever the surgeon considers convenient.

Once the first examination of the nasal pyramid has been made, the SM allows taking all the anthropometric measures the surgeon considers useful.

Surgical planning follows with the evaluation of the risk points. These are peculiar for each patient and can influence or modify the authors surgical strategy, i.e. secondary nose, abnormal osteal structures, complex nasal tip, etc.

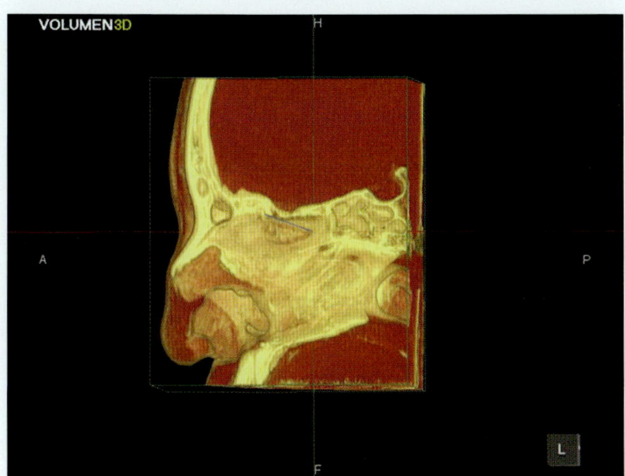

Fig. 17: Nasal septum perforation
Courtesy: Image has been produced by the aid of the software Alma IT Systems (Barcelona, Spain)

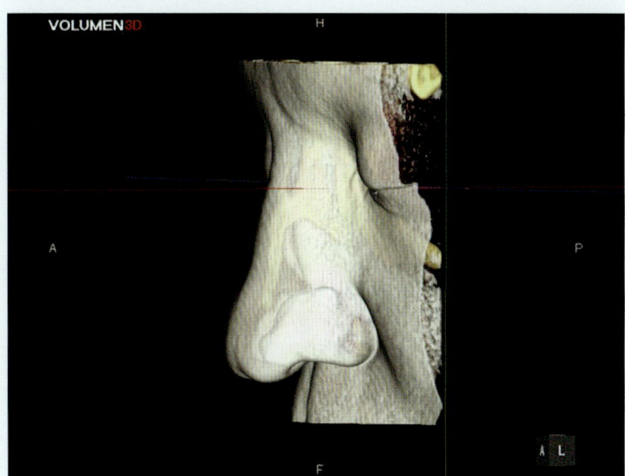

Fig. 18: With special windows, it is possible to evaluate the distribution of cartilaginous elements
Courtesy: Image has been produced by the aid of the software Alma IT Systems (Barcelona, Spain)

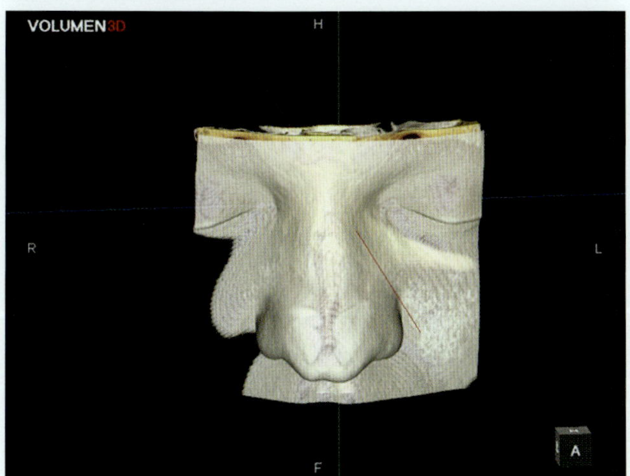

Fig. 19: Facial 3D reconstructions are very useful to explain the anatomy
Courtesy: Image has been produced by the aid of the software Alma IT Systems (Barcelona, Spain)

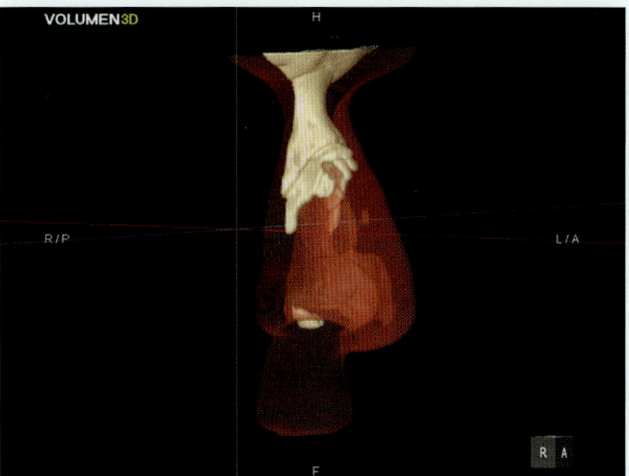

Fig. 20: Close-up view of osteocartilaginous structures
Courtesy: Image has been produced by the aid of the software Alma IT Systems (Barcelona, Spain)

The SM also allows evaluating the nasal soft tissue, like fat and muscles. Thickness of subcutaneous tissue can influence, sometimes, the surgical strategy due to the cartilage grafts' visibility in the skin or due to the inefficacy of the work in a nasal tip with a very thick skin.

At this moment, it is useful to study the upper lateral cartilages, nasal septum and columella morphology.

Projection, width and length of the nasal pyramid are three sizes that will be evaluated all together due to the tight relation between the three parameters. SM will be useful to evaluate the nasal dorsum structures, bones and cartilages, and to calculate the excess to be removed or the defect to be filled. In frontal, oblique and lateral views, it is possible to decide where to perform the lateral osteotomies, if needed, according to the osteal morphology and preview fractures.

Once established—the dorsal projection and the width of the pyramid—it is mandatory to plan the total length of the nose and the nasolabial angle. In the nasolabial angle, the authors are able to clearly look at all structures to be modified, like columella, nasal spine and septum.

In the basal view, it will be possible to evaluate the length of the columella and of the nasal lobule, the width of the nasal orifice and the width of the nasal ala.

Surgical model is very useful also in functional operations. It allows to study, in detail, the internal valve, turbinates, septum and the whole internal nasal cavity with a complete understanding of all the structures to modify.

Reduction Rhinoplasty

The nasal pyramid can be reduced in all its structures—both osteal and cartilaginous. The amount of tissue to remove has to be evaluated according to: total length of the nose, length/projection ratio, nasolabial angle, upper lip height.

Augmentation Rhinoplasty

Nasal dorsum, tip or both, can need increasing their size in terms of projection, width or length, according to the facial anthropometric measures.

To improve nasal dorsum projection, adequate solutions can include the use of autologous cartilage grafts—costal, septal or auricular. Bone grafts can also be considered but have a great quote of reabsorption.

Increasing the projection of the tip is performed in different steps according to the desired result and the anatomy of the patient. Shortly, to obtain tip projection, one of the easiest and first procedures consists of conservative modifications (i.e. suturing) of the domal cartilages. If it is not enough, a strut cartilage graft is put on the nasal spine and between the two inferior lateral cartilages in order to create a support and an augmentation of the tip. As last option, if needed, a small cartilage graft can be sutured over the domal cartilage. Grafts above the domal cartilages, in few years, can become visible through the skin (unless it is very thick), so the graft has to be cut very carefully in size.

CHAPTER

97 A Color Atlas of Septorhinoplasty

Sonna Ifeacho, Rajib Dasgupta, Guy Kenyon

PREOPERATIVE PLANNING

Patient Selection

The key to successful outcomes in rhinoplasty and septorhinoplasty is careful patient selection.

Managing the patient's expectation is of paramount importance. Patients undergoing septorhinoplasty must have realistic expectations of what can be achieved with surgery. Details of past trauma, previous surgery and the relevant past medical history should all be meticulously recorded prior to surgery.

Clinical Examination

The clinical examination seeks to combine the patient's concerns with an objective assessment of the nose and face. The face as a whole must be assessed from an esthetic and symmetry point of view to identify sources of generalized asymmetry and deformity that may impact the nose. For example, there may be an apparent, but not true, distortion of the nasal profile in asymmetrical hemifacial microsomia or a perceived over-projection of the nose relative to a retrognathic mandible.

General facial esthetics are assessed using fixed bony points and ideal facial proportions. A symmetrical face when viewed with the Frankfort plane parallel to the floor face is divided into equal horizontal thirds:

- From radix to nasion (Fig. 1)
- From nasion to columella
- From collumella to menton

The face is further assessed for symmetry by dividing it into vertical fifths:

- From the outer ear to the ipsilateral lateral canthus of the eye
- From the lateral canthus to the ipsilateral medial canthus
- From the ipsilateral medial canthus to the contralateral medial canthus
- From the medial canthus to the ipsilateral lateral canthus
- From the lateral canthus to the ipsilateral outer ear (Fig. 2)

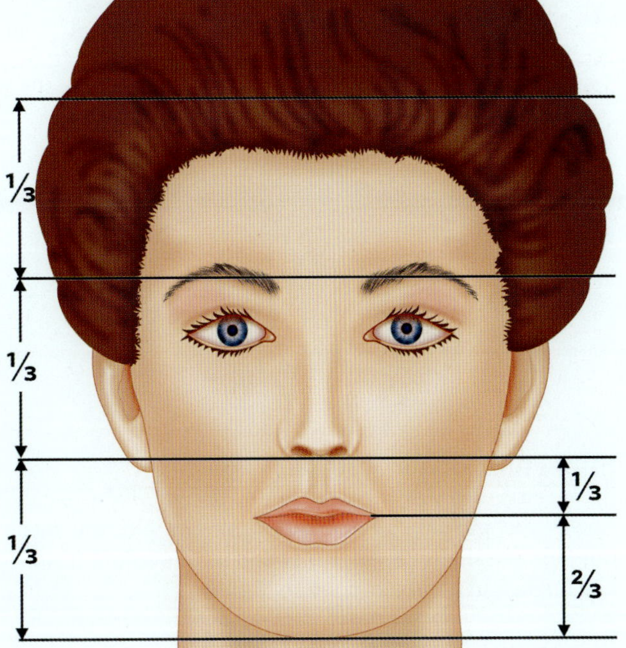

Fig. 1

This initial examination will provide a generalized assessment of the individual's facial esthetics, skin quality and identify gross facial asymmetry that may give an illusion of nasal asymmetry. Operating on the latter may result in unsatisfactory results due to poor preoperative planning.

Nasal examination follows the basic principles of inspection and palpation. The following are key areas to assess:

Inspection of the Frontal View

Follow the brow-tip esthetic (also known as the dorsal esthetic) line on each side and assess for smoothness. Assess the width of the nose, deviation of the dorsum and assess the nasal tip for bulbosity or asymmetry (Fig. 3).

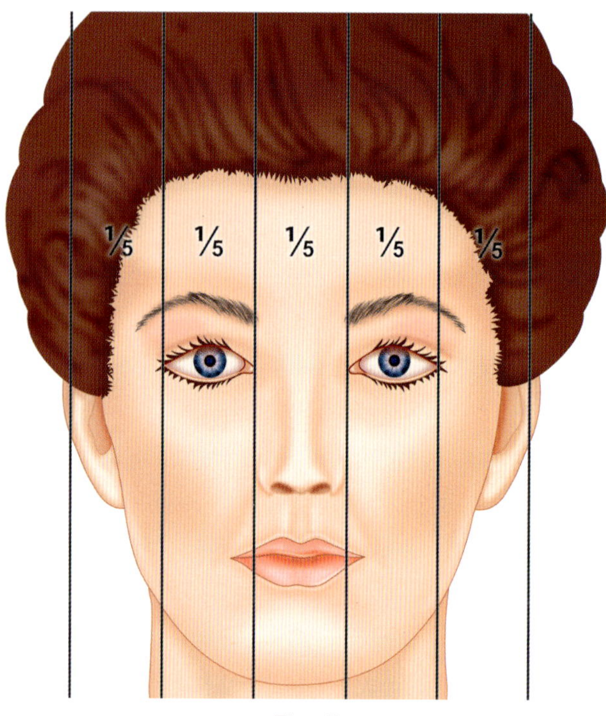

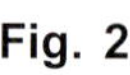

Fig. 2

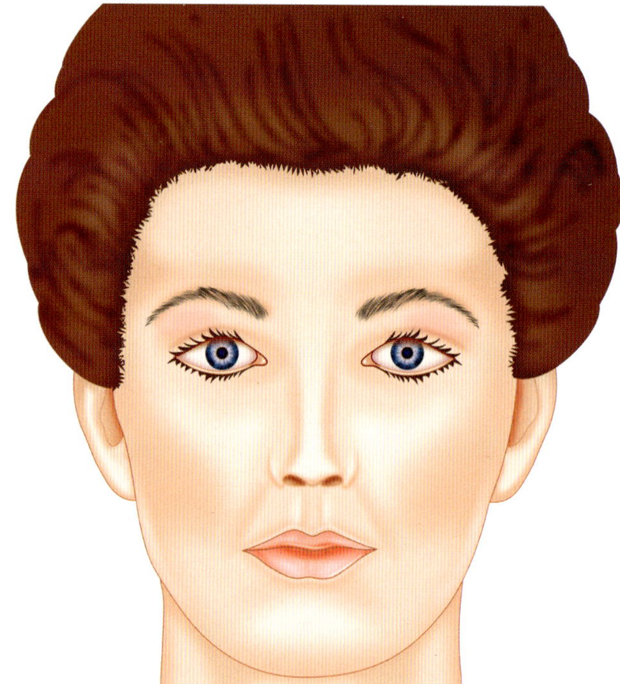

Fig. 3

Inspection of the Lateral View

Assess the position of the nasofrontal angle, the nasal dorsum, nasal length, tip projection and rotation, nasolabial angle and degree of columella show.

Inspection of the Basal View

Inspection of the nose in the caudal and cranial planes provides further information. From the basal view the alar base should be equal to the intercanthal distance. Tip asymmetry is also assessed (Fig. 4).

Assessment of the Skin

Assess the skin for thickness. Very thick skin is sebaceous and will hide minor irregularities of the underlying bony and cartilaginous framework. Thin skin is less forgiving and must be handled with great care during surgery. Palpate the nose for superficial irregularities.

- Assess the dorsum of the nose with respect to deviations. Divide the nose into horizontal thirds to locate the cause of the deviation. Deviations of the upper third are usually due to a problem with the nasal bones, middle third deviations due to septal or upper lateral cartilage (ULC) deviation or asymmetry and lower third deformity are due to deformities of the lower lateral cartilages (LLC) caudal septum or alar base.

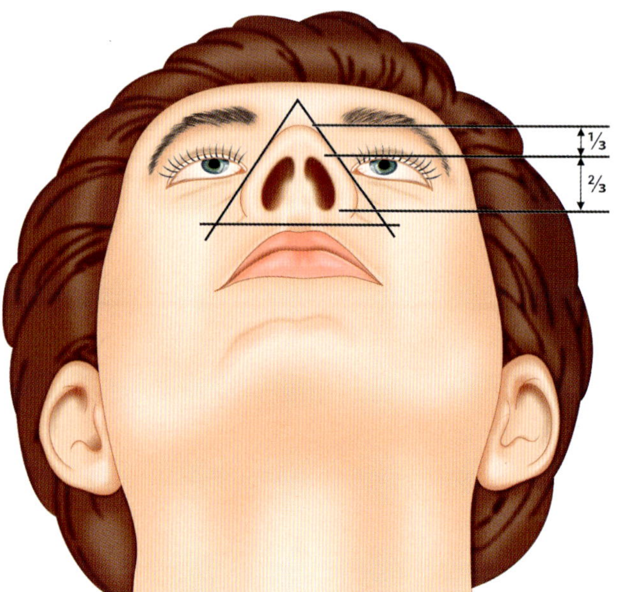

Fig. 4

- Tip projection: Apply Goode's formula (Fig. 5). Assess for over or under-projection.
- *Dorsum*: Assess from the front and while standing behind the patient.

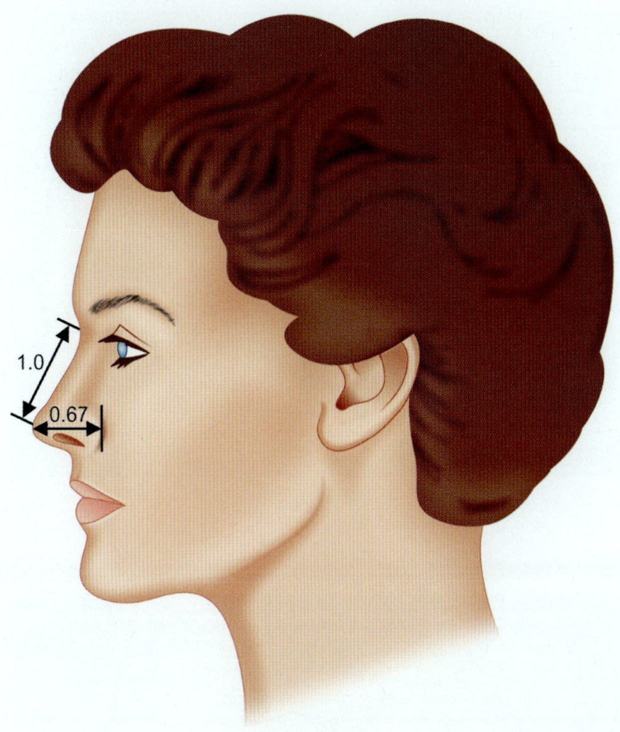

Fig. 5

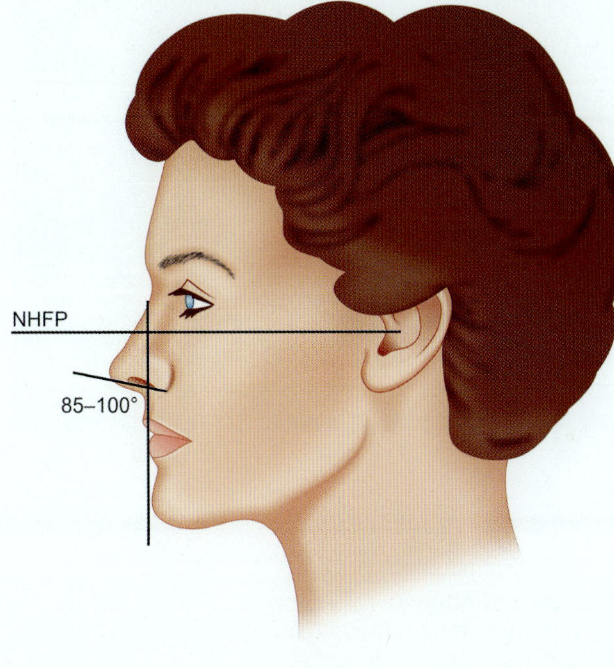

Fig. 6

- *Tip-defining points*: Medial crura-, supra- and infra-tip-defining points. Assess the size and shape of the alar cartilage, asymmetry, bifidicity and rotation.
- *Assess the nasolabial angle* (Fig. 6).
- *Assess columella show*: This should be approximately 3–5 mm.
- *Assess the alar base*: It should be equal to the intercanthal distance.
- *Inspect the internal nose*: The septum by palpation of the anterior margin if necessary and by direct vision using anterior rhinoscopy and then nasendoscopy. Assess the turbinates, the internal valve and assess the nose for any alar collapse. Nasendoscopy adds further information regarding the more posterior septum, postnasal space and turbinates.

Lopez et al. have published a stepwise approach to assessment for rhinoplasty, highlighting the likely surgical correction needed for various deformities.[1]

Clinical Photographs

Standardized preoperative photographs aid planning and postoperative comparative assessment. The lateral photographs must be taken in the Frankfort plane if a false sense of over or under-projection of the nose is to be avoided.[2] The standard views required are frontal, lateral, profile, lateral obliques (left and right) and basal views.[3,4] The bird's eye view is another helpful view.[5] Attention to patient positioning, lighting and accurate color printing is essential for producing photographs that are an accurate replication of the patient's face.[6]

Consent

The procedure to obtain consent for a septorhinoplasty starts at the first consultation and culminates in a preoperative appointment where the necessary consent forms are signed. It is important to ensure that the sources of patient's dissatisfaction are understood and that these are addressed. If they cannot be addressed then the reasoning behind this should be explained to the patient. Agreement at this stage and a written plan of the proposed procedure (which the patient should understand) avoids potential embarrassment, at least, and litigation, at worse. Providing as much information as possible is crucial to obtain informed consent. Written information in the form of a leaflet is a useful adjunct to promote retention and understanding of information; there is published evidence to suggest this is more useful amongst the female population.[7]

Some of the points that should be discussed during the consent process are:[5]

- Bleeding
- Infection
- Nasal blockage

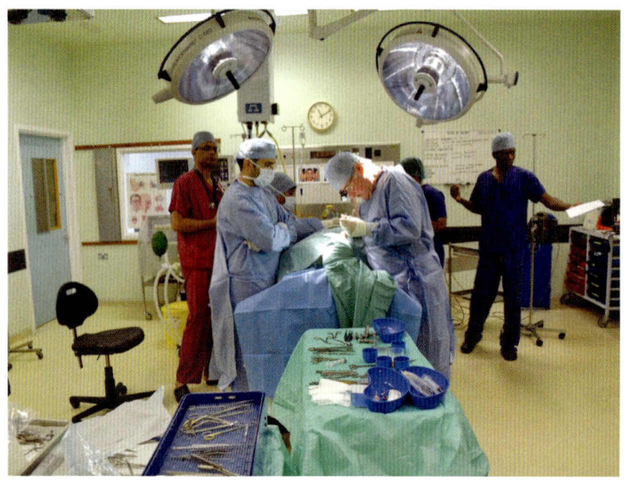

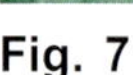

Fig. 7

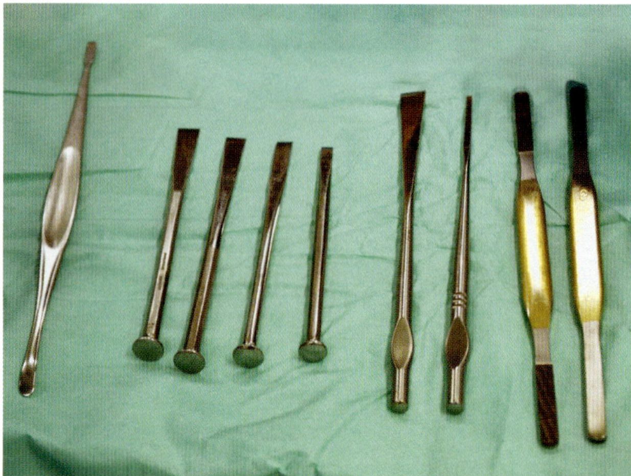

Fig. 8

- Septal hematoma
- Septal perforation
- Graft migration/extrusion/resorption
- Skin necrosis
- Scars (keloid, hypertrophic and pigmentatory changes)
- Dissatisfaction
- Failure
- Possibility of further procedures
- Bruising
- Time off work
- Dressings and splints, and the length of their application.

SETUP OF THE OPERATING THEATER

General Theater Layout

Photograph shows an optimum theater setup that is acceptable to the surgeon, anesthetist and theater nurse. The equipment trolley and theater nurse's positions promote smooth passage between the surgeon and the nurse—who should be aware of the normal stages of the operative process and who should be able to anticipate the surgeon's needs (Fig. 7).

Instruments (Figs 8 and 9)

The basic instruments required are:

- Alar retractors
- Sharp dissecting scissors
- An Aufricht's retractor

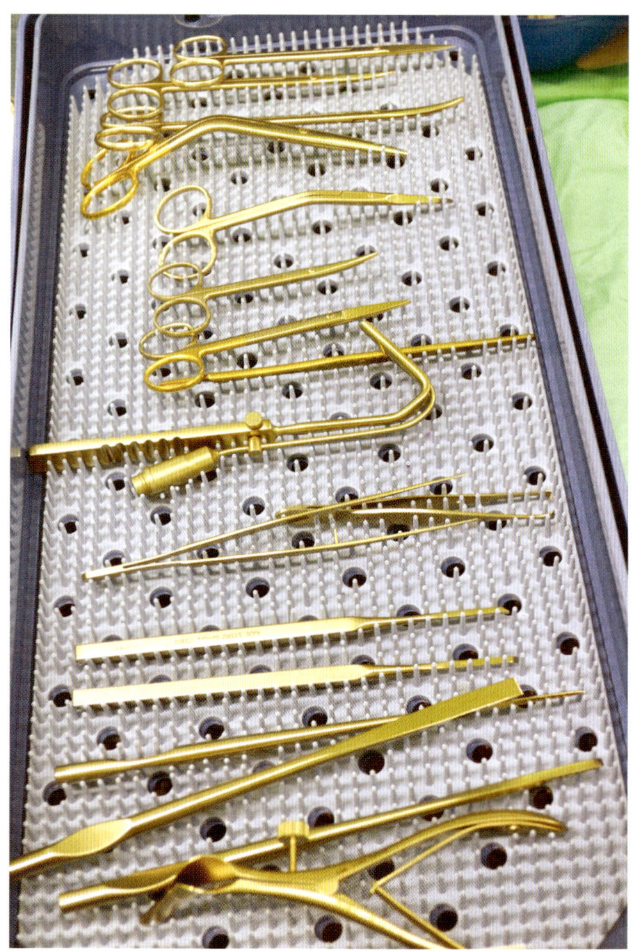

Fig. 9

- A range of osteotomes
- Rasps
- Tissue holding forceps
- Needle holders
- Suture cutting scissors.

Mounting Clinical Photographs

The preoperative clinical photographs (all views) must be displayed in the operating theater in an easily accessible location so the photographs may be referred to during the procedure. They serve as a general reminder of the preoperative status, but can also provide guidance for specific areas e.g. intraoperative assessment of the nasal tip. This is particularly helpful once intraoperative swelling has intervened and once the nasal bones have been fractured and repositioned, and the original anatomy has been altered (Fig. 10).

Theater Lighting

Visualization during rhinoplasty is of great importance. Therefore it is beneficial to use both a headlight and the overhead theater lights. Individual preferences vary but a battery operated headlight and loupes permits greater ease of movement around the operating table and is the senior authors preferred option (Figs 10 to 13).

Position of the Patient and Surgeon

It is traditional to stand at the right hand side of the patient. The patient lies prone, on a headrest, at elbow height with a degree of upward head tilt to aid visualization and reduce bleeding from venous congestion (Figs 14 and 15).

Patient Preparation (Fig. 16)

The patient requires eye protection, there are several options including Lacrilube© ointment, eye tape or eye pads (Figs 17 and 18).

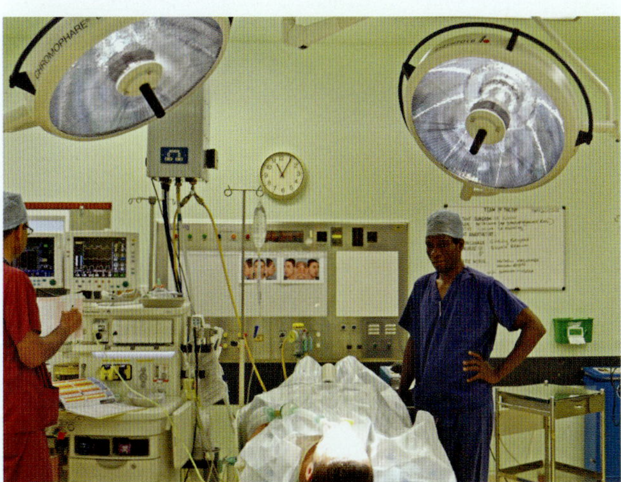

Fig. 10

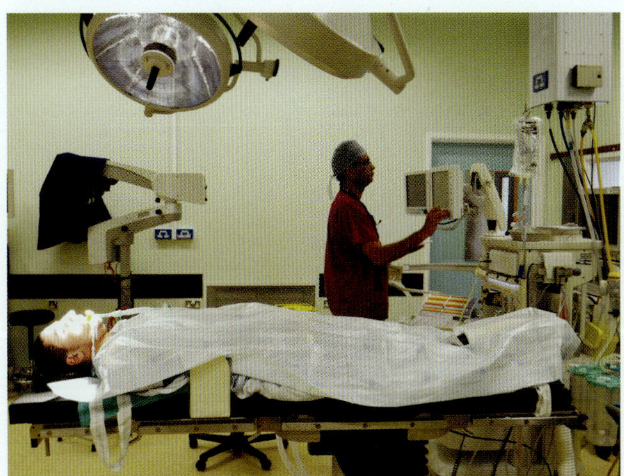

Fig. 11

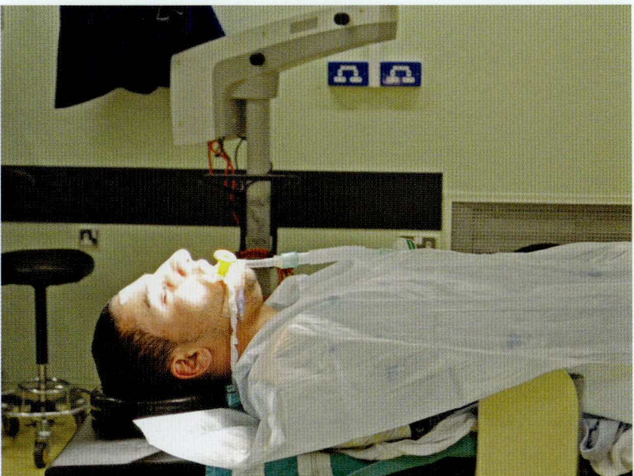

Fig. 12

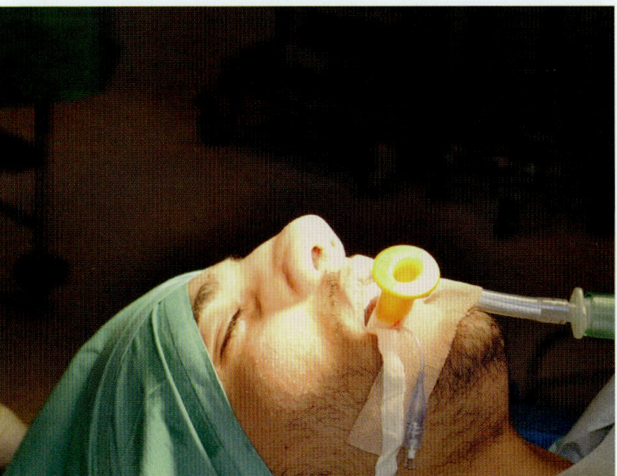

Fig. 13

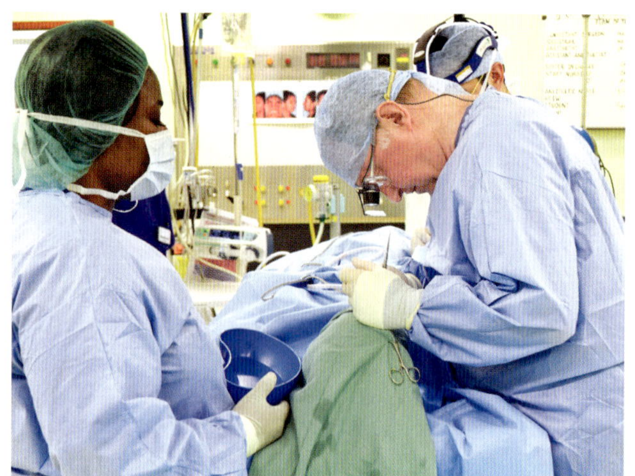

Fig. 14

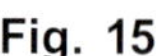

Fig. 15

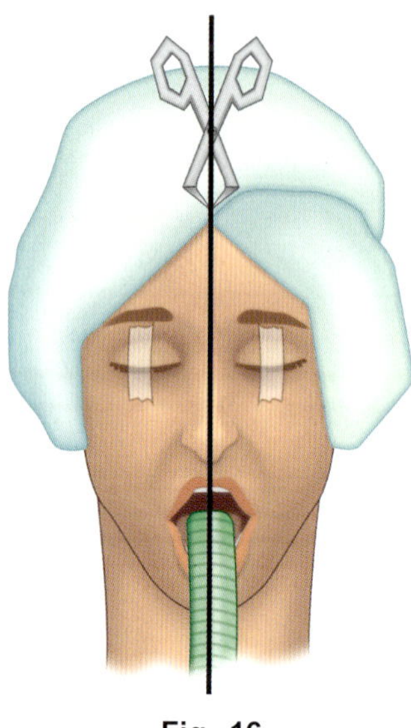

Fig. 16

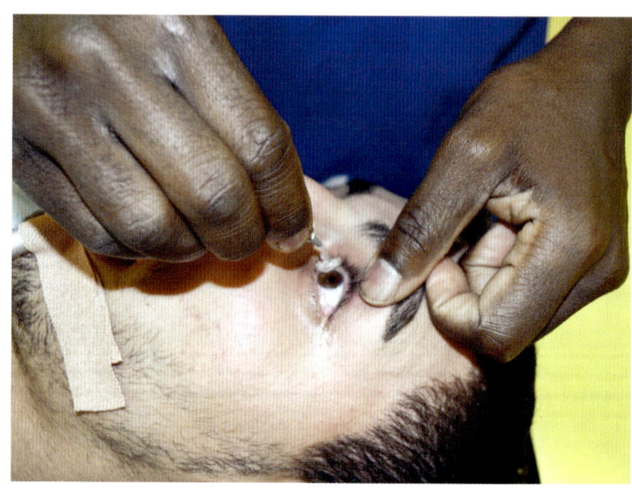

Fig. 17

The nasal skin and surrounding areas are prepared using a water-based skin preparation solution that is nontoxic to the cornea of the eyes (Figs 19 and 20).

It is imperative that, as far as possible, the orientation of the patient is preserved. Therefore the head should not be tilted at setup and the drapes should be secured so that they cross in the midline (Figs 21 and 22). In like manner the endotracheal tube should be centrally placed.

A bipolar diathermy is setup with the cable and diathermy forceps resting on the operating table and secured to the drapes with the sucker.

SURGICAL STEPS

Local Anesthetic

Adequate infiltration of local anesthetic affords dissection with minimal bleeding and swelling. Lignocaine with adrenaline in dental cartridges is the senior authors preferred choice of local anesthetic (2% lignocaine and 1:80000 adrenaline). Infiltration of local anesthetic into the correct tissue planes promotes hemostasis of the surgical field and improved visualization. It also contributes to pain control in the early postoperative period.

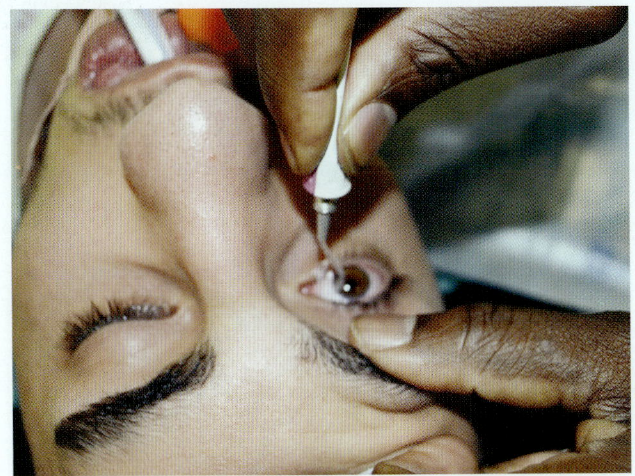

Fig. 18

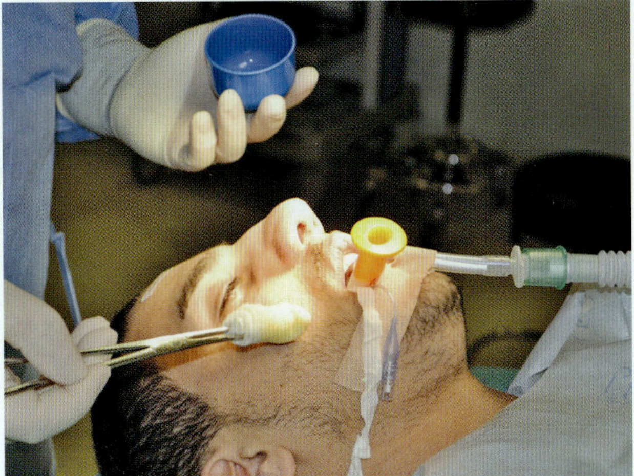

Fig. 19

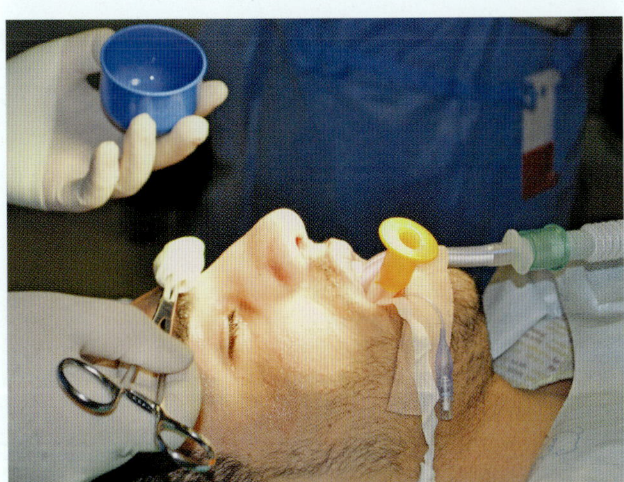

Fig. 20

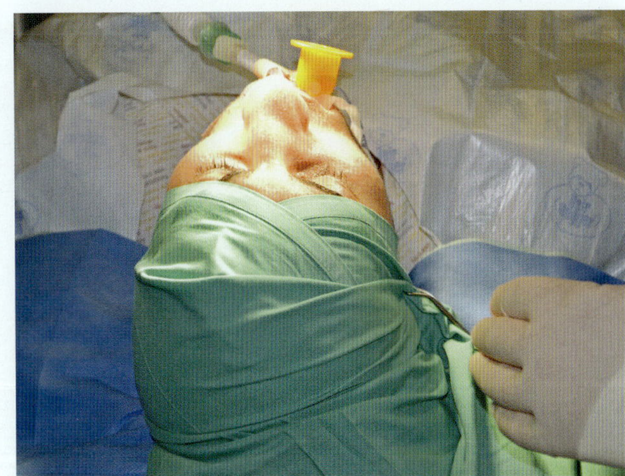

Fig. 21

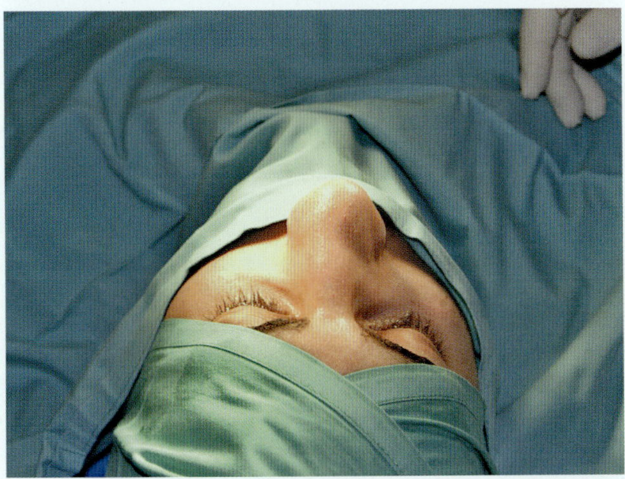

Fig. 22

Local anesthetic is injected into the proposed site of incision for the septoplasty (Killian's or hemitransfixion) with a more widespread subperichondrial infiltration to the remainder of the septum (Fig. 23). Infiltration produces a degree of hydrodissection which aids flap elevation during the septoplasty. Further infiltrations are performed in the mid-columella region, (Fig. 24) marginal incision sites (Figs 25 and 26), intranasally to the dorsum of the nose (Fig. 27) and externally at the sites of any proposed osteotomies (Fig. 28).

The photographs below depict the points of infiltration. Care must be taken not to inject excessive amounts. In total 6 mL of local anesthetic volume should suffice. It is imperative that sufficient time is given for the anesthetic to take effect. During this waiting period the clinical photographs are reviewed and the necessary surgical steps are

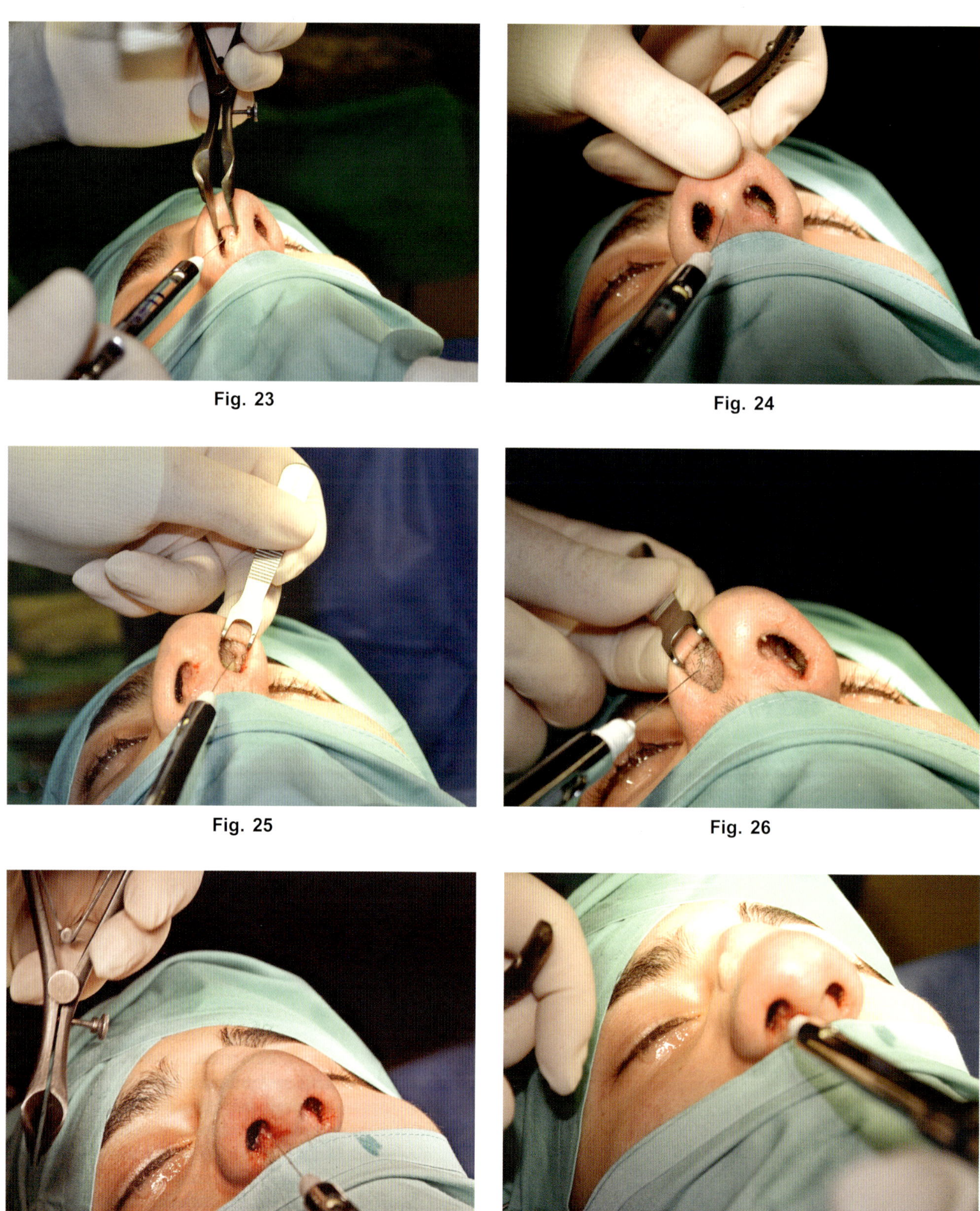

Fig. 23

Fig. 24

Fig. 25

Fig. 26

Fig. 27

Fig. 28

visualized in the mind. It is often helpful to discuss these points with nursing staff or surgical trainees since they can then appreciate what is anticipated and where appropriate prepare for this.

Vibrissae Trimming

Many surgeons appear to inject the local anesthetic and then reach almost immediately for a scalpel. However, the local anesthetic needs time to act and this time can be profitably spent removing the nasal vibrissae since they frequently act to obstruct a good view of the nasal vestibule and they may obscure the incision line if a marginal incision is to be performed. Scissors that are not required for any other steps of the rhinoplasty are to be preferred and if these are coated with Vaseline or passed over a Jelonet dressing they will be sticky and hence catch the nasal vibrissae as they are trimmed. Care must be taken not to cut skin as this may predispose to infection or contribute to unwanted scarring (Figs 29 to 31).

Septoplasty

The septoplasty is normally the first surgical step in septorhinoplasty and, if the surgery is being performed following trauma, this part of the operation is often the most difficult part of the entire procedure. It is preferable to perform a septoplasty through a hemitransfixion incision. The mucosa is incised using a no. 15 blade on the same side as the leading edge of the septum and a mucoperichondrial flap is then elevated and the septum exposed—dissection must be in the subperichondrial plane. The bony-cartilaginous junction is identified and a chondrotomy is undertaken just anterior and parallel to that the perpendicular plate of the ethmoid. The cartilage is freed posteriorly and is also divided inferiorly toward the maxillary crest. A "swing-door" of the quadrilateral cartilage is then created. It is important to leave dorsal and caudal struts as supporting structures. The bony maxillary crest can then be dissected free of mucosa so that it can, if necessary, be removed. For this maneuver it is considerably easier to commence the mucosal dissection posteriorly and work forward toward the maxillary spine since the mucosa is not so adherent posteriorly. This approach minimizes the risk of mucosal tears. Selective cartilage and bone excision is then undertaken and, if required, bone or cartilage can be harvested to use during the reconstructive procedure.

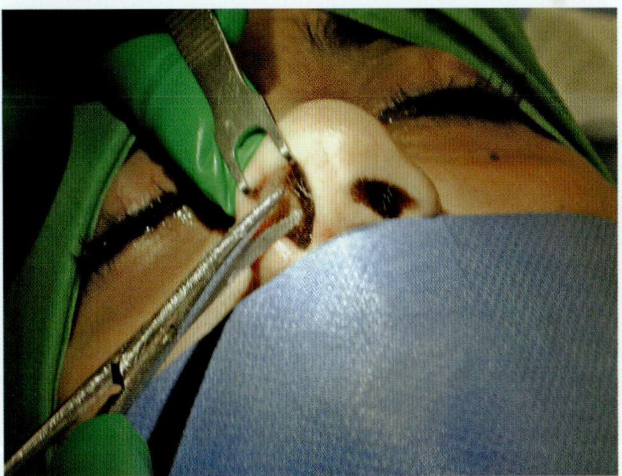

Fig. 30

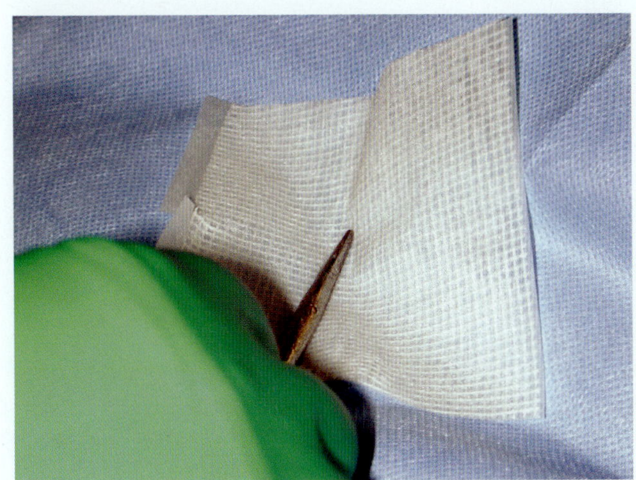

Fig. 29

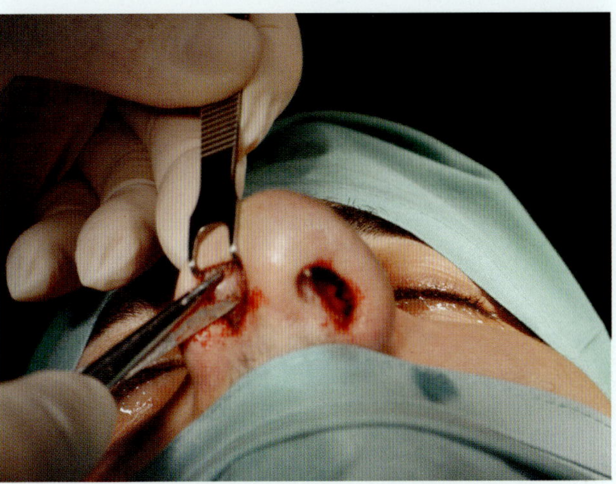

Fig. 31

If the caudal septum is deviated then this must normally be repositioned. Excision is not recommended unless the preoperative photographs suggest that the columella is truly "hanging". An assessment of the ala-columella esthetics therefore needs to be made if excision is to be accomplished without adverse postoperative sequelae.[8] It is important to anchor the anteroinferior part of the septum to the maxillary spine in order to ensure adequate fixation of this part of the septum.[9] This can be accomplished by suturing with a suture such as 3/0 PDS.

Rhinoplasty: Endonasal versus External Exposure

The nasal skeleton may be approached by a variety of differing incisions (trans-collumellar, marginal, intercartilaginous and transcartilaginous) and there is frequently a robust discussion regarding the merits of an "open" as opposed to a "closed" approach—in truth such arguments are sterile since both can damage the skin and supporting mechanisms of the nose. While the added "insult" of an external skin incision is real it is somewhat over-rated since, if the incision is closed carefully, the wound is only rarely visible. The real risks of the external approach are of increased soft tissue swelling and of some transient numbness of the nasal tip, which can last up to 6 months. The patient should therefore be warned of this during the consenting process if an external approach is contemplated.

The external approach is to be preferred in patients who have had trauma and is also very helpful in those in whom the middle third is deformed, as insertion of grafts to correct deviation here is otherwise difficult. It is also to be recommended in revision cases.

Endonasal Approach

The endonasal approach to the nose normally starts with an intercartilaginous incision on each side using a no. 15 blade. This incision follows the caudal border of the ULC and is normally continued over the septal angle (the anterosuperior corner of the quadrilateral cartilage) such that it then joins a hemitransfixion incision at the caudal margin of the nasal septum (Figs 32 to 34).

The skin and the soft tissues of the SMAS are then elevated over the ULCs and the bony pyramid on each side and are joined over the dorsum such that the whole skin envelope is raised from the underlying tissues. Sharp dissection using the scalpel blade and McIndoe, or other similar scissors, is required to effect this. It is important during this dissection that every attempt is made to remain

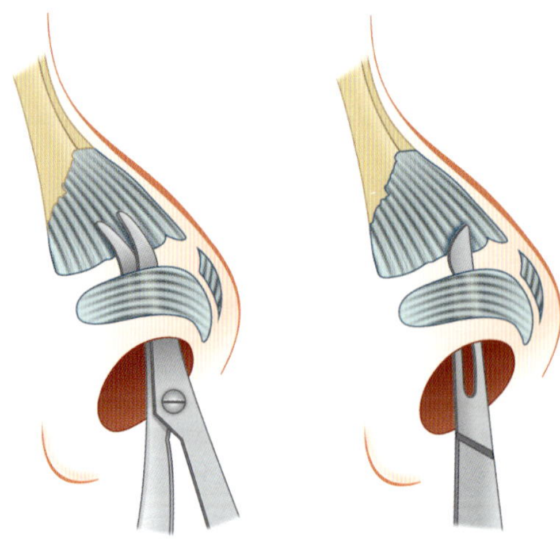

Fig. 33

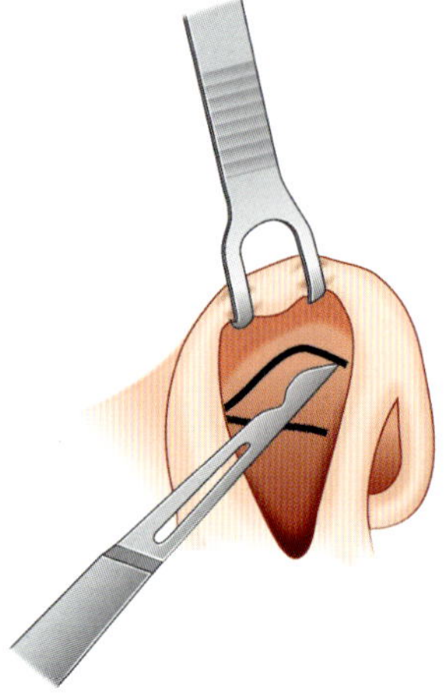

Fig. 32

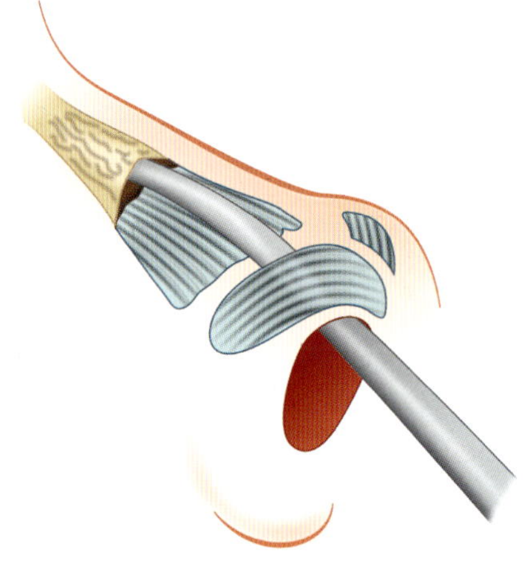

Fig. 34

close to the underlying bones and cartilages. The skin over the keystone area is the thinnest of the dorsum and particular care must be taken in this area, especially where there has been previous trauma. The soft tissues are elevated to provide a midline tunnel exposing the ULCs, the keystone area and the bony vault. It is important not to extend this dissection too far laterally as the soft tissues play a supporting role and prevent the nasal bones collapsing when they are in-fractured. A Howarth's elevator is then used to elevate the periosteum from the dorsal aspect of the nasal bones and a small postage stamp shaped piece of ribbon gauze can then be temporarily inserted to reduce any minor bleeding. The gauze also acts to remove any small pieces of adherent soft tissues from the underlying nasal skeleton.

External Approach

Skin Marking

The columella incision is either a stepped or inverted 'V' incision. The external approach is joined to a marginal incision on each side and the incisions are then joined to lift the skin of the lower third of the nose before elevation is developed over the ULCs and the bony pyramid in a manner that is entirely similar to the endonasal approach.
Columella incision: The columella incision is marked out using either a stepped (Gunter) or inverted 'V' incision.[10] The incision is marked over the narrowest aspect of the columella. A Gunter incision has one arm which is vertically placed and is easily camouflaged. It has proved reliable in over X cases for such cases over a number of years with only 3% visible at 6 months (Kenyon—unpublished data) (Fig. 35).

Marginal incisions (Fig. 36): This should be done with great care as mistakes here are difficult to rectify. The caudal border of the LLC is identified by elevating the vestibular rim. If there is doubt as to the position of the leading edge then the caudal margin of the lower lateral can be palpated using a blunt instrument. An incision is made using a knife and the lower edge of the cartilage is identified. The margin is at the junction of the nonhair and hair bearing skin margin and is usually readily identified, especially when wearing loupes. It runs closer to the vestibular rim as it is developed medially and care should be taken to avoid transgressing the skin edge toward the nasal tip.
Columella flap elevation: A no. 15 blade is used to incise the skin having first marked it with a marker pen. Elevation of the columella skin by sharp dissection is then undertaken taking care not to notch the medial crura of the underlying LLC, which will support the incision during healing and help prevent a depressed scar. If an assistant gently holds the tip elevated by insertion of an alar retractor to the domes of the lower laterals the dissection can proceed by lifting the skin under direct vision and by the use of a single skin hook. An alternative to sharp dissection is a pair of converse scissors. The paired columella arteries are usually encountered and are cauterized using bipolar diathermy (Figs 37 to 42).
Dorsal nasal flap elevation/SMAS layer elevation: The columella flap is joined to the marginal incisions. The skin is then elevated in continuity from the lateral crura of the LLCs staying in the supraperichondrial layer. Once the cephalic margins of the lower laterals are identified an Aufricht's retractor is inserted and further dissection is readily accomplished in the midline (and then laterally) using scissors and sharp dissection up to the nasion.

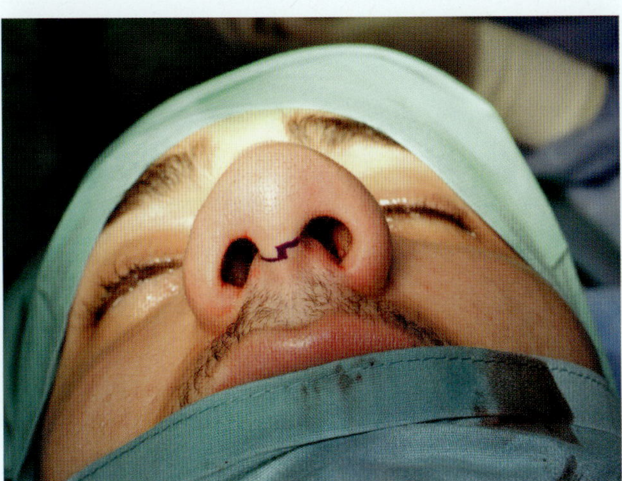

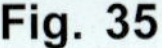

Fig. 35

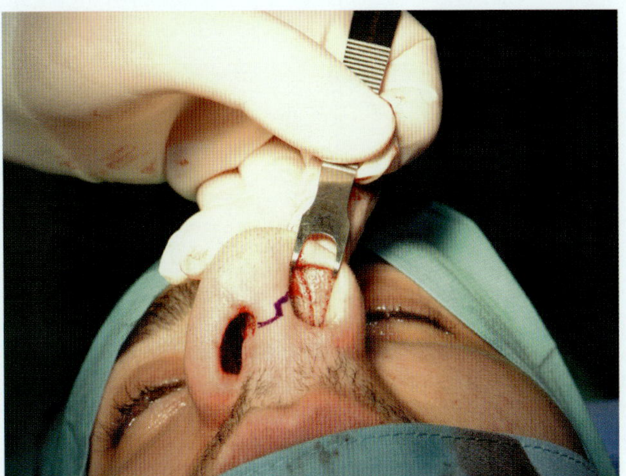

Fig. 36

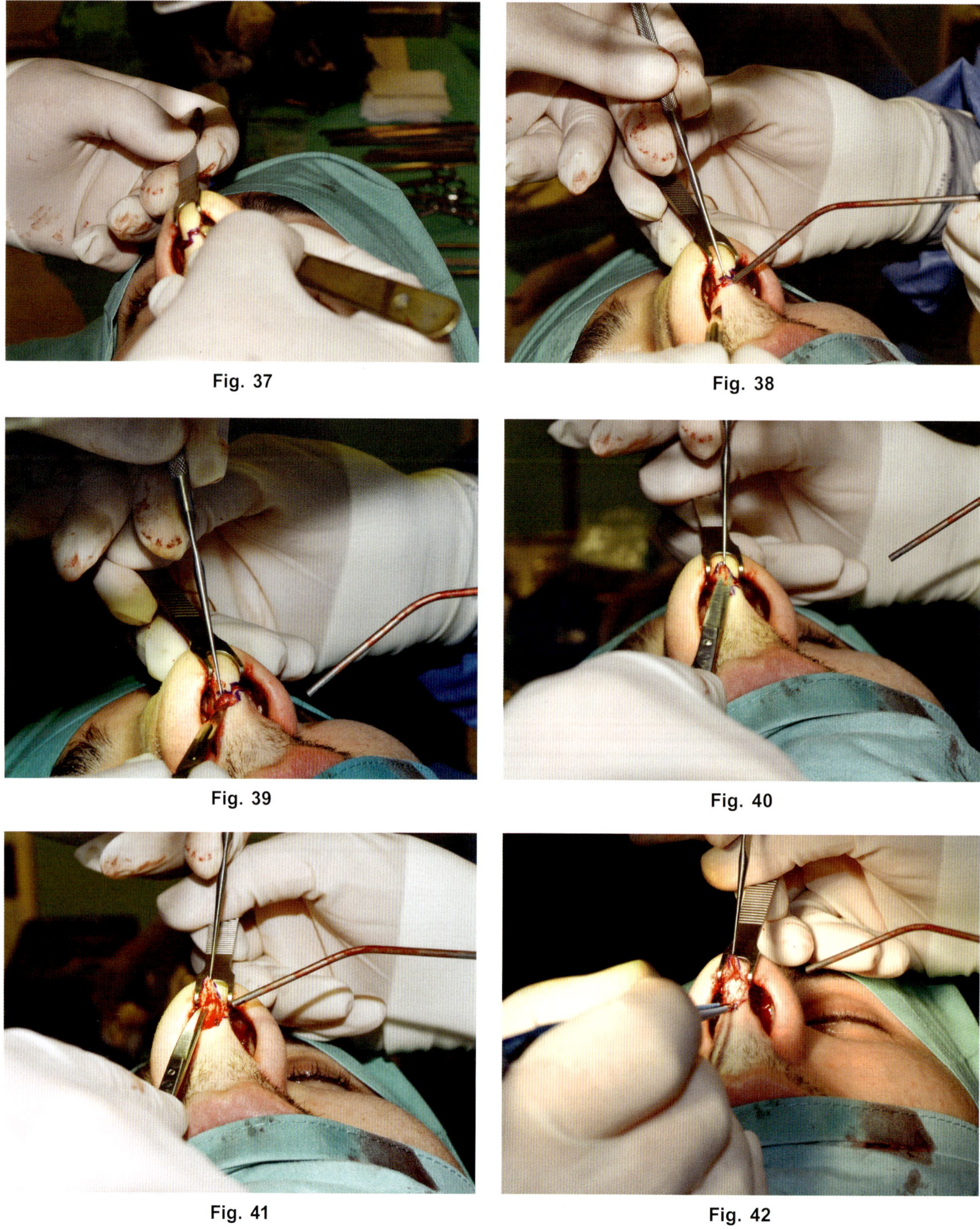

Fig. 37

Fig. 38

Fig. 39

Fig. 40

Fig. 41

Fig. 42

This dissection is entirely similar in effect to the endonasal approach (Figs 43 to 47).

Hump Reduction

A dorsal hump is formed either of cartilage or bone, and is in most instances a mixture of the two. Full exposure allows identification of the appropriate site of reduction. Using a no. 15 blade the cartilaginous hump is reduced initially. Prior to doing this, it is necessary to separate the ULCs from the dorsal septum. In an endonasal approach, an incision is made through the mucosa beneath the ULC and then through the junction between the upper lateral and dorsal septum. It is imperative that the dissection is kept as close as possible to the upper part of the cartilaginous septum to avoid leaving a T-shaped segment. In an open approach rhinoplasty, it is easy to dissect the upper laterals from the dorsal septum under direct vision. Particularly, if it is anticipated that spreader graft will be required it is important to leave within "mucosal trench" between the upper lateral and the septum so that the graft will lie parallel to the dorsum and create a satisfactory dorsal esthetic line.

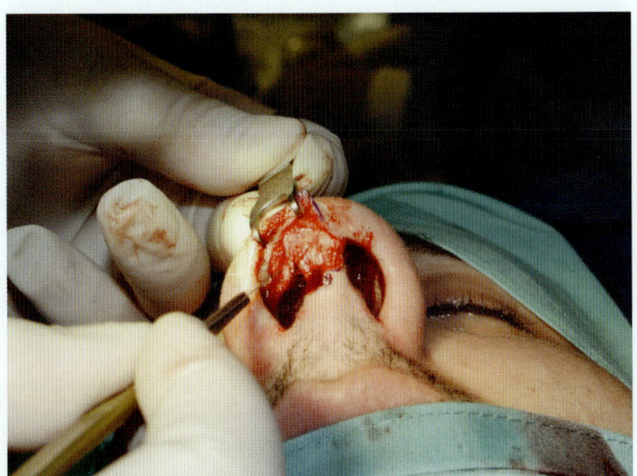

Fig. 43

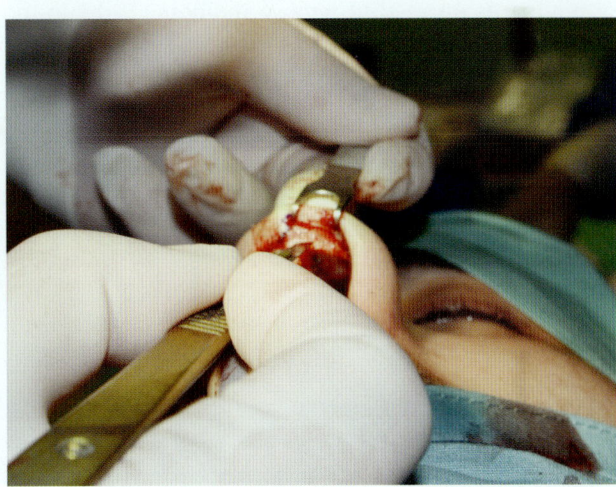

Fig. 44

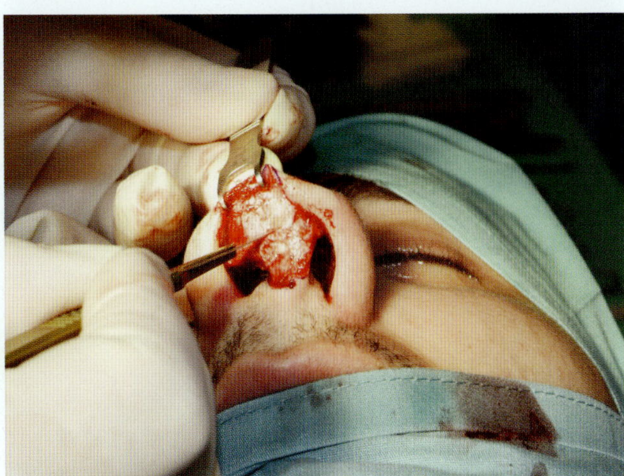

Fig. 45

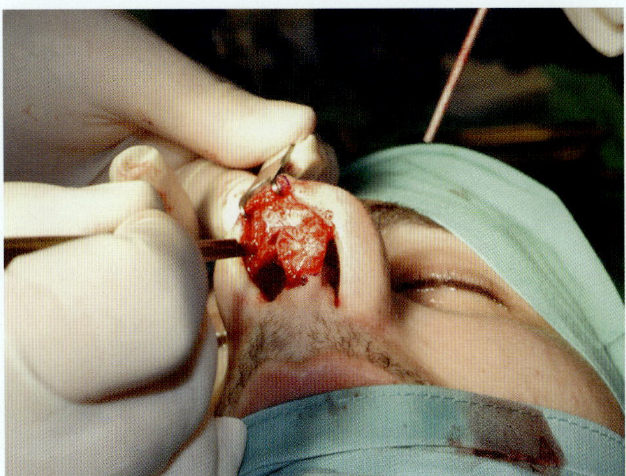

Fig. 46

Once the cartilaginous elements of the dorsum have been separated, the cartilaginous dorsum can be lowered up to the keystone area. The ULCs can then be lowered sequentially inline with the new dorsum but it is probably better to delay doing this initially until the bony hump has been removed. It is particularly important to realize that is Aufricht's elevator is being inserted under the skin, the ULCs can be elevated as the skin is raised. The danger is that the ULCs can be over-resected once the skin is elevated and the surgeon should be aware of this possibility and be as conservative as possible when lowering the ULCs.

Once the cartilaginous dorsal is satisfactory, the bony hump is then identified at the keystone area and a 7 mm osteotome is inserted to remove the bone. If the hump is symmetrical then the osteotome is kept level as the hump reduction proceeds. If the bones are skewed then an asymmetrical removal should be attempted leaving a slightly greater bony height to the bone that is the more vertically placed (Fig. 48). If this is not done then there will be residual asymmetry after an in-fracture has been performed (Figs 49 and 50).

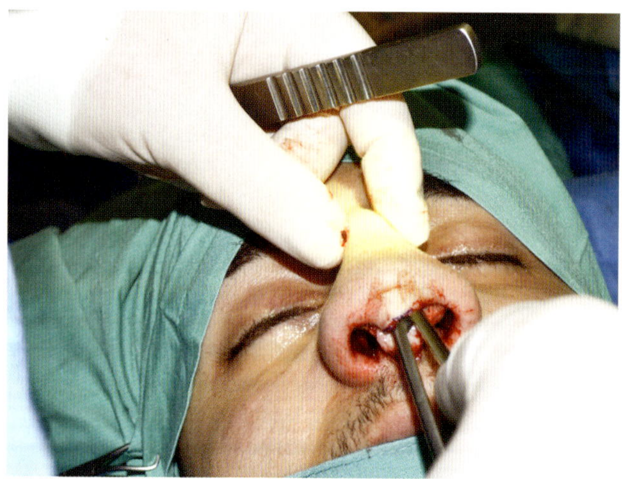

Fig. 47

After the bony hump has been divided from the underlying bones a fine artery forceps is inserted to grasp the caudal end of the excised hump. After an initial cephalic movement, to free any soft tissue strands, the forceps are pulled caudally to remove the hump from the attached soft tissues (Figs 51 to 53).

A rasp is then used to smooth the dorsal surface of the bones. In doing this the surgeon should keep the elbow elevated and use small strokes of the rasp in order to smooth the bone while avoiding trauma to the overlying skin. Initially a number 1 or 2 rasp is used and the final smoothing is undertaken with a number 5 or 6. A rasp cleaned of all debris and everted may serve to remove all minor bony fragments from the underlying skin at the end of this process. All fragments must be removed and it is also helpful to wash the affected area with some saline from a syringe with a quill attached in order to ensure that all minor pieces of debris are removed (Figs 54 and 55).

Overzealous rasping can cause detachment of the ULCs from the bone above. Bilateral disarticulation produces an inverted V deformity with a poor esthetic outcome, and unilateral disarticulation also produces disfigurement with asymmetry in the middle third of the nose. In each case a spreader graft is then required to correct the deformity (vide infra). Once the hump has been reduced further adjustments to the septum and ULCs may also be necessary.

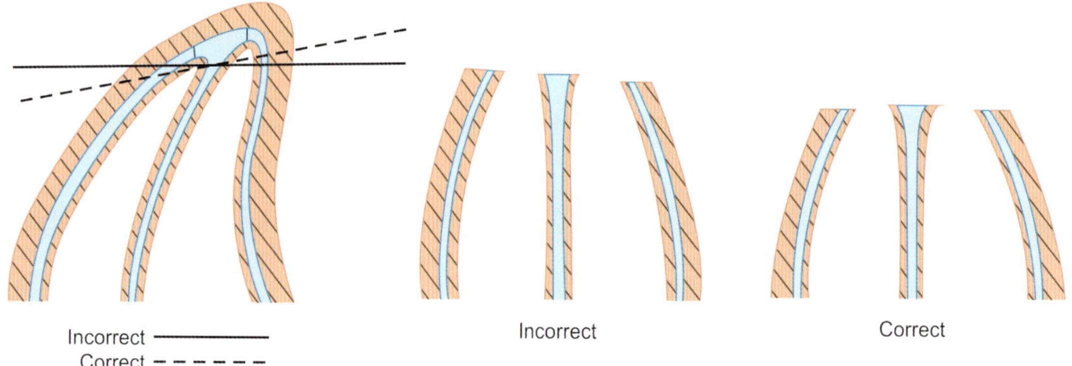

Fig. 48

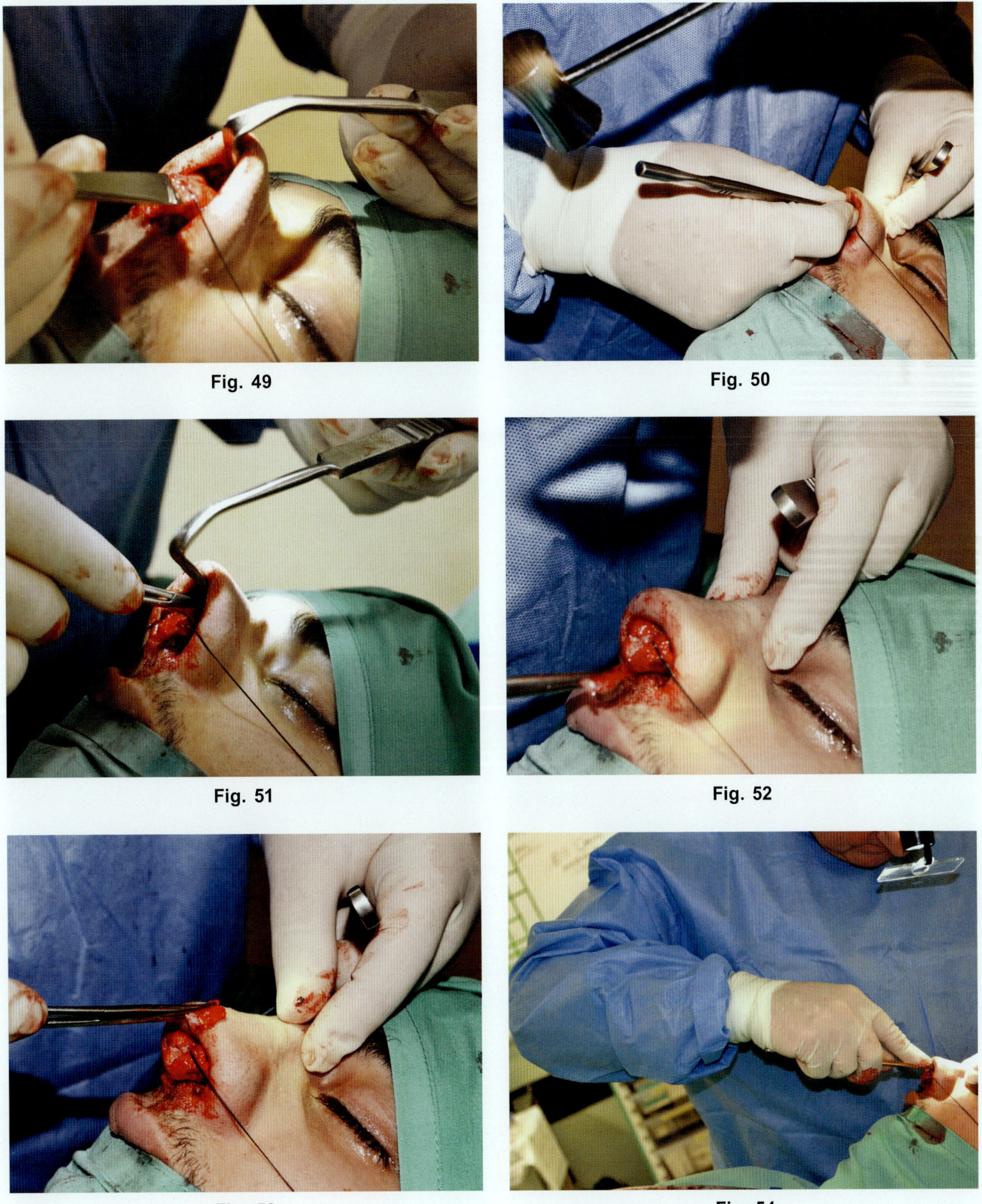

Fig. 49

Fig. 50

Fig. 51

Fig. 52

Fig. 53

Fig. 54

Osteotomies: Medial and Lateral

Medial Osteotomy

Medial or paramedian osteotomies are not always required if an "open book" deformity is created after dorsal hump reduction.[11] If they are required then it should be remembered that the bone above the intercanthal line is too thick to fracture with accuracy and the osteotomy should not continue above this line—continuation in a cephalad direction also risks breaching the skull base. If the osteotomy creates a cephalic fracture in the thicker part of the frontonasal junction then, after in-fracture, there is also the risk that cephalic margin of the bone moves laterally, so creating a "rocker" deformity (Fig. 56).

To effect the osteotomies place a sharp 4 mm osteotome at the junction of the nasal bones and the septum and use a controlled double tap technique to progressively incise the nasal bones. The position of the osteotome should be continually monitored via external palpation as the osteotome moves under the skin. So it is imperative an assistant performs the tapping of the osteotome. The osteotomy should fade laterally at the upper end and should end when the note of the tap changes which signifies that denser bone has been reached (Figs 57 and 58).

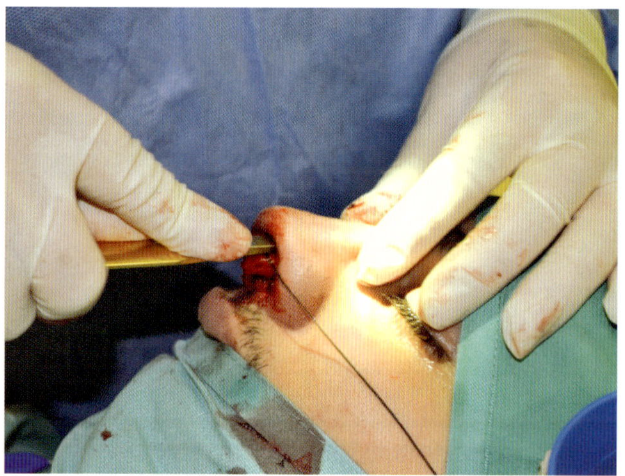

Fig. 55

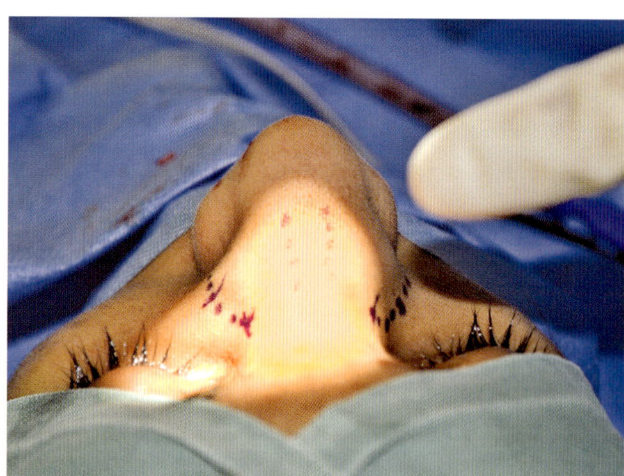

Fig. 56

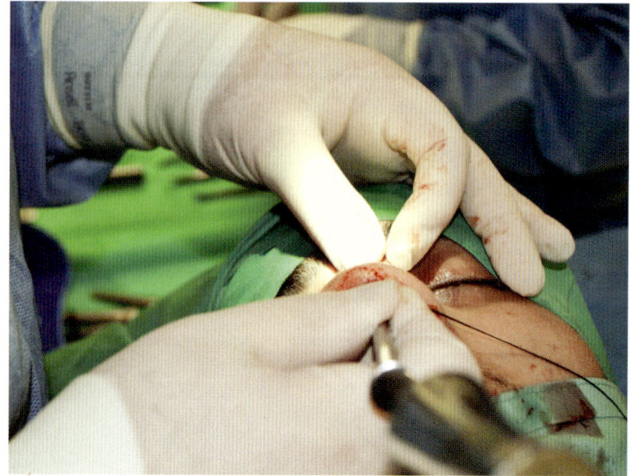

Fig. 57

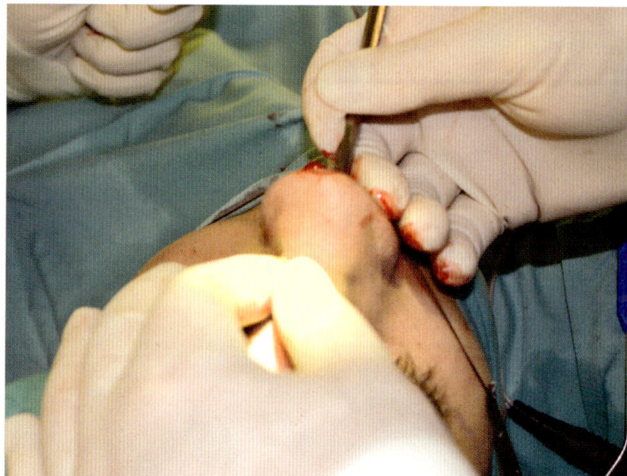

Fig. 58

Lateral Osteotomy (Fig. 59)

The lateral osteotomies can be marked on the skin to aid accurate results. Lateral osteotomies are used to close an open book deformity following hump reduction, correct asymmetrical lateral wall deformity or narrow a widened vault.[12,13] Stab skin incisions are made using a no. 11 blade, marking points near the pyriform aperture and midway between the medial canthus and the nasion. Using a controlled double tap technique and a 2 mm osteotome bony perforations are created initially heading cephalically and posteriorly just above the pyriform aperture, then heading toward the ipsilateral medial canthus in a high-low-high manner[13] (Figs 60 to 66). It is of great importance that a triangular piece of bone above the pyriform 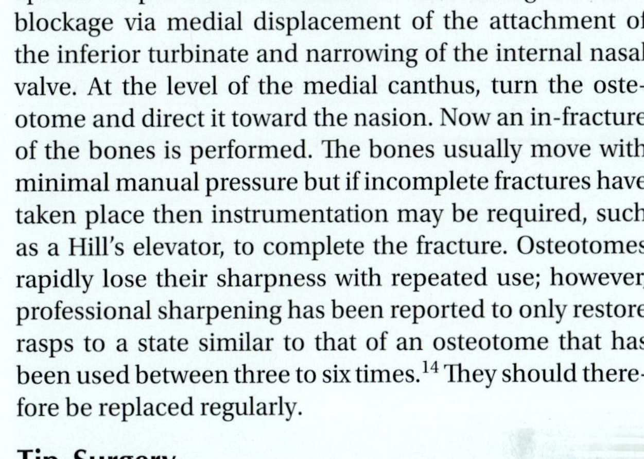 aperture is preserved to reduce the risk of iatrogenic nasal blockage via medial displacement of the attachment of the inferior turbinate and narrowing of the internal nasal valve. At the level of the medial canthus, turn the osteotome and direct it toward the nasion. Now an in-fracture of the bones is performed. The bones usually move with minimal manual pressure but if incomplete fractures have taken place then instrumentation may be required, such as a Hill's elevator, to complete the fracture. Osteotomes rapidly lose their sharpness with repeated use; however, professional sharpening has been reported to only restore rasps to a state similar to that of an osteotome that has been used between three to six times.[14] They should therefore be replaced regularly.

Tip Surgery

Alterations of the nasal tip generates considerable anxiety in the neophyte surgeon and a basic understanding of the underlying anatomy is necessary if the desired effects are to be achieved. In this respect understanding the anatomy and the relevant connections of the LLCs to the skin and the surrounding structures is imperative.

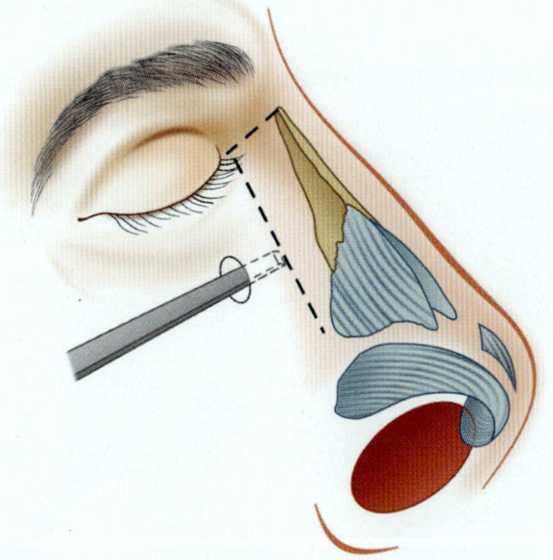

Fig. 59

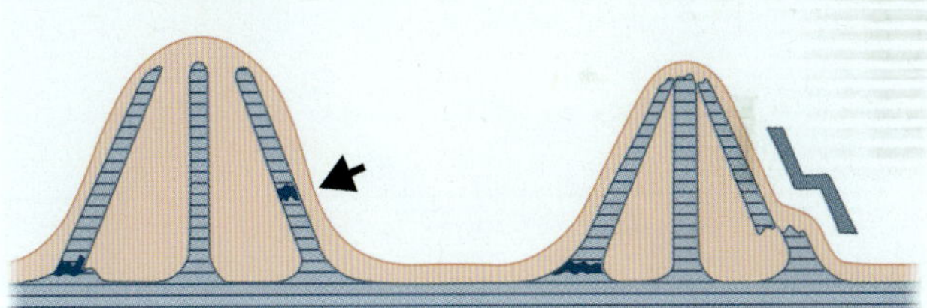

Fig. 60

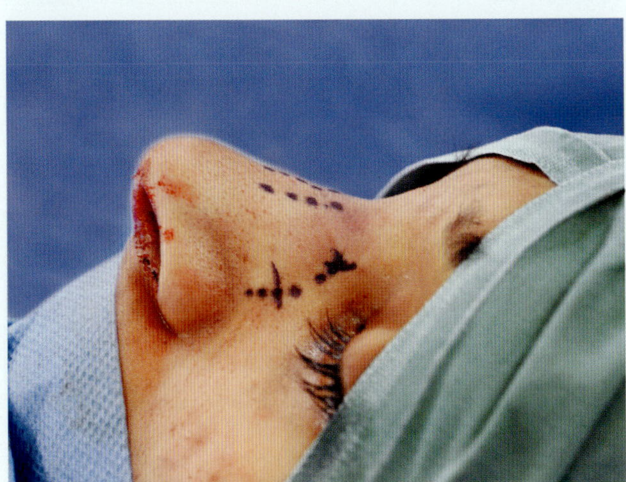

Fig. 61

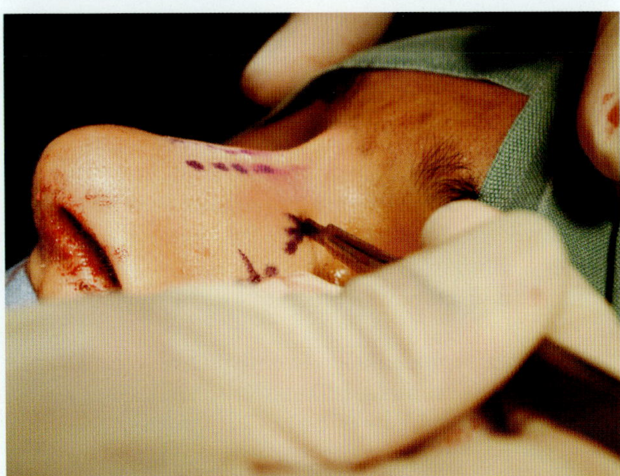

Fig. 62

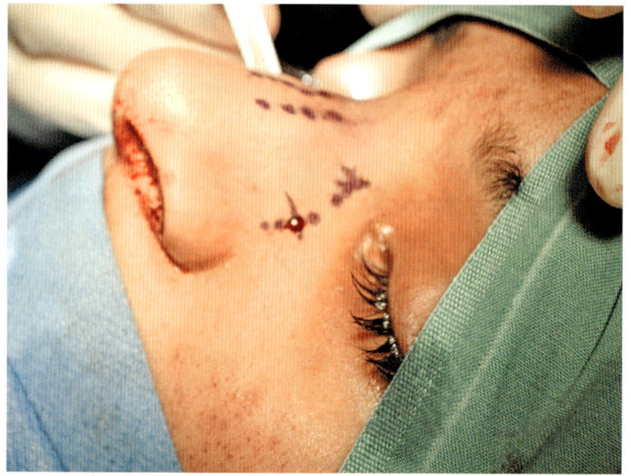

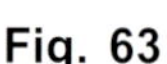

Fig. 63

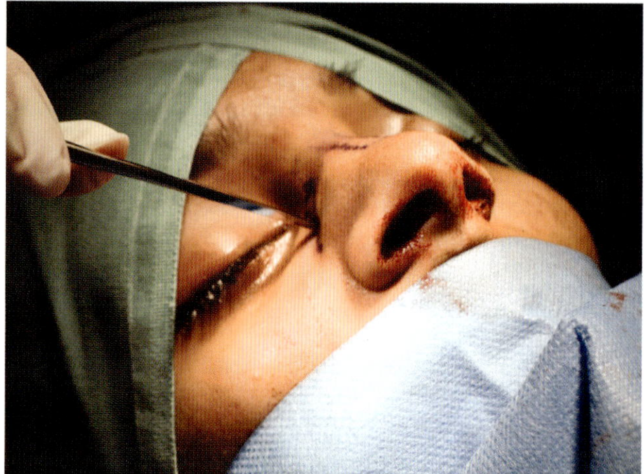

Fig. 64

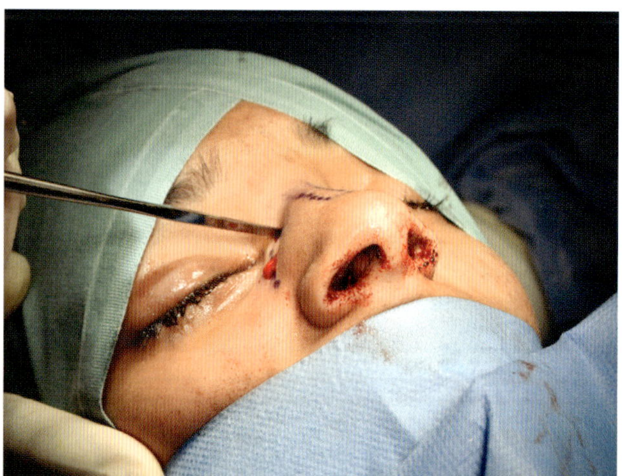

Fig. 65

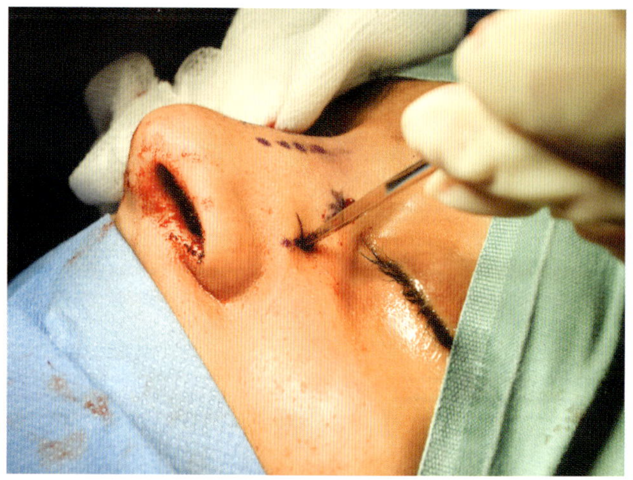

Fig. 66

The LLCs themselves consist of medial, intermediate and lateral crura. Together with the accessory cartilages (which are of little practical importance) they form the framework for the nasal tip and the shape and position of these cartilages, and the thickness of the overlying skin, are the factors which determine the appearance of the tip.

While the shape is dependent on the size, strength and curvature of the cartilages, their position is determined by the fibrous attachments to the adjacent anatomical structures. The lateral crural complexes are supported by:

- The suspensory ligament of the tip which rests on the septal angle. The ligament joins the cephalic margins of the lateral crura as they diverge from one another in the supra tip area. Lowering of the dorsum in this area reduces this support.
- The fibrous connections of the lateral crura to the ULCs. This support is compromised by an intercartilaginous incision.
- The abutment with the pyriform aperture gives support to the tip and resists backward movement.

The Tripod Concept

The tripod concept was popularized by Anderson.[15] The tripod is envisaged with the lower leg representing the medial crura and with each upper leg formed by the lateral crural complex on each side. The tip of the tripod corresponds to the nasal tip.

Shortening or removal of the lower leg should move the tip downward and backward:

- Shortening of the upper legs should move the tip upward and backward
- Shortening of all three legs should result in backward an upward movement of the tip
- Lengthening of the lower leg should move the tip upward and forward
- Lengthening the lower leg and shortening the upper leg should accentuate upward movement of the tip

TIP MODIFICATION

Many techniques have been described to modify the tip cartilages and the profusion of descriptions can be confusing. Basically there are six different reasons for modifying the tip:

1. Changing tip projection
2. Altering tip rotation
3. Decreasing the distance between the tip-defining points
4. Reducing tip fullness
5. Creating a supra-tip break
6. Altering the relationship between the columella and alar rims.

Changing Tip Projection

Increasing Projection

In practice this is one of the most frequently required and desired maneuvers.

Where there is a moderate degree of flare of the medial or intermediate crura a limited amount of tip projection can be achieved by suturing the medial walls of the domes to each other. This is simple to effect using an open approach and gives a 2–3 mm of additional projection—a modest amount.

Vertical transfixion of the lateral crura and dissection off the underlying vestibular skin with closure of the lateral segments of the domes with a horizontal mattress suture (the Goldman tip) also increases tip projection. The senior author has never undertaken this as the disadvantage of this approach are that it may predispose to collapse of the alar rim and may give a pinched appearance to the tip. In addition a single tip-defining point is produced in a more cephalad position than normal with increased infralobular show, which are rarely desired outcomes.

An alternative is that a columella strut of autologous cartilage can be inserted. A rectangular cartilage graft is sutured between the medial crura of the LLCs. This can be effected either through a transfixion incision as part of an endonasal approach or insertion as part of an open approach rhinoplasty is easier. A strut can improve tip support and projection and also help to straighten the caudal septum or the medial crura of the LLCs.

A pocket is dissected between the soft tissue that lies between the medial crura to house the strut of cartilage, which then sits above and in the plane of the anterior nasal spine. Sutures are used to secure the strut in place. A notch in the lower end of the graft helps the lower end to sit astride the nasal spine and avoids movement; more dramatically the graft can be stabilized against the underlying nasal spine using a K wire. The long-term results of this graft have recently been emphasized.[16] The objection to the strut is that it tends to widen the columella and it also limits the mobility of the nasal tip.

A tip graft will also produce tip projection.[17] A flat shield shaped graft is used which is notched at the center leaving the corners 6–8 mm apart to form two tip-defining points. Shield grafts have to be secured by suturing, and for these reasons are more readily used during open rhinoplasty.

Decreasing Projection

A complete transfixion incision destroys the support provided by the attachments of the feet of the medial crura to the caudal septum allowing the feet to settle toward the premaxilla. The shorter the medial crura and the further the feet are from the premaxilla, the more the tip can move backward. Interruption of the suspensory ligament eliminates the support provided by the dorsal septum and also allows backward movement of the LLCs.

However, the strength and stability of the lateral crura is important. If these are strong and firmly adherent to the pyriform aperture then they will resists backward movement of the tip. In such circumstances, if the vestibular skin is mobilized and the crura vertically transacted, then they will move backward. The overlying segments can be re-sutures with 4/0 Vicryl rapide in order to re-establish support of the lateral alar wall.

The medial crura can also be transacted and re-sutured if they are too long. The transaction is normally performed midway between the tip-defining points and the columella-lobular angle after undermining vestibular skin in that area.

Reducing tip projection tends to result in flaring of the alar. This may be desirable in a narrow nose but when there is a normal contour the increased flaring then has to be reduced, either by bilateral crural incision or by alar based resection.

Altering Tip Rotation

The elements that resist rotation of the tip are:

- The fibrous attachments of the ULCs to the lateral crura
- The abutment of the lateral crural complex to the pyriform aperture or long ULCs
- The caudal septum
- A high septal angle
- Adherence of the skin to the lateral crura, ULCs and nasal bones.

The resistance offered by the attachments of the lateral crura to the ULCs is eliminated by an inter-cartilaginous incision or by resection of the cephalic margin of the lateral crus. When rotation is desired a portion of the cephalic margin of the lateral crura is usually resected (Fig. 67). High attachments of the lateral crus to the pyriform suture will cause resistance to rotation, which rarely may have to be reduced by transection of the lateral crus. In spite of this the tip may still not rotate if the caudal end of the septum interferes with upward movement of the medial crura. Trimming of the septum anteriorly will therefore allow rotation. The skin attachment cephalad to the tip will resist upward movement of the LLCs and any rotation will therefore involve undermining and redraping of the skin of the lower dorsum.

In particular terms, rotation of the LLCs can normally be achieved by removal of some of the cephalic margins. This can be done endonasally through a cartilage splitting incision or fashioning a rim incision. The cartilage is then dissected free from the overlying skin and everted, often on a Hill's Elevator or other such instrument, such that it can be trimmed in situ. A senior also prefers a rim incision in this respect since this gives the full exposure to the whole of the LLC and allows us a direct inspection of the whole structure rather than a part thereof (Figs 68 and 69).

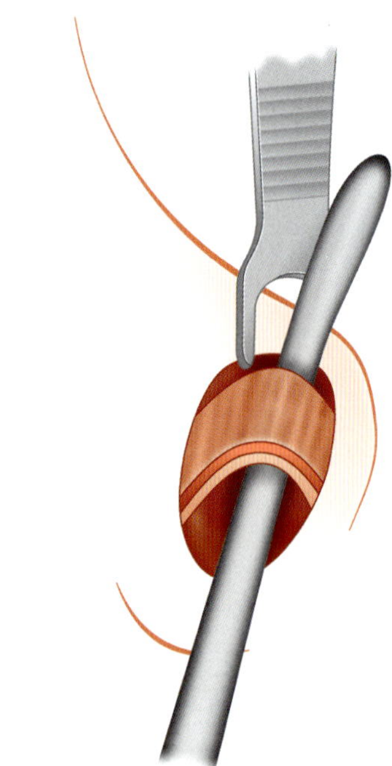

Fig. 68

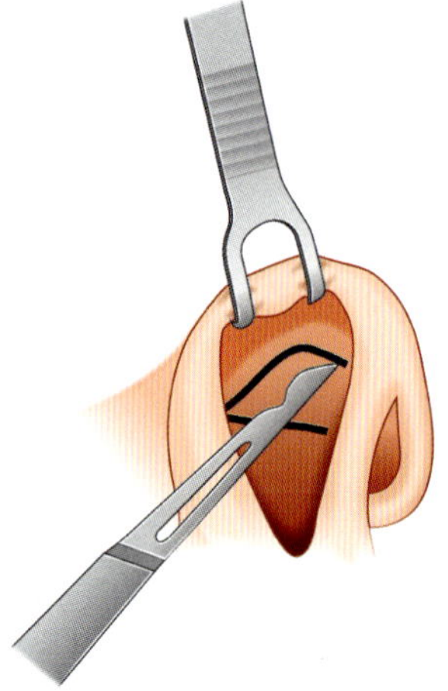

Fig. 67

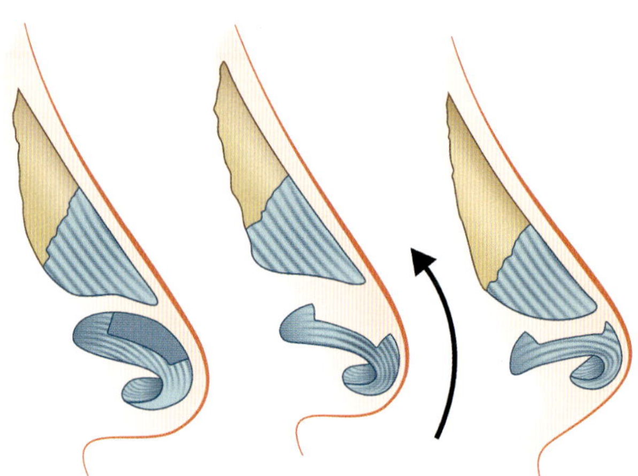

Fig. 69

In open approach rhinoplasty removal of the cephalic margin of the lower lateral is relatively simple as this structure is immediately visible.

Whichever way is chosen it is important to realize that the resection of the upper border of the LLC defiles some of the important support mechanisms for the lateral crus.

Resection should always be conservative and it is a good maxim always to "leave more than you take away".

A more important problem is rotation of the tip downward to increase the length of the nose. The forces resisting this the adherence of the skin to the underlying framework, fibrous attachments of the lower to the ULCs and adherence of the mucosa and vestibular skin to the nasal bones, upper and LLCs and septum. This can be overcome by an extended spreader graft.

Decreasing the Distance between the Tip-Defining Points

If the nose appears wide because of an increase distance between the tip-defining points, suturing the medial walls of the domes toward each other with permanent sutures will reduce the gap.

In certain cases the distance can also be reduced by resection of the cephalic margins of the medial wall of the domes and the anterior medial crura. This is because, as the cartilages curve away from the dome area toward the columella (the intermediate crura), they flare such that the caudal margins are separated. Resection of the cephalic rim eliminates this abutment and allows the tip-defining points to move closer together (Figs 70 to 74).

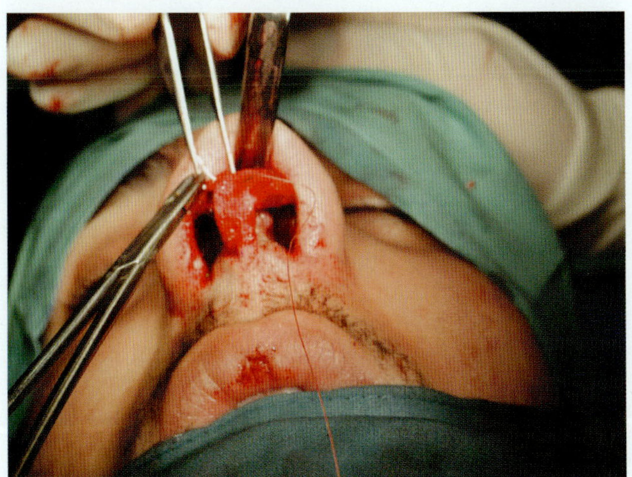

Fig. 70

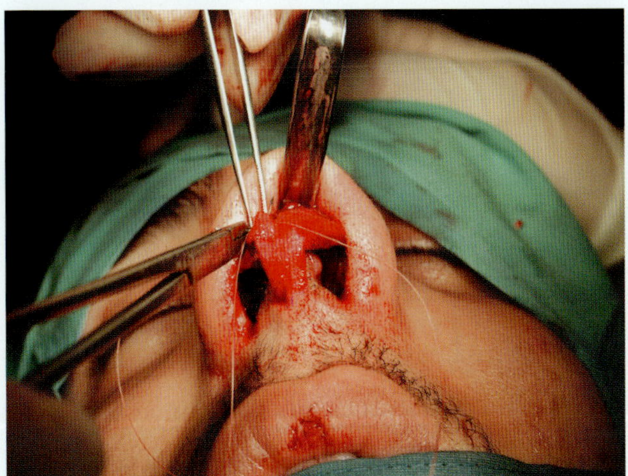

Fig. 71

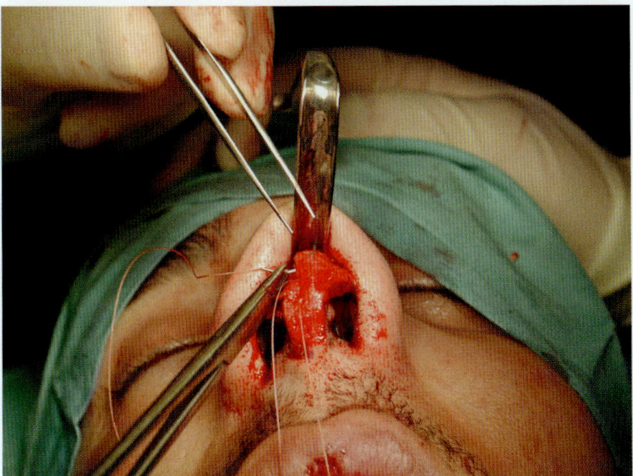

Fig. 72

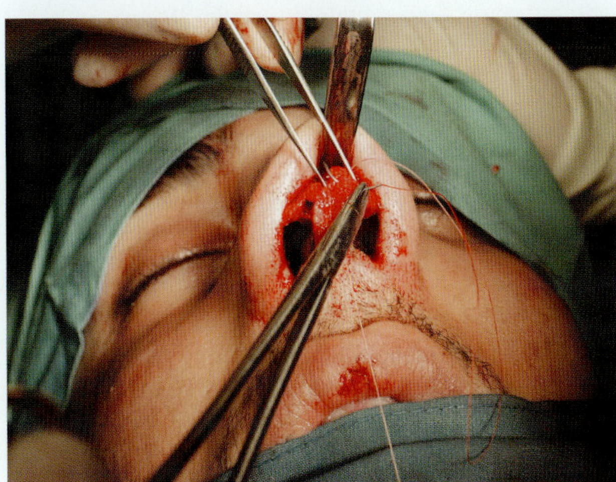

Fig. 73

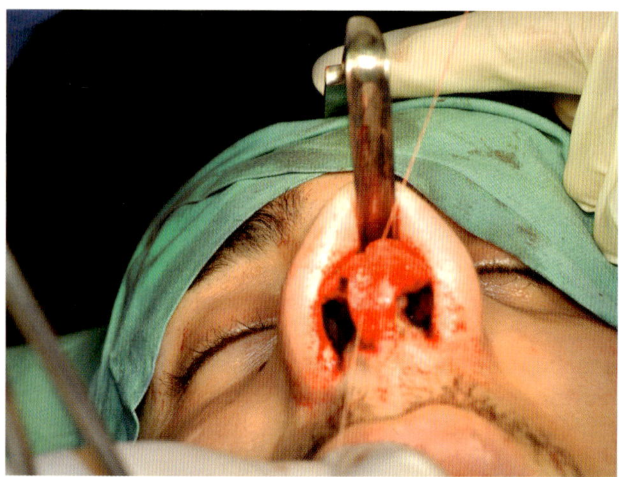

Fig. 74

Reducing Tip Fullness

Decreasing fullness of the tip usually requires partial resection and/or weakening of the lateral crura. Resection of the cephalic segments of the lateral crura will decrease tip fullness but the remaining caudal segments may remain flared giving the nose a bulbous appearance. To overcome this, the lateral crura can be attenuated by interdigitating incisions which are made through the cartilage only avoiding damage to the underlying vestibular lining. The risk is that the lateral crura may subsequently collapse on inspiration.

A better way to reduced flare is to place 5/0 sutures in the dome area. This can be done on both sides and if it is also necessary to narrow the distance between the tip-defining points then, if one suture is left long on each side and then tightened, the desired effect can be achieved. Any such maneuver can cause medial migration of the lateral crus and cause alar intrusion to the airway.

Creating a Supra-Tip Break

It is usually desirable, especially in female patients, to create a break immediately above the tip. This is accomplished by lowering the dorsal septum just above the septal angle.

The skin in this area is thicker than that which covers the intermediate dorsum. If it is very thick then it is possible to remove some fat and loose tissue on the under surface of the skin. However this must be done with great care and only that tissue which is loosely attached should be removed in order to avoid damaging the underlying dermis. Dimpling or even necrosis of the skin may then result.

Altering the Alar-Columellar Relationship

The relationship between the alar and columella is most frequently described from the lateral view but it is also important to look at the nose from the front and to ensure that this relationship is correct. Gunter et al. have written of an analysis of several hundred patients and have found that it is possible to divide the end of the nose by three horizontal planes through, respectively, the tip-defining points, the highest point of the alar rims and the columella lobular angle.[18]

The same relationship was found on the lateral view but they found that the most common and valuable finding was that the outline of the nostril should simulate a complete oval. The alar rooms form the upper half of this oval and the lower half is formed by the columella rim at the junction of the external skin with the vestibular skin.

A line drawn through the most anterior and posterior points of the oval represents the long axis of the nostril and divides it into an upper and lower half. By using the distance from this long axis to alar rim superiorly (AB) and the columella rim inferiorly (BC) they have categorized alar-columella relationships into one of six groups. Class one is normal and shown opposite. In this diagram the alar rim (AB) and the columella (BC) are both equal.

In the literature the common method described for correction of an abnormality in this area is resection of part of the membranous columella or part of the caudal septum together with resection of the caudal margins of the medial crura. To this these authors have added partial removal of the medial crus on each side with suturing of the ages together and insertion of composite grafts and removal of tissues at the alar rims. The paper should be consulted for details regarding these removers which allow infinite adjustments of the alar-columella relationships.

SPECIALIST TECHNIQUES

Spreader Grafts

Spreader grafts were first described by Sheen in 1984, and act as spacers in the internal nasal valve region. This region is bounded medially by the caudal septum and laterally by the inferior turbinate.[19] Spreader grafts improve nasal airflow in the internal valve area and are also useful in correcting middle nasal vault asymmetry. They also restore the dorsal esthetic lines.

Spreader grafts are placed in a subperichondrial pocket that lies between the ULCs and the septum. A pocket is created in a horizontal plane starting from the anterior septal angle and heading in a cephalic direction and ending at the keystone area. This pocket can be created by sharp dissection using a no. 15 blade scalpel and can be further developed using a Freer's elevator. The ULCs are dissected free from the septum preserving, as far as possible, the underlying mucoperichondrium. A rectangular cartilage graft of approximately 1–3 mm thickness and 2–3 cm length that extends from the keystone area to the anterior septal angle is then inserted and the grafts are secured in situ with horizontal mattress sutures (5/0 Vicryl rapide) above and below.

Alar Batten, Alar Strut and Rim Grafts

The terms alar batten and alar strut grafts are used interchangeably with some confusion. Batten grafts were first described by Toriumi in 1997 and are cartilage grafts used to augment the alar rim and hence alter the elasticity of the external nasal valve.[20] A batten graft is placed deep to the lateral crus in the space between the lateral crus and the vestibular mucosa. Maximum support is achieved by placing the alar graft over the bone of the pyriform aperture. They are best secured with sutures and in order to maintain position, and it is easier to insert these utilizing an open approach rhinoplasty.

A strut is placed over the lateral crus to reinforce it and to prevent collapse and a pinched look. This graft is particularly useful if the lateral crus is naturally concave to the nasal vestibule and is producing a deformity in the supra-alar crease. A gentle curve to the graft aids optimal placing and an external approach rhinoplasty permits the best access for this graft. If the deformity of the underlying cartilage is severe then excision of the concave part of the lateral crus and reversing it and reattaching it prior to attaching an overlying graft will facilitate correction. The graft should not be too thick or excessive rigidity and thickening of the alar is achieved which is undesirable.

Alar rim grafts, also known as alar contour grafts, are placed in the most caudal aspect of the nasal ala in an effort to prevent a pinched nose appearance. They can be inserted through a stab incision.

Dorsal Augmentation

The dorsum of the nose may be altered using onlay grafts.[21] These may formed from autologous cartilage sources such as the septum, upper or LLCs, conchal bowl or costal cartilage. Alternatively irradiated homograft cartilage can be used.

A newer technique of using cartilage that has been diced and wrapped in fascia can remain malleable in the early postoperative period should further correction be necessary.[22] Autologous soft tissue may also be used, such as subcutaneous fat, temporalis fascia or SMAS or even hard tissue such as bone.[23] The latter is associated with rather high levels of reabsorption. Research is needed into the long-term behavior of materials such as processed fascia lata (Tutoplast©) and synthetic materials such as silicone, Gore-Tex© (expanded polytetrafluorethylene) or Medpor© (high density polyethylene). All such materials have their proponents and early studies have suggested favorable outcomes using these materials.[24] However, in most instances long-term outcomes are not known.

Closure and Dressings

The aim of early postoperative care including the use of dressings is for:

- Reduction of swelling by the elimination of dead space
- Maintenance of a patent nasal airway
- Stabilizing the osteotomized nasal bones
- Protection from external trauma
- Pain control.

Intranasal incisions are best closed using 3/0 Vicryl rapide (Fig. 75). Closure is important in order to avoid asymmetry during healing. In external approach rhinoplasty the skin is closured with an absorbable mattress suture such as 5/0 Vicryl (Figs 76 to 82). The marginal and hemitransfixion incisions are also closed with a nonabsorbable suture (4/0 Vicryl rapide) (Figs 84 and 85).

At then end of the procedure, the nasal cavity and dorsal skin is gently cleansed to avoid disturbing the new position of the nasal bones, and any grafts. Intranasal packs (e.g. Merocel©) soaked with an antibiotic ointment and then inflated with antibiotic solution provides extra internal support for up to 6 hours as the patient gently recovers full consciousness (Figs 85 to 88).

Friars Balsam/Benzoin compound tincture is lightly painted over the skin lateral to the dorsum of the skin to ensure the skin tape dressing remains in situ until the follow-up appointment (Fig. 89). Skin tapes (Steristrips) are applied in a horizontal fashion from the radix to the nasal tip with a long U-shaped strip placed to

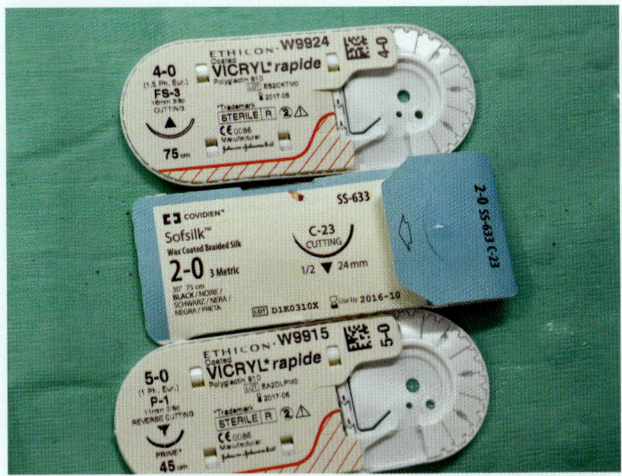

Fig. 75

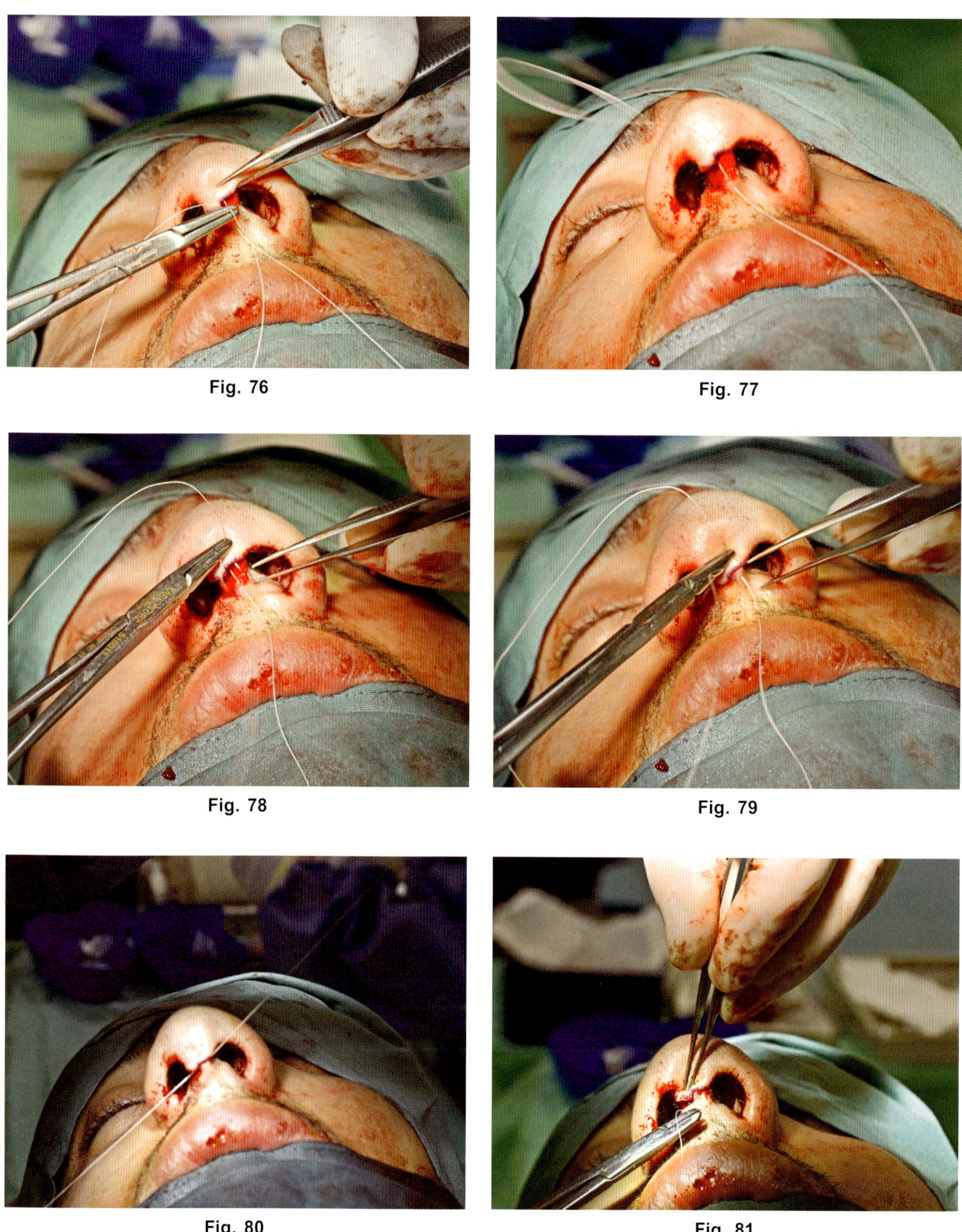

Fig. 76

Fig. 77

Fig. 78

Fig. 79

Fig. 80

Fig. 81

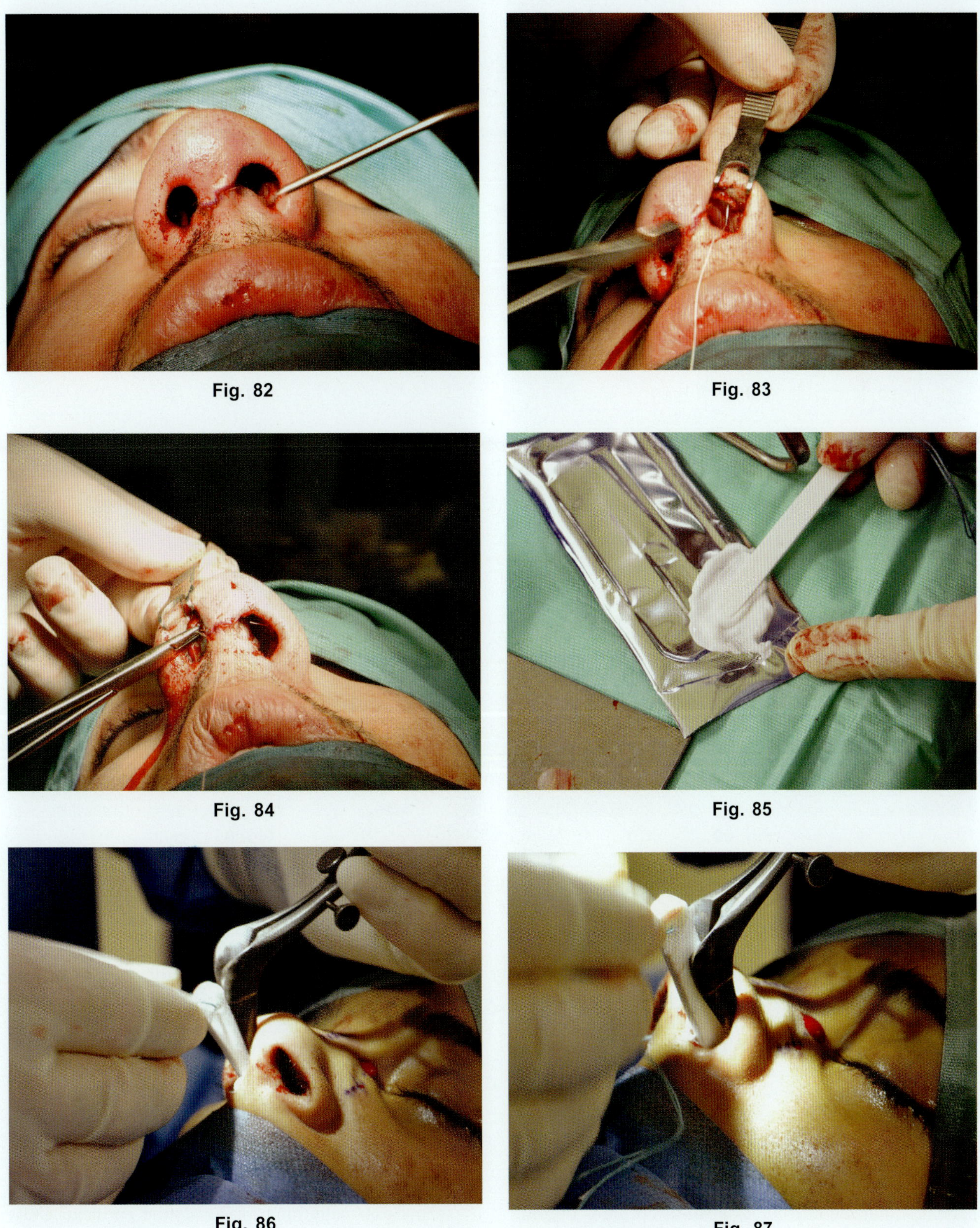

Fig. 82

Fig. 83

Fig. 84

Fig. 85

Fig. 86

Fig. 87

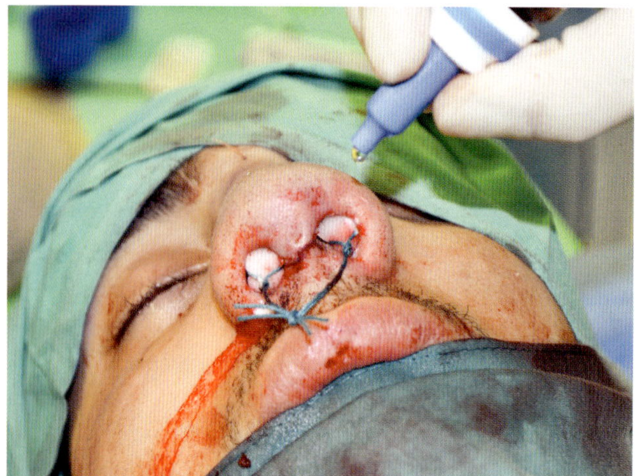
Fig. 88

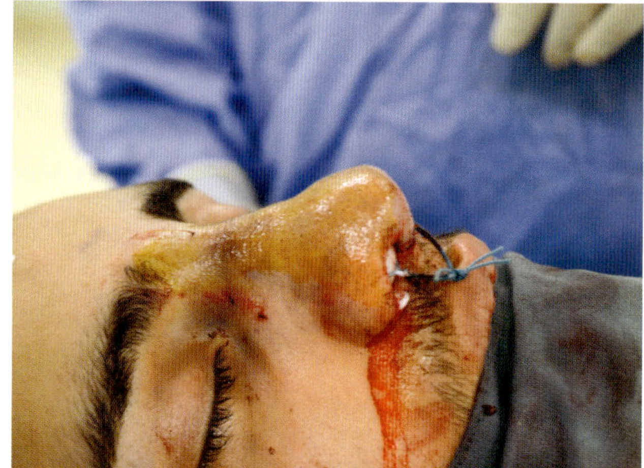
Fig. 89

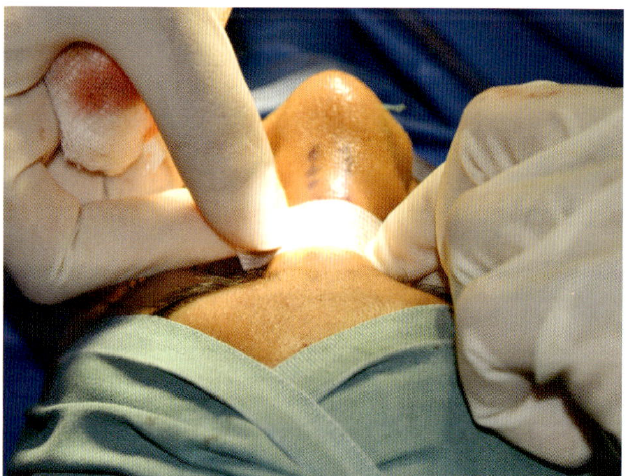
Fig. 90

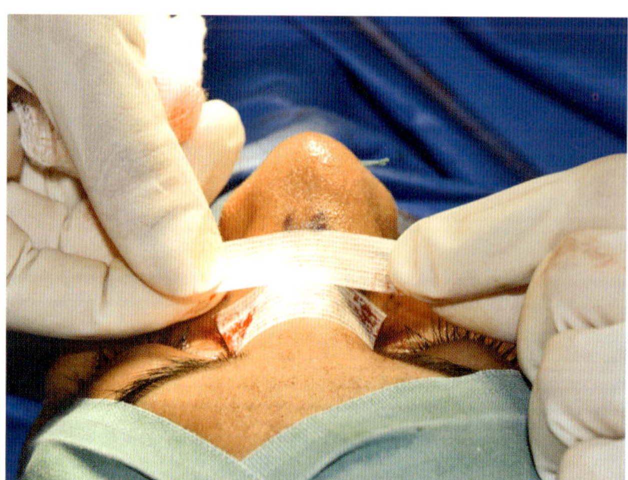
Fig. 91

support the nasal tip (Figs 90 to 96). A piece of transparent Transpore© tape is then applied to add further soft tissue protection. Finally, a plaster of Paris cast is cut and shaped to fit the patient, moistened with warm water and carefully molded to fit the dorsum of the nose. The plaster cast must lie over the dorsum of the nose and the sites of the lateral astronomies (Figs 97 and 98). Flesh-colored micropore tape secures the plaster in place.

A temporary bolster dressing placed over the inferior aspect of the nose to absorb any minor nasal bleeding or secretions in the immediate postoperative period. The patient should be nursed 30° head-up in order to minimize tissue edema (Figs 99 and 100).

POSTOPERATIVE CARE

Patients may be discharged the same day after a suitable period of observation.

- *Analgesia*: It has been reported that postoperative pain is at its worst during the first 3 days.[25] Suitable analgesics in clued paracetamol and a nonsteroidal anti-inflammatory such as voltarol.
- *Antibiotics*: There are no published guidelines on the use of antibiotics in this patient group. However, a survey reported 72% of surgeons prescribed antibiotics in the intraoperative and postoperative period.[26] This seems especially appropriate if free cartilage grafts have been inserted.

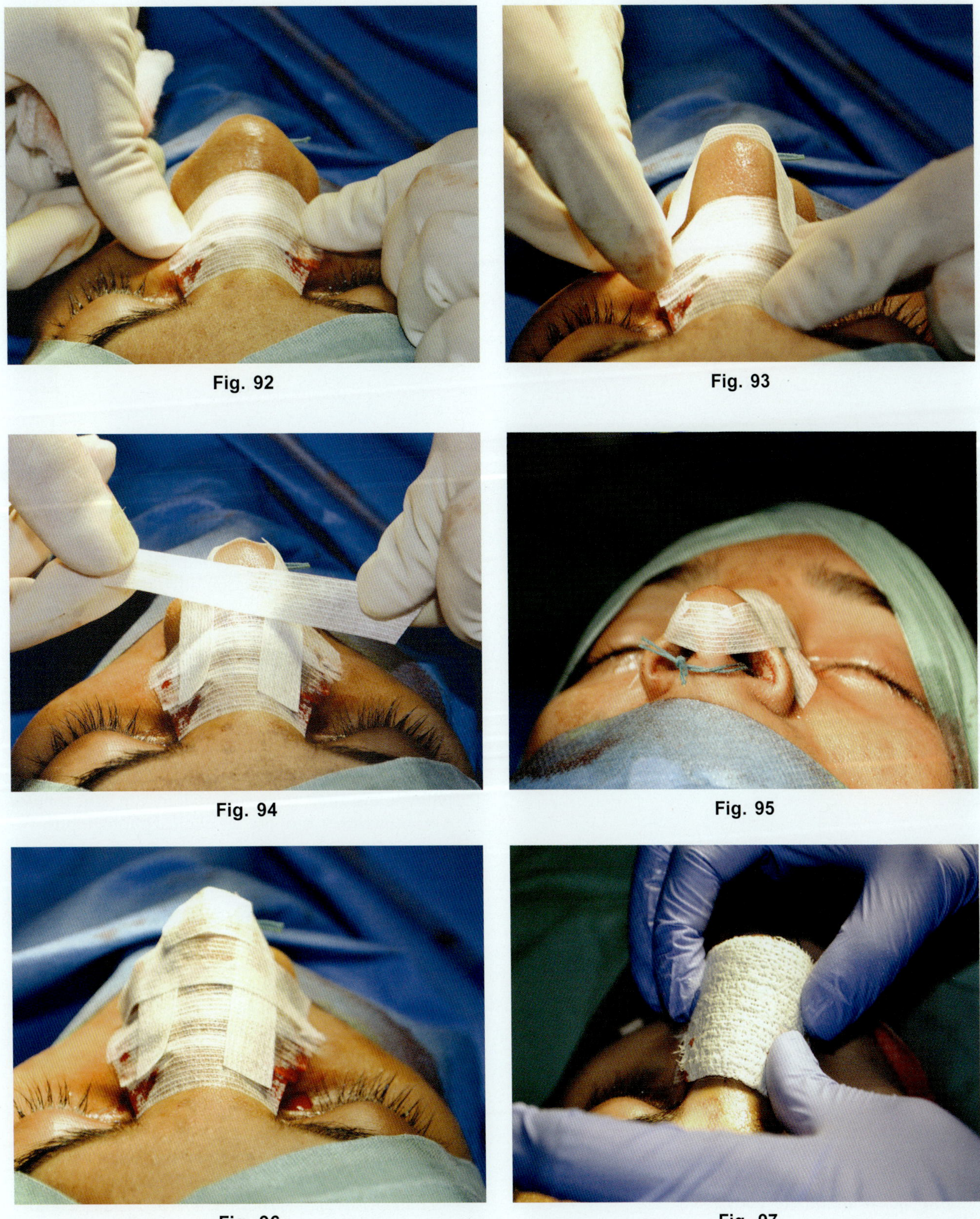

Fig. 92

Fig. 93

Fig. 94

Fig. 95

Fig. 96

Fig. 97

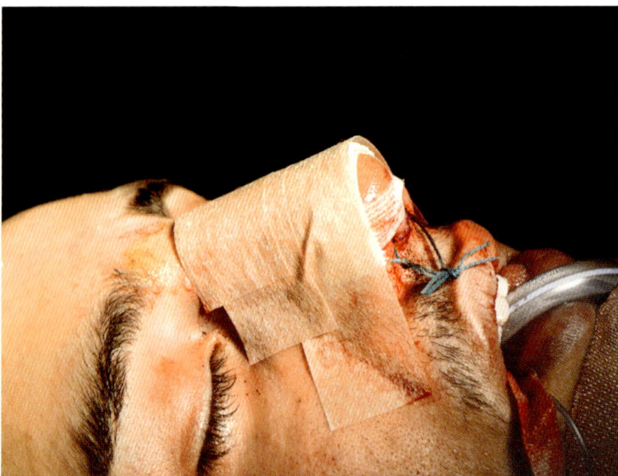

Fig. 98

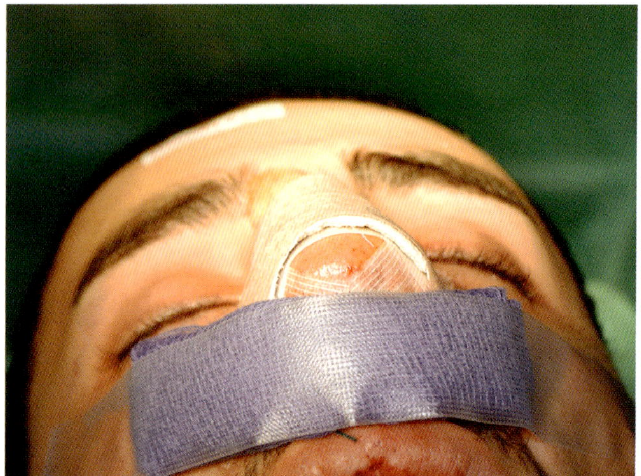

Fig. 99

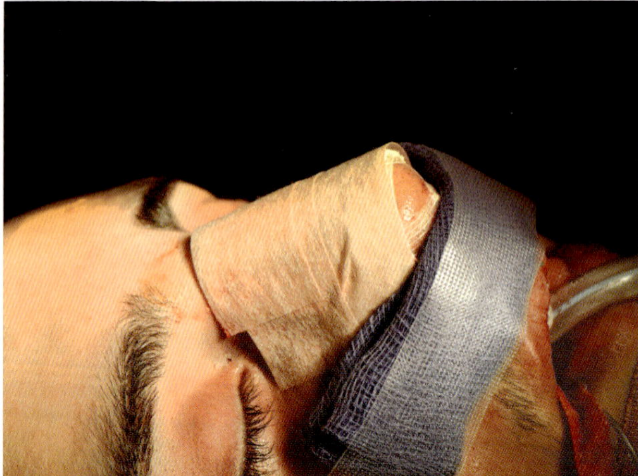

Fig. 100

- *Low dose oral steroids*: There is conflicting data on the use of steroids, but short courses are beneficial in patients with no medical contraindications.[26] A single dose of steroid is beneficial to reduce periorbital edema and ecchymosis for up to 2 days postoperatively.[27] Three doses provide a benefit for up to a week.[28] Further evidence shows that postoperative edema is reduced for up to 2 weeks when a single intraoperative dose is followed up by a 5 day oral course.[29] There is evidence to suggest a trend toward long-term reduction of edema and bruising when steroids are given for 3 days.[30] The senior author ensures that the patient is given intraoperative Dexamethasone (8 mg) and that this is followed by the same drug in a dose of 2 mg qds by mouth for 5 days.
- *Saline nasal drops*: These have been reported to significantly reduce the symptoms associated with the stasis of secretions and crust formation which occurs as a result of the reduced mucociliary function in the first three postoperative weeks.[31,32]
- *Ephedrine nasal drops*: It helps to advance nasal patency in the early postoperative period. These are routinely prescribed.
- Antibiotic ointment helps to prevent secondary infection of the crusting that inevitably forms around the nares.
- The patient should be advised not to blow nose and to try and sneeze through an open mouth in order to try and avoid separation of the tissue flaps. Removal of sutures and plaster of Paris occurs at 1 week. The patients are then reviewed at 1 month and then at 4 months with postoperative clinical photographs.

REFERENCES

1. Lopez MA, Michaelson PG, Westine JG. A systematic approach for preoperative rhinoplasty planning. Am J Otolaryngol. 2008;29(4):265-9.
2. Ahluwalia S, Veer V, Kenyon GS. Lateral photography of the nasal tip: what is acceptable and can it be improved? Plast Reconstr Surg. 2010;126(5):250e-2e.
3. Krugman ME. Photoanalysis of the rhinoplasty patient. Ear Nose Throat J. 1981;60(7):328-30.
4. Staffel JG. Photo documentation in rhinoplasty. Facial Plast Surg. 1997;13(4):317-32.
5. LaNasa JJ, Smith O, Johnson CM. The cephalic view in nasal photography. J Otolaryngol. 1991;20(6):443-5.
6. Galdino GM, DaSilva And D, Gunter JP. Digital photography for rhinoplasty. Plast Reconstr Surg. 2002;109(4):1421-34.

7. Makdessian AS, Ellis DA, Irish JC. Informed consent in facial plastic surgery: effectiveness of a simple educational intervention. Arch Facial Plast Surg. 2004;6(1):26-30.
8. Rettinger G. Risks and complications of rhinoplasty. Laryngorhinootologie. 2007;86(Suppl 1):S40-54.
9. Gunter JP, Rohrich RJ, Friedman RM. Classification and correction of alar-columellar discrepancies in rhinoplasty. Plastic Reconstr Surg. 1996;97:643-8.
10. Kenyon GS, Kalan A, Jones NS. Columelloplasty: a new suture technique to correct caudal septal cartilage dislocation. Clin Otolaryngol Allied Sci. 2002;27(3):188-91.
11. Gunter JP, Rohrich RJ. External approach for secondary rhinoplasty. Plast Reconstr Surg. 1987;80(2):161-74.
12. Most SP, Murakami CS. Nasal osteotomies: anatomy, planning, and technique. Facial Plast Surg Clin North Am. 2002; 10(3):279-85.
13. Rohrich RJ, Minoli JJ, Adams WP, et al. The lateral nasal osteotomy in rhinoplasty: an anatomic endoscopic comparison of the external versus the internal approach. Plast Reconstr Surg. 1997;99:1309-12.
14. Murakami CS, Larrabee WF. Comparison of osteotomy techniques in the treatment of nasal fractures. Facial Plast Surg. 1992;8:209-19.
15. Bloom JD, Ransom ER, Antunes MB, et al. Quantifying the sharpness of osteotomes for dorsal hump reduction. Arch Facial Plast Surg. 2011;13(2):103-8.
16. Anderson JR. A personal technique of rhinoplasty. Otolaryngol Clin North Am. 1975;8:599-62.
17. Rohrich RJ, Hoxworth RE, Kurkjian TJ. The role of the columellar strut in rhinoplasty: indications and rationale. Plast Reconstr Surg. 2012;129(1):118e-25e.
18. Sheen JH. Achieving more tip projection by the use of a small autogenous vomer or septal cartilage graft. A preliminary report. Plast Reconstr Surg. 1975;56(1):35-40.
19. Sheen JH. Spreader graft: a method of reconstructing the roof of the middle nasal vault following rhinoplasty. Plast Reconstr Surg. 1984;73:230-9.
20. Toriumi DM, Josen J, Weinberger M, et al. Use of alar batten grafts for correction of nasal valve collapse. Arch Otolaryngol Head Neck Surg. 1997;123:802-8.
21. Lee MR, Unger JG, Rohrich RJ. Management of the nasal dorsum in rhinoplasty: a systematic review of the literature regarding technique, outcomes, and complications. Plast Reconstr Surg. 2011;128(5):538e-50e.
22. Erol OO. The Turkish delight: a pliable graft for rhinoplasty. Plast Reconstr Surg. 2000;105:2229-41.
23. Toriumi DM, Larrabee WF, Walike JW, et al. Demineralized bone: implant resorption with long-term follow-up. Arch Otolaryngol Head Neck Surg. 1990;116:676-80.
24. Reiffel AJ, Cross KJ, Spinelli HM. Nasal spreader grafts: a comparison of medpor to autologous tissue reconstruction. Ann Plast Surg. 2011;66(1):24-8.
25. Szychta P, Antoszewski B. Assessment of early postoperative pain following septorhinoplasty. J Laryngol Otol. 2010;124 (11):1194-9.
26. Cochran CS, Ducic Y, DeFatta RJ. Current concepts in the postoperative care of the rhinoplasty patient. South Med J. 2008;101(9):935-9.
27. Kara CO, Gökalan I. Effects of single-dose steroid usage on edema, ecchymosis, and intraopertive bleeding in rhinoplasty. Plast Reconstr Surg. 1999;104:2213-8.
28. Kargi E, Hoşnuter M, Babucçu O, et al. Effect of steroids on edema, ecchymosis, and intraoperative bleeding in rhinoplasty. Ann Plastic Surg. 2003;51:570-4.
29. Hoffman DF, Cook TA, Quatela VC, et al. Steroids and rhinoplasty. A double-blind study. Arch Otolaryngol Head Neck Surg. 1991;117:990-3.
30. Hatef DA, Ellsworth WA, Allen JN, et al. Perioperative steroids for minimizing edema and ecchymosis after rhinoplasty: a meta-analysis. Aesthet Surg J. 2011;31(6):648-57.
31. Tomooka LT, Murphy C, Davidson TM. Clinical study and literature review of nasal irrigation. Laryngoscope. 2000;110:1189-93.
32. Shone GR, Yardley MP, Knight LC. Mucociliary function in the early weeks after nasal surgery. Rhinology. 1990;28: 265-8.

CHAPTER

98 Augmentation Rhinoplasty

Yong Ju Jang, Ji Heui Kim

INDICATIONS FOR THE SURGERY

Dorsal augmentation is a surgery that is performed for the purpose of elevating the nasal dorsum using an autologous tissue or an alloplastic implant when the nasal dorsum has been lowered by a congenital cause, trauma, inflammation, or reduction rhinoplasty.

SPECIFIC PREOPERATIVE EVALUATION

Analyzing and Making Reference of the Preoperative Photographs of the Patient

Length of the Nose

Determining the length of the implant also determines the length of the nose. Thus, it is important to make the correct decision regarding the suitable length of the patient's nose. For patients with a round shaped face and small eyes and mouth, a shorter nose is more suitable than a longer nose. Conversely, for patients with an elongated and angled face, a long and elevated nose with a clear definition is more suitable than a small nose. Likewise, harmony of the nose with the overall surrounding structure is important. Also, excessive augmentation and lengthening of the nose can always result in disasters, such as the extrusion of the implant. Therefore, any request by the patient for an excessive augmentation must be rejected outright.

Hump

It is advisable to properly remove even the slightest hump and then perform dorsal augmentation. In most cases, more problems are caused by inadequate removal rather than from an excessive removal of the hump. Thus, the removal of the hump (whether it is a bony hump or cartilage hump) should be accurately ascertained if a nasal dorsum is to take correct shape (Figs 1A and B).

The Relationship to the Chin

Although a close relationship exists between the chin and the nasal tip surgery and between the chin and dorsal augmentation, it is often disregarded. The chins of Koreans are generally retruded so that if just a dorsal augmentation is performed, it would in many cases make the chin look even more retruded. If patients with a low nasal dorsum and tip as well as a pre-existing microgenia or retrognathia

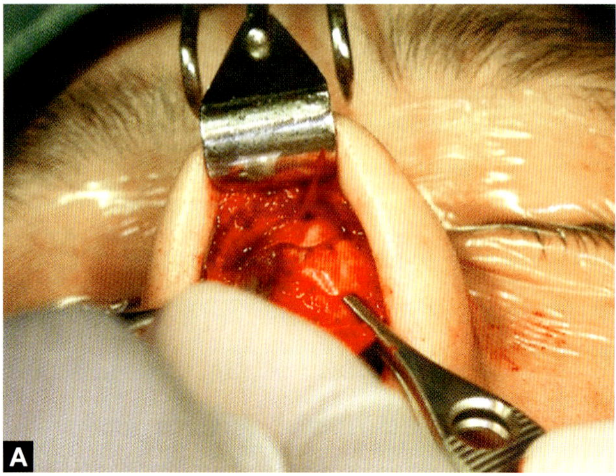

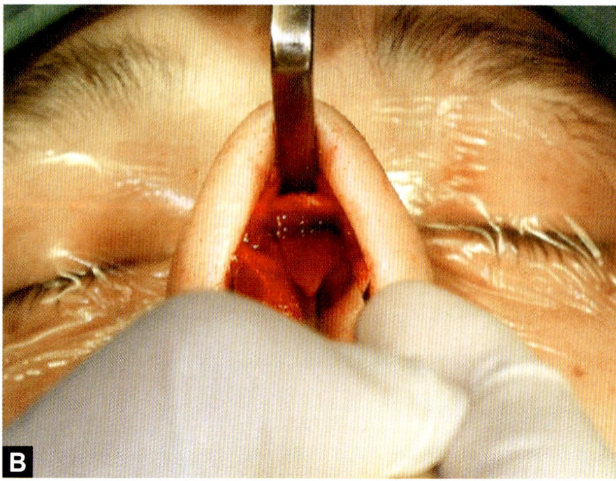

Figs 1A and B: (A) A cartilage hump and; (B) Bony hump being removed

undergo surgery to elevate the low nasal dorsum and tip, it will result in the lip and chin being repositioned relatively further backward. Thus, to maintain the symmetry of the face, it is desirable to perform genioplasty concurrently or subsequently (Figs 2A and B).

Verifying Physiological or Anatomical Problems within the Nasal Cavity

Should septal deviation, turbinate hypertrophy, or sinusitis exist within the nasal cavity, the patient may complain of an increased nasal obstruction despite being highly satisfied cosmetically. Thus, it is advisable to always be fully aware of any problems within the patient's nasal cavity prior to surgery. Particular attention is required when there is infection within the nasal cavity as the risk of infection following dorsal augmentation increases in such a case. In addition, in case the patient is diagnosed with chronic inflammation due to allergic rhinitis so that blowing or touching the nose is unavoidable, there is a high risk that scarring will occur at the incision area or that the implant will migrate. In such a case, medication, such as antihistamine, needs to be prescribed.

Considering the Occupation and the Circumstances Surrounding the Patients

The general population or housewives generally prefer a natural looking but slightly augmented nose while entertainers or those working in service-oriented fields prefer robust looking features and relatively high nose. Therefore, deciding the extent of dorsal augmentation based on patient's occupation can reduce possible discontent that may arise later on.

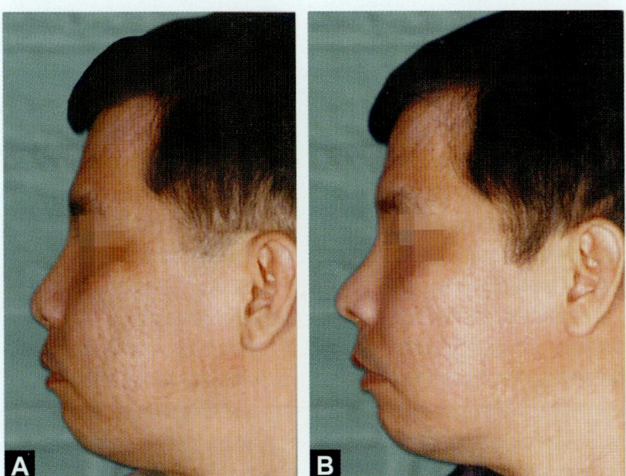

Figs 2A and B: (A) A preoperative image of a patient with a micrognathia and; (B) An image showing a patient whose chin seems more drawn back following tip projection surgery

ANESTHETIC CONSIDERATIONS

Before selecting the types of anesthesia to be used, the surgeon must make it a standard practice to examine the following factors.

The Condition of the Patient

Most patients prefer general to local anesthesia because of their fear of surgery and pain. However, most rhinoplasty can usually be performed using conscious sedation or local anesthesia. Nevertheless, if patients express excessive fear of surgery or pain, if the patient is a child, when there is a severe case of saddle nose, in case of a total reconstructive surgery of the nose, or when harvesting costal cartilage, the inhalational general anesthesia is recommended. As some patients react negatively to the inhalational general anesthesia because of mistaken popular belief that in may adversely affect the memory function, doctors need to provide proper guidance for patients.

Familiarity of the Anesthesia to the Surgeon

There is always the possibility of the unexpected happening as a result of anesthesia. Thus, it is always best for the surgeon to select the anesthesia that he is familiar with as it is the fastest means for the surgeon to properly and rapidly respond to an emergency situation.

SURGICAL STEPS

Various implant materials have been used for dorsal augmentation. Materials used in rhinoplasty can be divided largely between biologic tissues (autologous and homologous tissue) and the alloplastic materials. In the rhinoplasty for Caucasian, use of alloplastic implant, especially silicone, on the nasal dorsum has been condemned. In Asian rhinoplasty, however, alloplastic implants still play a role due to the differing anatomical characteristics of Asians, such as thick skin and poorly developed cartilaginous framework, compared with Caucasians. Alloplastic implants generally need to be biocompatible, nontoxic, chemically safe, and nonimmunogenic. They must also not induce infection, cancer or produce toxic substances within the body. Additionally, during recovery, these implants should maintain their original size, shape, and hardness. At present, the most commonly used alloplastic implants that meet these conditions are silicone, Gore-Tex, and Medpor.

Autologous Tissue

The advantage of autologous material for the dorsal augmentation of the nose cannot be questioned as these implants are well-tolerated and carry the least risk of infection. However, if any autologous tissue other than septal cartilage is selected, the additional operative time required to harvest the graft and donor site morbidity become limiting factors. Common autologous tissues used for dorsal augmentation include septal cartilage, conchal cartilage, costal cartilage, fascia, and dermofat.

Septal Cartilage

As it is easy to harvest and shape the septal cartilage, it can be used to moderately elevate the nasal dorsum, to camouflage a partial concavity on the dorsum, and for nasal tip surgery. Since Asian patients have relatively small noses, it is practically difficult to harvest enough amount of cartilage, leaving at least 1-cm width of the L-strut, suitable for a full-length dorsal graft (Fig. 3).

Technique of harvesting the septal cartilage

- After incising the mucosa, use a Freer elevator to perform dissection on one side of the nasal septum. During the elevation of the mucoperichondrium, if the cartilage takes on a blue-gray color and the hemorrhage is minor, it can be determined that the dissection is successful (Figs 4A and B).
- At junction area between the cartilaginous area of the cartilaginous septum and the bony septum, apply proper pressure to the elevator and separate the septal cartilage and the junctional area of the perpendicular plate, vomer of the ethmoid bone. When separating the septal cartilage with the perpendicular plate, try to preserve the upper 10 mm belonging to the keystone area (Figs 5A and B).
- While preserving about 10-mm width of the L-strut septal cartilage, apply full-thickness incision on the cartilage parallel to the nasal dorsum—a distance of about 10 mm from the dorsum of the nasal septum (Figs 6A and B).
- After applying a full-thickness incision vertically, 10 mm from the caudal margin of the nasal septum, dissect the perichondrium on the opposite side (Figs 7A and B).
- While dissecting the perichondrium from the opposite side, using a Freer elevator, separate the connection between the septal cartilage and the partially attached vomer and maxillary crest (Figs 8A and B).

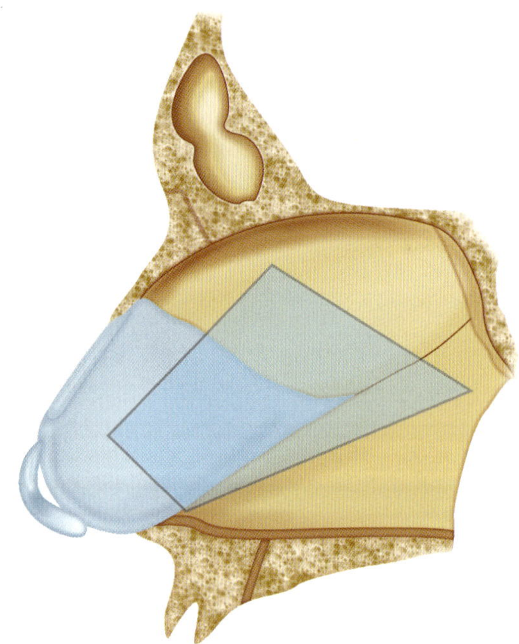

Fig. 3: Septal cartilage harvest area

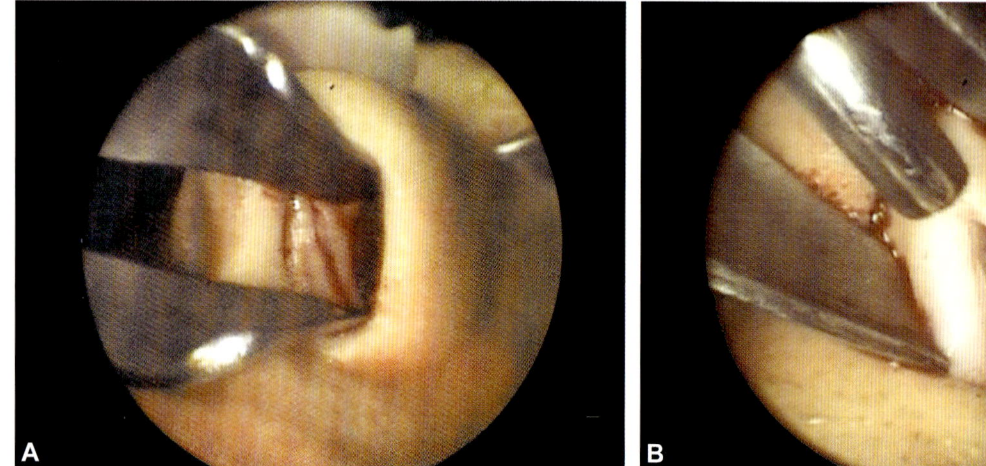

Figs 4A and B: (A) Modified Killian incision; (B) Elevation of the mucoperichondrium

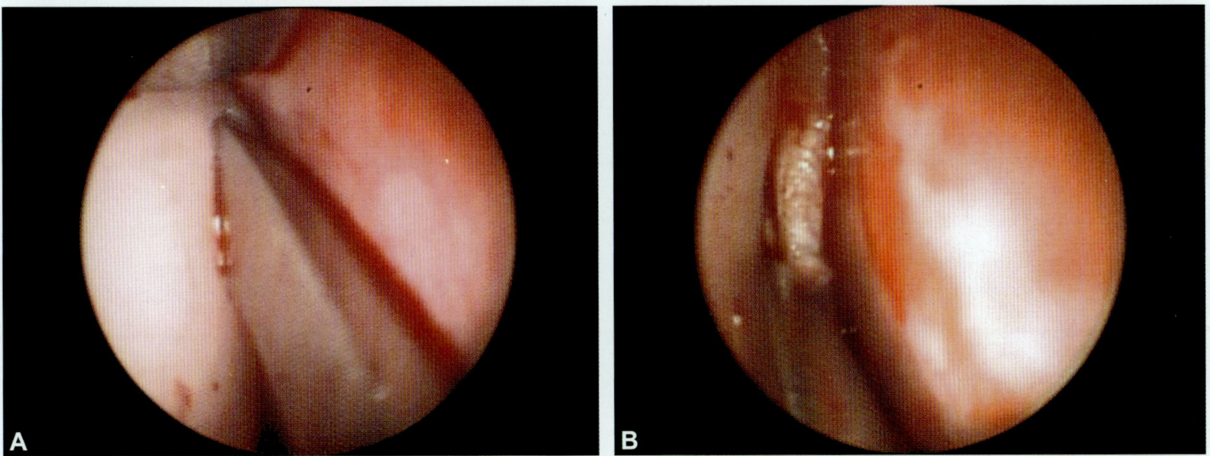

Figs 5A and B: (A) Separating the septal cartilage and the perpendicular plate; (B) Vomer

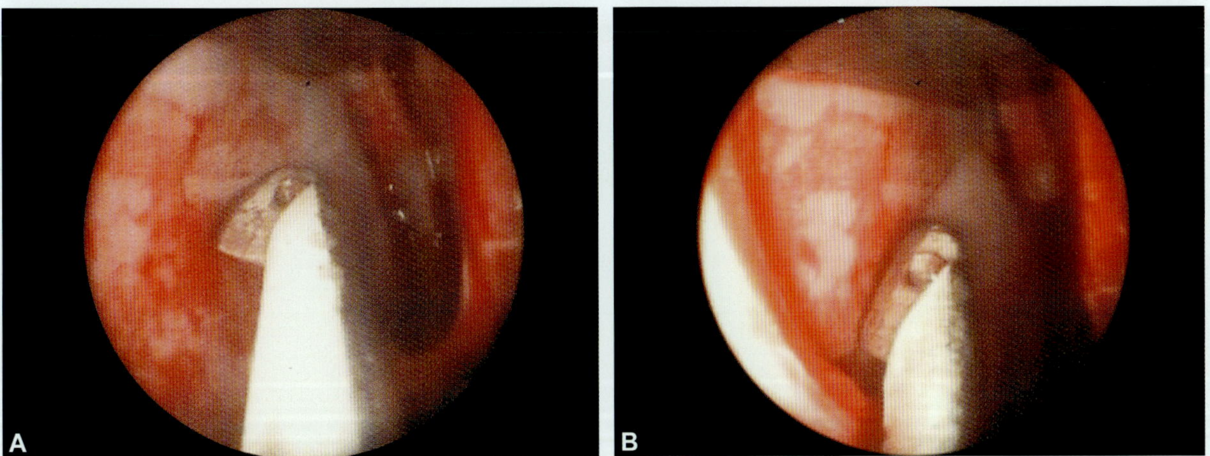

Figs 6A and B: Using D-knife, perform a full-thickness incision parallel to the nasal dorsum while keeping a 1-cm cartilage strut

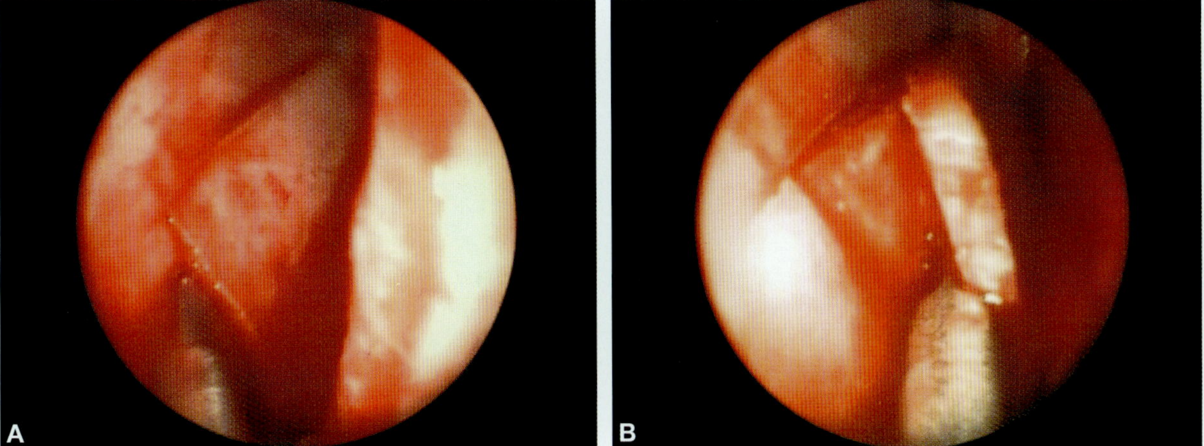

Figs 7A and B: (A) Maintaining a 10-mm distance from the caudal most part of the septum, perform a full-thickness incision parallel to the caudal margin of the septum and then; (B) Dissect out perichondrium on the opposing side

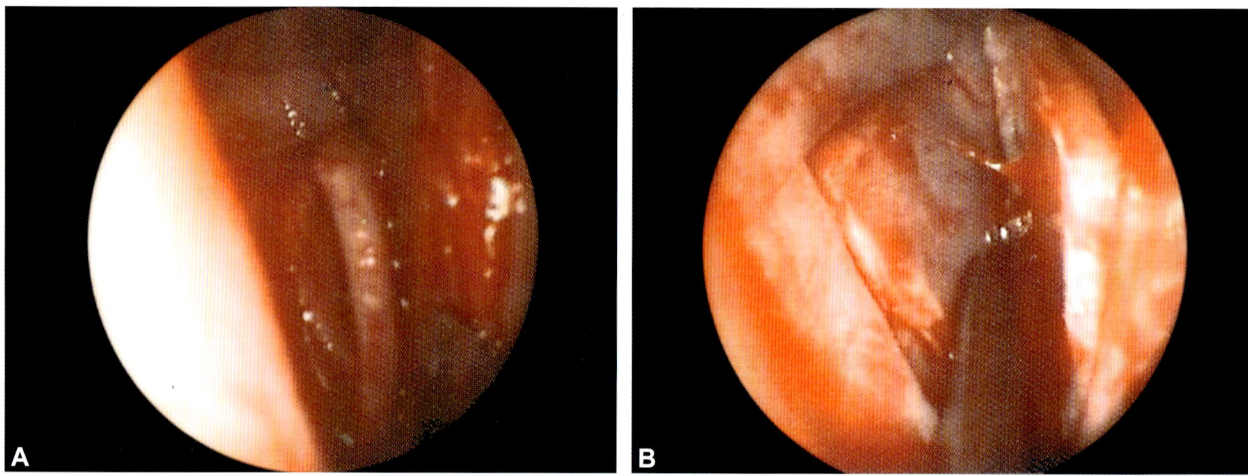

Figs 8A and B: (A) Dissect the perichondrium on the opposite side through the incision area and; (B) Detach the connection to the vomer and maxillary crest

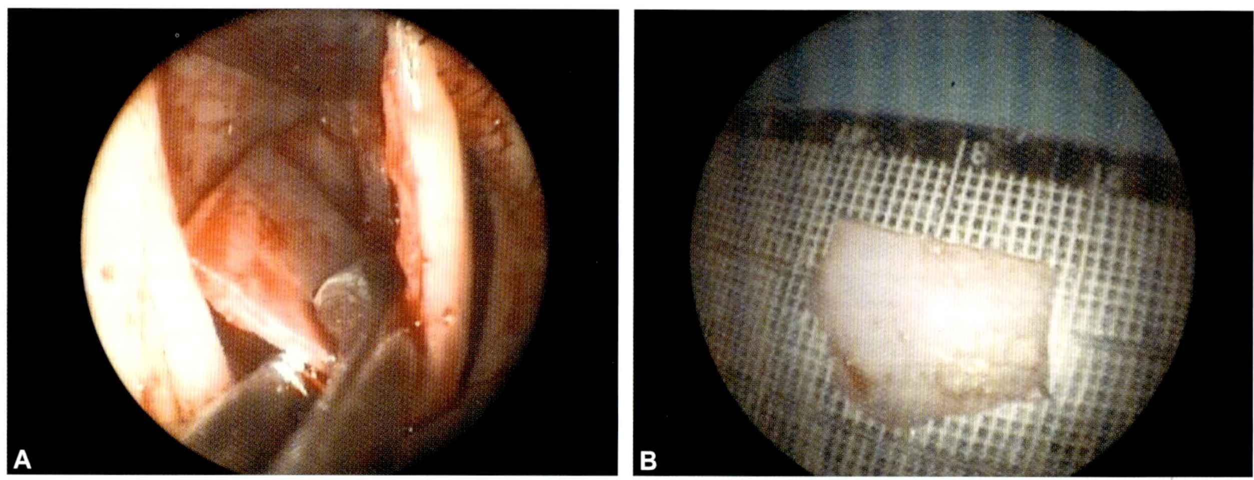

Figs 9A and B: (A) Harvesting the septal cartilage with care using nasal forceps; (B) Photo of an extracted septal cartilage

- Harvest the separated septal cartilage with care using a nasal forceps (Figs 9A and B). After suturing the incision site, perform a through-and-through running quilting suture with vicryl or PDS in the area from which the septum is harvested.

Trimming the septal cartilage (Figs 10A and B)

To perform an augmentation using a nasal septum, as much cartilage as possible must be harvested. And, it is useful to also harvest the bony part. When trimming the cartilage, the absorption rate can be reduced by sparing one side of the perichondrium when the cartilage is used by folding it into a shape of a hinge. First of all, after overlapping the cartilage slices two-fold to obtain a certain level of thickness, stack the remaining cartilage and bony part layer upon layer while suturing them in order to determine the thickness (see Fig. 27). However, the edge of the implant must be made as slim as possible if a protrusion free nasal dorsum is to be created.

Augmentation using a septal cartilage

Although it is difficult to augment the nasal dorsum significantly with a septal cartilage, it is a suitable material for minor augmentation or when the patient is seeking a dorsal augmentation using the autologous tissue. However, to use the septal cartilage to perform augmentation, a relatively large quantity of septal cartilage to perform augmentation, a relatively large quantity of septal cartilage and bone need to be harvested. Also, if the size and width of the harvested cartilage is small, it can lead to

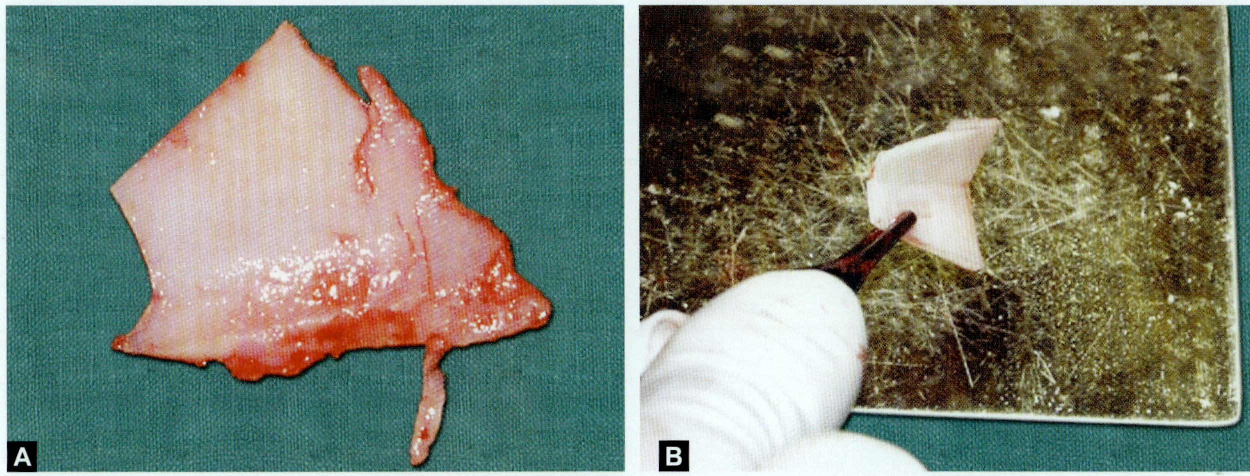

Figs 10A and B: Trimming the septal cartilage

the nasal dorsum looking narrow or protruding. Because the septal cartilage frequently migrates after being grafted, it is useful to fixate it to the nasal dorsum with a suture or needle and, more than anything else, it is important to dissect a proper-sized pocket (Figs 11A to D).

Various uses for septal cartilage

It is easy to harvest and carve the septal cartilage into a straight shape, which allows for it to be used for various purposes, such as tip graft, strut, and septal extension graft.

Conchal Cartilage

Unlike septal cartilage, conchal cartilage has an intrinsic curvature that hampers its routine use in a dorsal augmentation in its original shape. Rather, in surgery on Asian noses, conchal cartilage is more frequently used for nasal tip surgery, to camouflage a partial concavity, or to cover the tip of the silicone implant to prevent extrusion. In addition, the conchal cartilage is frequently too small to yield a cartilage piece suitable for one piece dorsal augmentation. To reduce the visibility and migration of the septal cartilages, and to overcome the limitation in the size, the authors prefer to place the septal cartilage onto the nasal dorsum after gentle crushing using a cartilage crusher. Also, when using conchal cartilage, it may be necessary to overlap pieces of cartilage in their opposite directions of curvature to neutralize their intrinsic curvature.

Technique of harvesting the conchal cartilage

The technique of harvesting the conchal cartilage can be divided largely between harvesting from the front of the ear. Each technique has its own merits and demerits. In the case of harvesting from the back of the ear, it has the advantage of hiding the scar from the frontal view but many pose difficulties for a beginner to accurately locate the area in the front of the ear using a needle. In harvesting from the front of the ear, it is easy to verify the location of the cartilage to be harvested so that harvesting the cartilage is simple. However, it can lead to problems, such as scarring. Whenever possible, harvesting the conchal cartilage with the perichondrium attached on one side can increase its survivability after being transplanted. Also, the crust of the helix, which is also called the support framework of the ear, must be left untouched. It is preferable that the cymba concha in the upper area and the cavum concha at the lower area be harvested separately (Figs 12A to C).

Application of the conchal cartilage

Because of its intrinsic curvature, it is difficult to use the conchal cartilage for dorsal augmentation. However, it can be used for tip graft, camouflage grafting, etc. The biggest advantage of a conchal cartilage is that it can be harvested in a composite graft so that the cartilage can be harvested with the skin. This composite graft can be applied usefully to correct an alar retraction (Figs 13A to C).

Costal Cartilage

Although costal cartilage is difficult to harvest and is associated with more serious donor site morbidity, such as pneumothorax, as well as the problem of warping, it is the most useful autologous cartilage for substantial augmentation or in patients who have experienced complications with alloplastic implants. Although strongly advocated by some surgeons of its routine use for Asian rhinoplasty, during the primary rhinoplasty, however, it is very difficult to persuade Asian women to use costal cartilage because the harvesting procedure leaves scars on the chest. One

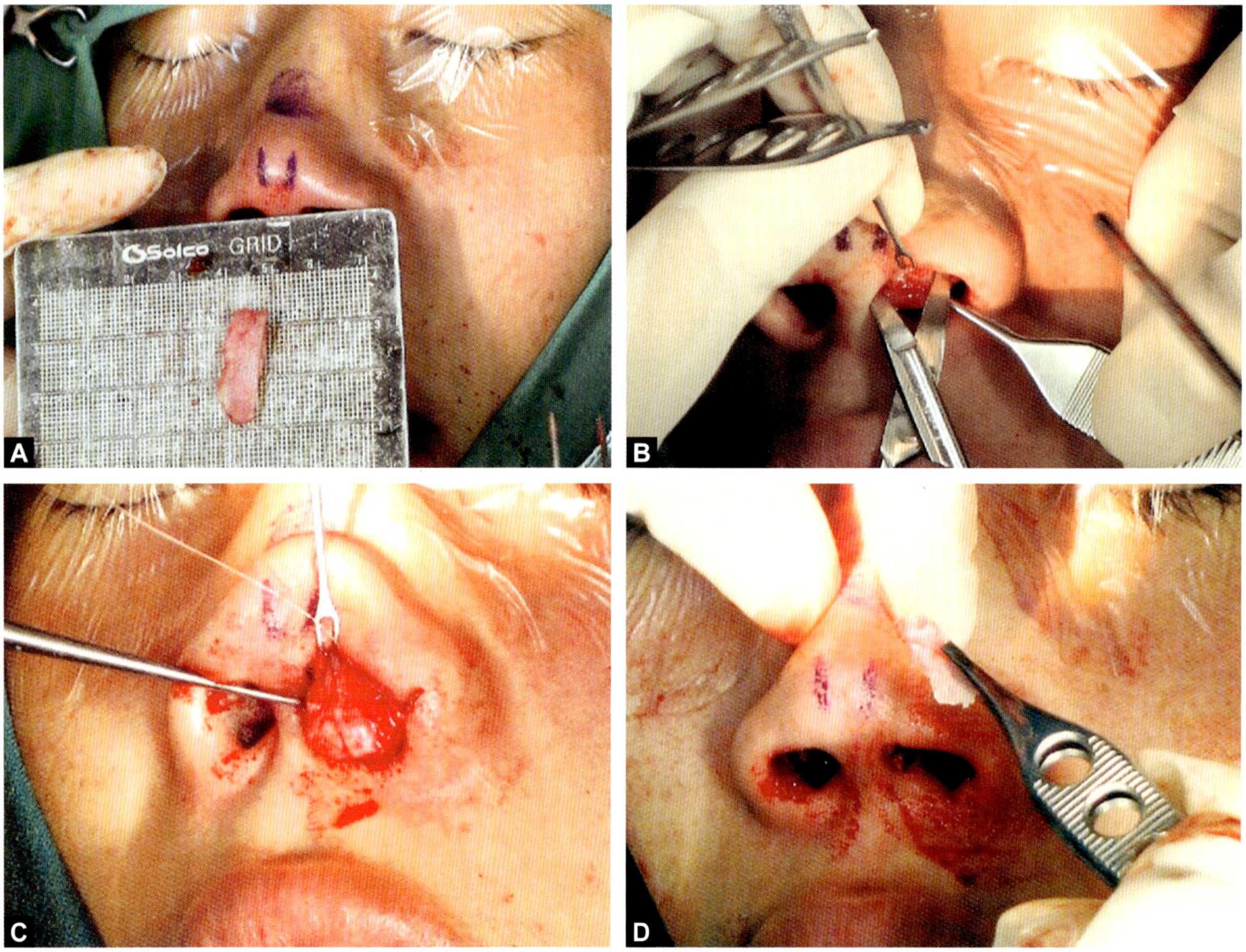

Figs 11A to D: Example of an augmentation being performed on a patient with a slight saddle nose using a septal cartilage. (A) After harvesting the septal cartilage, overlap it three-fold and trim it to match the depression area. After performing a marginal incision (B); undertake a cephalic resection and tip plasty (C). (D) Insert the septal cartilage graft and fixate it with a needle to prevent any movement

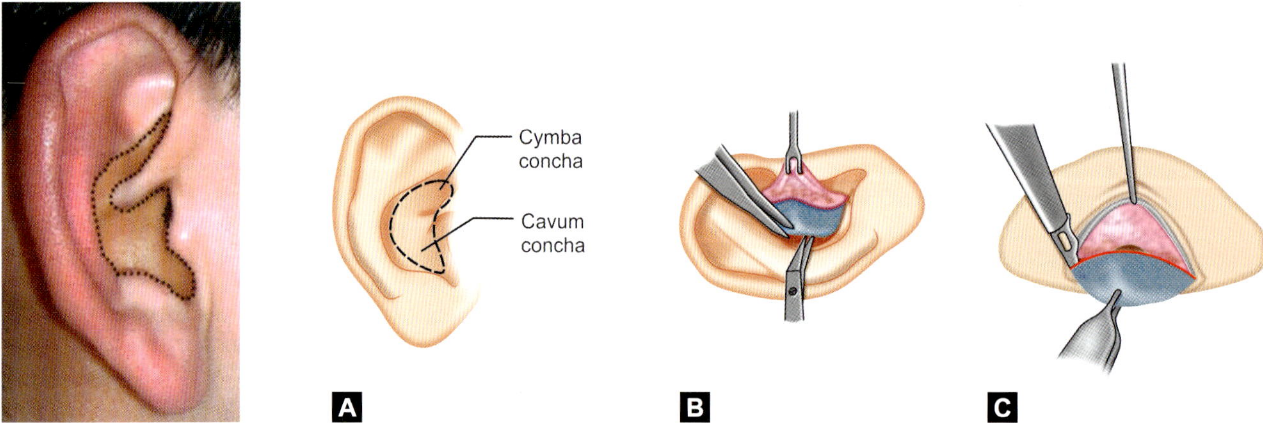

Figs 12A to C: (A) Region for harvesting the conchal cartilage; (B) Technique of harvesting from the front of the ear and; (C) From the rear

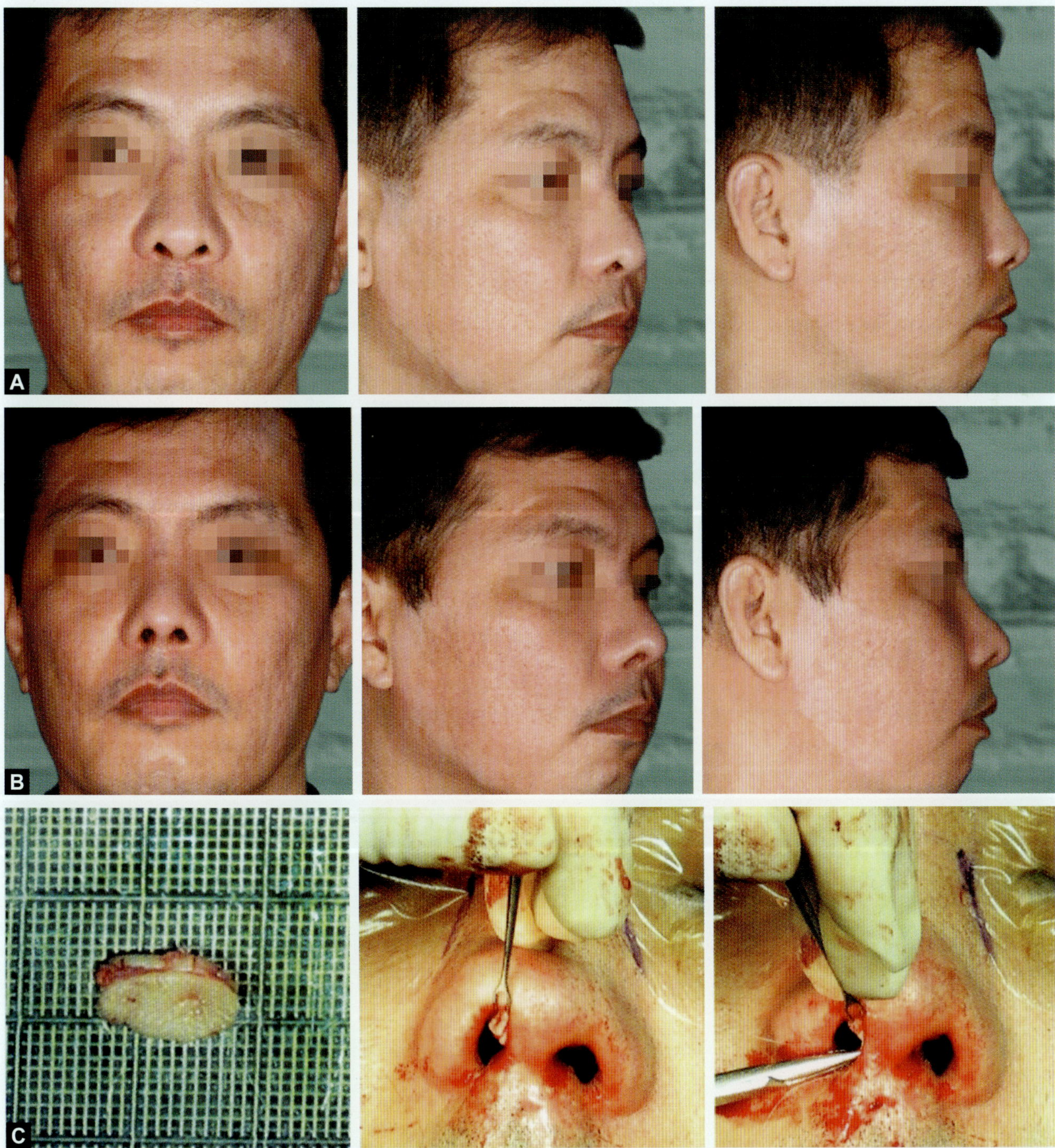

Figs 13A to C: (A) A patient presenting a blunt tip and alar retraction prior to surgery; (B) Appearance of the blunt tip and alar retraction improved using a composite graft (conchal cartilage and skin) and septal extension graft; (C) Photographs of the surgery

other critically important limitation of autologous tissue is that, except for only a few highly-experienced surgeons, most rhinoplasty surgeons have difficulty using these implants to form an esthetically pleasing nose, resulting in a high revision rate.

Techniques of harvesting the costal cartilage

- Select the location of the cartilage to be harvested. In case of a woman or when the breast is large, it is fine to harvest the fourth or fifth costal cartilage. But when harvesting in large quantity or in case of a beginner, it is preferable to harvest from the broad cartilage area of the sixth or seventh rib. Once the cartilage to be harvested is chosen, as it is often difficult to verify the exact position of the costal cartilage once it has been draped, it is advisable to premark the position while tracing from the eleventh costal cartilage onward. When there is an assistant who will harvest the cartilage during surgery, it is preferable for the cartilage to be harvested from the left. When the surgeon is operating from the right, harvesting the cartilage by himself, it is best to harvest the cartilage from the right.
- It is desirable for the size of the incision to be small but, when it is overly small, it can restrict the surgical exposure and, by forcing the skin to be overly retracted during the incision, often cause scarring. Thus, an incision line of about 3–4 cm is suitable. The incision should always be performed in concert with frequent efforts to verify the costal cartilage area with the fingers in order to accurately confirm the surgical plane. If this is difficult due to excessive amount of fat, using a needle to verify the location of the costal cartilage can be helpful. While doing this, damage to the skin must be minimized and, due to the restricted view, a thorough hemostasis is needed. Additionally, in case of patients with a thick fatty layer, excision part of the fatty tissue for re-insertion, after the cartilage is harvested, can prevent a postsurgical wound depression or seroma formation (Figs 14A and B).
- After the fascia of the external abdominal oblique muscle is exposed, do not excise the muscle but, rather carefully, dissect in between the muscle. While doing this, damage to the fascia and the muscle must be minimized in order to minimize the postoperative pain. In addition, as oozing can occur from the dissected muscle, a thorough hemostasis is necessary to obtain a good exposure and to prevent the occurrence of a postoperative hematoma (Figs 15A and B).
- Dissecting between the external abdominal oblique muscle will allow the perichondrium of the costal cartilage to be inspected. After exposing the superficial part of the perichondrium of the cartilage, make an incision line at the perichondrium with a knife and then perform dissection using a periosteal elevator or Freer elevator. All following manipulation must be performed on the inside of the perichondrium for it to be safe. Dissecting the perichondrium at the superficial part of the cartilage is relatively easy but the upper and lower area is so firmly attached that it is best to dissect this area carefully, a la slowly stripping the onion. And, although it is proper to dissect the whole length of the cartilage, rather than forcefully perform dissection while the surgical exposure is poor, it is better to dissect just two third of the radius. In particular, the surgeon must be particularly careful not to exert too much force while dissecting in order

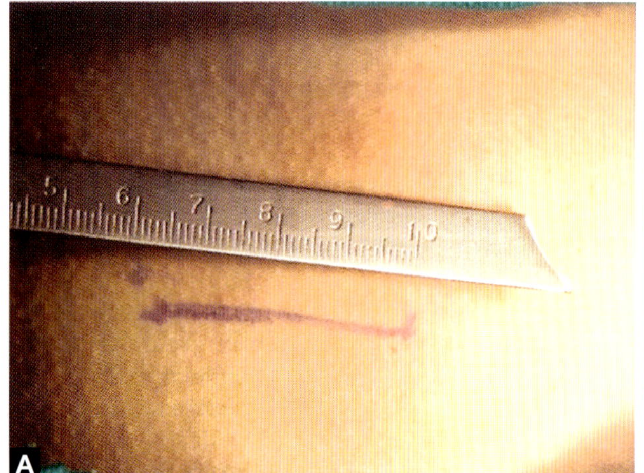

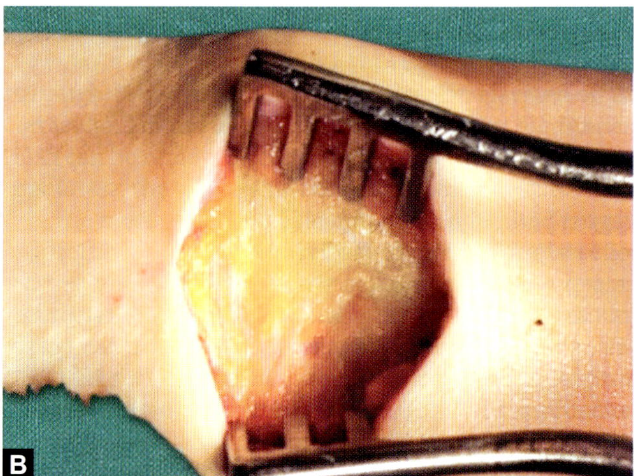

Figs 14A and B: (A) After marking the incision line at the seventh costal cartilage area; (B) Dissect all the way down the fatty layer of the superficial fascia

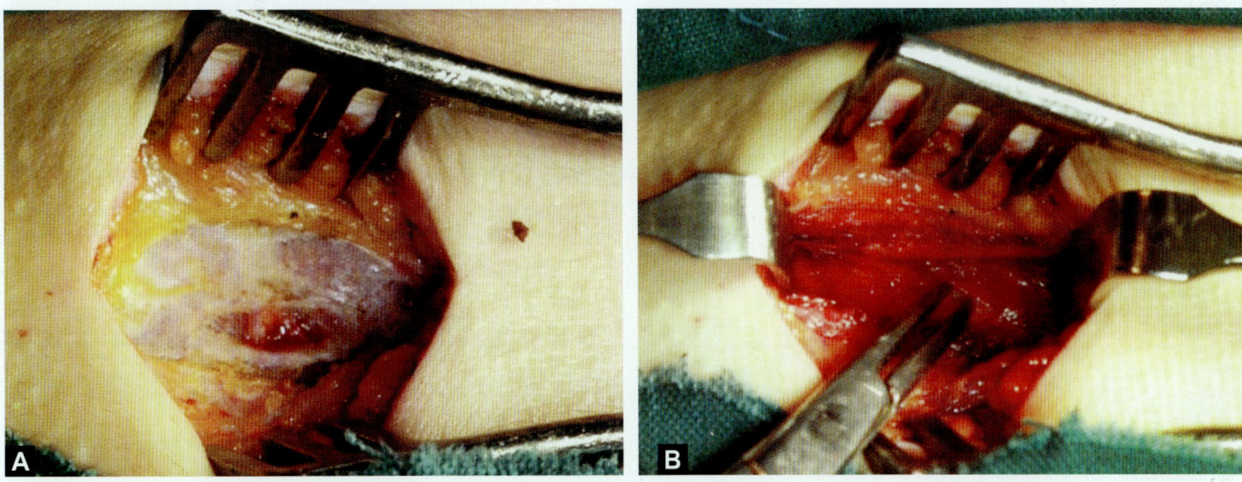

Figs 15A and B: (A) After the fascia of the external abdominal oblique muscle is exposed; (B) Use a mosquito forceps to carefully spread the muscles by dissecting in between the muscles

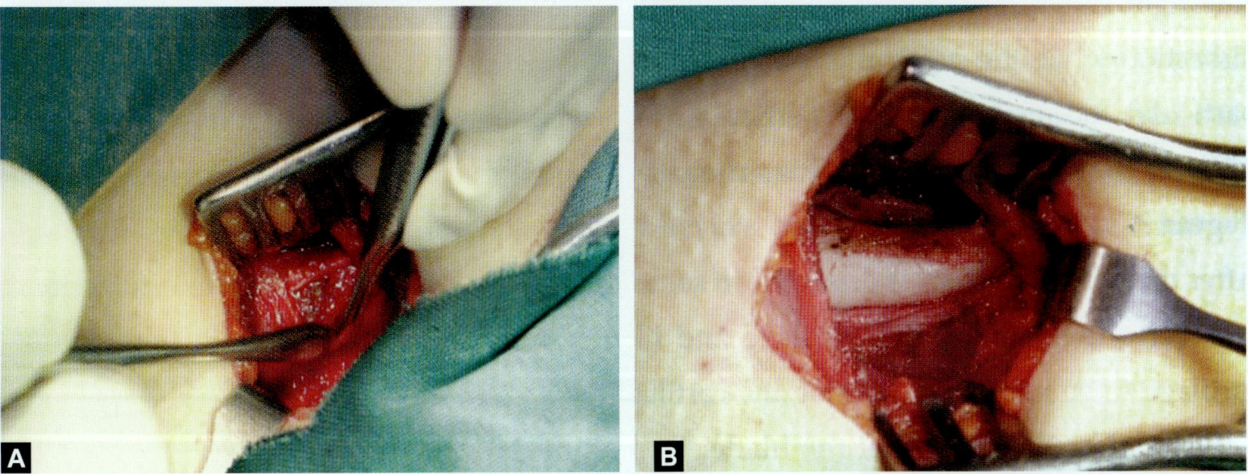

Figs 16A and B: (A) Surgical photos showing a perichondrium being dissected and; (B) After the dissection is performed

to prevent the surgical instrument from entering too deeply and tearing the pleura (Figs 16A and B).

- After the perichondrium is dissected to some extent, make a partial incision line at the junction between the bone and the cartilage, and likewise make an incision at the edge of the cartilage to be harvested. Cutting the cartilaginous area in increments rather than at once can prevent pleural damage by the blade. By hooking one side of the Dorian elevator to the cartilage and lifting up the costal cartilage by dissecting it from one side, the cartilaginous area attached to the perichondrium will fall off naturally, enabling it to be harvested. It is important that the edge of the Dorian elevator be inserted in a careful manner so that it does not stick to the pleura. The risk of damaging the pleura is greatest during this maneuver (Figs 17A and B). The pleura can be torn slightly when a particularly string force is exerted during the dissection so that the instrument enters too deeply. In such a case, the torn area can be sutured while the lung is expanded. However, if the tear is too large, first insert a nelaton catheter into the thoracic cavity and, while the suction is placed in position, suture the circumference of the nelaton catheter with a vicryl 3-0 so that the perimeter of the nelaton can be closed in a pulse-string shape. Then, if the suture is swiftly performed as the nelaton is being removed, the chest tube need not be inserted after surgery (Figs 18A and B).
- After the costal cartilage is harvested, it is deemed essential that a saline solution should be poured in and the chest pressed down to verify the existence of air

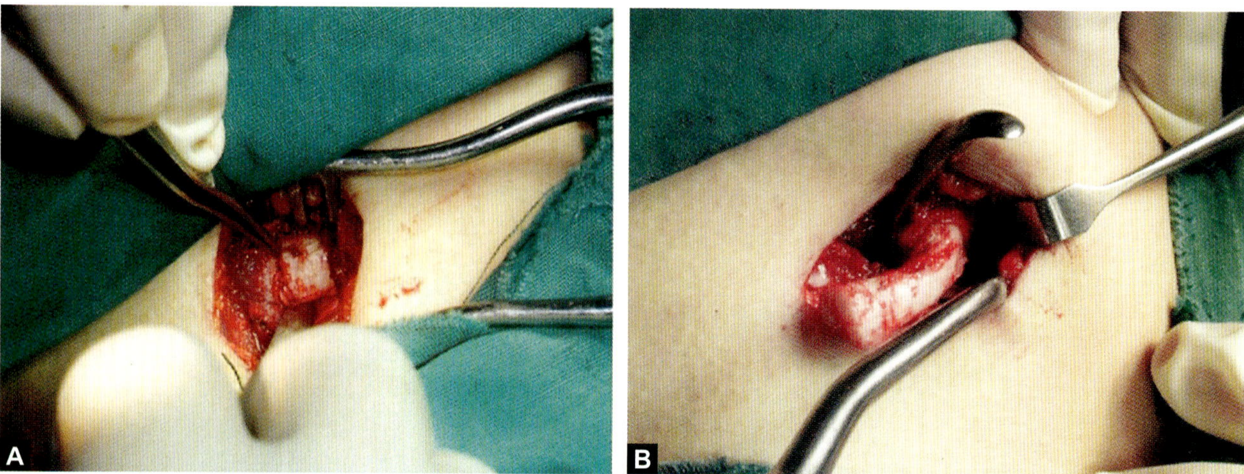

Figs 17A and B: (A) Photos of a cartilage being excised using a knife and then; (B) Being lifted using a Dorian elevator

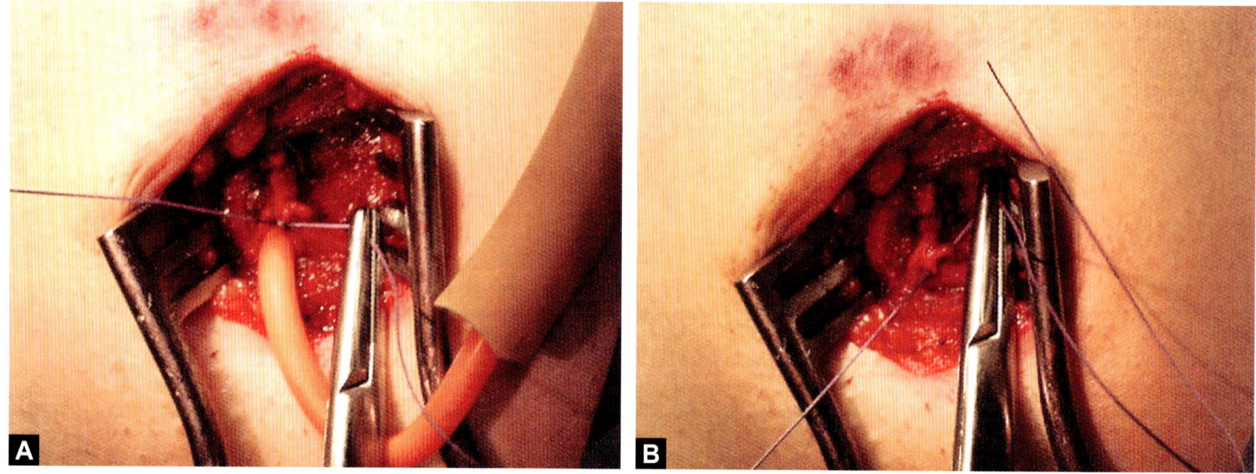

Figs 18A and B: (A) After connecting a suction to the nelaton, perform a purse-string suture around the nelaton and then; (B) Suture the laceration area rapidly while pulling out the nelaton

bubbles due to pneumothorax followed by saline irrigation and hemostasis. If needed, bone wax can be used for the hemostasis (Figs 19A and B). When repairing the cartilage harvest area, each layer must be sutured separately and if there isn't any particularly severe oozing, placement of a drain is not necessary and the stitch-out is usually performed on the seventh day.

Trimming the costal cartilage

Warping, graft visibility, and unnatural looking noses are common complications of augmentation using costal cartilage (Figs 20A and B). To avoid warping, it is best to soak the cartilage in saline solution to let the maximal warping occur, and perform careful carving after a certain time elapsed (Fig. 21A). To reduce the risk of warping, the authors prefer to use costal cartilage in a laminated form (Fig. 21B). So, harvested costal cartilage was cut into several vertical strips and placed in saline solution during initial warping.

Dorsal augmentation using a costal cartilage

Costal cartilage is one of the best autologous implants, in cases where a substantial amount of augmentation is needed, where a previous graft is causing a rejection or infection, or where a patient requests for an augmentation using an autologous implant (Figs 22A to C).

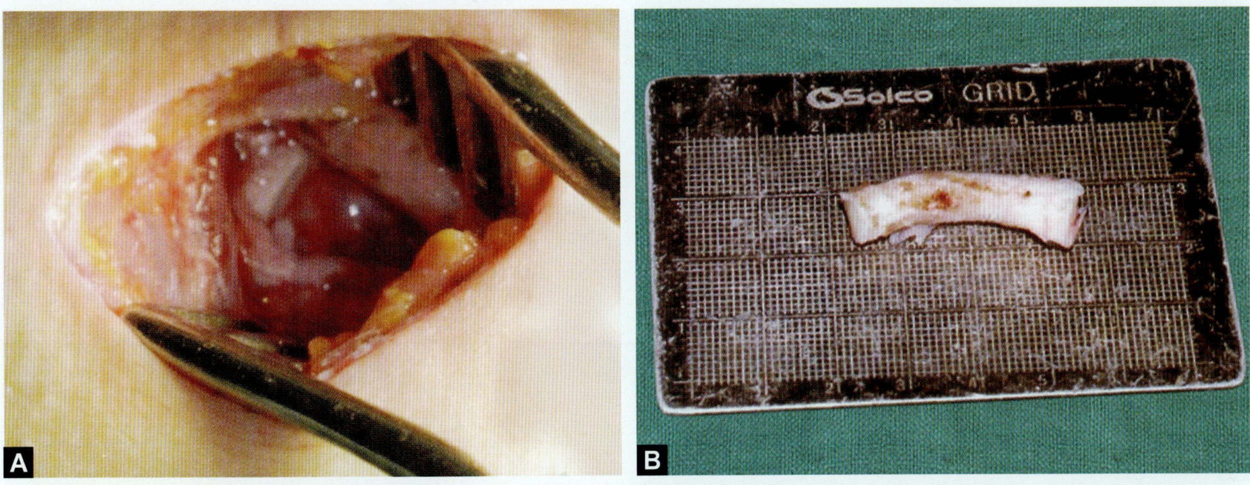

Figs 19A and B: (A) An image showing the wound filled with saline solution after the costal cartilage has been harvested to check for air bubbles and; (B) A harvested costal cartilage

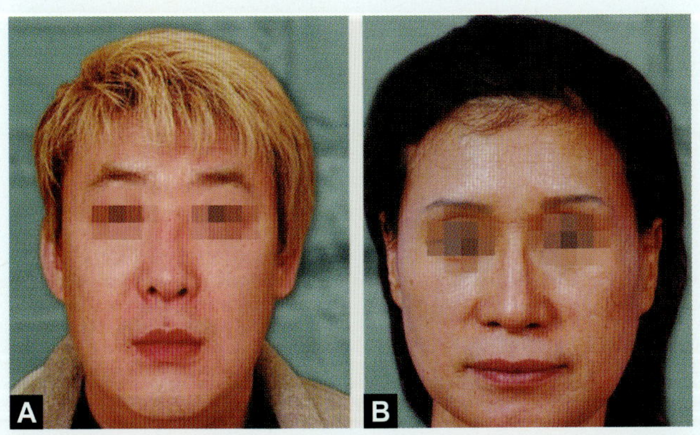

Figs 20A and B: Patients showing cartilage warping (A); and visible graft contour (B), years after dorsal augmentation using autologous costal cartilage

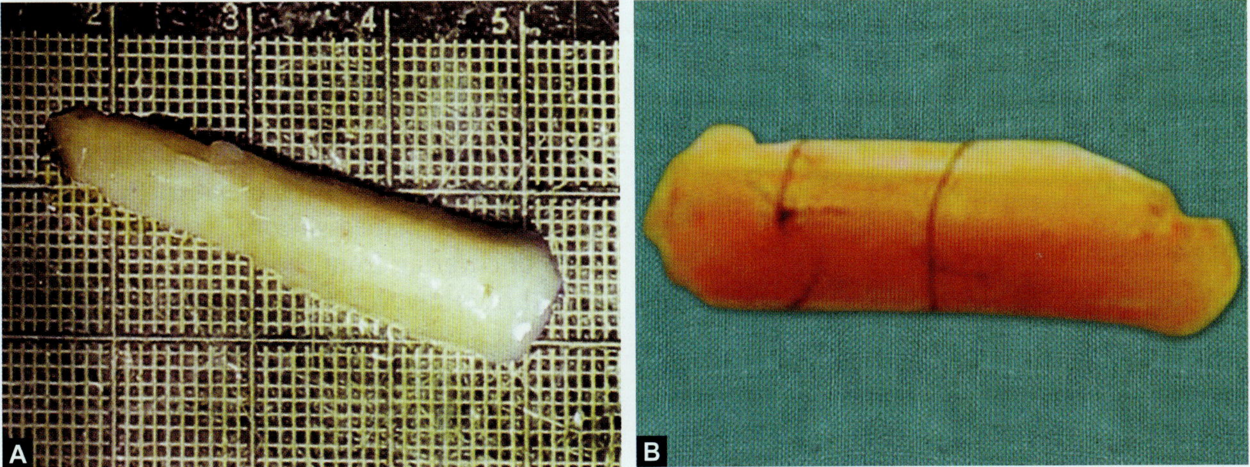

Figs 21A and B: (A) To avoid warping, it is best to soak the cartilage in saline solution to let the maximal warping occur, and to perform careful carving after a certain time has elapsed; (B) Laminated costal cartilage graft for nasal dorsum

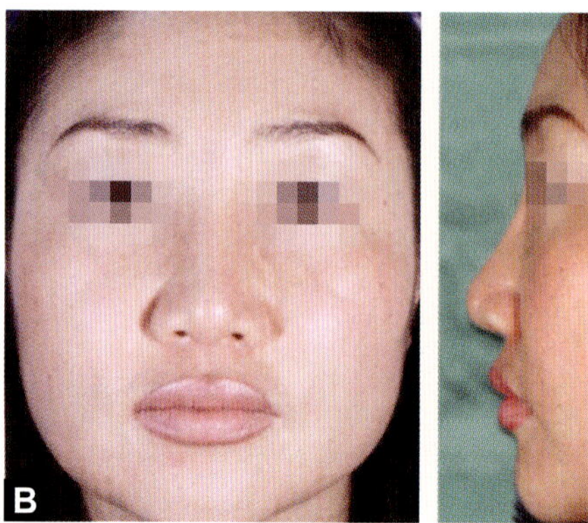

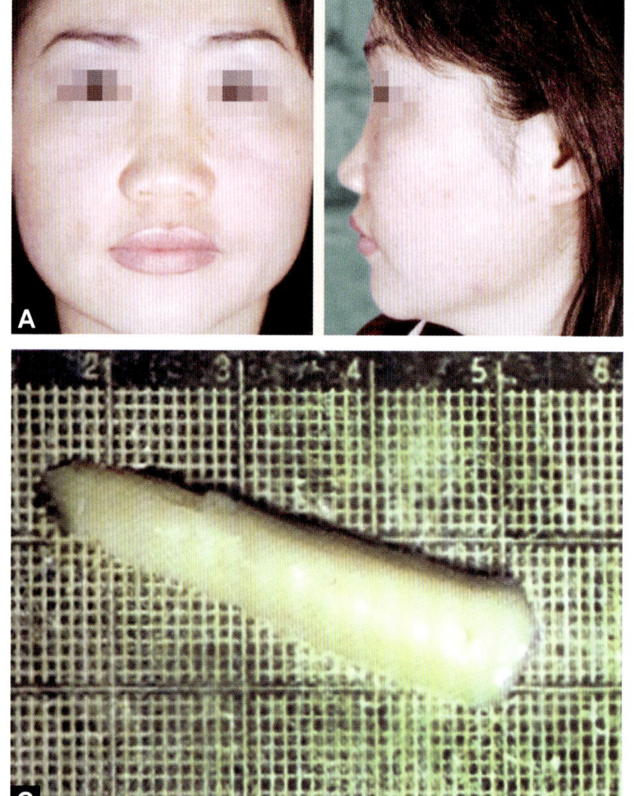

Figs 22A to C: A case where a patient with a lowered nasal dorsum requested for an autologous implant surgery and received a dorsal augmentation and nasal tip surgery using the costal cartilage; (A) Preoperative; (B) Postoperative and; (C) Extracted costal cartilage

Application of the conchal cartilage

The greatest advantage of a costal cartilage is an autologous implant that is relatively solid and has a low rate of resorption. Therefore, it can be used variously, in areas requiring hardness and volume. It is particularly useful in cases where a strong tip support is needed due to the contracture of the nose resulting from a previous surgery or accident and when a strong tip projection is needed (Figs 23A and B).

Autologous Fascia

Autologous fascia, including temporalis fascia, can be used in rhinoplasty as radix graft or dorsal onlay grafts. However, harvesting autologous fascia requires an additional incision and hence, is associated with additional morbidity. Furthermore, it is not always possible to harvest sufficient fascia of reasonable thickness, because harvested fascia shrinks in volume as it dries, and when wet, it is hard to manipulate. Comparing with the temporalis fascia, fascia lata can provide a sufficient amount of connective tissue with significant thickness suitable for dorsal augmentation. However, harvesting this tissue also requires additional incision distant from the main operative field. Nonetheless, in rhinoplasty, fascia lata could be used for dorsal augmentation, especially in secondary rhinoplasty for the correction of a failed alloplastic implant. One other advantage of fascia is that this material, placed right underneath the skin and over the crushed or morselized cartilage, or used after wrapping up the morselized cartilage, can nicely camouflage the irregular contour of diced cartilage or crushed cartilage, maximizing the full use of the small pieces of autologous tissues left behind after other procedures, and making it an alternative method of dorsal augmentation (Fig. 24).

Studies have shown that diced cartilage-fascia wrapped grafts survived and demonstrated normal cartilage survival.

Dermofat

Dermofat, harvested from various locations, can also be used in dorsal augmentation. Although dermofat can be harvested in great quantities, its absorption is difficult to predict, making it unsuitable for substantial dorsal augmentation. However, dermofat can be useful for

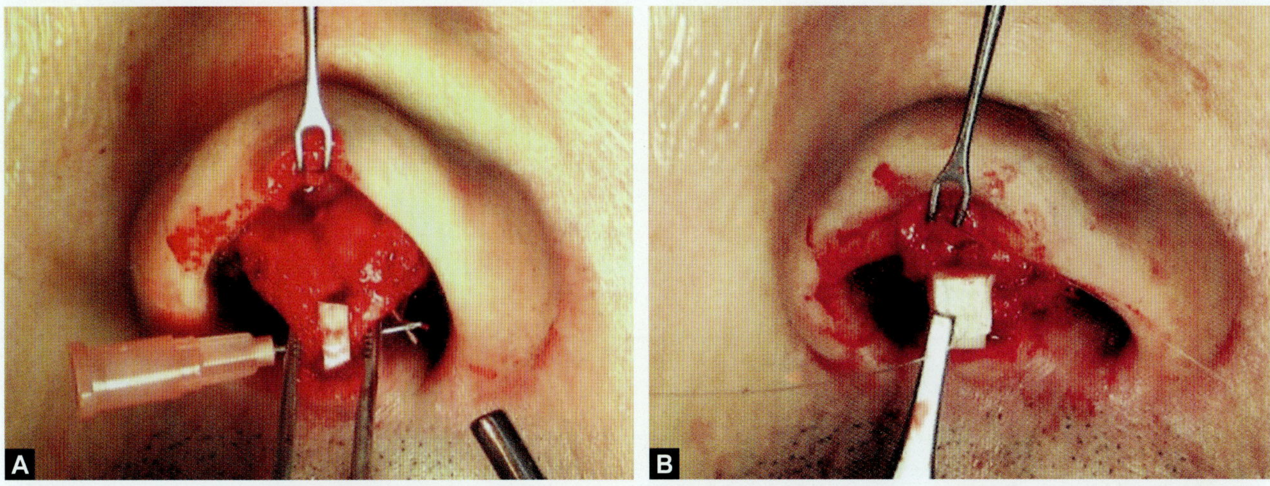

Figs 23A and B: Columellar strut and tip graft from a costal cartilage

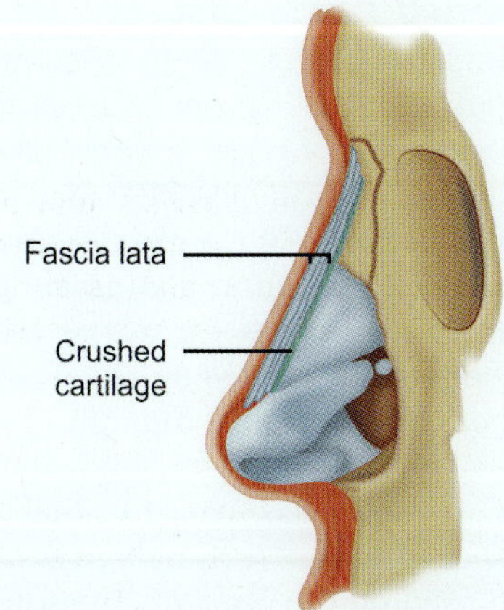

Fig. 24: Dorsal augmentation using fascia with crushed cartilage

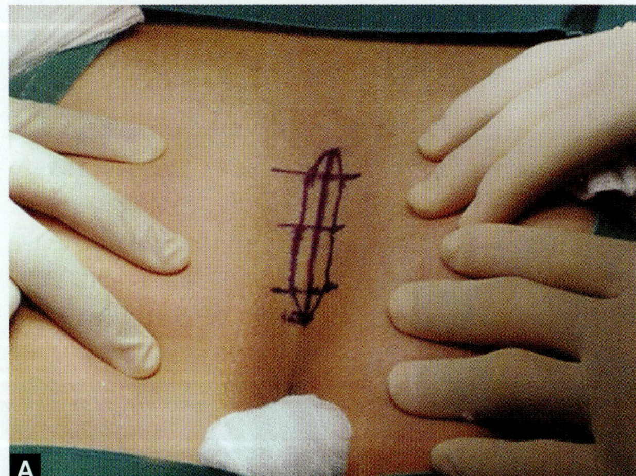

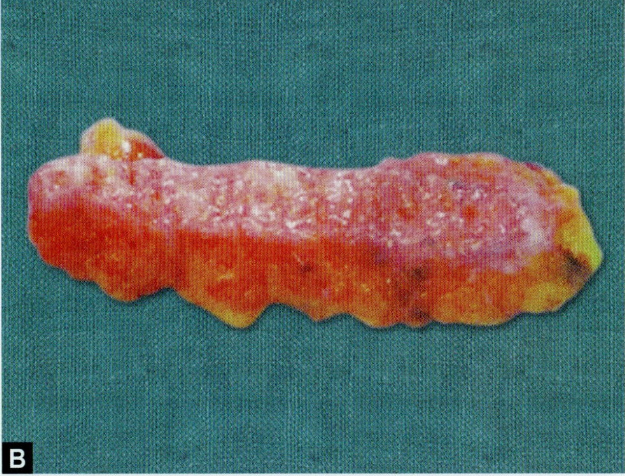

Figs 25A and B: (A) Harvesting dermofat from coccygeal area and; (B) Harvested dermofat

patients with thin skin or contracture of the nose due to complicated primary rhinoplasty.

Harvesting the dermofat

Though it is possible to harvest the dermis-fat from various regions, it is mostly harvested from the buttock below the coccyx or from the inguinal area (Figs 25A and B). However, although this area offers the advantage that the dermofat can be harvested in large quantity, it also has the disadvantage that the surgical area will be broad and performing dressing after surgery will be difficult. It is best to minimize the incision during harvesting and the damage to the dermofat from forceps if the absorption rate is to be reduced. Also, this area being in frequent friction, the skin suture should be performed with the greatest precision to prevent the dehiscence of the skin. Furthermore,

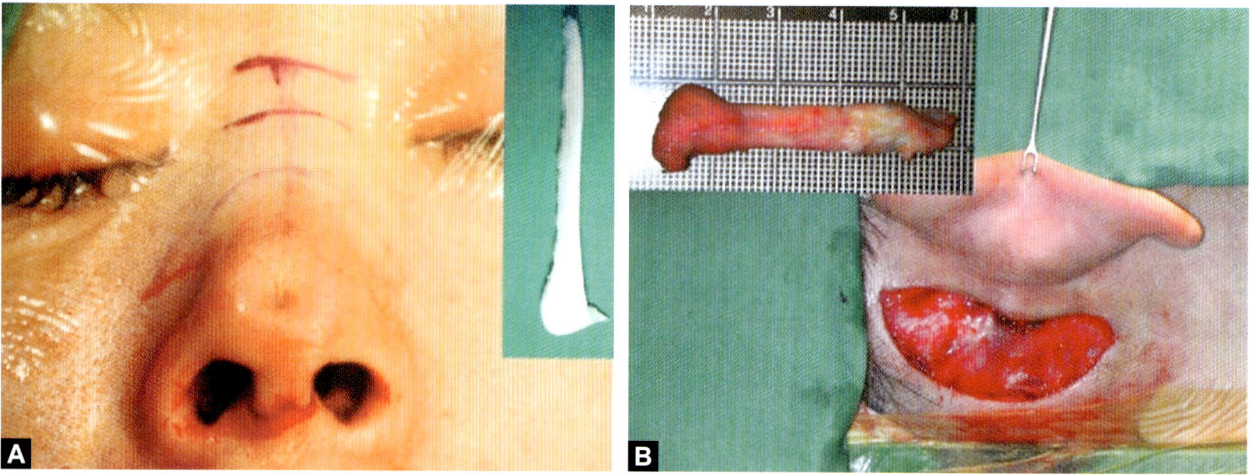

Figs 26A and B: Postauricular dermofat and Gore-Tex was used to perform a dorsal augmentation as well as tip surgery

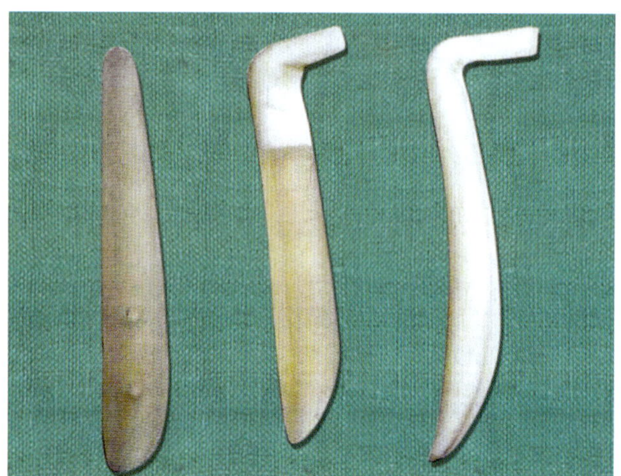

Fig. 27: Various shapes of prefabricated silicone implants

a thorough hemostasis is of an utmost importance. In the case of the author, the use of a postauricular dermofat is usually favored because of such advantages as the donor site being within the same surgical field of head and neck area, and that it is easy to perform disinfection with limited scarring (Figs 26A and B).

Homologous Tissue or Tissue Allograft

Homologous Costal Cartilage

Homologous costal cartilage can be used in revision rhinoplasties requiring structural reconstruction of the nasal framework, but in which patients resist harvesting their own costal cartilage.

Tutoplast Processed Fascia Lata

Tutoplast processed fascia lata (TPFL) is commercially available homograft fascia that has been successfully used as human tissue grafts for physical support procedures, such as slings for stress incontinence, filler material, facial paralysis or congenital ptosis. The author has used TPFL in rhinoplasty for dorsal and radix onlay grafts. TPFL can be used for smoothening grafts for dorsal irregularity following correction of a deviated nose, as additional graft material when an inadequate amount of septal or conchal cartilage is available for dorsal augmentation, in patients who dislike using of alloplastic material for dorsal augmentation, for complicated revision surgery in which silicone has been used on the dorsum. The soft contour of TPFL means that it can be nicely blended with the overlying skin soft tissue envelope.

Silicone

Nasal dorsal augmentation with silicone rubber is the most popular rhinoplasty procedure in Eastern Asia. Due to its stable chemical structure, silicone has several advantages including its lack of tissue reaction and ease of handling. Moreover, the availability of readymade products makes application convenient and the relative hardness of silicone makes it suitable for fashioning the desired nasal shape for Asians with a thick skin. The skin of Asians is thicker than that of Caucasians, so there is a lower risk of an implant extrusion after surgery. The prefabricated products can be divided largely into L-and I-shaped implants (Fig. 27). Because the nasal tip area is an area that is always exposed to exterior stimulation, the use of L-shaped silicone carries a higher risk of extrusion, regardless of the thickness of nasal subcutaneous tissue in Asians. Thus, a placement of I-shaped implant at the nasal dorsum area, and tip plasty using an autologous material (septal cartilage, conchal cartilage) at the nasal tip area, is the preferable surgical method.

Trimming the Silicone

- In most cases, problem arises from trying to remove too much quantity all at once using a #15 blade or #11 blade, so that the desired length fails to materialize or the silicone becomes torn so that a new silicone becomes needed. Therefore, if the surgeon is a novice, he should give up trying to carve the silicone cleanly all at once but rather concentrate on trimming the silicone slowly and with care. Also, he should prefabricate the silicone to some extent and keep it sterilized.
- Most readymade products are 4.5–5.0 cm × 8–10 mm in size and the decision regarding the length of the silicone should be based on the distance between the nasion or nasal root to the supratip area. Also, it should preferably be about 3.5–4.0 cm long, about 8 mm wide, and the edge should be made as thin as possible. At this point, it is convenient to have the line, between the eyelashes of the upper eyelid and the supratarsal fold, act as a starting point of augmentation.

Method of Inserting the Silicone

To insert the silicone, an open rhinoplasty approach or an endonasal approach is used. As with other implants, when inserting silicone, one must be mindful of the following aspects:

- The subperiosteal placement of silicone implant may lead to the resorption of the underlying nasal bone by exerting too much pressure. However, if it is inserted above the periosteum, the implant can shift when touched and become visible. Therefore, the implant must be inserted within the subperiosteal space and, even with the risk of bone resorption, in reality that is not a problem because a relatively thick fibrous capsule gets formed around the implant (Figs 28A and B).

  To create a precise pocket, make a small incision at an area 5–6 mm lateral to the midline of the keystone area using a Joseph knife and then insert a periosteal elevator into the subperiosteal space, and gradually create a pocket towards the midline.
- The size of the pocket should be made slightly larger than the implant, with just enough space for the implant and a surgical tool holding the implant to be jammed through. Also, a space needs to be created evenly on either side. If not, and one side is made larger than the other, the implant can break away from the center and, if a hematoma occurs within the pocket, the implant can incline towards one side.
- The nasal dorsum and the base of silicone should be trimmed to the point that they almost adhere closely together. Otherwise, the implant will become detached and a seesaw phenomenon occurs after surgery, causing a hematoma to form and the implant to become deviated and show through the skin.

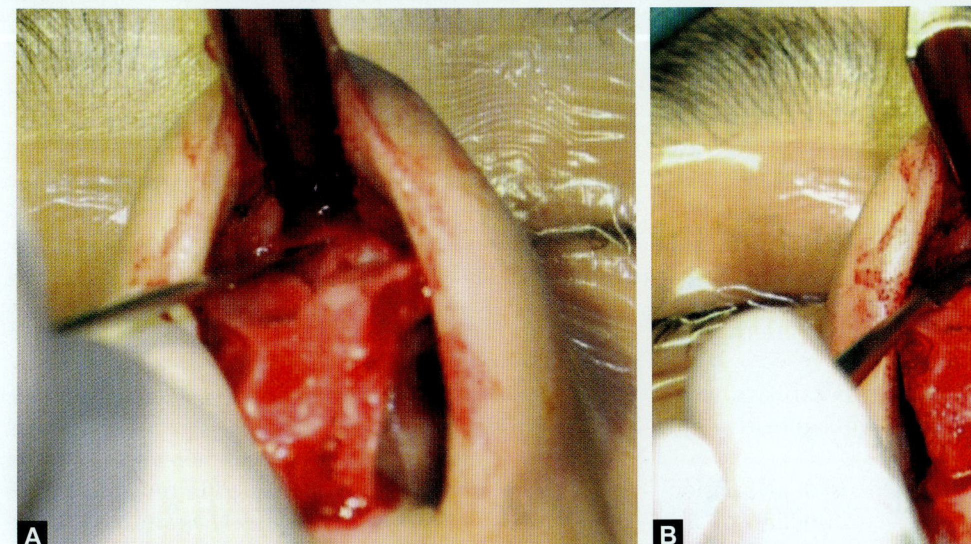

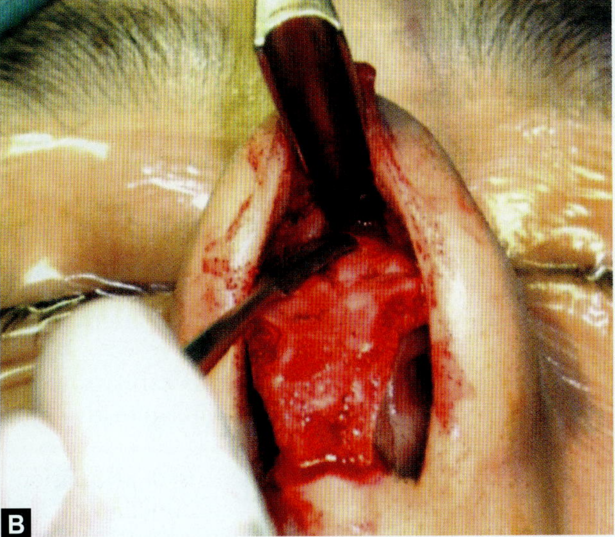

Figs 28A and B: After incising the junctional area between the bone and the cartilage with a Joseph knife (A); carefully perform dissection with an elevator (B)

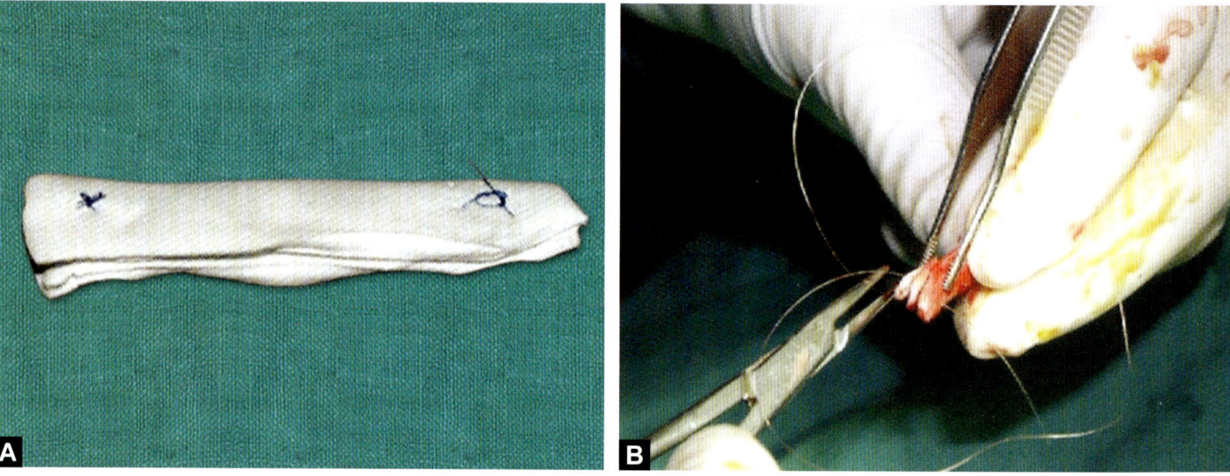

Figs 29A and B: (A) Method of suturing a Gore-Tex sheet together and; (B) Additionally fastening the sheets to the area requiring partial insertion of Gore-Tex

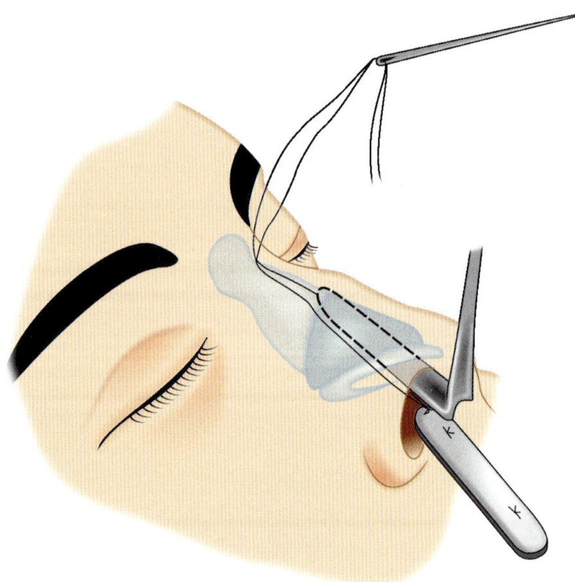

Fig. 30: Method of inserting a sheet-shaped Gore-Tex using a thread

- Deviated nose must be corrected prior to inserting the silicone.
- It is preferable to use an autologous cartilage when operating on the nasal tip to avoid inflammation and silicone extrusion.

Gore-Tex

Gore-Tex (expanded polytetrafluoroethylene:ePTFE), next to silicone, is the most widely used alloplastic implant in Asian noses and currently, its use is on the increase. Gore-Tex implants are porous inducing the surrounding tissue to grow inward through the pore, and have the advantages of increased stability and lower incidence of capsule formation. In addition, the risk of extrusion is lower with Gore-Tex than with silicone. The soft texture of Gore-Tex reduces patient discomfort and the occurrence of unnatural visible graft contours through the skin. One important disadvantage of Gore-Tex is that it decreases in volume after insertion. In addition, it is more difficult to remove a Gore-Tex implant than a silicone implant.

Method of Trimming and Inserting Gore-Tex According to Each Individual Type

- Sheet-shaped Gore-Tex
  - *Trimming a sheet-shaped Gore-Tex*: Sheet-shaped Gore-Tex is 2 mm thick and usually, according to the intended degree of augmentation, a sheet 8 mm wide should be multilayered with two-fold (4 mm) to three-fold (6 mm) and used. While doing this, suture both ends with nylon or PDS to prevent the sheet from opening up and then the supratip side must be trimmed as thin as possible into a triangular shape while the end of the nasion area must also be trimmed and made as thin as possible (Figs 29A and B).
  - *Technique of inserting a sheet-shaped Gore-Tex*: Because Gore-Tex sheet, unlike silicone, is soft and has a low solidity, care must be taken to prevent it from folding while it is being inserted. Method of insertion can be divided largely between two types as shown in the Figures 30 and 31, and it is all right for the surgeon to choose the method of his choice. Only, make sure to feel for the nasal dorsum

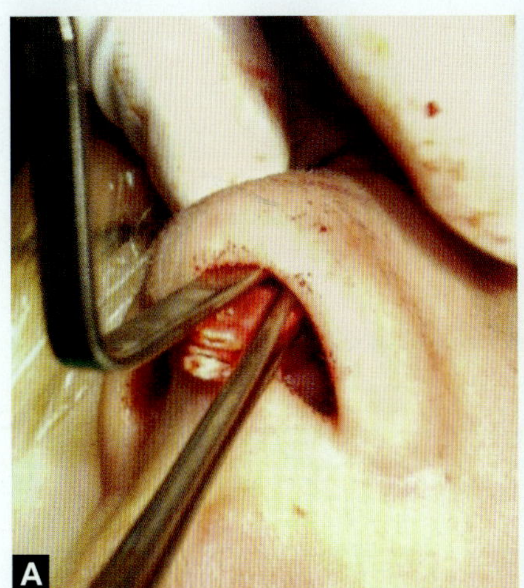

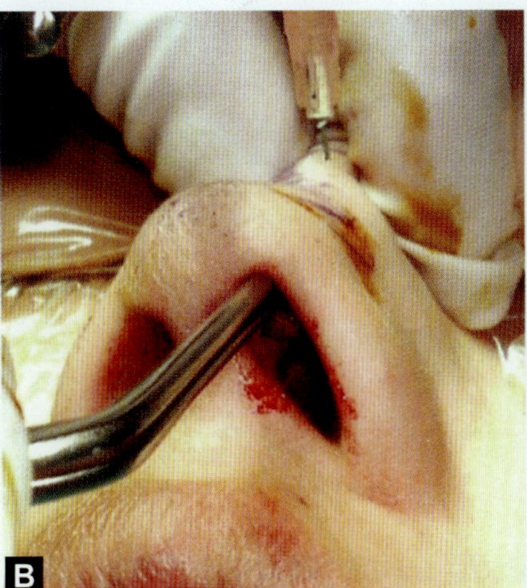

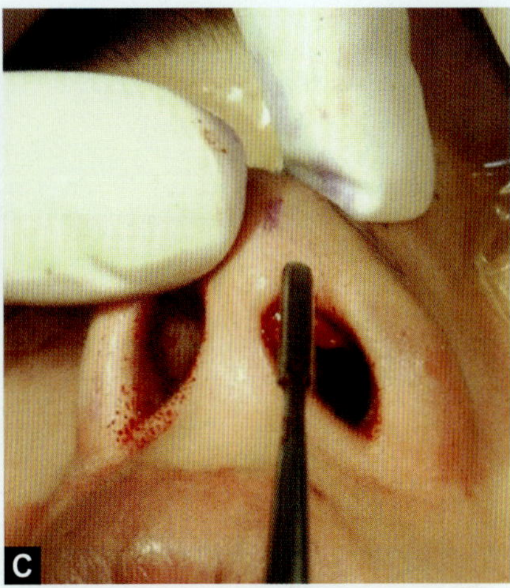

Figs 31A to C: (A) Method of inserting a sheet-shaped Gore-Tex using a bayonet forceps. After grasping the front part of a sheet-shaped Gore-Tex with a bayonet forceps, start inserting it in a slightly lifting manner; (B) When the implant reaches the correct position, fixate it to the bone by penetrating a needle through the skin of the nasal dorsum and the implant so that it does not slip away from the desired location when the forceps is withdrawn; (C) Subsequently, the nasal dorsum must be felt with fingers to check for any bent areas and then use an elevator to straighten it. As occasion demands, it is sometimes sutured to the lower lateral cartilage to make it secure

with fingers for any bent area after the implant is inserted and do not forget to use an elevator to straighten it out. In the case of Gore-Tex, although there is a lesser risk of extrusion than silicone, an autologous tissue must always be used at the nasal tip.

- Block-shaped (Reinforced) Gore-Tex
  - *Trimming*: Unlike the sheet-shaped Gore-Tex, the block-shaped Gore-Tex has a certain level of hardness, so it is easy to carve with a blade. Similar to silicone, a block-shaped Gore-Tex needs to be pretrimmed to approximately match the patient's nose using an appropriately sized block (a rectangular parallelopipedon which is about 3–5 mm thick, 8–10 mm wide, 5–6 cm long). Then, it must be prepared for surgery by gas sterilization. During surgery, a blade should be used to adjust it to the patient's nasal dorsum and then applied to the patient. Currently, there are readymade nasal augmentation products in the market which are relatively easy to carve and use.

    In most cases, either a #15 blade or #11 blade is used for trimming. And, because the block-shaped Gore-Tex has a softer quality than silicone, instead of forcing the blade, it is best to trim it in a softly twirling manner. In addition, when trimming the dorsal part of the implant, it is useful to use a razor that is rolled in a carved shape (Figs 32A and B).

    As in trimming silicone, the decision regarding the length should be based on the distance between the nasion or nasal root to the supratip and preferably should be about 3.5–4.0 cm long, and about 8 mm wide. Also, the edge should be as thin as possible.
  - *Insertion technique*: The insertion technique of a block-shaped Gore-Tex, same as in inserting silicone, can either be an open rhinoplasty approach (Figs 33A to D) or an intranasal approach (Figs 34A to P).

NEW TECHNIQUES IN THE SURGERY

Crushed Cartilage-TPFL Grafting

Crushed cartilage-TPFL grafting to the nasal dorsum was used in patients who disliked the use of alloplastic material for dorsal augmentation, and in revision surgery cases involving complications following the use of silicone implants on the nasal dorsum. All rhinoplasties were performed via an external approach after making a transcolumellar incision. Intravenous antibiotics, usually a second generation cephalosporin, were injected 1 hour prior to incision. TPFL was rehydrated in a saline solution for at least 5 minutes before use (according to the manufacturer's instructions) and then cut to the desired size. The technique used has been

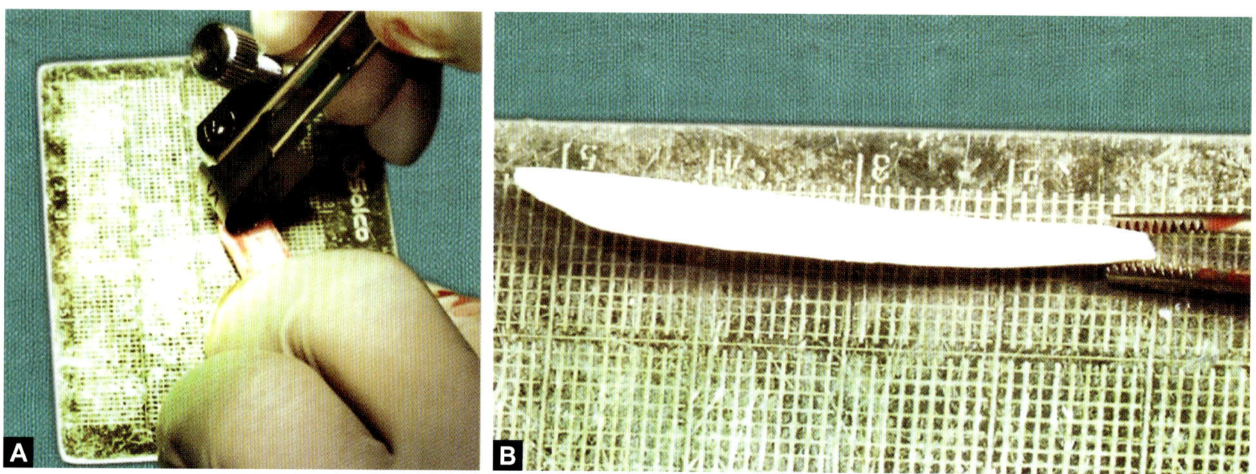

Figs 32A and B: Trimming a block-shaped Gore-Tex

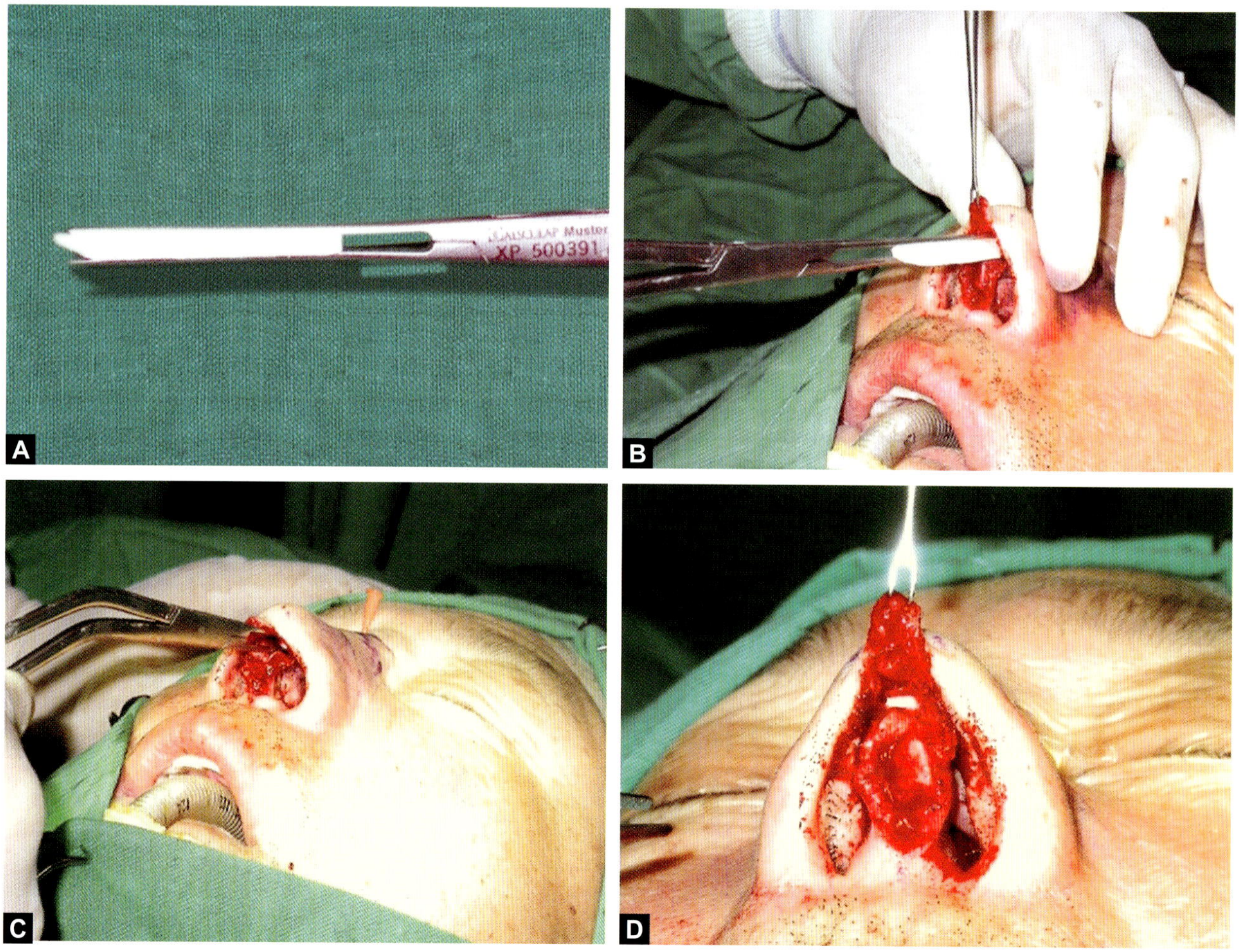

Figs 33A to D: After grasping the Gore-Tex with the bayonet-shaped forceps capable of clamping (A); insert the Gore-Tex into the dissected pocket (B). (C) To prevent the implant from slipping out with the forceps when it is withdrawn, fixate it with a needle; (D) The fastened needle can be maintained until the casting is removed after surgery. Cut or adjust the position of the implant so that the end of the implant is positioned at the supratip break area

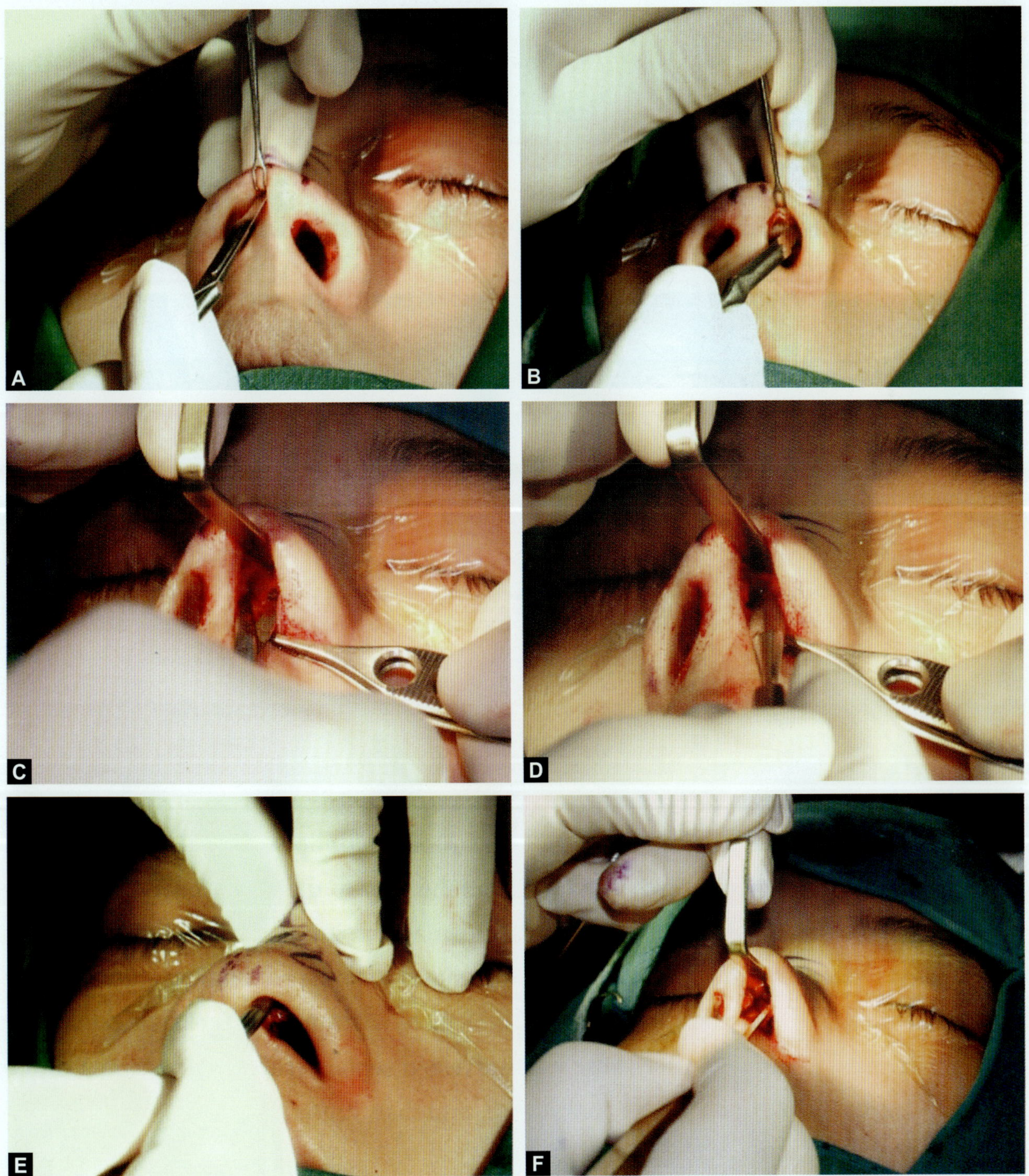

Figs 34A to F

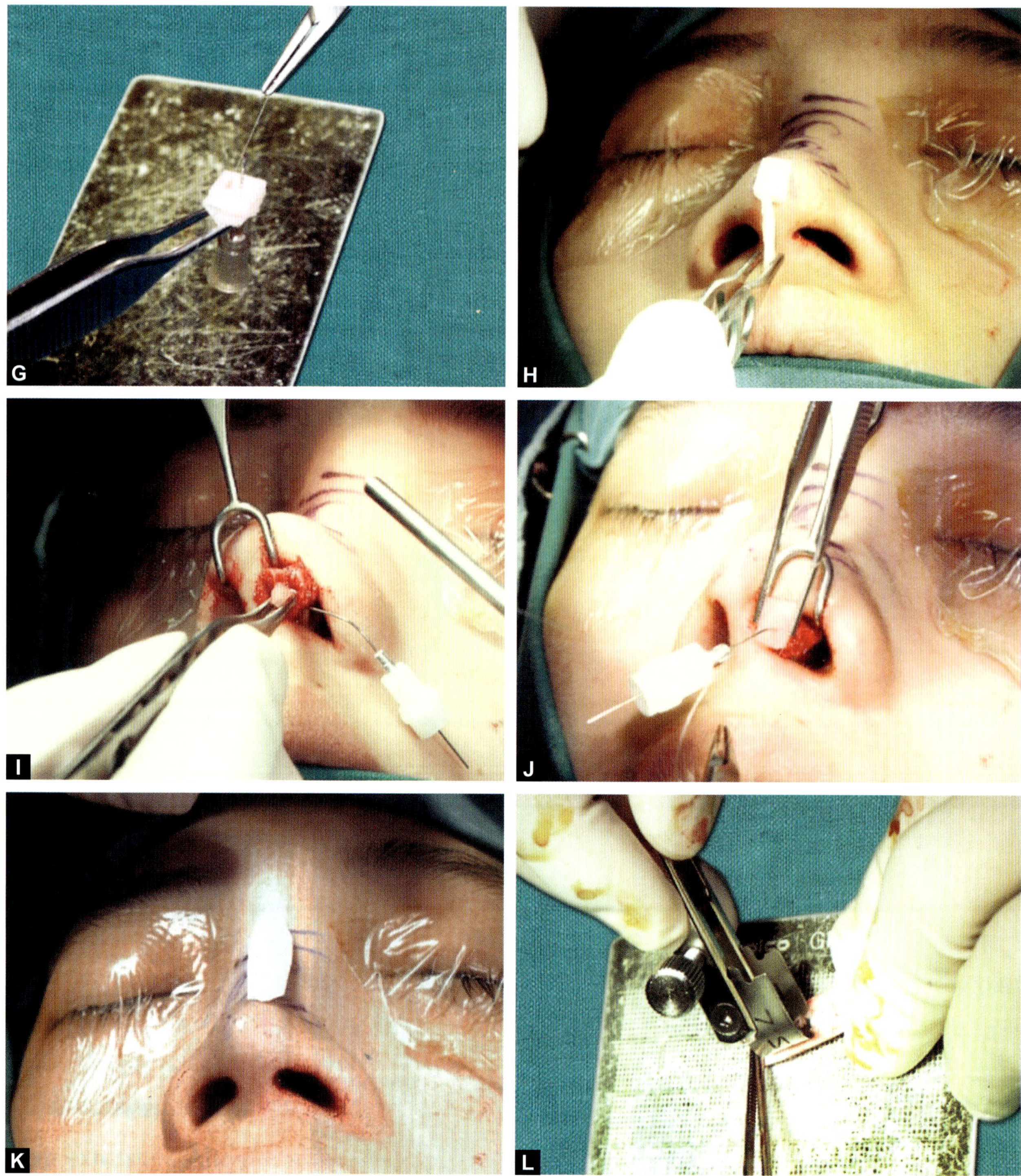

Figs 34G to L

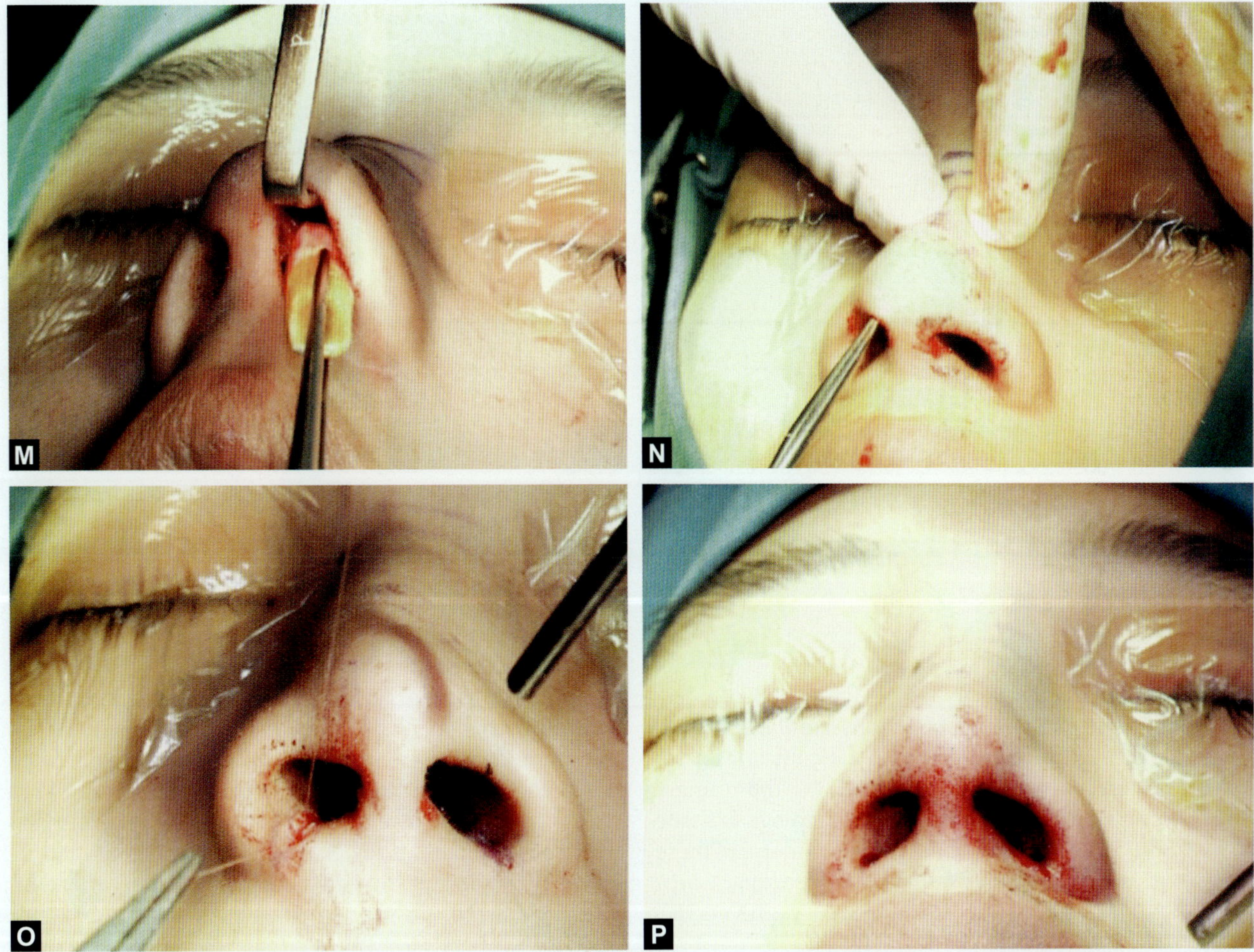

Figs 34A to P: Technique of performing a Gore-Tex augmentation rhinoplasty using an intranasal approach

previously published.[6] Cartilage was preferentially used for tip surgery and reconstruction of the septal cartilage framework. Any remaining cartilage fragments or bones were gently crushed using a cartilage crusher. The crushed cartilage and/or bone were then placed onto the nasal dorsum under direct vision, considering a differential augmentation along the length of the dorsum (see Fig. 24). A stack of multilayered (two or three layers) TPFL at the desired thickness was inserted onto the dorsum. When further augmentation of the nasal dorsum was required, a little more remaining crushed cartilage was inserted deep to the TPFL. The nose was then taped and external nasal splinting, using Aquaplast (WFR/Aquaplast Corp, Wyckoff, NJ), was placed for 6 days after the surgery to prevent lateral displacement of the fascia and crushed cartilage complex. Postoperative antibiotics were prescribed for 2 weeks after the operation.

Silicone Sheeting

The author has used silicone sheeting for nasal dorsal augmentation, which is more versatile but without an increased risk of complications (Figs 35A and B). In trimming the silicone, it should preferably be about 3.5–4.0 cm long and about 8 mm wide, and the edge should be as thin as possible. To insert the silicone, an open rhinoplasty approach or an endonasal approach is used. The size of the pocket should be made slightly larger than the implant, with just enough space for insertion of the implant and a surgical tool holding the implant at the same time.

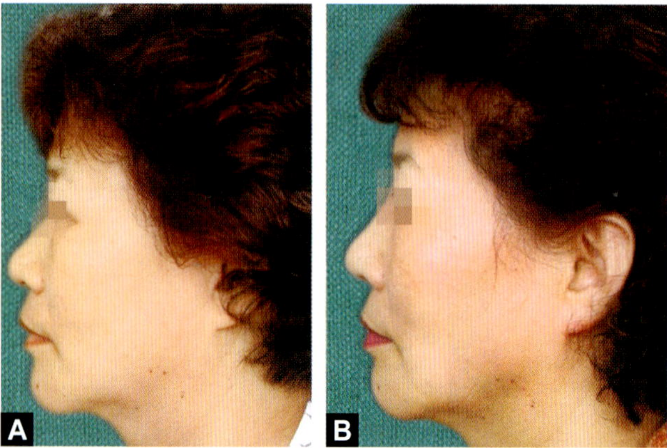

Figs 35A and B: (A) Patient before and; (B) After undergoing dorsal augmentation using silicone sheeting

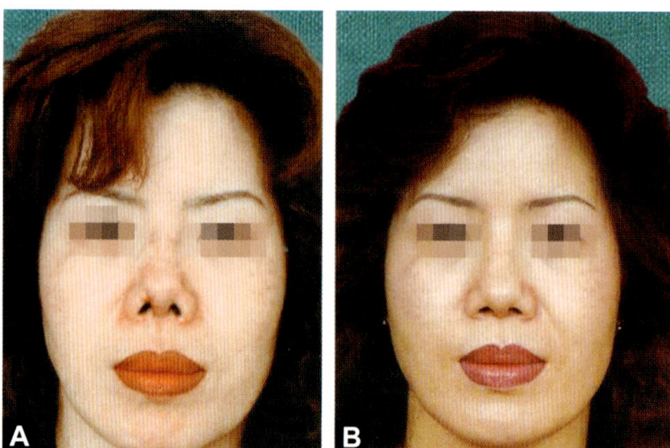

Figs 36A and B: (A) Patient before and; (B) After undergoing rhinoplasty using Tutoplast processed fascia lata for management of contracted nose caused by infection due to silicone implant

COMPLICATIONS

Autologous Cartilage

Although autologous cartilage has the lowest risk of infection among graft materials, autologous cartilage including costal cartilage is associated with a significant risk of revision surgery, with rates as high as 15.5%. The primary reasons for this high revision rate is that autologous tissue is usually used to treat more difficult cases and use of these implants is associated with unpredictable scarring, warping and, at times, visible graft contours (see Figs 20A and B).

Homologous Costal Cartilage

The use of homologous costal cartilage in rhinoplasty has shown conflicting results regarding the degree of resorption and warping. In the authors' own experience, a significant number of patients had unpredictable complications, such as resorption, warping, and graft visibility, when this cartilage was used as full-length dorsal graft. The high complication rate associated with homologous cartilage may limit its utility for dorsal augmentation.

Homologous Fascia

Although TPFL has very low risks of infection, displacement and extrusion, but an unpredictable degree of resorption could be a problem.

Silicone

Revision rhinoplasty after silicone implants may be needed for implant deviation, floating, displacement, extrusion, impending extrusion, and infection. Early infections can be prevented by the use of aseptic techniques and prophylactic antibiotics. Infection can also be treated by implant removal, antibiotic administration, and delayed reinsertion. Extrusion of the implant can occur through the nasal skin or mucosa, with tension over the implant being the most common cause of extrusion. The most likely cause of implant displacement is supraperiosteal placement of implants. Thus, implant displacement can be reduced by placing it immediately below the periosteum (Figs 36A and B).

Gore-Tex

Reports of a delayed inflammation are increasing and outcome data are not adequately accumulated to date. One must be cautious when using Gore-Tex in the presence of inflammation within the nasal cavity (sinusitis, vestibulitis, and active acne). Moreover, when performing operations that may create microcommunication with the nasal cavity (e.g. osteotomy or septal reconstruction), there is an increased risk of infection. It has been recommended that patients be treated with antibiotics prior to inserting the Gore-Tex as well as after surgery, and it is essential to soak the Gore-Tex in saline solution containing Betadine or antibiotics before use. Also, before handling the Gore-Tex, surgical personnel should wash their gloves to remove powder or other foreign substances. It has been reported that infection rate in primary surgery is 1.2%, while infection rate in secondary surgery is 5.4%.

SPECIAL INSTRUMENTS USED FOR THE SURGERY

Figures 37 to 40 show the instruments used for the surgery.

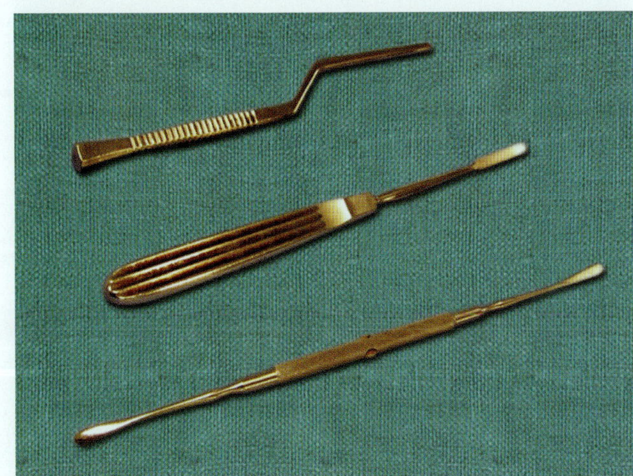

Fig. 37: Gouge (right), Joseph nasal knife (middle), and Freer septum elevator (left)

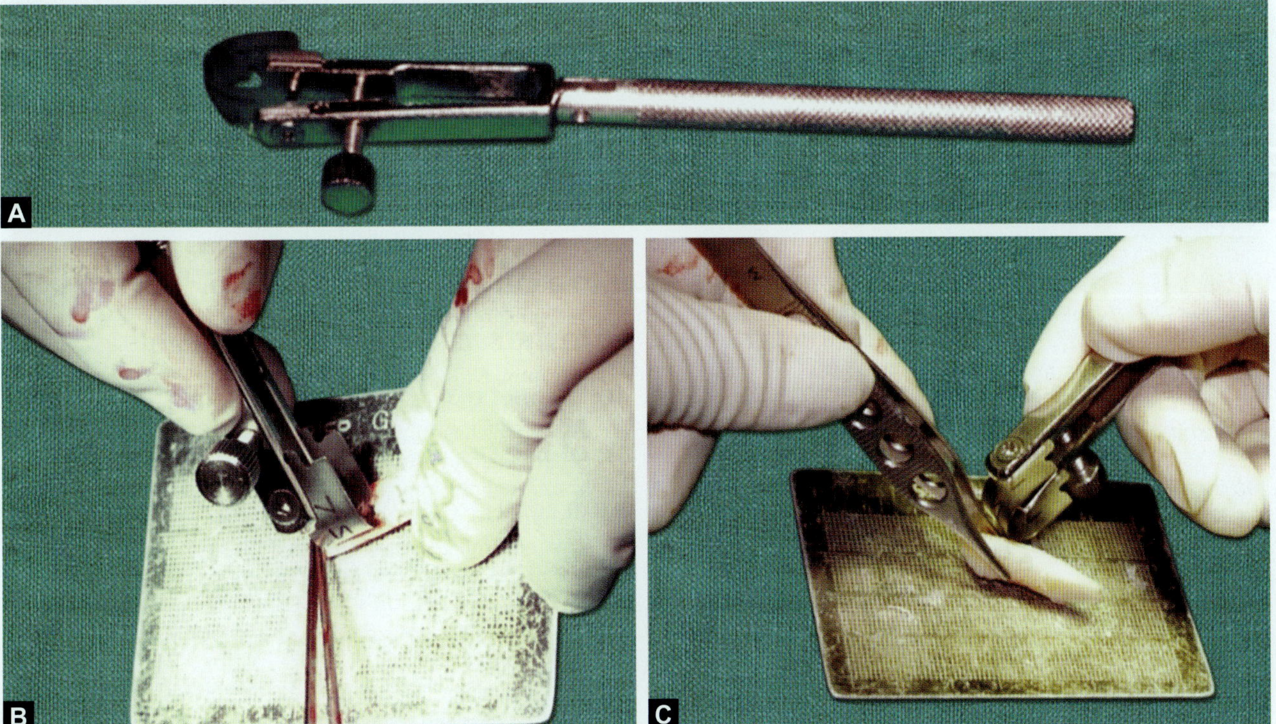

Figs 38A to C: Razor blade

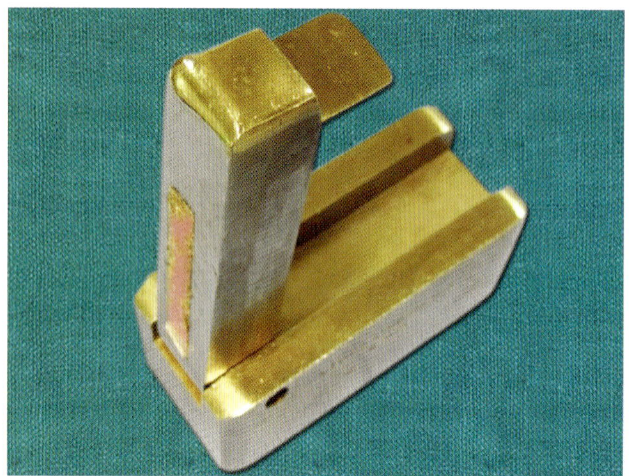

Fig. 39: Cartilage crusher

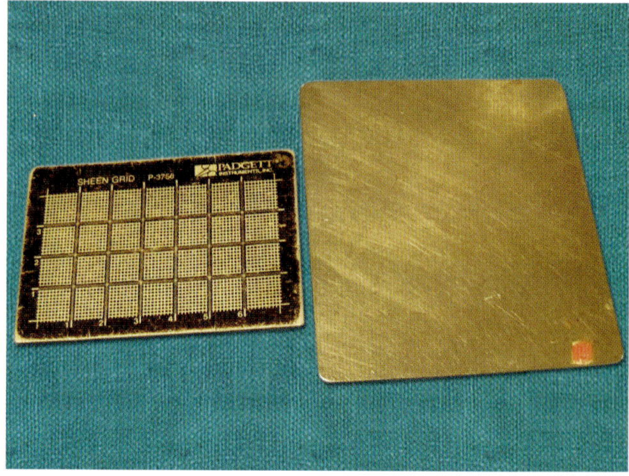

Fig. 40: Grid

BIBLIOGRAPHY

1. Baeck SI, Joung DH, Min YG. Rhinoplasty. In Min YG (Ed). Clinical Rhinology, 1st edition. Seoul: Ilchokak Publishing Co; 1997. pp. 507-63.
2. Bateman N, Jones NS. Retrospective review of augmentation rhinoplasties using autologous cartilage grafts. J Laryngol Otol. 2000;114(7):514-8.
3. Byrd HS, Andochick S. Copit S. et al. Septal extension graft: a method of controlling tip projection shape. Plast Reconstr Surg. 1997;100(4):999-1010.
4. Daniel RK, Calvert JW. Diced cartilage grafts in rhinoplasty surgery. Plast Reconstr Surg. 2004;113(7):2156-71.
5. Erlich MA, Parhiscar A. Nasal dorsal augmentation with silicone implants. Facial Plast Surg. 2003;19(4):325-30.
6. Ghoniem GM. Allograft sling material: is it the state of the art? Int Urogynecol J Pelvic Floor Dysfunct. 2000;11(2): 69-70.
7. Godin MS, Waldman SR, Johnson CM Jr. Nasal augmentation using Gore-Tex: a 10-year experience. Arch Facial Plast Surg. 1999;1(2):118-21.
8. Guerrerosantos J. Nose and paranasal augmentation: autogenous, fascia, and cartilage. Clin Plast Surg. 1991;18 (1):65-86.
9. Jang YJ, Song HM, Yoon YJ, et al. Combined use of crushed cartilage and processed fascia lata for dorsal augmentation in rhinoplasty for Asians. Laryngoscope. 2009;119 (6):1088-92.
10. Jang YJ, Wang JH, Sinha V, et al. Tutoplast-processed fascia lata for dorsal augmentation in rhinoplasty. Otolaryngol Head Neck Surg. 2007;137(1):88-92.
11. Lewis RP, Schweitzer J, Odum BC, et al. Sheets, 3-D strands, trimensional (3-D) shapes, and sutures of either reinforced or nonreinforced expanded polytetrafluoroethylene for facial soft-tissue suspension, augmentation, and reconstruction. J Long Term Eff Med Implants. 1998;8(1):19-42.
12. Maas CS, Gnepp DR, Bumpous J. Expanded polytetrafluoroethylene (Gore-Tex soft-tissue patch) in facial augmentation. Arch Otolaryngol Head Neck Surg. 1993;119(9): 1008-14.
13. Maas CS, Monhian N, Shah SB. Implants in rhinoplasty. Facial Plast Surg. 1997;13(4):279-90.
14. McCurdy JA Jr. The Asian nose: augmentation rhinoplasty with L-shaped silicone implants. Facial Plast Surg. 2002;18 (4):245-52.
15. Slavin SA, Rees TD, Guy CL, et al. An investigation of bacteremia during rhinoplasty. Plast Reconstr Surg. 1983;71 (2):196-8.
16. Stucker FJ, Shaw G. Ephrat M. Biologic tissue implants. In: Papel ID (Ed). Facial Plastic and Reconstructive Surgery, 2nd edition. New York: Thieme; 2002. pp. 73-8.
17. Tham C, Lai YL, Weng CJ, et al. Silicone augmentation rhinoplasty in an oriental population. Ann Plast Surg. 2005;54 (1):1-5.
18. Toriumi DM, Swartout B. Asian rhinoplasty. Facial Plast Surg Clin North Am. 2007;15(3):293-307.
19. Wang JH, Lee BJ, Jang YJ. Use of silicone sheets for dorsal augmentation in rhinoplasty for Asian noses. Acta Otolaryngol Suppl. 2007;(558):115-20.
20. Welling DB, Maves MD, Schuller DE, et al. Irradiated homologous cartilage grafts. Long-term results. Arch Otolaryngol Head Neck Surg. 1988;114(3):291-5.
21. Yang SJ, Kim BS, Kim JH. Secondary augmentation rhinoplasty with dermofat graft. J Korean Soc Plast Reconstr Surg. 1998;25:152-60.
22. Yeo NK, Jang YJ. Rhinoplasty to correct nasal deformities in postseptoplasty patients. Am J Rhinol Allergy. 2009;23(5):540-5.

CHAPTER

99 The Surgical Management of the Crooked Nose

Yakup Cil

INTRODUCTION

The primary goal of the crooked nose management is straightening the nose symmetrically without collapse or relapse. Collapse or relapse occurs frequently due to weak structural support. Conventional septal surgery may not be adequate to prevent recurrences. The aim of this chapter is to present the author and associates' current principles of correcting the crooked nose with iliac bone graft.[1]

OPERATIVE TECHNIQUE

Indications

Iliac bone graft is indicated for the patients who have crooked nose; if their cartilaginous septum is seriously destructed and/or their deformity includes both upper lateral cartilage and cartilaginous septum.

Preoperative Planning

Successful management of the crooked nose surgery is best achieved through careful analysis of the problem and clear communication with the patient regarding expectations of surgery. The crooked nose should be considered as an osseocartilaginous unit in which all components may potentially play a role. The external examination concludes with an assessment of the shape and position of the nasal bones and the upper and lower lateral cartilaginous vault. Photographic documentations should be performed in all cases before surgery.

Patients

Treatments of the crooked nose with iliac bone graft were performed in the author and associates' clinic since February 2005. All the patients had severely distorted septum with cosmetic nasal problems. All surgeries were performed under general anesthesia.

Case Presentation for Technique

Twenty-three-year-old male who had crooked nose due to blunt trauma at childhood is presented here (Fig. 1). Clinical examination revealed osseocartilaginous deviation with severely distorted septum.

Step 1

The patient under general anesthesia, the nasal septum and the external nose were infiltrated with 1% xylocaine with 1:100,000 epinephrine. Time has been allowed for the vasoconstrictive effect of the infiltration solution to take place and number-15 blade was used to perform nasal incision for open rhinoplasty approach. Nasal structures were exposed through standard transcolumellar incision and two marginal incisions. The hump resection with mucosal preservation was performed primarily to conserve the vertical nasal height. Then, septal dissection began between medial cruras of both lower lateral cartilages, and septum was separated from two mucoperichondrial flaps (Fig. 2).

Step 2

After septal separation, iliac bone donor site's skin area was infiltrated with 1% xylocaine with 1:100,000 epinephrine. A block of bone 3 × 2 × 0.5 cm in size was harvested from right iliac crest medial wall (right or left could be used) with electrical saw (Fig. 3).

Step 3

The bone graft was shaped as L-strut by electrical saw and thinned by abrasion (Fig. 4).

Step 4

The septum was resected leaving a 0.8–1 cm dorsal and caudal L-strut. Deviated caudal portion of the septal cartilage was straightened by medialization. L-strut bone graft was stabilized by the nasal septal cartilage (Fig. 5). Lateral and medial osteotomies were performed. Residual irregularities on the dorsum were camouflaged with Turkish delight and operation was completed.[2]

Postoperative Care

After nasal packing, external bandage and cast plaster were applied. The packing was removed after 4 days. The plaster nasal splint was replaced with another one at 7 days postoperatively. The second splint was removed 1 week after. Donor site was closed appropriately with mini Hemovac drain, which was removed within 3 days

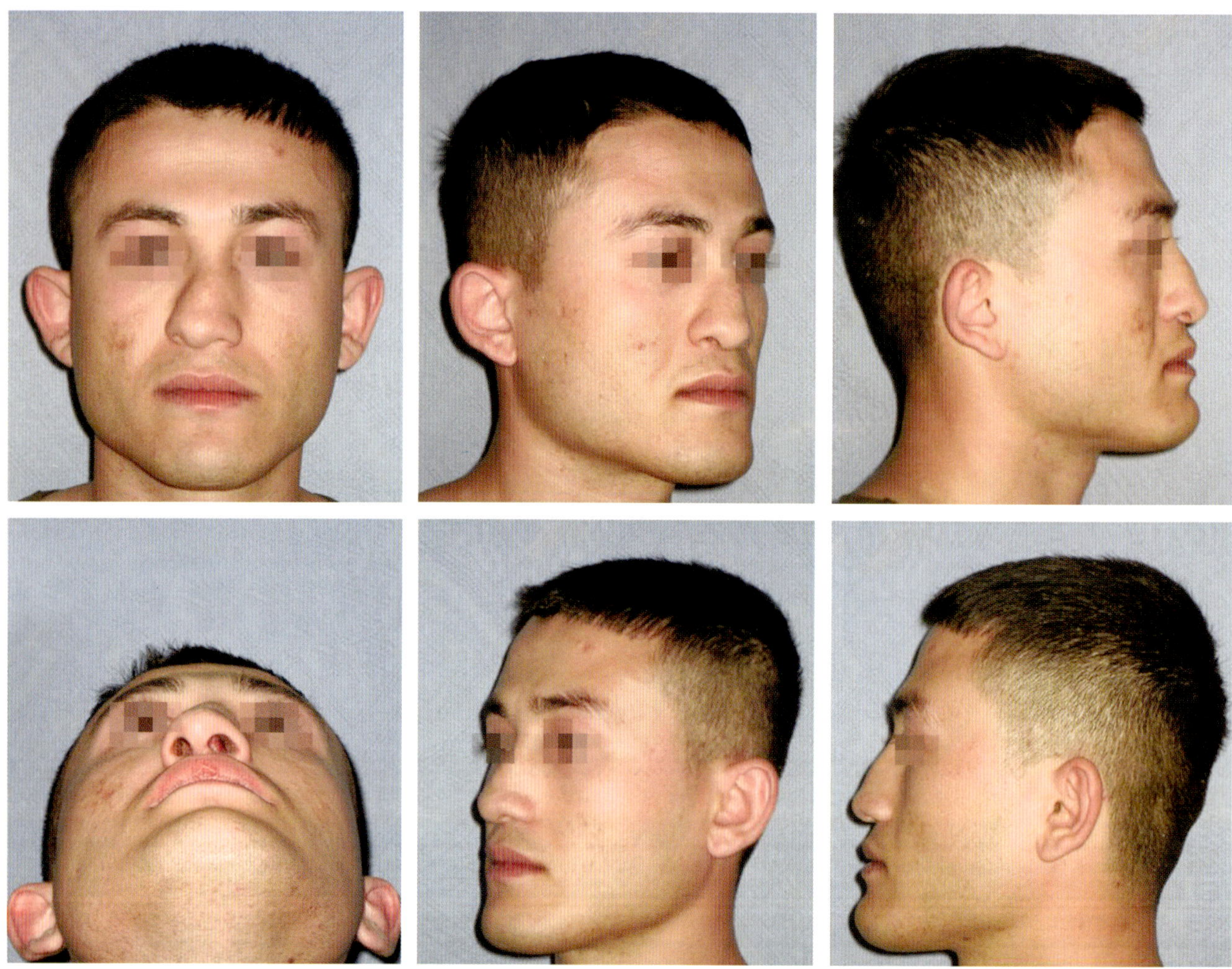

Fig. 1: Preoperative view of the patient with crooked nose

postoperatively. Patient had a straight nose with a natural appearance at 13-month follow-up (Figs 6 and 7).

Results

The mean operation time was 4 hours (3–4.5 hours). All patients healed uneventfully. The grafts have shifted in any case, and have not developed unsightly irregularities over time. Absorption of the grafts was not seen in the follow-up (Fig. 8). All patients had a straight nose with a natural appearance at follow-up.

Alternative Bone Graft Sources for L-Strut Frame

Radial and fibular bone may also be used for crooked nose treatment. Bone graft was harvested from the lateral side of radial bone and L-strut framework was prepared with this graft (Fig. 9). Lateral antecubital nerve, flexor, and extensor muscles were protected during bone graft harvesting procedure.

Fibular bone graft was accessed from the lateral leg region, and bone graft was taken from the lateral side of fibular bone for L-strut framework (Fig. 10). Lateral muscles were protected during bone graft harvesting procedure.

Discussion

Various techniques have been described for the correction of the crooked nose. Problems can be localized in the upper (bony) and lower (cartilaginous) portions or both (osteocartilaginous).[3] According to these localizations, surgical algorithm for the management of the crooked nose may differ. Only the osteotomies may be performed,

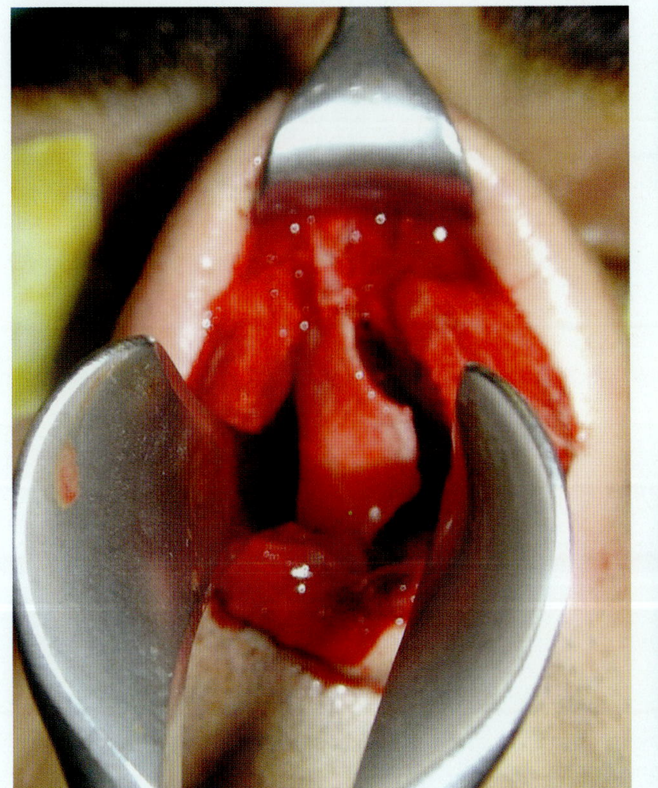

Fig. 2: Deviated nasal septum, intraoperatively

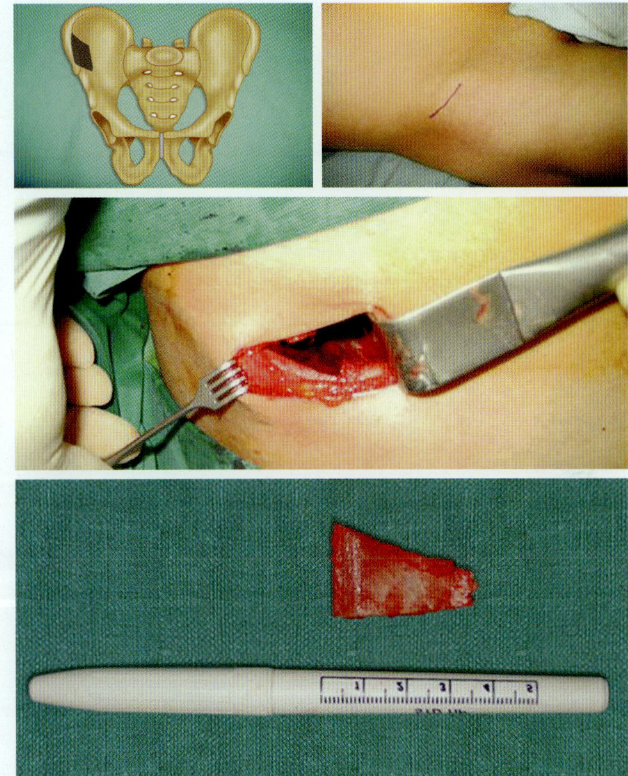

Fig. 3: Bloc bone graft was taken from iliac crest

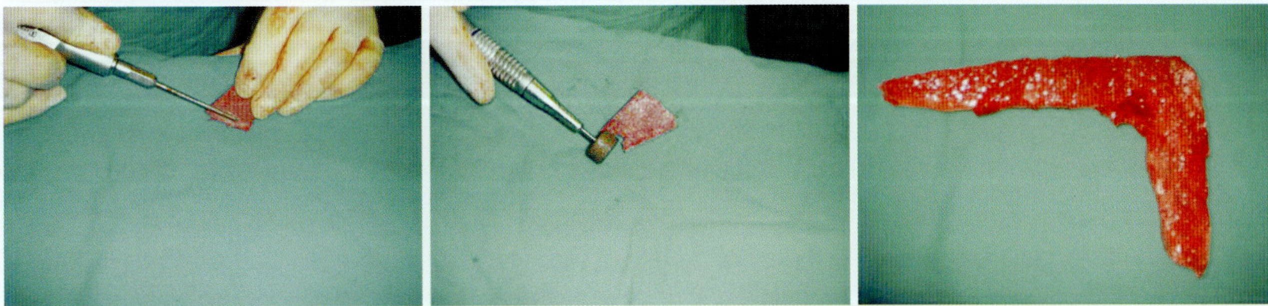

Fig. 4: The bone graft was shaped as L-strut by electrical saw and thinned by abrasion

if bony deviation is present.[4] Dorsal hump resections,[5] a variety of modified osteotomies,[6-8] septal cartilage manipulations,[9] suture correction,[10] and spreader grafts[11,12] have been recommended. However, the problem still challenges with high recurrence and revision rates because of unpredictable behavior of cartilage even after correction. Besides straightening the septum, maintaining its support is also crucial for long lasting results. Conventional septal surgery may not be adequate to prevent recurrences. To prevent redeviation, the author and associates aimed to use rigid iliac bone grafts instead of flexible and relatively weak cartilage to maintain the support of the corrected deformity.

The most popular method to maintain long-term support is reinforcement of corrected septum with spreader grafts.[11,13] The spreader grafts restore the integrity of septal L-struts. These splinting grafts resist the memory of the septal cartilage and prevent relapse of the curvature.[14]

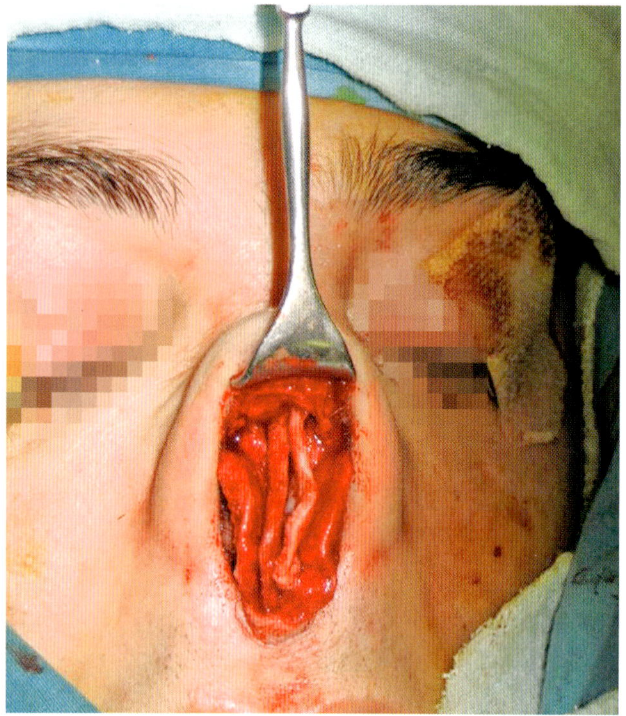

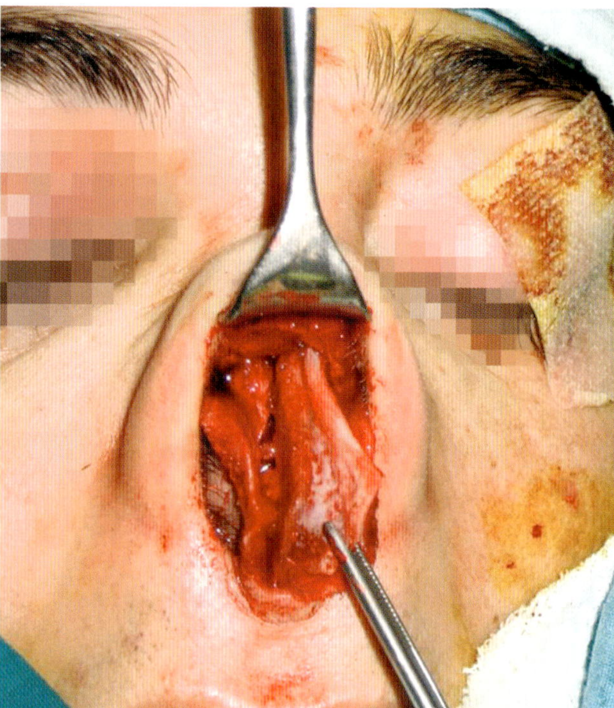

Fig. 5: Deviated septal cartilage was straightened by medialization and L-strut bone graft was stabilized by the nasal septal cartilage

Unilateral spreader graft,[3] unilateral spreader-extension grafts,[11] asymmetric spreader grafts[4] were also described. However, the graft obtained from severely deviated cartilaginous septum is relatively weak and cannot produce adequate support. Bony-cartilaginous spreader stents may also fail even if they are combined.[4] It is also technically difficult to harvest long and straight pieces of spreader grafts from a severely distorted osseocartilaginous septum. In addition, flexible cartilage has unpredictable tendency to retain its curvature attributed to its memory. A more rigid framework is necessary against deforming forces during the healing period. Some authors[12] have preferred using alloplastic materials as spreader grafts in respect of more rigid stabilization. The author and associates considered to use an autolog material that is more rigid from cartilage and more reliable than alloplasts. Medial side of iliac crest provides a source of straight bone when shaped properly. L-strut shaped medial crest graft supports the realigned caudal-dorsal septum despite the cartilaginous memory of the previous position. There was no significant contour deformity at the donor site.

In conclusion, L-strut iliac bone graft could be very usable in selected patients who have crooked nose.

Surgical Tips

- Clear communication with the patient regarding his or her expectations from the surgery.
- Careful analysis of the nasal problem.
- Open rhinoplasty approach is preferable.
- Deviated portion of the septal cartilage should be straightened by medialization before L-strut bone graft stabilization.
- The bone graft should be harvested from medial iliac region in order to minimize donor site morbidity.
- Shaping the bone graft as L-strut framework should be done carefully.
- Camouflage grafts could be used for dorsal smoothness, and hide minor residual deviations.

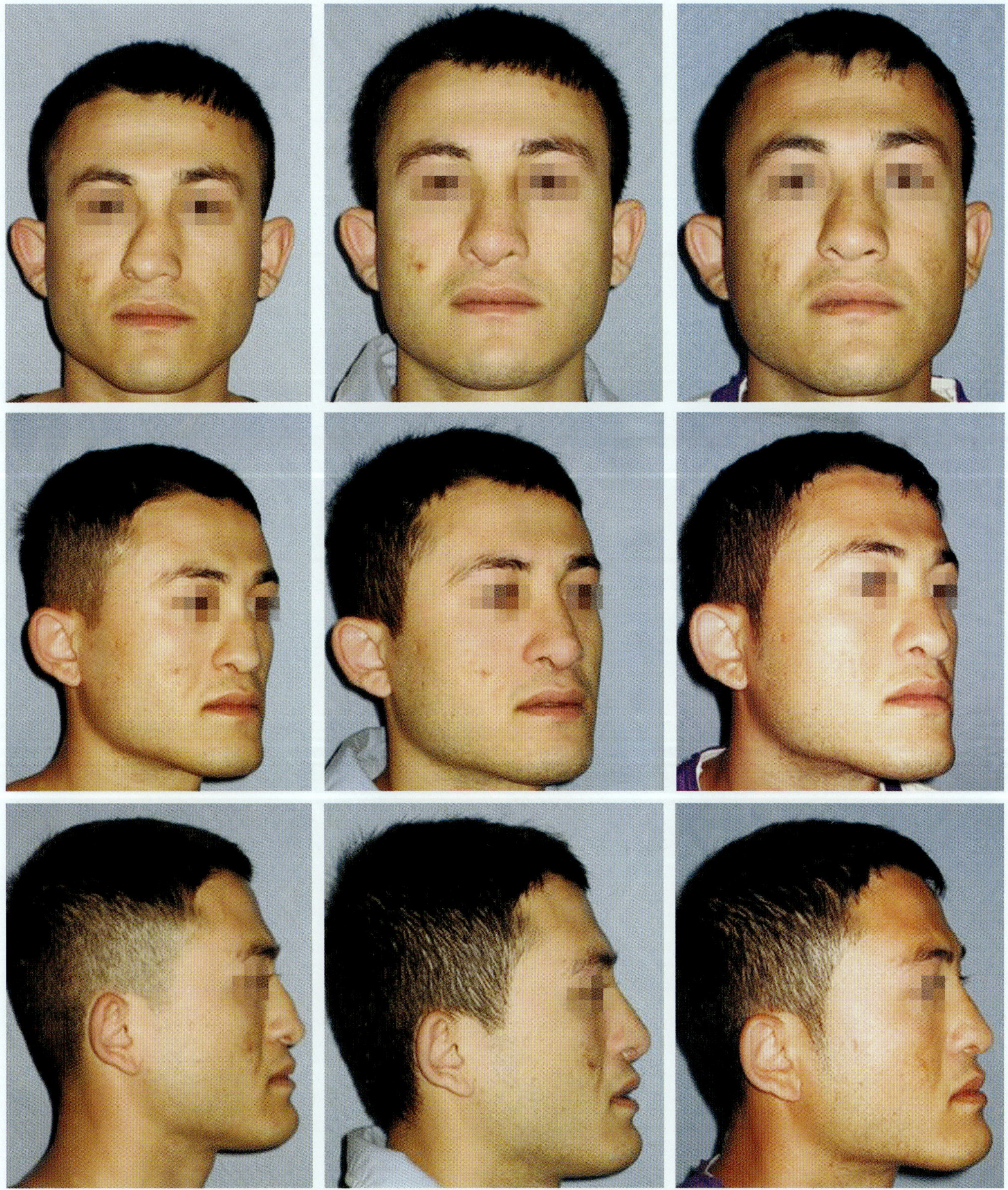

Fig. 6: Preoperative (left), postoperative 1 month (middle), 13 months (right) view of patient

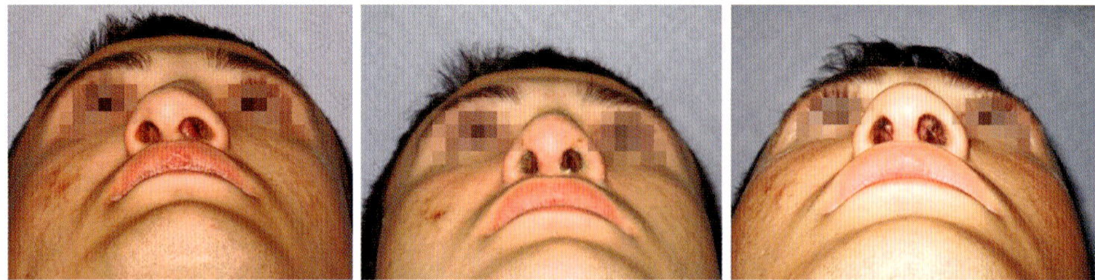

Fig. 7: Preoperative (left), postoperative 1 month (middle), 13 months (right) inferior view of patient

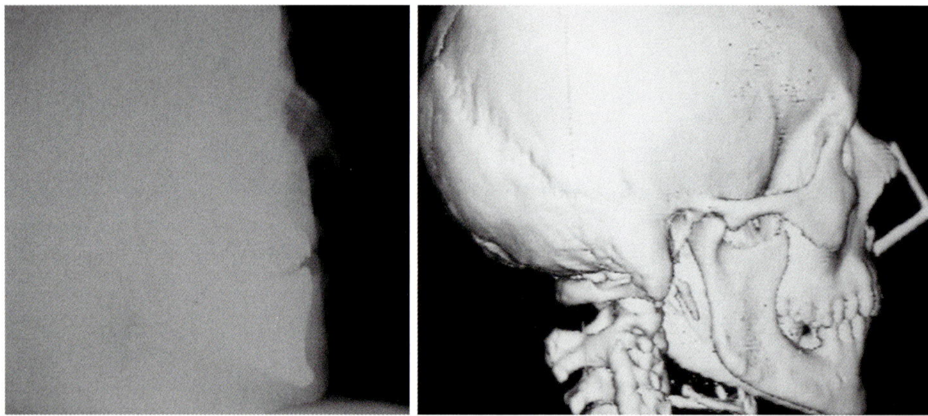

Fig. 8: Radiologic appearances of L-strut bone graft

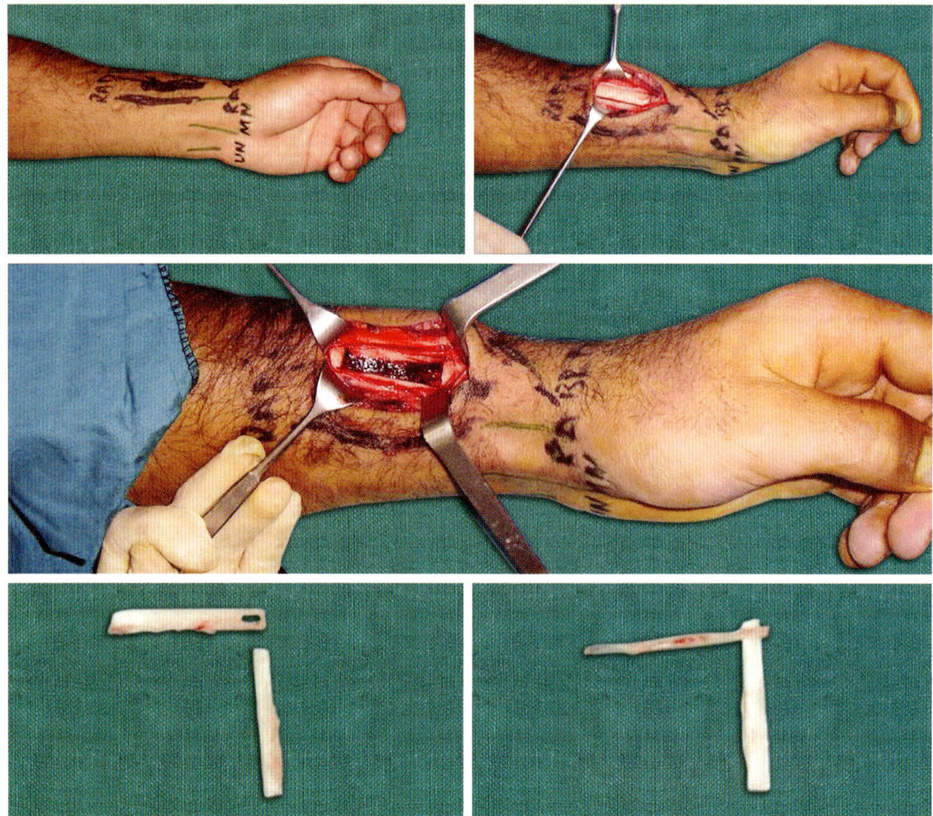

Fig. 9: Radial bone graft alternative to L-strut graft source (RA: Radial artery; UN: Ulnar nerve; MN: Median nerve)

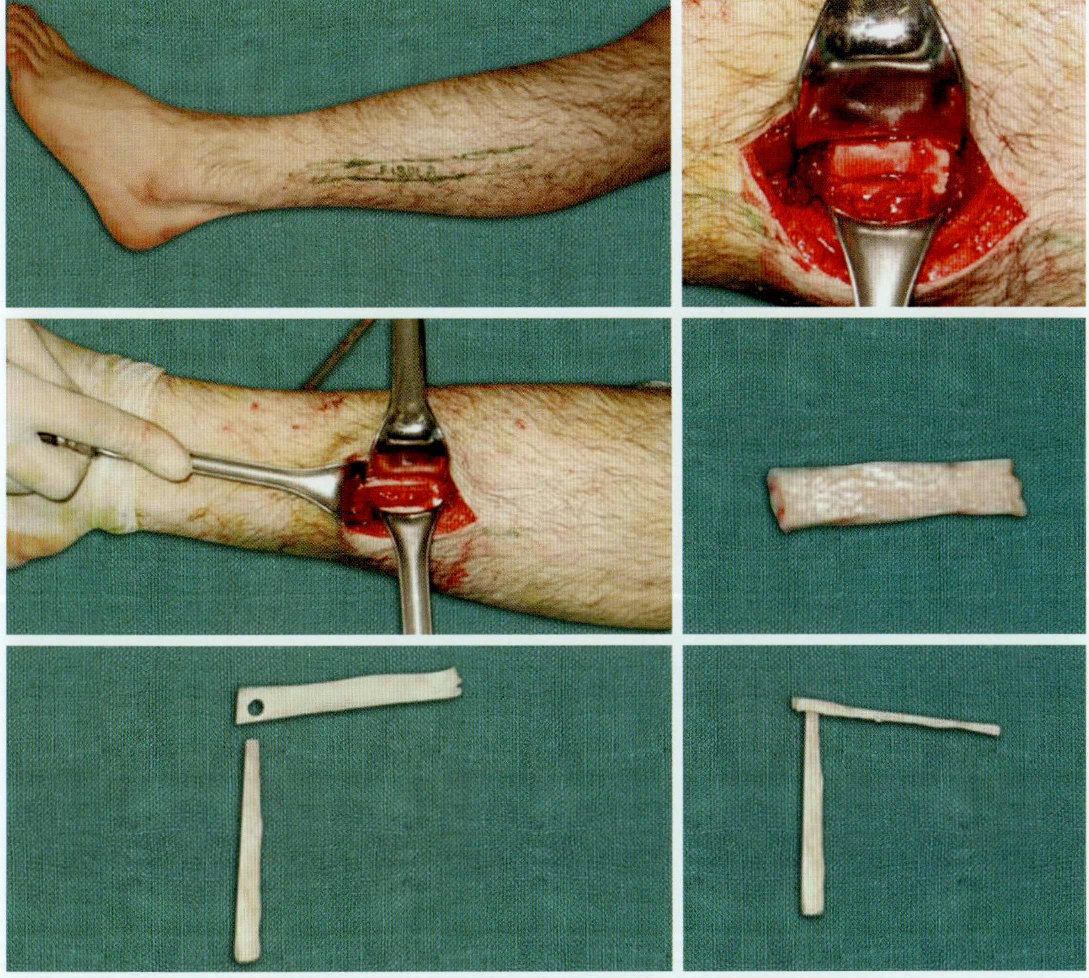

Fig. 10: Fibular bone graft alternative to L-strut graft source

REFERENCES

1. Cil Y, Ozturk S, Kocman AE, et al. The crooked nose: the use of medial iliac crest bone graft as a supporting framework. J Craniofac Surg. 2008;19(6):1631-8.
2. Erol OO. The Turkish delight: a pliable graft for rhinoplasty. Plast Reconstr Surg. 2000;105(6):2229-41.
3. Boccieri A, Pascali M. Septal crossbar graft for the correction of the crooked nose. Plast Reconstr Surg. 2003;111(2):629-38.
4. Rohrich RJ, Gunter JP, Deuber MA, et al. The deviated nose: optimizing results using a simplified classification and algorithmic approach. Plast Reconstr Surg. 2002;110(6):1509-23.
5. Constantian MB. An algorithm for correcting the asymmetrical nose. Plast Reconstr Surg. 1989;83(5):801-11.
6. Jameson JJ, Perry AD, Ritter EF. High septal osteotomy in rhinoplasty for the deviated nose. Ann Plast Surg. 2006;56(1):40-5.
7. Bracaglia R, Fortunato R, Gentileschi S. Double lateral osteotomy in aesthetic rhinoplasty. Br J Plast Surg. 2004;57(2):156-9.
8. Fanous N. Unilateral osteotomies for external bony deviation of the nose. Plast Reconstr Surg. 1997;100(1):115-23.
9. Park DH, Kim TM, Han DG, et al. Endoscopic-assisted correction of the deviated nose. Aesthetic Plast Surg. 1998;22(3):190-5.
10. Calderón-Cuéllar LT, Trujillo-Hernández B, Vásquez C, et al. Modified mattress suture technique to correct anterior septal deviation. Plast Reconstr Surg. 2004;114(6):1436-41.
11. Byrd HS, Salomon J, Flood J. Correction of the crooked nose. Plast Reconstr Surg. 1998;102(6):2148-57.
12. Mendelsohn M. Straightening the crooked middle third of the nose: using porous polyethylene extended spreader grafts. Arch Facial Plast Surg. 2005;7(2):74-80.
13. Guyuron B, Uzzo CD, Scull H. A practical classification of septonasal deviation and an effective guide to septal surgery. Plast Reconstr Surg. 1999;104(7):2202-9.
14. Kim DW, Toriumi DM. Management of posttraumatic nasal deformities: the crooked nose and the saddle nose. Facial Plast Surg Clin North Am. 2004;12(1):111-32.

CHAPTER

100 Surgical Techniques in Open Rhinoplasty Procedures

Tamer Seyhan

HISTORY

Historically, the first rhinoplasty procedure was performed by using a midline dorsal external incision in the 1850s.[1] Subsequently, Jacques Joseph popularized the endonasal approach for rhinoplasty in the 1930s.[2] In a 1948 issue of "Plastic and Reconstructive Surgery," Rethi, a Hungarian surgeon, described the transcolumellar incison (vertical V) and renewed interest in the external (open) rhinoplasty approach.[3] It was Goodman, who devoted the entire issue of the "Canadian Journal of Otolaryngology" to the external (open) rhinoplasty approach and increased interest in the external approach among North Americans during the 1970s.[4] Although the controversy of "open versus closed" rhinoplasty approach is still an ongoing issue among surgeons, the external approach has gained proponents increasingly.[5,6] Younger surgeons perform open rhinoplasty more frequently than older surgeons.[6]

INDICATIONS FOR THE SURGERY

Proponents of the open rhinoplasty approach cite supporting points in favor of the open technique.[6] First of all, direct visualization of the nasal cartilages and handling and grafting of the nasal cartilages are easier with the open approach rhinoplasty than the closed approach rhinoplasty. Management of a deviated bony and cartilaginous septum and management of nasal septal spurs are easier in the open approach rhinoplasty. Finally, low revision rates for primary open rhinoplasty have been reported.[7,8] Except for the difficulty of secondary revision procedures, following open rhinoplasty, the disadvantages of the open approach are minimal, such as prolonged tip edema, extended operation time and scarring. With respect to the final transcolumellar scar, it is acceptable in most cases. In the beginning of my practice, the ratio of open-to-close approaches was 50:50. After 10 years of experience and approximately 1,000 rhinoplasties that ratio was 90:10, favoring the open approach. In addition to the aforementioned advantages, the author believes that the longevity of the results of an open approach exceed the closed approach. Although the choice of open or closed approach rhinoplasty is generally related to the surgeon's preference, management of some conditions requires an open approach. Such conditions generally corrected with the open approach are summarized in Table 1.

Table 1: Medical conditions generally corrected with an open rhinoplasty approach

Revision rhinoplasties
Severe alar and upper lateral cartilage deformities
Severe nasal valve problems
Severe septal deformities and septal perforations
Nasal deformity with severe breathing problems
Cleft lip nose deformity

The author prefers the closed approach for "simple" cases that require simple tip and dorsal surgery.

SPECIFIC PREOPERATIVE EVALUATIONS

A specific preoperative evaluation is necessary for the patient who demands a rhinoplasty. Patient expectations are noted and those which are surgically correctable or require secondary and other operations should be discussed openly with the patient. The patients with body dysmorphic disorder and unrealistic expectations should be identified during the preoperative interview.[9-12] Cosmetic surgery should not be performed in such patients, who are then referred to a psychiatrist. A detailed history should be obtained and a physical examination of the patient should be performed and all findings recorded in a printed examination form or as computer data. Important points of this form are demonstrated below (Table 2). Also, signed informed consent should be obtained from the patient. An informed consent form for rhinoplasty can easily be found on the internet (Appendage 1).

ANESTHETIC CONSIDERATIONS

The majority of operations, except minor revisions, are performed under general anesthesia, supplemented with 7 mL of 0.5% bupivacaine and 3 mL of physiologic serum

Table 2: Some important points taken into consideration during the examination of a rhinoplasty patient

Brief history	*Prior nasal trauma or nasal surgery?*
Identifying the body-dysmorphic patient	If some clues are detected during the interview, use a screening questionnaire or refer for psychiatric counseling!
The use of herbal medicine (potential for increased bleeding)	Such as garlic, ginseng, ginger, ginkgo biloba and echinacea should be discontinued 2 weeks before surgery.
Questions in relation to hemorrhagic diatheses	Table 3
History of smoking	Patients should quit smoking for at least 4 weeks before surgery.
Allergies	Allergic rhinitis? Allergies to any medications or plaster?
Prior operations under general anesthesia	Any problems related to general anesthesia?
Primary complaint of the patient	Breathing (which of the areas? Right, left or both?), aesthetic concerns or both?
Nasal physical examination	Nasal skin (thin, thick and oily or mixed); nasofrontal angle; nasolabial angle; hump (cartilaginous, bony or both); nasal tip projection; nasal tip width; nasal tip asymmetry; upper lip height (narrow or long); nasal spine hypertrophy (yes or no); smiling deformity (yes or no); nasal radix (low or high [requires wedge excision]); alar base (narrow or large [requires wedge excision]); nostril asymmetry (yes or no); Examination of the nasal valve (Cottle test); speculum exam (septum, inferior and middle concha and concha bullosa?); nasal passage exam (prior and after vasoconstrictor, such as xylometazoline and oxymetazoline gut)
CT examination of paranasal sinuses	If history of severe headache, suspected concha bullosa or any reason that explains breathing problem on physical examination is not present.
Impression and any specific explanations to the patient	The probability of second or third operations, continuing breathing problems due to surgically insoluble problem (allergy)
Operation plan	Specific procedures based on the above findings (e.g., median osteotomy with wedge excision, alar base narrowing, nasal spine reduction, asymmetric spreader graft, spur resection, concha bullosa resection, functional endoscopic sinus surgery, concha resection or lateralization.
Surgical procedure	Gunter rhinoplasty diagrams[13]

Table 3: Clues for hemorrhagic diathesis during preoperative evaluation

- History of excessive bleeding after previous surgical or nonsurgical trauma.
- History of excessive bruising, epistaxis, intramuscular or intraarticular bleeding episodes.
- Family history remarkable for a coagulopathy.
- Petechiae, purpura and ecchymotic areas.
- History of menorrhagia (heavy and prolonged menstrual periods), severe preeclampsia, eclampsia and repeated abortus.
- Spontaneous abortus during previous pregnancies.

with epinephrine (1 : 100,000). Nasal packing soaked in oxymetazoline and xylometazoline is inserted in the nasal passages 5 to 10 minutes before surgery. A throat pack is then placed in the oropharynx after oral intubation, which reduces postoperative nausea from swallowed blood. The columella and nasal lobule are infiltrated first and then hydrodissection of the septal mucosa is infiltrated and hydrodissected with a local anesthetic. Infiltration to the lateral osteotomy site is performed 7 to 10 minutes before perforating lateral osteotomies. If turbinate surgery or radiofrequency ablation is planned under general anesthesia, topically decongest the turbinates with application of a decongestant on nasal pledgets. If a concha bullosa resection is performed under general anesthesia, the conchae are infiltrated with local anesthetic solution after vasoconstrictor-containing nasal packing.

SURGICAL STEPS

Surgical Technique

- The patient is prepped and draped. The back of the patient is elevated, and then adjusted in a manner such that the head of the patient is parallel to the floor (Fig. 1).
- Radiofrequency cauterization or anterior turbinoplasty is performed in case of hypertrophied turbinate. The author uses a 3.8, 140 watt MHz Surgitron EMC high frequency radiosurgical unit (Elman Corporation, Hewlett, NY, USA; Fig. 2A). Coagulation mode (partially rectified waves) is selected. The power is adjusted to 3. The Bayonette Turbinate Electrode needles are placed in the hypertrophic inferior turbinate approximately 2 to 3 mm into the turbinate tissue (Figs 2B to D). The current is used until visual blanching occurs at the hypertrophied site.

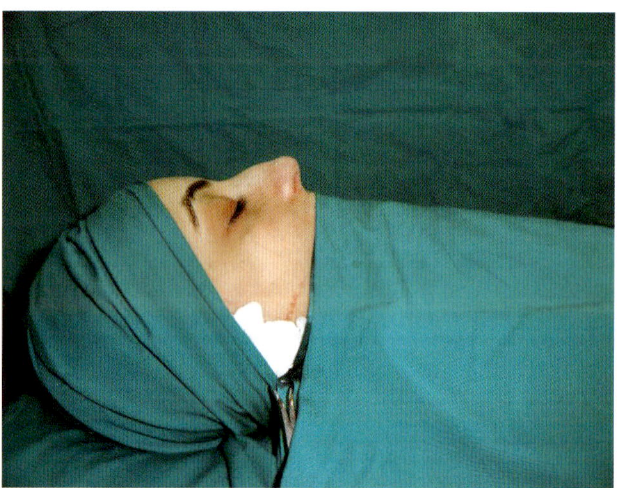

Fig. 1: Preoperative positioning of the patient

- A winged inverted-V incision of Goodman[4] is made using a No. 15 blade at the narrowest distance between the nostrils with special care not to damage the underlying medial crura. The columellar part of the marginal incision should be placed 1.5 to 2 mm inside the vestibulum. The alar part of the incision should be placed 1.5 to 2 mm inside the alar rim, at the apex and follow the cranial edge of the alar cartilages (Fig. 3A). The soft tissue envelope (the columellar skin over the incision, distal nasal skin over the upper and lower lateral cartilages and the skin over the bony pyramid) is raised subperichondrially and subperiosteally, using a skin hook and fine dissecting scissors (Figs 3B to E). The transected columellar arteries are coagulated with fine bipolar cautery. The elevation over the bony pyramid should not be very far laterally, but only to the area of the hump to be resected. Thick supratip subcutaneous tissues can be thinned very conservatively. The shape, size and volume of the alar cartilages are evaluated. As a rule, the excess cephalic part of the lateral crus of the alar cartilages is excised by leaving a 6 to 8 mm caudal strip of the cartilages (Fig. 3F). The management of other deformities of the lateral crura have been described before.[14]
- Approach a deviated quadrangular septum, bony septal spurs, deviated vomer and caudal septum with the tip split and dorsal split techniques.[4,15] Dorsal and

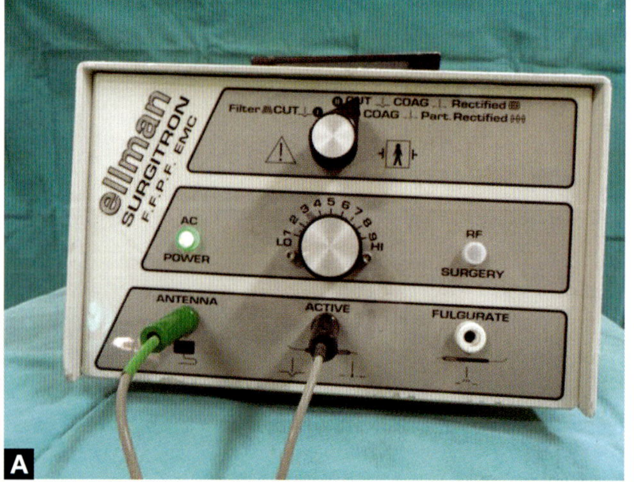

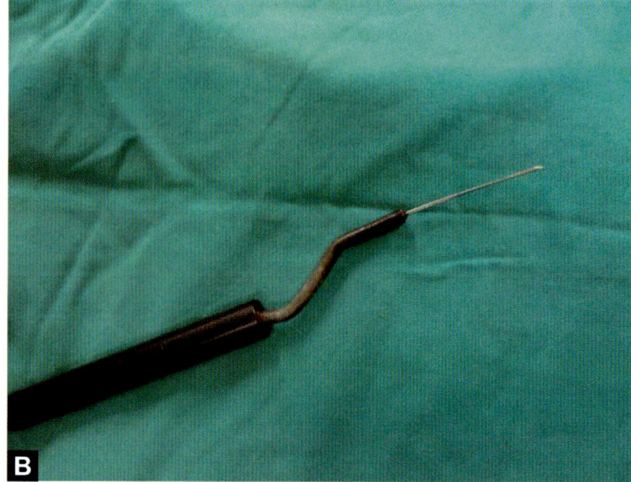

Figs 2A and B

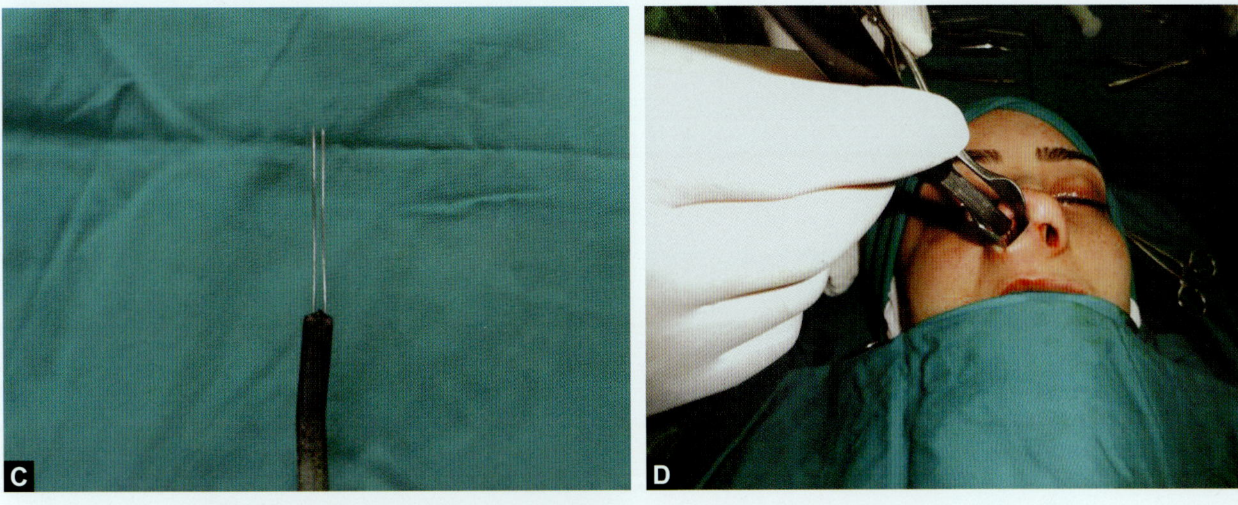

Figs 2A to D: The view of Surgitron EMC high frequency radiosurgical unit and the Bayonette Turbinate Electrode needles and its usage

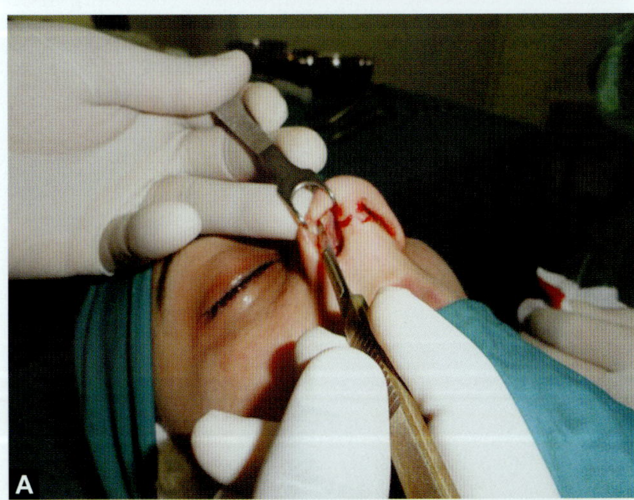

Fig. 3A: The view of winged-inverted V incision and marginal incision of columella and alae

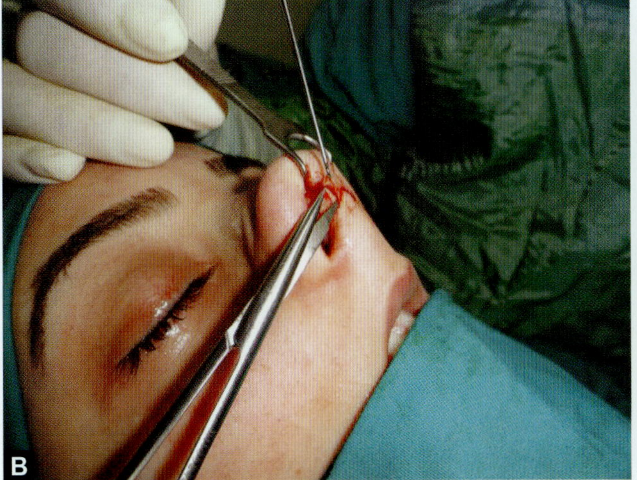

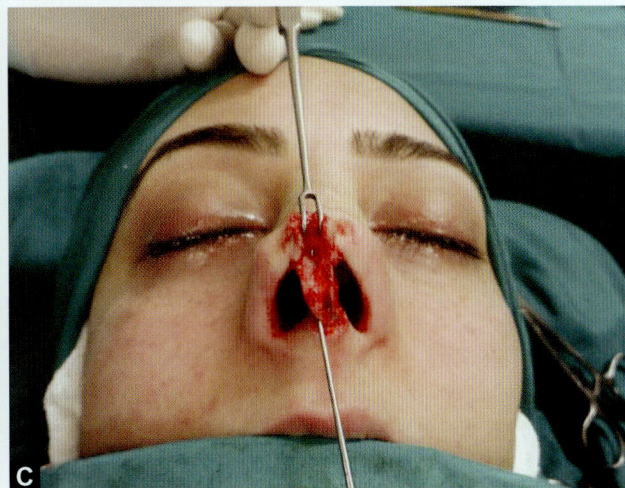

Figs 3B and C

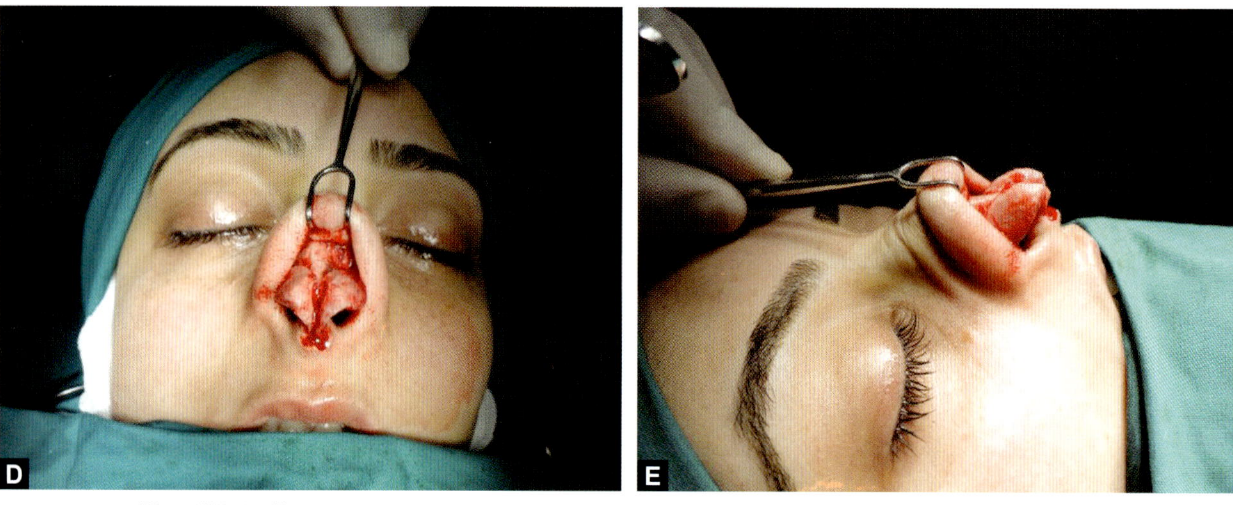

Figs 3B to E: Raising of the soft tissue envelope with fine dissecting scissors and skin hooks

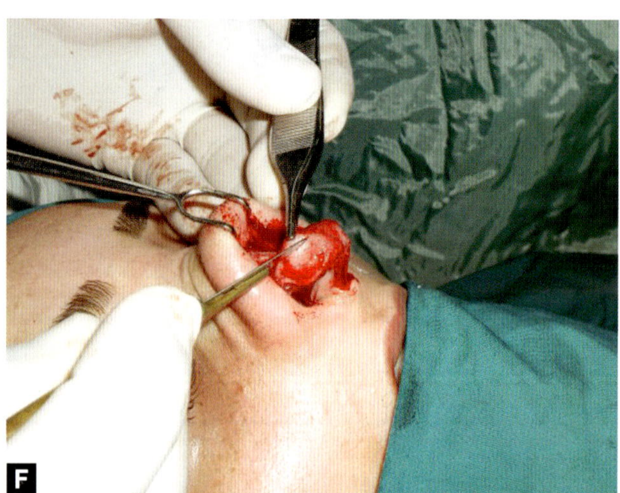

Fig. 3F: Excision of excess cephalic alar cartilages leaving a 6 to 8 mm caudal strip

base deviations of the septum are easily handled with these approaches. Also, placement of caudal strut grafts between the medial crura is easy with a tip split approach. The medial crura of the alar cartilages are separated to expose the septum and bilateral septal submucoperichondrial dissections are performed. Both sides of the cartilaginous and bony septum are exposed (Fig. 4A). The upper lateral cartilages are separated from the septum (Fig. 4B). The septum is detached from its base and from the bony septum. The deviated septal parts, including the septal spurs, are resected, leaving at least a 0.8 to 1 cm dorsal and caudal L-shaped strip of cartilage (Fig. 4C). Graft materials for the columellar strut and spreader grafts are harvested from the base of the septum without damaging the anterior nasal spine (Figs 4C and D). A reverse

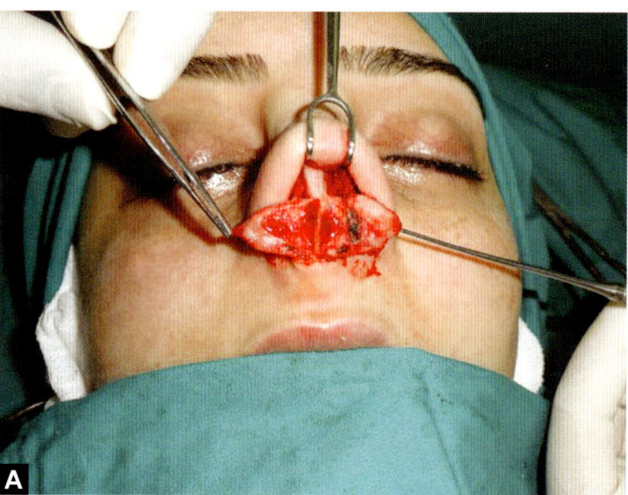

Fig. 4A: The view of the tip split approach

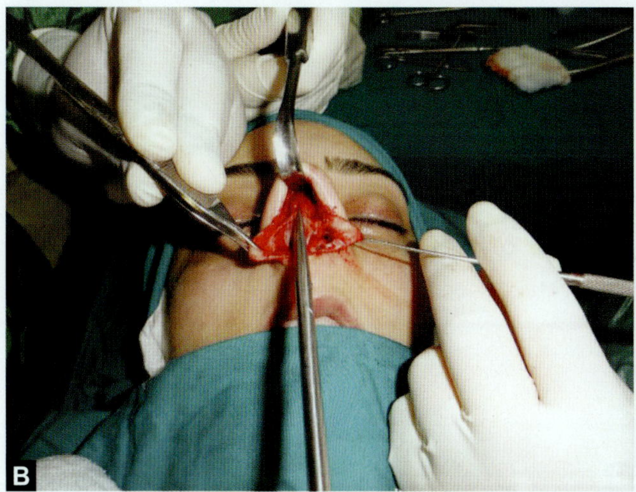

Fig. 4B: The view of the dorsal split approach

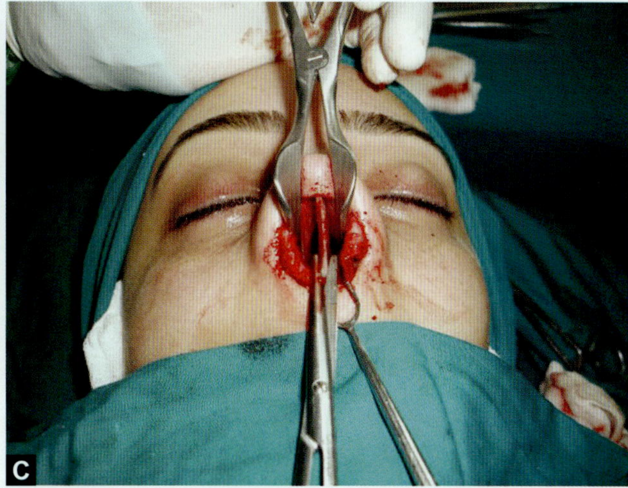

Fig. 4C: Resection of the deviated septal parts

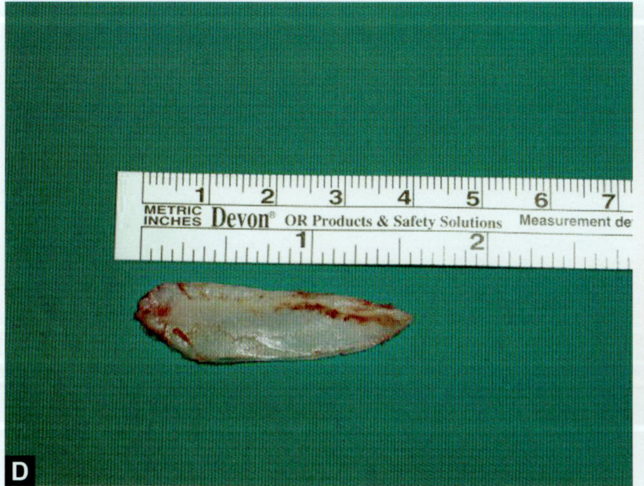

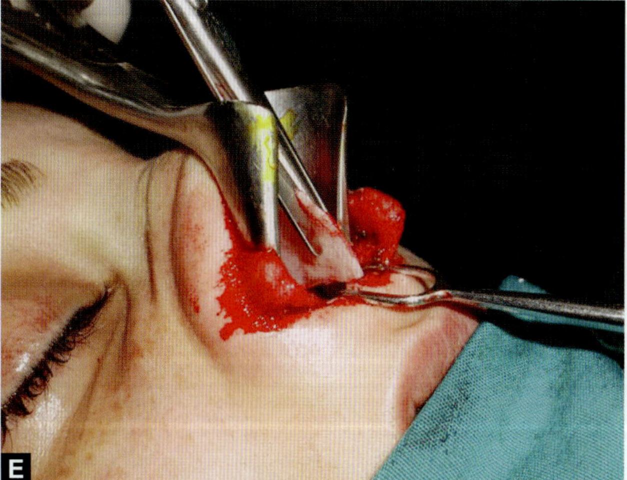

Figs 4D and E: (D) Harvested graft material from the base of the septum; (E) Tip rotation maneuver by resecting reverse triangular segment of the caudal septum

triangular segment of the caudal septum is resected to achieve tip rotation (Fig. 4E).

- The caudal end of the upper lateral cartilages are grasped with a clamp and pulled to facilitate the intra-mucosal dissection of the dorsal edges. The excess dorsal part of the upper lateral cartilages and septum are conservatively lowered before hump reduction (Figs 5A to C).
- The septal hump is lowered using a knife and the bony hump is lowered using a tungsten carbide rasp to open the roof. A straight rasp is used for the caudal hump and a curved rasp is used for lowering the radix (Figs 6A and B). Prefer not to use the hump osteotome for hump reduction.
- Use the transoral lateral osteotomy both for saddle nose deformity and nasomaxillary depression.[16] Perform external/percutaneous perforating lateral osteotomies with a 2 mm straight chisel to reduce post-operative ecchymoses and edema.[17] External/percutaneous perforating lateral osteotomies are begun at the midportion of the lateral osteotomy line after piercing with a 2 mm osteotome (Fig. 7A). The tip of the osteotome leans against the bone with pressure at an angle between 30° and 45° (Fig. 7B). Perforations are barely made through the bone. Adjacent punctures are placed a few millimeters apart and terminated at the level of the medial canthus. Digital pressure to the bony nasal pyramid at the canthal level produces a greenstick

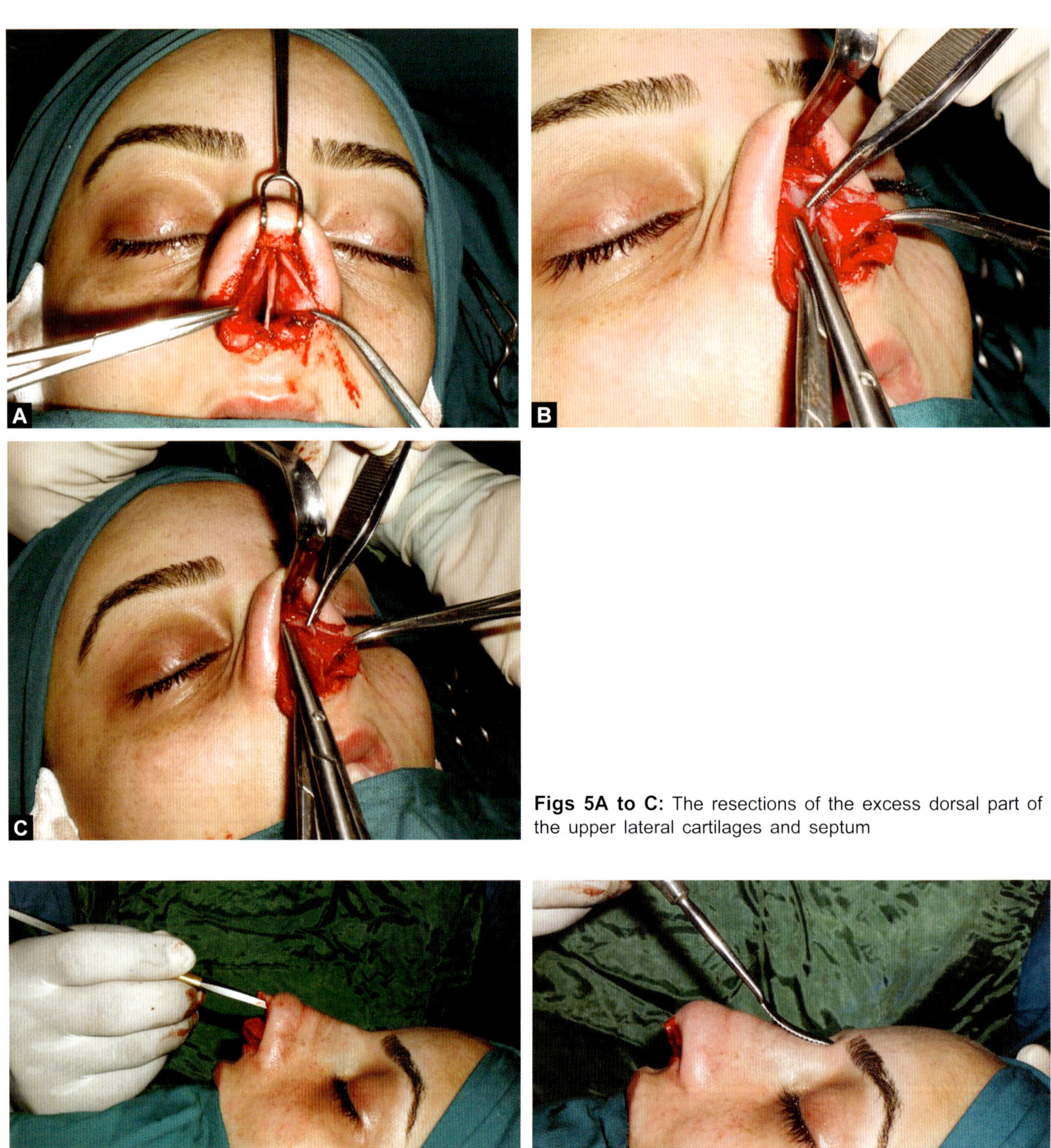

Figs 5A to C: The resections of the excess dorsal part of the upper lateral cartilages and septum

Figs 6A and B: A straight rasp used for the caudal hump and a curved rasp used for lowering the radix

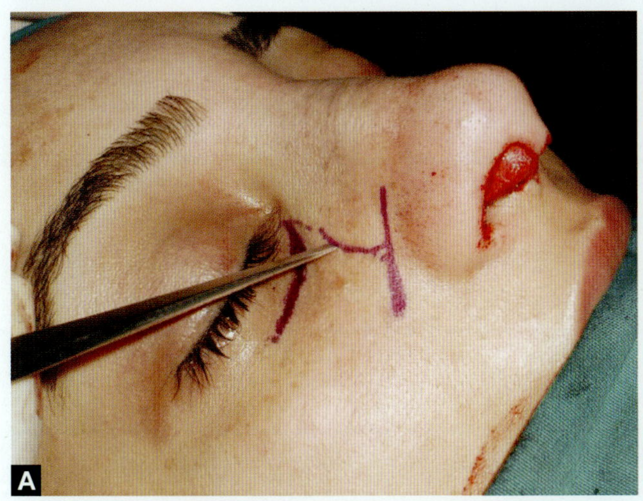

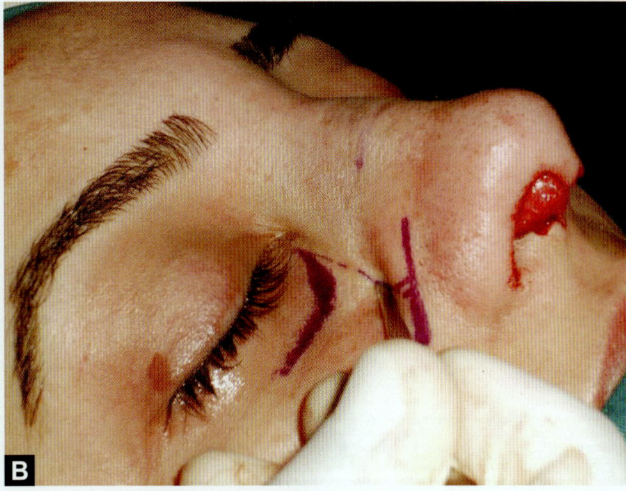

Figs 7A and B: The view of the external percutaneous perforating lateral osteotomy

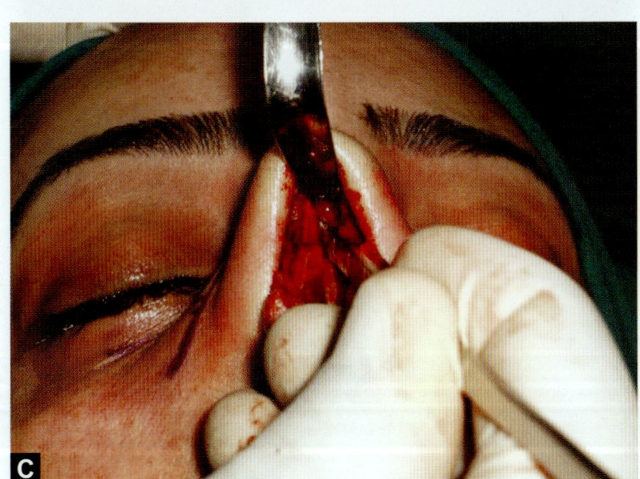

Fig. 7C: The view of 15° medial osteotomies of the nasal root with 5 mm sharp unguarded osteotomies

fracture. Fifteen-degree medial osteotomies of the nasal root are performed with 5 mm sharp unguarded osteotomes for patients with thick nasal bone or a deviated bony pyramid (Fig. 7C). Removal of the bone wedge between the nasal bone and the bony septum at the radix nasi region prior to the medial osteotomy is performed in patients who have a wide nasal root.

- The dorsal septum is straightened and nasal valve collapse is prevented using bilateral spreader grafts prepared from the septal graft (Figs 8A and B).
- A columellar strut graft is inserted between the medial crura of the alar cartilages and accurate alignment can be achieved by skewering the medial crura with No. 27 needles (Fig. 9A). The columellar strut graft provides columellar lengthening and supports the nasal tip (Fig. 9B). Horizontal mattress interdomal sutures, sandwiching the columellar strut are used to increase the lobular projection. Horizontal mattress transdomal sutures are used to narrow the lobular width (Figs 9C and D). Suture between the medial crura and septum is used if columella-lobular rotation is inadequate (Fig. 9E). Other suture techniques which can be used for the nasal tip have been described in detail before.[18]
- The transcolumellar incision is closed using 6 to 0 polypropylene suture and marginal incisions are closed using 5 to 0 rapid polyglactin 910 sutures (Figs 10A to C).

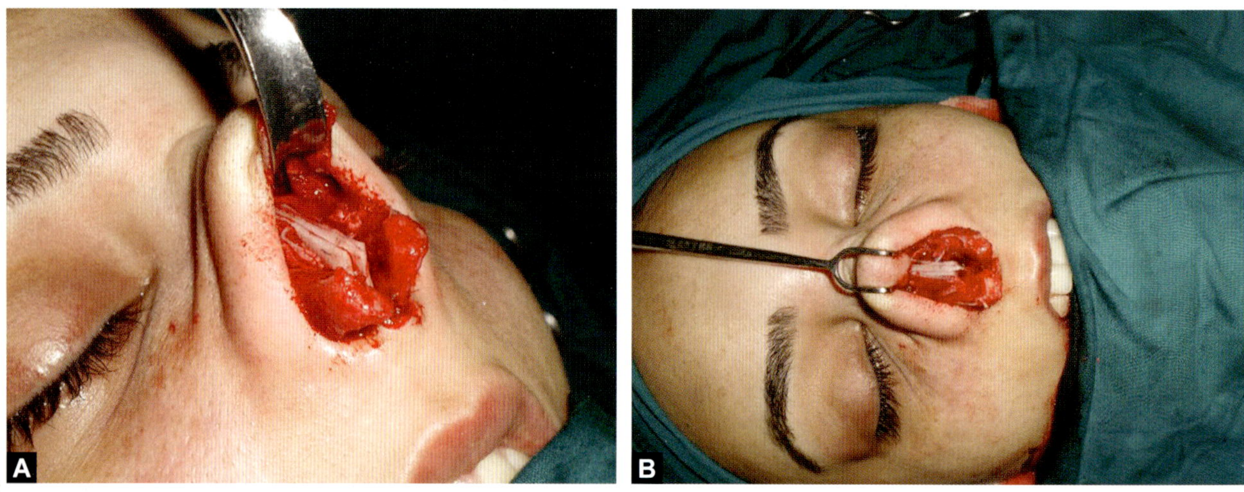

Figs 8A and B: The placement of bilateral spreader grafts

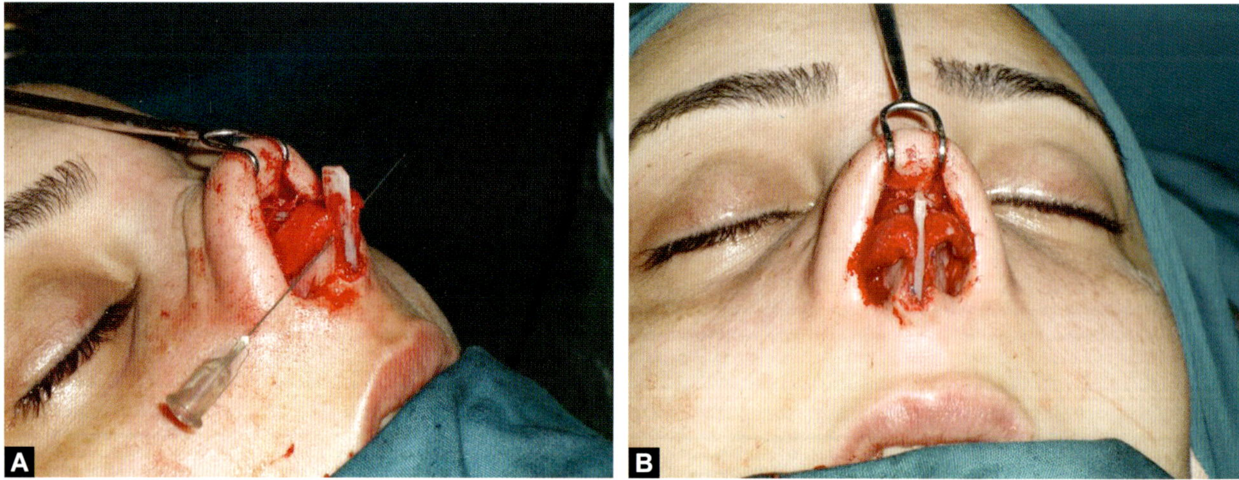

Figs 9A and B: (A) The view of a columellar strut between the medial crura. (B) The columellar strut is sandwiched between the medial and middle crura with sutures

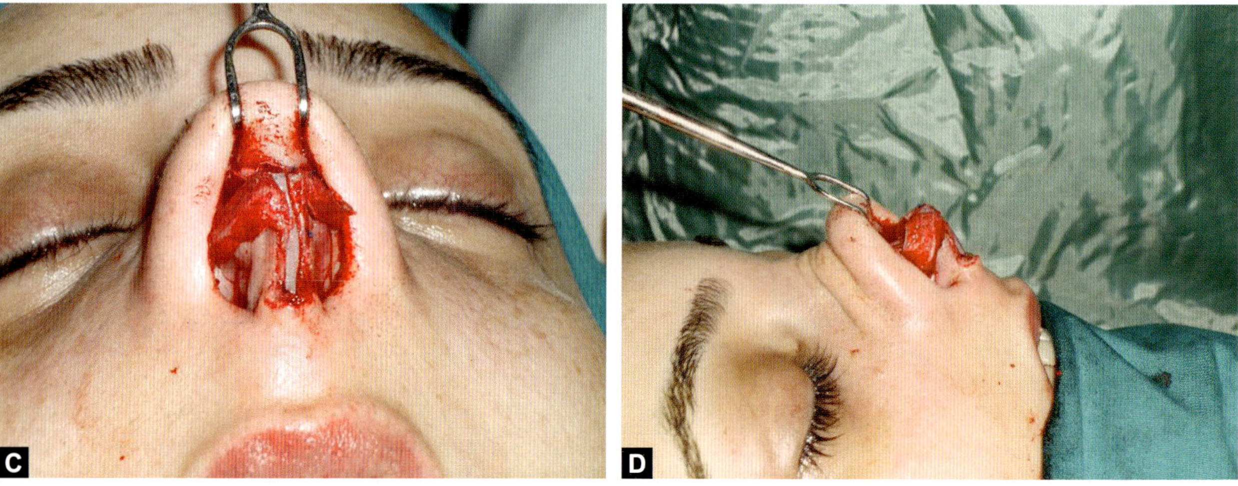

Figs 9C and D

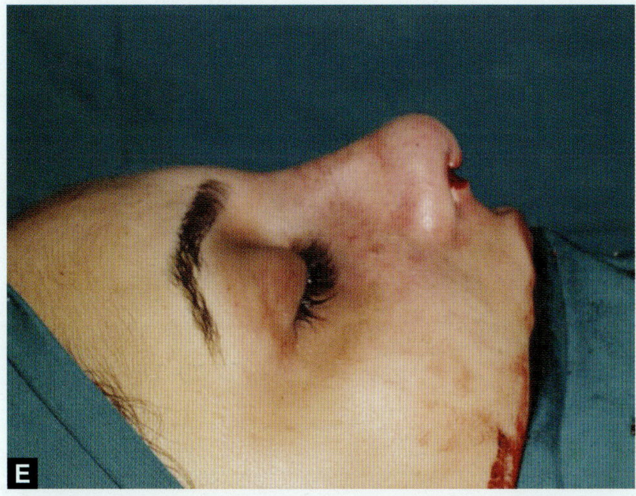

Figs 9C to E: (C and D) Interdomal and transdomal sutures used to increase lobular projection and narrow the lobular width. (E) Suture between medial crura and septum is used, if columellar-lobular rotation is inadequate. It was not used in this patient because the columellar-lobular rotation was adequate

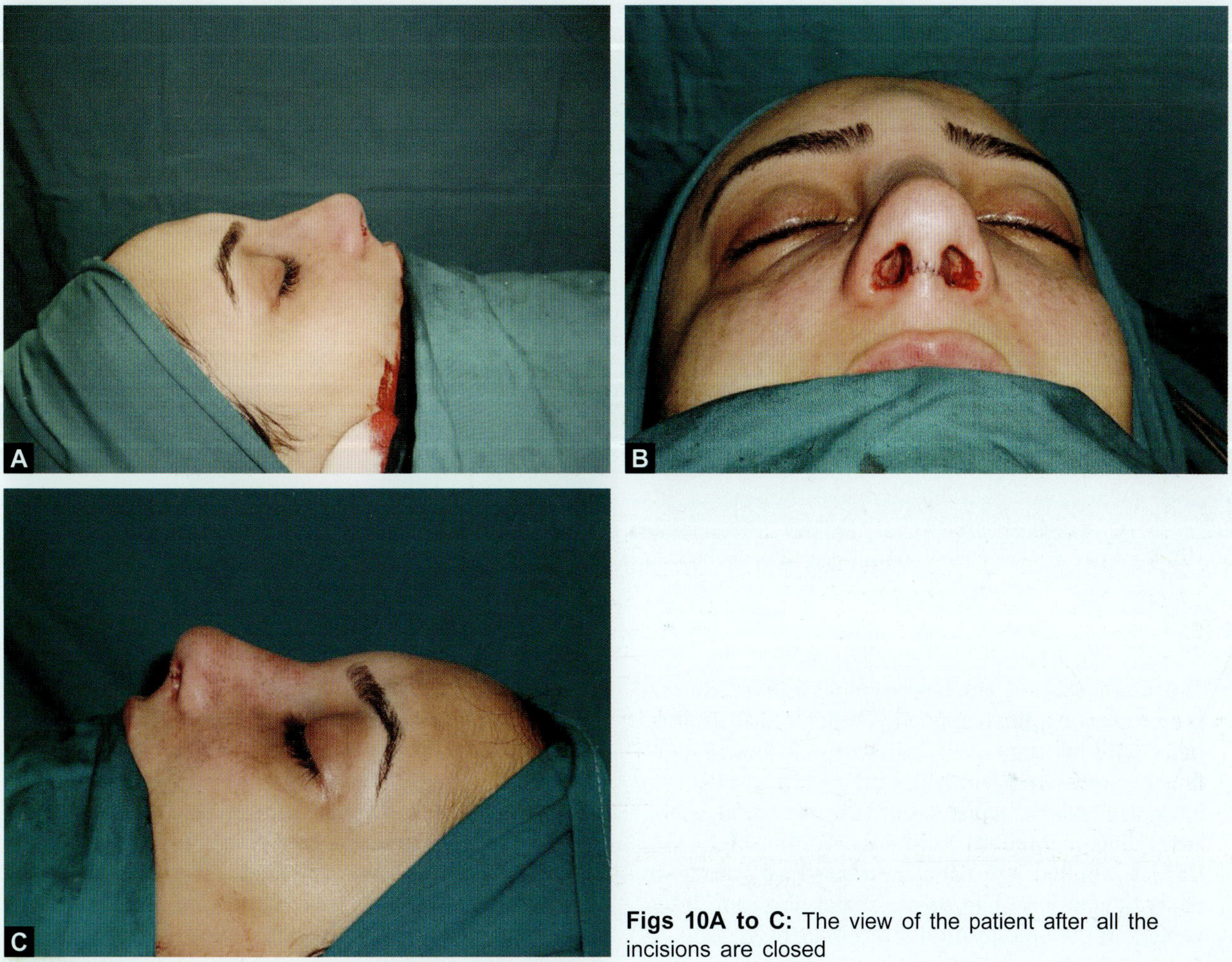

Figs 10A to C: The view of the patient after all the incisions are closed

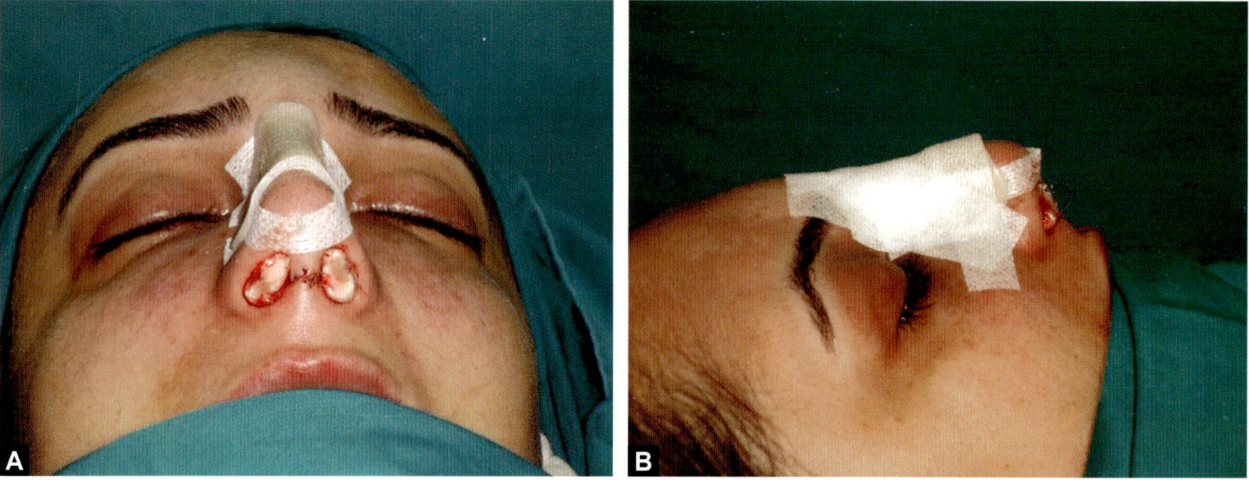

Figs 11A and B: The postoperative view of the patient after nasal packing and splinting

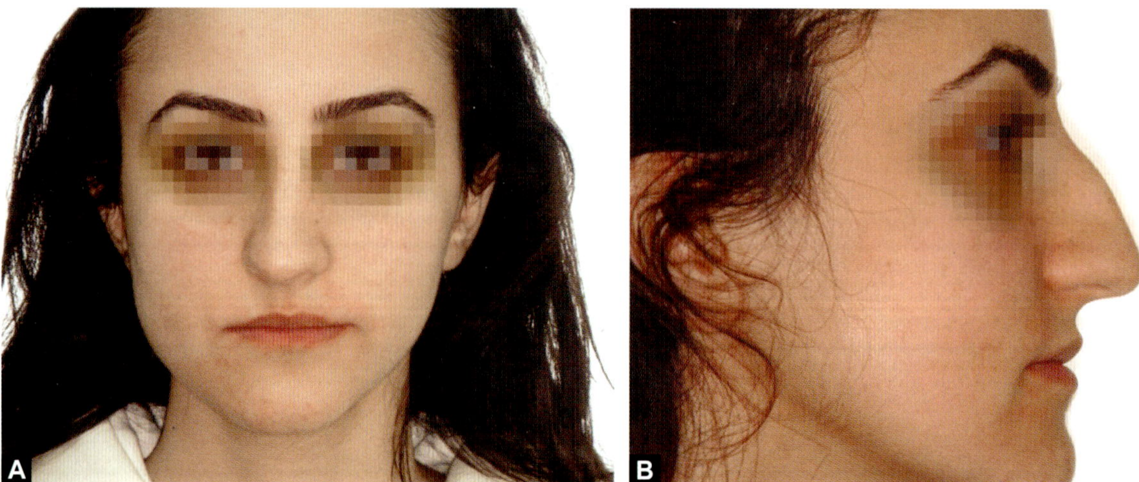

Figs 12A and B: The preoperative view of the patient

- The nose is draped with layered tapes and an external thermoplastic splint is applied. A split merocel impregnated with lidocaine-prilocaine cream in a clear glove finger is used as a nasal packing (Figs 11A and B).[19] An intranasal silastic septal splint (Bivalve Nasal Splint, large; Boston Medical Products, Westborough, MA, USA) is applied and fixed by transseptal sutures in patients who have had severe septal deviation intervention or undergone inferior turbinate resection.
- The septal splints and a dorsal nasal splint are removed after 10 days.
- The patient is reexamined following the operation at first, third, sixth month and 1 year after the operation (Figs 12A to D).
- In conclusion open approach in rhinoplasty provides a direct inspection of the osteocartilaginous vault and corrections of anatomical deformities by grafting and suturing techniques. Its disadvantages are minimal and for this reason it has become popular all over the world. The only absolute contradiction to open rhinoplasty is patient refusal regarding a potentially perceptible scar.

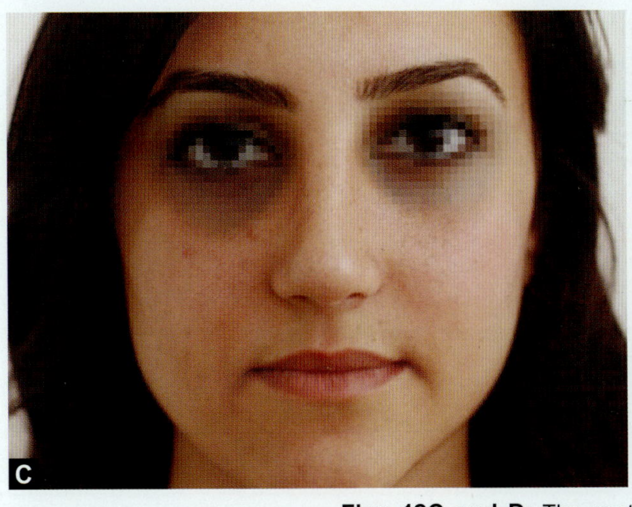

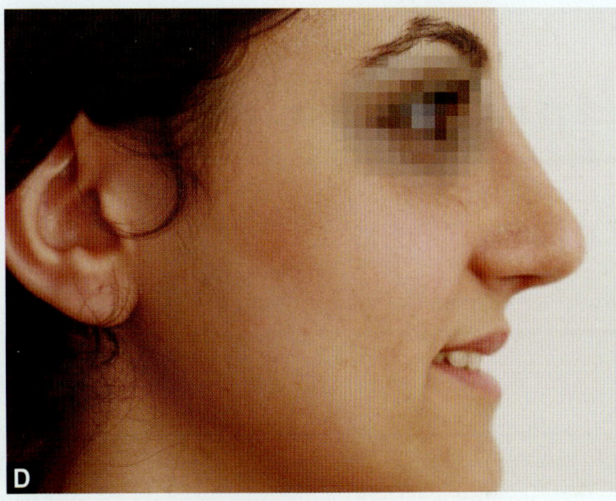

Figs 12C and D: The postoperative view of the patient

REFERENCES

1. McDowell F. History of rhinoplasty. Aesthetic Plast Surg. 1978; 1:321-48.
2. Joseph J. Nasen Plastik und Sonstige Gesichts Plastik. Leipzig, Germany: Verlag C. Kabitsch; 1931.
3. Rethi A. Right and wrong in rhinoplastic operations. Plast Reconstr Surg (1946). 1948; 3(3):361-70.
4. Goodman WS. External approach to rhinoplasty. Can J Otolaryngol. 1973; 2(3):207-10.
5. Gentile P, Bottini DJ, Nicoli F, et al. Open-tip approach: evolutions in rhinoplasty. J Craniofac Surg. 2008; 19(5):1323-9.
6. Adamson PA, Galli SK. Rhinoplasty approaches: current state of the art. Arch Facial Plast Surg. 2005; 7(1):32-7.
7. Kamer FM, McQuown SA. Revision rhinoplasty: analysis and treatment. Arch Otolaryngol Head and Neck Surg. 1988; 114(3):257-66.
8. Bagal AA, Adamson PA. Revision rhinoplasty. Facial Plast Surg. 2002; 18:233-44.
9. Veale D, De Haro L, Lambrou C. Cosmetic rhinoplasty in body dysmorphic disorder. Br J Plast Surg. 2003; 56(6):546-51.
10. Hodgkinson DJ. Identifying the body-dysmorphic patient in aesthetic surgery. Aesthetic Plast Surg. 2005; 29(6):503-9.
11. Andretto Amodeo C. The central role of the nose in the face and the psyche: review of the nose and the psyche. Aesthetic Plast Surg. 2007; 31(4):406-10.
12. Jakubietz M, Jakubietz RJ, Kloss DF, et al. Body dysmorphic disorder: diagnosis and approach. Plast Reconstr Surg. 2007; 119(6):1924-30.
13. Gunter JP. A Graphic Record of Intraoperative Maneuvers in Rhinoplasty: The Missing Link for Evaluating Rhinoplasty Results. Plast Reconstr Surg. 1989; 84(2): 204-12.
14. Whitaker EG, Johnson CM. The evolution of open structure rhinoplasty. Arch Facial Plast Surg. 2003; 5(4): 291-300.
15. Adamson PR. Rhinoplasty-Our Past. Fac Plast Surg. 1988; 5:93-6.
16. Seyhan T. Correction of major saddle nose deformities with nasomaxillary depression by using an intraoral and external open rhinoplasty approach. Aesthetic Plast Surg; 2010. [Epub ahead of print].
17. Gryskiewicz JM, Gryskiewicz KM. Nasal osteotomies: A clinical comparison of the perforating methods versus the continious technique. Plast Reconstr Surg. 2004; 113(5):1445-56.
18. Guyuron B, Behmand RA. Nasal Tip Sutures part II: the interplays. Plast Reconstr Surg. 2003; 112(4): 1130-45.
19. Seyhan T. A comfortable and practical nasal packing method: Tied merocel in clear glove finger impregnated with lidocaine-prilocaine cream. Plast Reconstr Surg. 2010; 125(3):111e-2e.

Appendage 1

Informed Consent – Rhinoplasty Surgery

INSTRUCTIONS

This is an informed consent document that has been prepared to assist your plastic surgeon inform you concerning rhinoplasty surgery, its risks, and alternative treatment.

It is important that you read this information carefully and completely. Please initial each page, indicating that you have read the page and sign the consent for surgery as proposed by your plastic surgeon and agreed upon by you.

GENERAL INFORMATION

Surgery of the nose (rhinoplasty) is an operation frequently performed by plastic surgeons. This surgical procedure can produce changes in the appearance, structure and function of the nose. Rhinoplasty can reduce or increase the size of the nose, change the shape of the tip, narrow the width of the nostrils or change the angle between the nose and the upper lip. This operation can help correct birth defects, nasal injuries and help relieve some breathing problems.

There is not a universal type of rhinoplasty surgery that will meet the needs of every patient. Rhinoplasty surgery is customized for each patient, depending on his or her needs. Incisions may be made within the nose or concealed in inconspicuous locations of the nose in the open rhinoplasty procedure. In some situations, cartilage grafts, taken from within the nose or from other areas of the body may be recommended in order to help reshape the structure of the nose. Internal nasal surgery to improve nasal breathing can be performed at the time of the rhinoplasty.

The best candidates for this type of surgery are individuals who are looking for improvement, not perfection, in the appearance of their nose. In addition to realistic expectations, good health and psychological stability are important qualities for a patient considering rhinoplasty surgery. Rhinoplasty can be performed in conjunction with other surgeries.

ALTERNATIVE TREATMENT

Alternative forms of management consist of not undergoing the rhinoplasty surgery. Certain internal nasal airway disorders may not require surgery on the exterior of the nose. Risks and potential complications are associated with alternative surgical forms of treatment.

RISKS OF RHINOPLASTY SURGERY

Every surgical procedure involves a certain amount of risk and it is important that you understand these risks and the possible complications associated with them. In addition, every procedure has limitations. An individual's choice to undergo a surgical procedure is based on the comparison of the risk to potential benefit. Although the majority of patients do not experience the following complications, you should discuss each of them with your plastic surgeon to make sure you understand the risks, potential complications and consequences of rhinoplasty.

Bleeding

It is possible, though unusual, to experience a bleeding episode during or after surgery. Intraoperative blood transfusions may be required. Should post-operative bleeding occur, it may require an emergency treatment to drain the accumulated blood or blood transfusion. Hypertension (high blood pressure) that is not under good medical control may cause bleeding during or after surgery. Accumulations of blood under the skin may delay healing and cause scarring. Do not take any aspirin or anti-inflammatory medications for ten days before or after surgery, as this may increase the risk of bleeding. Nonprescription "herbs" and dietary supplements can increase the risk of surgical bleeding. Hematoma can occur at any time following injury. If blood transfusions are necessary to treat blood loss, there is the risk of blood-related infections such as hepatitis and HIV (AIDS). Heparin medications that are used to prevent blood clots in veins can produce bleeding and decreased blood platelets.

Infection

Infection is unusual after surgery. Should an infection occur, additional treatment including antibiotics, hospitalization or additional surgery may be necessary.

Scarring

All surgery leaves scars, some more visible than others. Although good wound healing after a surgical procedure is expected, abnormal scars may occur within the skin and deeper tissues. Scars may be unattractive and of different color than the surrounding skin tone. Scar appearance may also vary within the same scar. Scars may be asymmetrical. There is the possibility of visible marks in the skin from sutures. In some cases scars may require surgical revision or treatment.

Damage to Deeper Structures

There is the potential for injury to deeper structures, including nerves, tear ducts, blood vessels, muscles and lungs (pneumothorax) during any surgical procedure. The potential for this to occur varies according to the type of rhinoplasty procedure being performed. Injury to deeper structures may be temporary or permanent.

Change in Skin Sensation

It is common to experience diminished (or loss) of skin sensation in areas that have had surgery. There is the potential for permanent numbness within the nasal skin after rhinoplasty. The occurrence of this is not predictable. Diminished (or loss) of skin sensation in the nasal area may not totally resolve after rhinoplasty.

Asymmetry

The human face is normally asymmetrical. There can be a variation from one side to the other in the results obtained from rhinoplasty. Additional surgery may be necessary to attempt to revise asymmetry.

Skin Discoloration/Swelling

Some bruising and swelling normally occurs following rhinoplasty. The skin in or near the surgical site can appear either lighter or darker than surrounding skin. Although uncommon, swelling and skin discoloration may persist for long periods of time and, in rare situations, may be permanent.

Seroma

Fluid accumulations infrequently occur in between the skin and the underlying tissues. Should this problem occur, it may require additional procedures for drainage of fluid.

Pain

You will experience pain after your surgery. Pain of varying intensity and duration may occur and persist after rhinoplasty. Chronic pain may occur very infrequently from nerves becoming trapped in scar tissue.

Allergic Reactions

In rare cases, local allergies to tape, suture materials and glues, blood products, topical preparations or injected agents have been reported. Serious systemic reactions including shock (anaphylaxis) may occur to drugs used during surgery and prescription medications. Allergic reactions may require additional treatment.

Delayed Healing

Fracture disruption or delayed wound healing is possible. Some areas of the nose may not heal normally and may take a long time to heal. Areas of skin may die. This may require frequent dressing changes or further surgery to remove the non-healed tissue. **Smokers have a greater risk of skin loss and wound healing complications.**

Skin Sensitivity

Itching, tenderness, or exaggerated responses to hot or cold temperatures may occur after surgery. Usually this resolves during healing, but in rare situations it may be chronic.

Nasal Septal Perforation

Infrequently, a hole in the nasal septum will develop. The occurrence of this is rare. Additional surgical treatment may be necessary to repair the nasal septum. In some cases, it may be impossible to correct this complication.

Nasal Airway Alterations

Changes may occur after a rhinoplasty or septoplasty operation that may interfere with normal passage of air through the nose.

Surgical Anesthesia

Both local and general anesthesia involve risk. There is the possibility of complications, injury and even death from all forms of surgical anesthesia or sedation.

Substance Abuse Disorders

Individuals with substance abuse problems that involve the inhalation of vasoconstrictive drugs such as cocaine are at risk for major complications including poor healing and nasal septal perforation.

Skin Contour Irregularities

Contour irregularities may occur. Residual skin irregularities at the ends of the incisions or "dog ears" are always a possibility and may require additional surgery. This may improve with time, or it can be surgically corrected.

Sutures

Most surgical techniques use deep sutures. You may notice these sutures after your surgery. Sutures may spontaneously poke through the skin, become visible or produce irritation that requires removal.

Unsatisfactory Result

Although good results are expected, there is no guarantee or warranty expressed or implied, on the results that may be obtained. You may be disappointed with the results of rhinoplasty surgery. This would include risks such as asymmetry, loss of function, structural malposition, unacceptable visible or tactile deformities, unsatisfactory surgical scar location, poor healing, wound disruption, and loss of sensation. It may be necessary to perform additional surgery to attempt to improve your results.

Shock

In rare circumstances, your surgical procedure can cause severe trauma, particularly when multiple or extensive procedures are performed. Although serious complications are infrequent, infections or excessive fluid loss can lead to severe illness and even death. If surgical shock occurs, hospitalization and additional treatment would be necessary.

Cardiac and Pulmonary Complications

Surgery, especially longer procedures, may be associated with the formation of, or increase in, blood clots in the venous system. Pulmonary complications may occur secondarily to both blood clots (pulmonary emboli), fat deposits (fat emboli) or partial collapse of the lungs after general anesthesia. Pulmonary and fat emboli can be life-threatening or fatal in some circumstances. Air travel, inactivity and other conditions may increase the incidence of blood clots traveling to the lungs causing a major blood clot that may result in death. It is important to discuss with your physician any past history of blood clots or swollen legs that may contribute to this condition. Cardiac complications are a risk with any surgery and anesthesia, even in patients without symptoms. *If you experience shortness of breath, chest pains, or unusual heart beats, seek medical attention immediately.* Should any of these complications occur, you may require hospitalization and additional treatment.

ADDITIONAL ADVISORIES

Skin Disorders/Skin Cancer

Rhinoplasty is a surgical procedure to reshape of both internal and external structure of the nose. Skin disorders and skin cancer may occur independently of a rhinoplasty.

Long-Term Results

Subsequent alterations in nasal appearance may occur as the result of aging, weight loss or gain, sun exposure, pregnancy, menopause, or other circumstances not related to rhinoplasty surgery. Future surgery or other treatments may be necessary.

Female Patient Information

It is important to inform your plastic surgeon if you use birth control pills, estrogen replacement, or if you believe you may be pregnant. Many medications including antibiotics may neutralize the preventive effect of birth control pills, allowing for conception and pregnancy.

Intimate Relations after Surgery

Surgery involves coagulating of blood vessels and increased activity of any kind may open these vessels leading to a bleed, or hematoma. Activity that increases your pulse or heart rate may cause additional bruising, swelling, and the need for return to surgery and control bleeding. It is wise to refrain from sexual activity until your physician states it is safe.

Smoking, Second-Hand Smoke Exposure, Nicotine Products (Patch, Gum, Nasal Spray)

Patients who are currently smoking, use tobacco products, or nicotine products (patch, gum, or nasal spray) are at a greater risk for significant surgical complications of skin dying, delayed healing and additional scarring. Individuals exposed to second-hand smoke are also at potential risk for similar complications attributable to nicotine exposure. Additionally, smoking may have a significant negative effect on anesthesia and recovery from anesthesia, with coughing and possibly increased bleeding. Individuals who are not exposed to tobacco smoke or nicotine-containing products have a significantly lower risk of this type of complication. Please indicate your current status regarding these items below:

________ I am a non-smoker and do not use nicotine products. I understand the risk of second-hand smoke exposure causing surgical complications.

________ I am a smoker or use tobacco/nicotine products. I understand the risk of surgical complications due to smoking or use of nicotine products.

It is important to refrain from smoking at least 6 weeks before surgery and until your physician states it is safe to return, if desired.

Mental Health Disorders and Elective Surgery

It is important that all patients seeking to undergo elective surgery have realistic expectations that focus on improvement rather than perfection. Complications or less than satisfactory results are sometimes unavoidable, may require additional surgery and often are stressful. Please openly discuss with your surgeon, prior to surgery, any history that you may have of significant emotional depression or mental health disorders. Although many individuals may benefit psychologically from the results of elective surgery, effects on mental health cannot be accurately predicted.

Medications

There are many adverse reactions that occur as the result of taking over-the-counter, herbal, and/or prescription medications. Be sure to check with your physician about any drug interactions that may exist with medications which you are already taking. If you have an adverse reaction, stop the drugs immediately and call your plastic surgeon for further instructions. If the reaction is severe, go immediately to the nearest emergency room. When taking the prescribed pain medications after surgery, realize that they can affect your thought process and coordination. Do not drive, do not operate complex equipment, do not make any important decisions, and do not drink any alcohol while taking these medications. Be sure to take your prescribed medication only as directed.

PATIENT COMPLIANCE

Follow all physician instructions carefully; this is essential for the success of your outcome. It is important that the surgical incisions are <u>not</u> subjected to excessive force, swelling, abrasion, or motion during the time of healing. Personal and vocational activity needs to be restricted. Protective dressings and splints should <u>not</u> be removed unless instructed by your plastic surgeon. Successful postoperative function depends on both surgery and subsequent care. Physical activity that increases your pulse or heart rate may cause bruising, swelling, fluid accumulation and the need for return to surgery. It is wise to refrain from intimate physical activities after surgery until your physician states it is safe. It is important that you participate in follow-up care, return for aftercare, and promote your recovery after surgery.

HEALTH INSURANCE

Most health insurance companies exclude coverage for cosmetic surgical operations or any complications that might occur from cosmetic surgery. If the procedure corrects a breathing problem or marked deformity after a nasal fracture, a portion may be covered. *Many insurance plans exclude coverage for secondary or revisionary surgery*. Please carefully review your health insurance subscriber-information pamphlet.

FINANCIAL RESPONSIBILITIES

The cost of surgery involves several charges for the services provided. The total includes fees charged by your doctor, the cost of surgical supplies, anesthesia, laboratory tests and possible outpatient hospital charges, depending on where the surgery is performed. Depending on whether the cost of surgery is covered by an insurance plan, you will be responsible for necessary co-payments, deductibles and charges not covered. Additional costs may occur should complications develop from the surgery. Secondary surgery or hospital day surgery charges involved with revisionary surgery would also be your responsibility.

ADDITIONAL SURGERY NECESSARY

There are many variable conditions that may influence the long-term result from rhinoplasty surgery. Secondary surgery may be necessary to obtain optimal results. Should complications occur, additional surgery or other treatments may be necessary. Even though risks and complications occur infrequently, the risks cited are particularly associated with rhinoplasty surgery. Other complications and risks can occur but are even more uncommon. The practice of medicine and surgery is not an exact science. Although good results are expected, there is no guarantee or warranty expressed or implied, on the results that may be obtained. In some situations, it may not be possible to achieve optimal results with a single surgical procedure.

DISCLAIMER

Informed-consent documents are used to communicate information about the proposed surgical treatment of a disease or condition along with disclosure of risks and alternative forms of treatment(s), including no surgery. The informed-consent process attempts to define principles of risk disclosure that should generally meet the needs of most patients in most circumstances.

However, informed-consent documents should not be considered all inclusive in defining other methods of care and risks encountered. Your plastic surgeon may provide you with additional or different information which is based on all the facts in your particular case and the current state of medical knowledge.

Informed-consent documents are not intended to define or serve as the standard of medical care. Standards of medical care are determined on the basis of all of the facts involved in an individual case and are subject to change as scientific knowledge and technology advance and as practice patterns evolve.

It is important that you read the above information carefully and have all of your questions answered before signing the consent on the next page.

CONSENT FOR SURGERY/PROCEDURE or TREATMENT

1. I hereby authorize DR. .... and such assistants as may be selected to perform the following procedure or treatment:

RHINOPLASTY SURGERY

I have received the following information sheet:

INFORMED CONSENT—RHINOPLASTY SURGERY

2. I recognize that during the course of the operation and medical treatment or anesthesia, unforeseen conditions may necessitate different procedures than those above. I therefore authorize the above physician and assistants or designees to perform such other procedures that are in the exercise of his or her professional judgment necessary and desirable. The authority granted under this paragraph shall include all conditions that require treatment and are not known to my physician at the time the procedure is begun.
3. I consent to the administration of such anesthetics considered necessary or advisable. I understand that all forms of anesthesia involve risk and the possibility of complications, injury, and sometimes death.
4. I acknowledge that no guarantee or representation has been given by anyone as to the results that may be obtained.
5. I consent to be photographed or televised before, during, and after the operation(s) or procedure(s) to be performed, including appropriate portions of my body, for medical, scientific or educational purposes, provided my identity is not revealed by the pictures.
6. For purposes of advancing medical education, I consent to the admittance of observers to the operating room.
7. I consent to the disposal of any tissue, medical devices or body parts, which may be removed.
8. I consent to the utilization of blood products should they be deemed necessary by my surgeon and/or his/her appointees and I am aware that there are potential significant risks to my health with their utilization.
9. I authorize the release of my Social Security number to appropriate agencies for legal reporting and medical-device registration, if applicable.
10. I understand that the surgeons' fees are separate from the anesthesia and hospital charges, and the fees are agreeable to me. If a secondary procedure is necessary, further expenditure will be required.
11. I realize that not having the operation is an option.
12. IT HAS BEEN EXPLAINED TO ME IN A WAY THAT I UNDERSTAND:
    a. THE ABOVE TREATMENT OR PROCEDURE TO BE UNDERTAKEN
    b. THERE MAY BE ALTERNATIVE PROCEDURES OR METHODS OF TREATMENT
    c. THERE ARE RISKS TO THE PROCEDURE OR TREATMENT PROPOSED

I CONSENT TO THE TREATMENT OR PROCEDURE AND THE ABOVE LISTED ITEMS (1 - 12).

I AM SATISFIED WITH THE EXPLANATION.

____

______________________________ Patient or Person Authorized to Sign for Patient.

Date: ____________________ Witness: ____________________

CHAPTER

101 Rhinoplasty for Cleft Nasal Deformity

C Thomas

INTRODUCTION

There is significant improvement in the results of cleft lip repair in the present decade but nasal deformity is the greatest corrective challenge and which is more obvious once the lip has been repaired.

The nasal deformity varies in

- Unilateral cleft lip
- Bilateral cleft lip

UNILATERAL CLEFT LIP NASAL DEFORMITY

The nasal deformity has characteristic features, but the severity varies and is related to the extent of the lip deformity and alveolar cleft.

Etiology

It may be the result of the following:

- Tissue deficiency of the cleft lip
- Deficiency of the maxilla
- Abnormal muscular pull on the nasal structures.

Components

Defects of the

- Alar cartilage
- Nasal septum
- Columella
- Nasal tip
- Entire nasal pyramid
- Abnormal orbicularis muscle attachments
- Hypoplastic maxilla.

Pathologic Anatomy

- Nasal tip is deflected toward the cleft side.
- The dome on the cleft side is retrodisplaced.
- The angle between the medial and lateral crura is excessively obtuse.
- Alar buckles inward on the cleft side.
- Alar-facial groove on the cleft side is absent.
- Real or apparent maxillary deficiency.
- Circumference of the naris is greater on the cleft side.
- Naris on the cleft side is retrodisplaced.
- Columella is shorter in the anteroposterior dimension on the cleft side.
- Medial crus is displaced on the cleft side.
- Columella is positioned obliquely with its base toward the non-cleft side.
- Absence of the nasal floor.
- Hypertrophy of the inferior turbinate on the cleft side.
- *Vestibular web*: Within the cleft side of interior nostril.

BILATERAL CLEFT LIP NASAL DEFORMITY

It is a characteristic nasal deformity which is usually symmetric, hence reconstruction is much easier than that of a unilateral cleft lip nasal deformity.

Etiology: Several Hypotheses

- Lateral traction on the alar bases and lowering of the ala due to abnormal muscle insertions
- Overgrowth of the mesoderm at the vomeropremaxillary suture due to lack of restraint by the nonunited orbicularis oris muscle
- Incorporation of prolabium into the lip repair.

Pathologic Anatomy

- A short columella with encroachment of the lip tissue, especially in a protruded premaxilla
- Medial crura of the alar cartilages are displaced inferiorly with lowering of the alar domes
- Alar domes are laterally displaced on a hypoplastic maxilla resulting in a widened nostril sill
- Prominent vestibular skin webs and buckling of the lateral crura produce a collapsed nasal contour
- The caudal septum and underdeveloped anterior nasal spine are displaced inferiorly or laterally depending on the degree and asymmetry of the cleft.

MANAGEMENT

Neonatal splintage prior to lip repair may be helpful to correct these deformities but difficult to practice because it needs prolonged nasal splintage and noncompliance by the parents.

SURGICAL CORRECTION

Timing of the Surgery

- *Primary rhinoplasty,* if nasal deformity is corrected along with the lip repair. Otherwise it is known as *secondary rhinoplasty,* which could be done during the school going age (5–6 years), early adolescence (10–12 years) or in adult age (above 18 years).
- *Primary rhinoplasty* can be done by closed approach, semi-open approach or open approach.

Primary Cheilorhinoplasty—Open Approach

- Proper reconstruction of the clefted musculoaponeurotic complex by a subperiosteal dissection and placing the muscles in their proper anatomic and physiologic orientation after detaching from their abnormal insertions with adequate mobilization.
- Muscle repair is the "key" for the establishment of a normal nasolabial complex.
- Primary rhinoplasty by delicate dissection and accurate repositioning of the lower alar cartilages during the primary lip repair enhances normal nasal shape and breathing.

Advantages

- Identification and proper repositioning of the lower alar cartilages by accurately placed sutures under direct vision.
- Approach of this procedure through the hidden rim incisions without any residual scars.
- Septal cartilage can be easily dislocated and relocated into normal position without any resection.
- Easy procedure comparable to the closed technique with a shorter operating time.
- It is a procedure of choice where there is no preoperative orthodontic treatment or nasoalveolar molding.

SURGICAL TECHNIQUE

Primary Rhinoplasty by Open Approach with Repair of Unilateral Complete Cleft Lip

The markings are made showing a modification of the Millard rotation-advancement technique and Harashina open rhinoplasty technique as shown in Figures 1 and 2. A triangular flap of 2 mm is incorporated at the advancement flap (Millard B flap) near the vermillion to break the scar and subsequent scar contraction. Addition points (philtral-columellar points) are also marked at the junction of the columellar and the philtrum on both the cleft and the non-cleft side. Millard C flap is drawn at the mucocutaneous junction of the rotation flap (Millard A flap) at the level of the philtral-columellar angle with its base in continuity with the mucosal lining of the septum as mucocutaneous

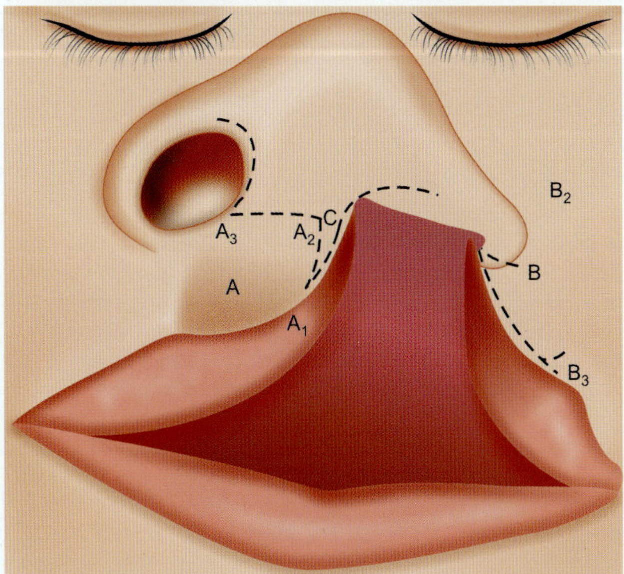

Fig. 1: Preoperative markings for unilateral complete cleft lip and palate repairs along with primary rhinoplasty by the open approach

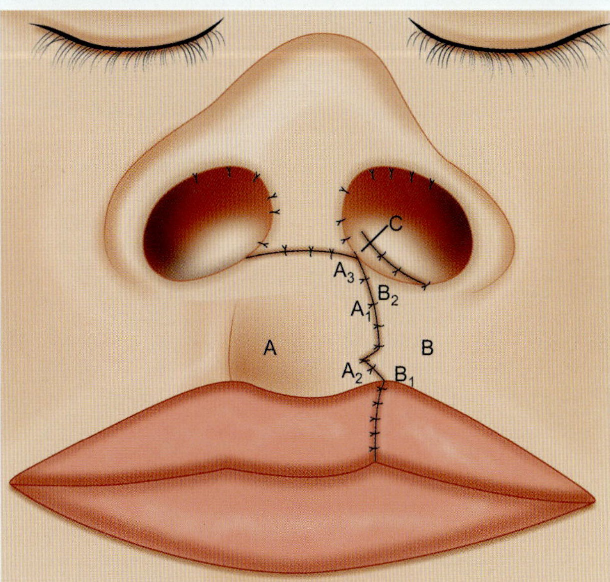

Fig. 2: Repair after the operation

flap. From the philtral-columellar points, the incisions are extended in the nose as standard rim incisions through the edge of the columella, extending through the inside margins of the nostril rim up to its middle on the cleft and non-cleft side.

Orbicularis oris muscles are radically mobilized from the vestibular nasal lining down to the edge of the bony cleft. The lateral nasal mucosa is elevated upward subperiosteally up to the inferior turbinate. The medial nasal septal mucosal flap is raised and extended posteriorly as a vomerine flap. Subperiosteal dissection of the cheek is performed widely from the anterior maxilla, respecting the inferior orbital nerve, to allow tension-free advancement of the soft tissue across the bony cleft. Columellar skin is dissected upward along the rim incision to expose the medial crura of the alar domes. Care is taken to free the fibrofatty tissue between the domes of the alar cartilage and to leave attached to the overlying skin. The nasal skin is dissected widely over the nasal skeleton to allow redraping over the reconstituted nasal tip. The nasal septum is dislocated from its base to provide a symmetrical appearance of the nostrils. Suturing begins with the repair of the anterior palate. The vomerine flap and lateral nasal mucosa are approximated to reconstruct a nostril tube. The C flap is incorporated into the nostril sill, which is an important step to avoid stenosis of the nostril. Lip repair is carried out in the conventional manner as in the Millard rotation-advancement technique. The length of the rotation flap A ($A_1 + A_2 + A_3$) is equal to the length of the advancement flap B (B_1 and B_2). The role of the triangular flap is mentioned earlier. Union of the orbicularis muscle from the cleft and non-cleft sides without tension should be given adequate emphasis.

The columellar skin is retracted with the skin hook. This maneuver tends to symmetrically align the alar cartilages. Four to five 5/0 Vicryl (Ethicon) sutures are used to suture the medial crura of the alar domes. The cranial edges of the lateral crura are sutured, securing the upward rotation of the lateral crura on the affected side (Figs 3 and 4). Finally, the nasal and the columellar incisions are sutured.

Transparent thin steri-strips are applied over the suture lines in the lip, followed by the application of the nostril conformers. Skin sutures and nostril conformers are removed after a week under a short general anesthesia.

Nostril conformers encourage proper nasal contours and keep the patency of the nostrils for breathing.

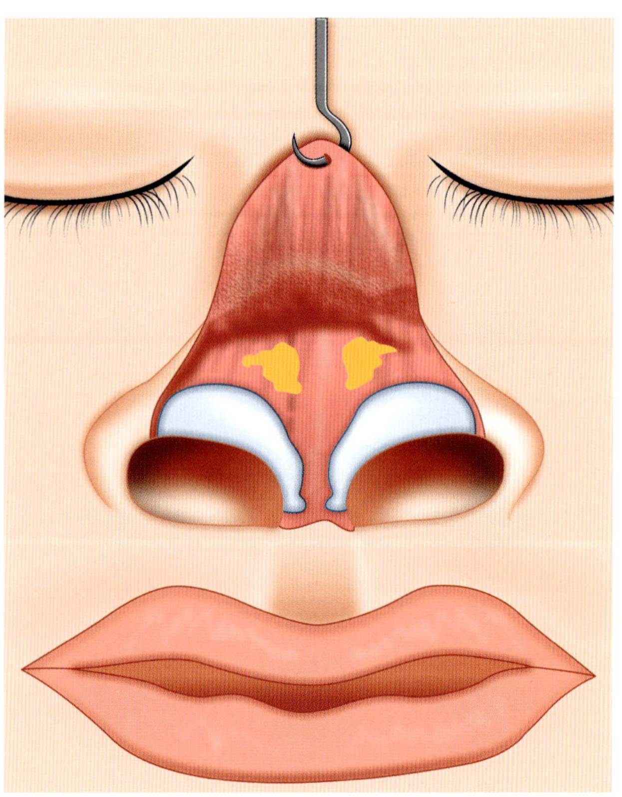

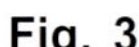

Fig. 3

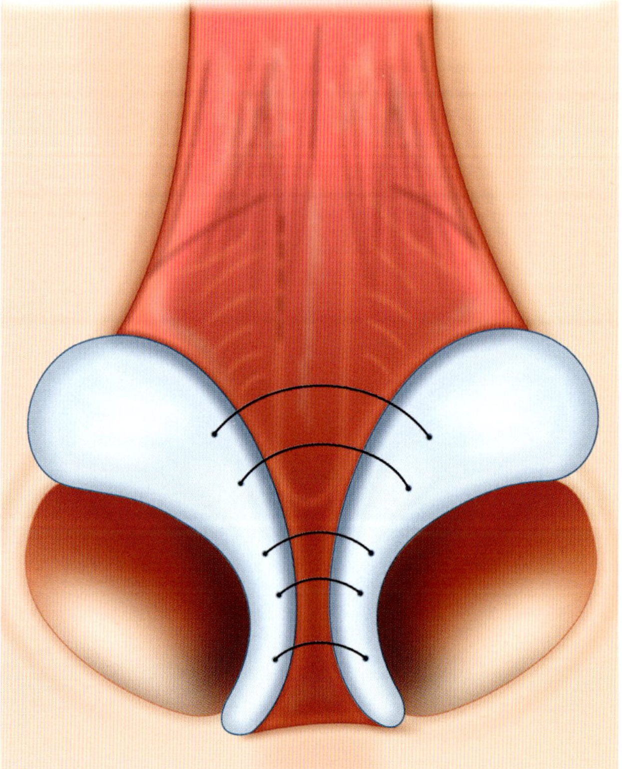

Fig. 4:

Surgical Technique—Unilateral Complete Cleft Lip

Figures 5 to 11 illustrate sequential operative steps of the surgery.

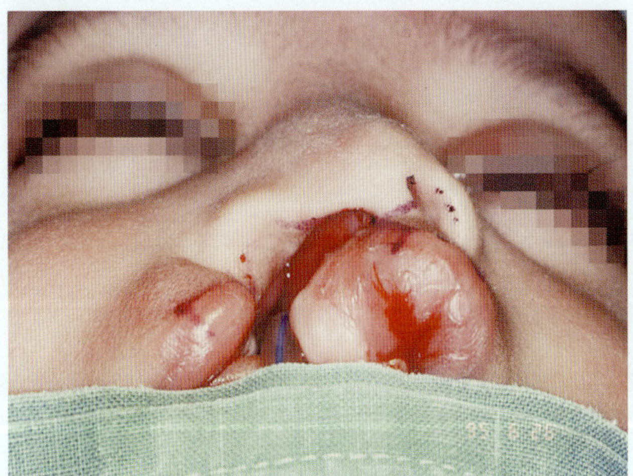

Fig. 5: Skin markings

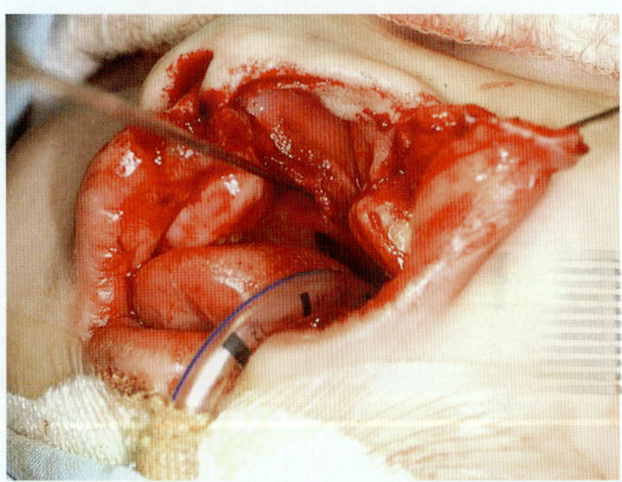

Fig. 6: After dissection with marginal incisions of nostrils

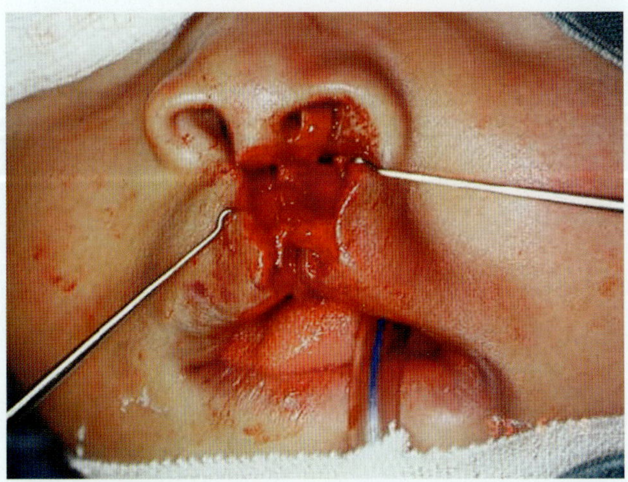

Fig. 7: Muscle repair with the C flap at the nostril sill

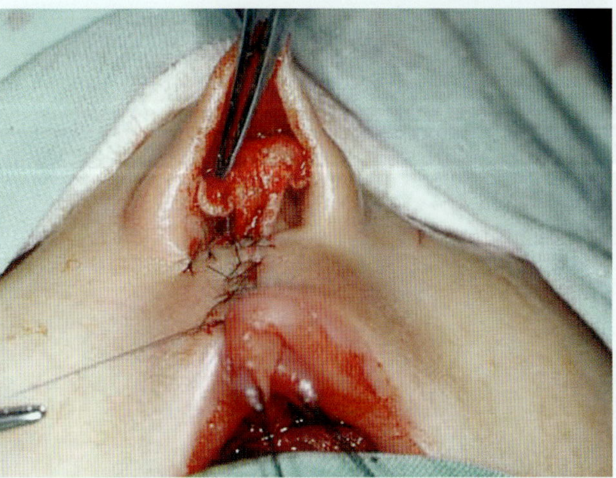

Fig. 8: Deformed lower alar cartilage at the cleft side

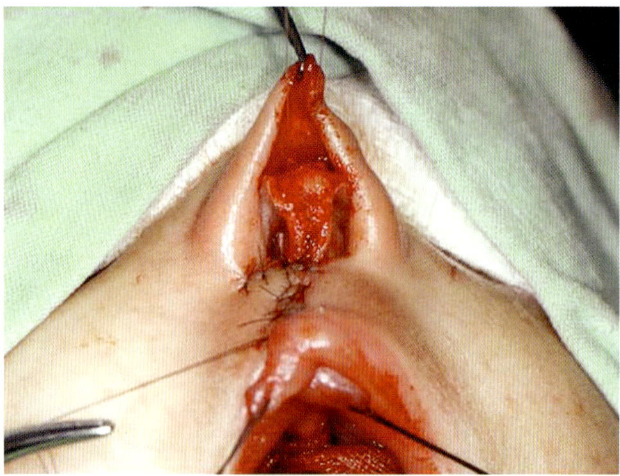

Fig. 9: Correction of the deformed lower alar cartilage with 5/0 Vicryl stitches

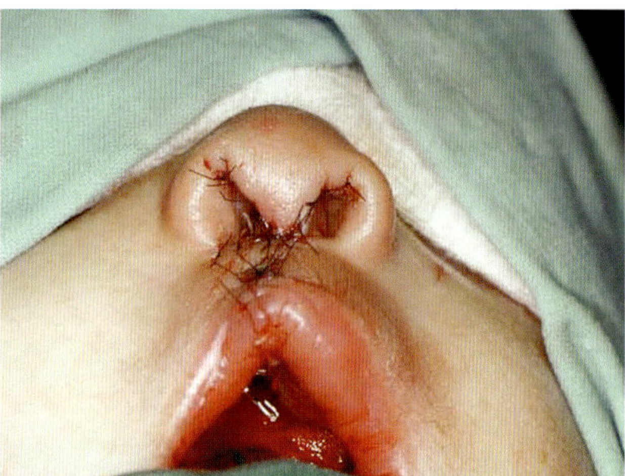

Fig. 10: Corrected symmetrical appearance of the nostrils

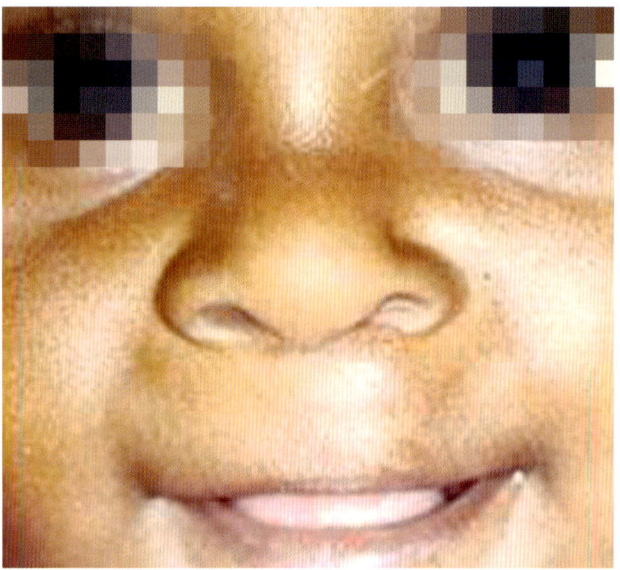

Fig. 11A: Postoperative frontal view after 1 year

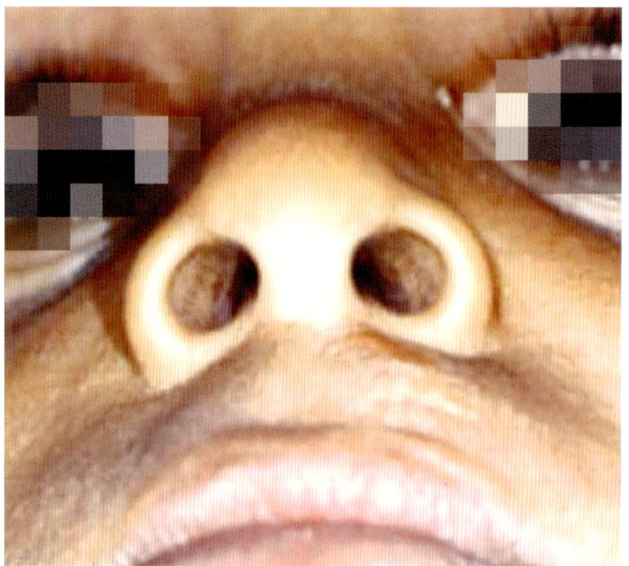

Fig. 11B: Postoperative nasal view after 1 year

Primary Rhinoplasty by Open Approach with Repair of Bilateral Complete Cleft Lip

Presurgical orthodontic correction by means of strapping is given to bilateral cleft lip with protruded premaxilla. The markings are made showing a modification of the Millard rotation-advancement technique and Harashina open rhinoplasty technique as shown in Figures 12 and 13. Additional points (philtral-columellar points) are also marked at the junction of the columella and the philtrum. The width of the prolabium is made the same as the width of the columella from the philtral-columellar points. These prolabial incisions are extended into the nose as standard rim incisions through the edges of the columella extending through the inside margins of the nostril rim up to its middle. The remaining prolabial skin is left attached to the skin of the membranous septum as two nasal septal mucosal flaps (Figs 12 and 13). Orbicularis oris muscles are radically mobilized from the vestibular

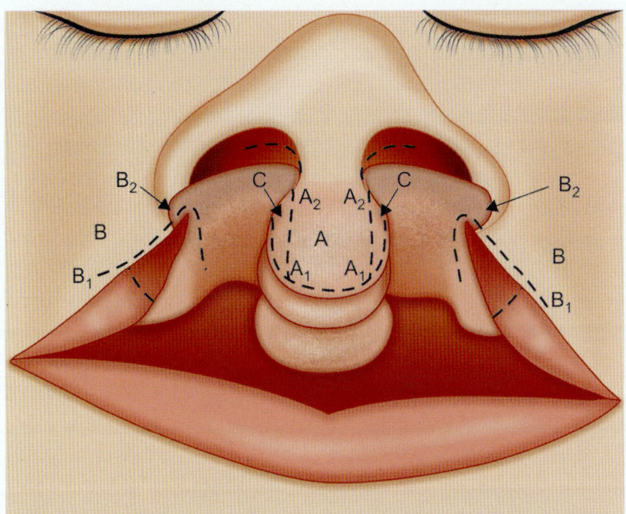

Fig. 12: Preoperative markings for bilateral complete cleft lip and palate repairs along with primary rhinoplasty by the open approach

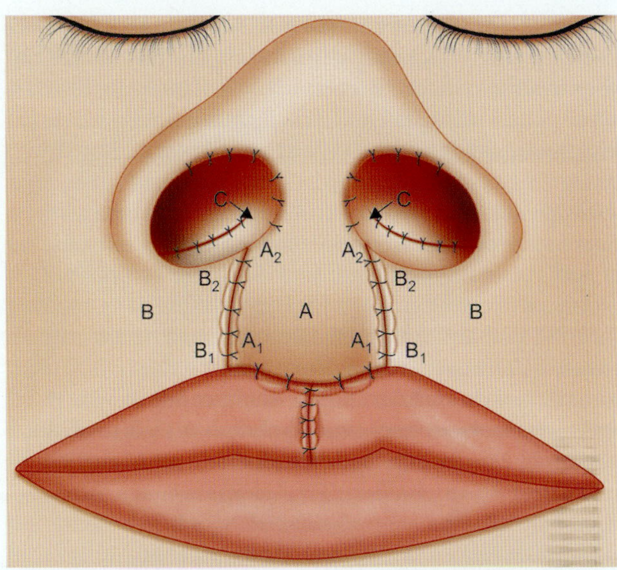

Fig. 13: Repair after the operation

nasal lining down to the edge of the bony cleft from the lateral lip elements. The lateral nasal mucosa is elevated upward subperiosteally up to the inferior turbinate. The medial nasal septal mucosal flap is raised and extended posteriorly as a vomerine flap. A central strip of the nasal septal mucosa at least approximately 1 cm in width is to be kept intact to preserve the blood supply of the premaxilla. Subperiosteal dissection of the cheek is performed widely from the anterior maxilla, respecting the inferior orbital nerve, to allow tension-free advancement of the soft tissue across the bony cleft (see Fig. 3).

The prolabial flap is reflected along with columellar skin by careful dissection especially at the base of the columella to dissect all fibrofatty soft tissue from the medial crura of the alar cartilages up to the dome and then from off the lateral crura, the septum, and upper lateral cartilages. Thus, the fibrofatty soft tissue is left attached to the elevated skin of the nose, which is dissected back to the dorsum of the nasal skeleton. The nasal skin is dissected widely over the nasal skeleton to allow redraping over the reconstituted nasal tip.

Suturing begins with the repair of the anterior palate. The vomerine flap and the lateral nasal mucosa are approximated to reconstruct a nostril tube on both sides. Lip repair is carried out in the conventional manner—first, the mucosa followed by the muscle repair. Union of the orbicularis oris muscle from both lateral elements across the premaxilla should be given adequate emphasis. The columellar skin is retracted with a skin hook, and this maneuver tends to symmetrically align the alar cartilages. Three to four 5/0 Vicryl (Ethicon) sutures are used to suture the medial crura and the alar domes. Cranial edges of the lateral crura are sutured securing the upward rotation of the lateral crus. The skin suturing is carried out with the prolabium to the lateral elements up to the philtral-columellar angle. Care should be taken to create an obtuse angle at the philtral-columellar junction by accurately placed sutures. The nasal and columellar skin incisions are sutured.

Cupid's bow of the philtral column is formed by the advancement of the vermillion flaps from both lateral elements. The length of flap A (A_1 to A_2) is equal to the length of advancement flap B (B_1 to B_2). Transparent thin steri-strips are applied over the suture lines in the lip followed by the application of the nostril conformers. Skin sutures and the nostril conformers are removed after a week under a short general anesthesia.

Nostril conformers encourage the proper nasal contours and keep up the patency of the nostrils for breathing.

Surgical Technique—Bilateral Complete Cleft Lip

Figures 14 to 18 illustrate sequential operative steps of the surgery.

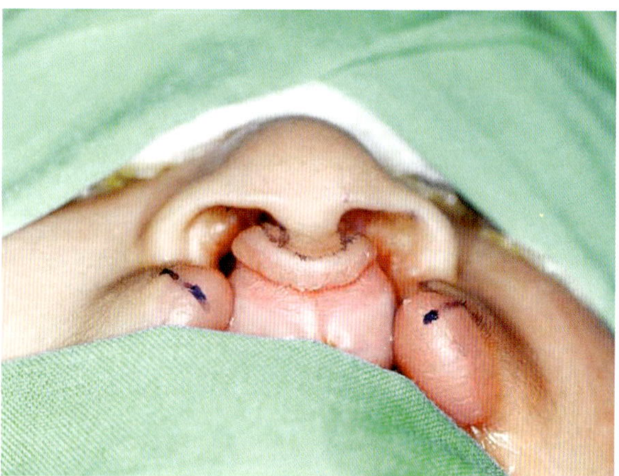

Fig. 14: Skin markings

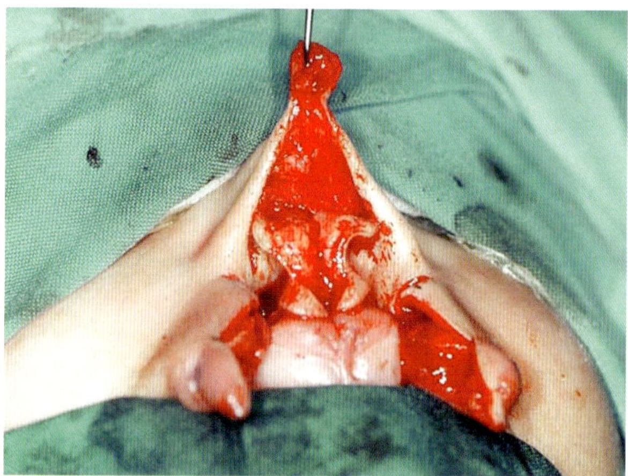

Fig. 15: After dissection, to show both lower alar cartilages by elevating the prolabium and columella by a skin hook

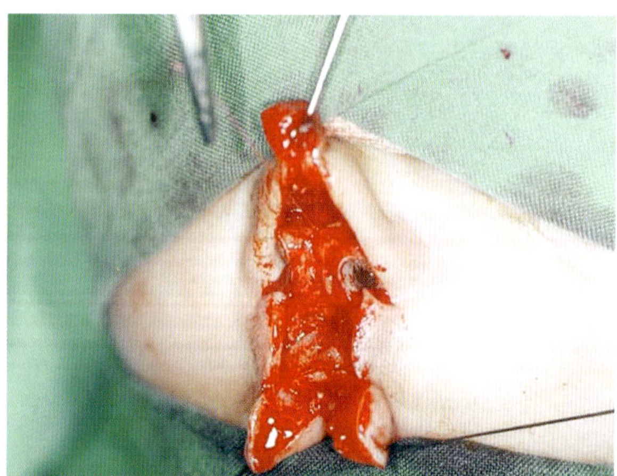

Fig. 16: Correction of the deformity of the lower alar cartilages and recreation of columella

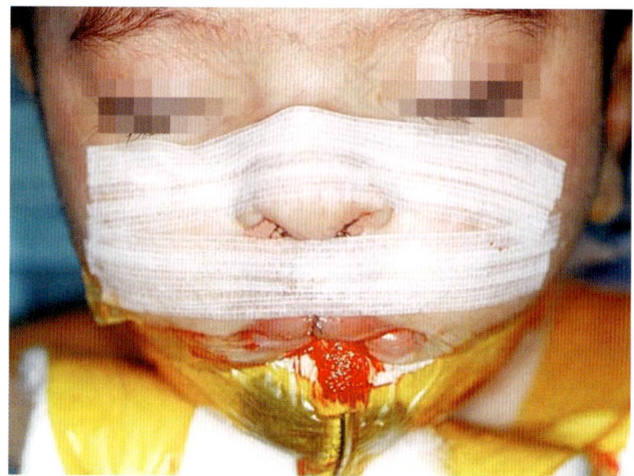

Fig. 17: Application of steri-strips at the end of the operation

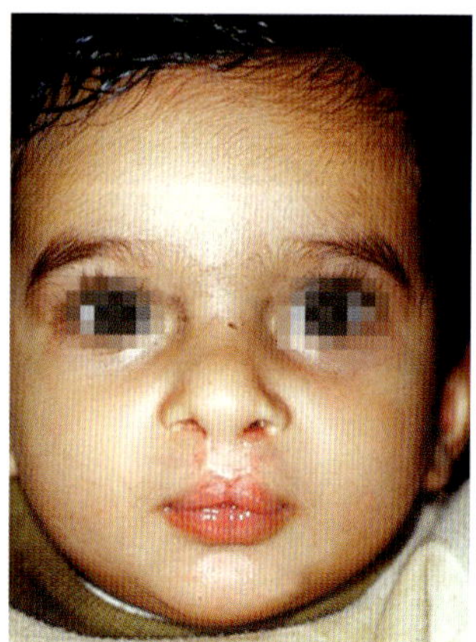

Fig. 18A: Postoperative frontal view after 1 year

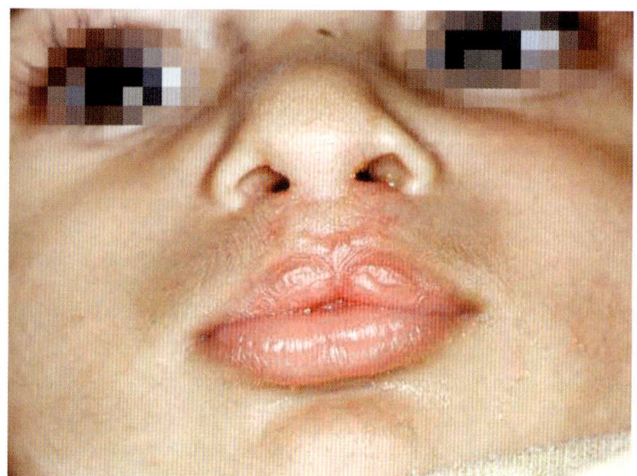

Fig. 18B: Postoperative nasal view after 1 year

NOSTRIL CONFORMERS (FIGS 19 TO 21)

Nostril conformers, recently introduced, encourage the proper nasal contours and keep up the patency of the nostrils for breathing.

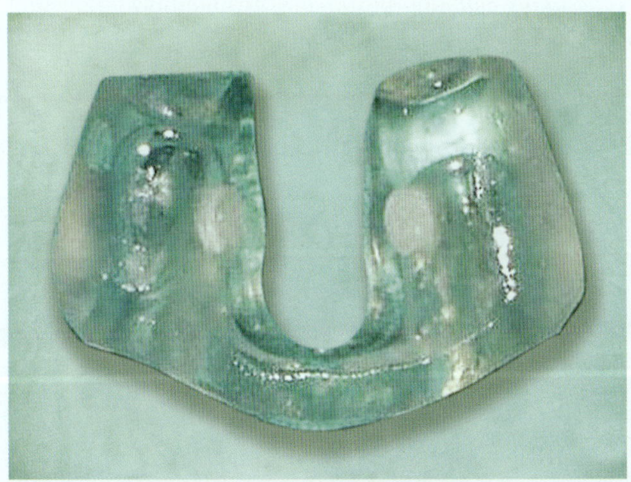

Fig. 19: Silicon nostril conformers

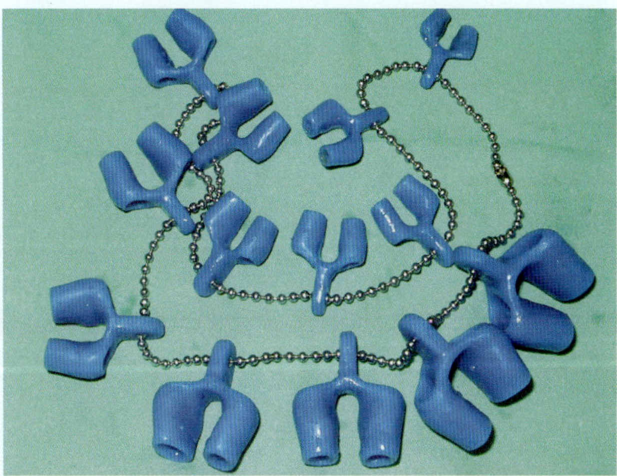

Fig. 20: Nostril conformers—sizing set

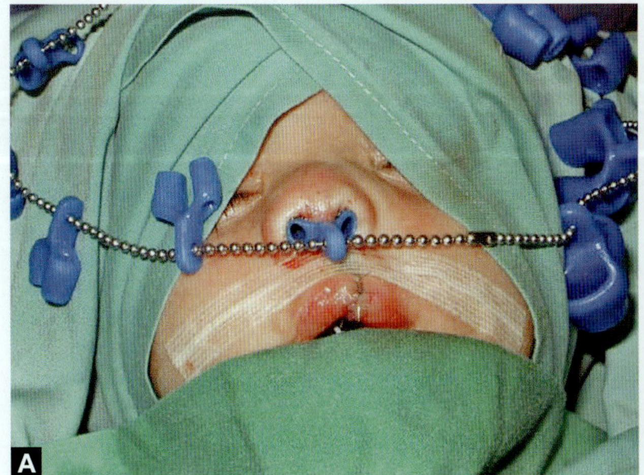

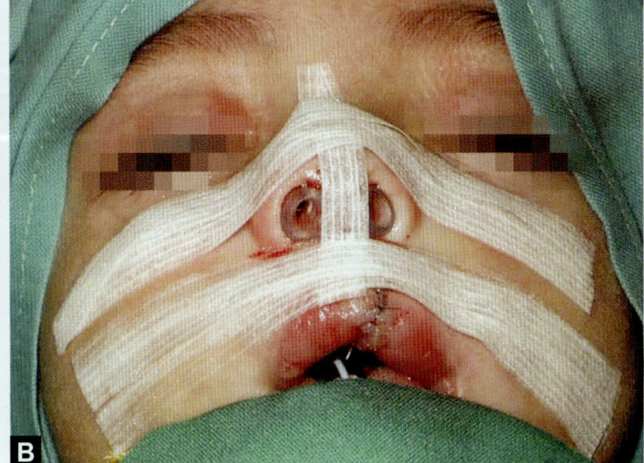

Figs 21A and B: Application of nostril conformers after cleft lip repair

PREOPERATIVE AND POSTOPERATIVE PHOTOGRAPHS OF CONSECUTIVE PATIENTS WITH LONG-TERM FOLLOW-UP

Unilateral Complete Cleft Lip (Figs 22A to G)

Directions for Figures

- *First column*: Preoperative anteroposterior and nasal views.
- *Middle column*: Postoperative anteroposterior and nasal views with 1 year follow-up of the same patient.
- *Last column*: Postoperative anteroposterior and nasal views over 12 years follow-up of the same patient.

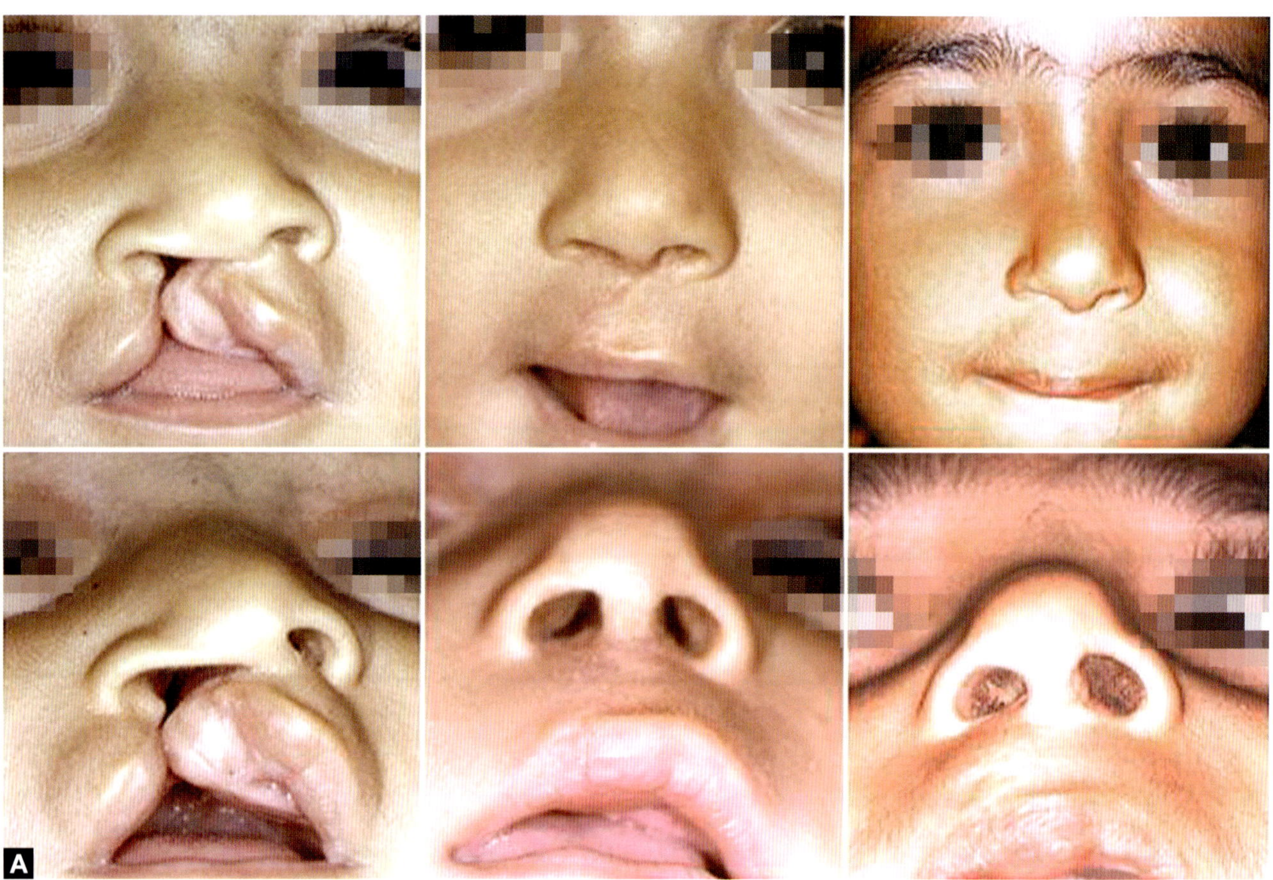

Fig. 22A

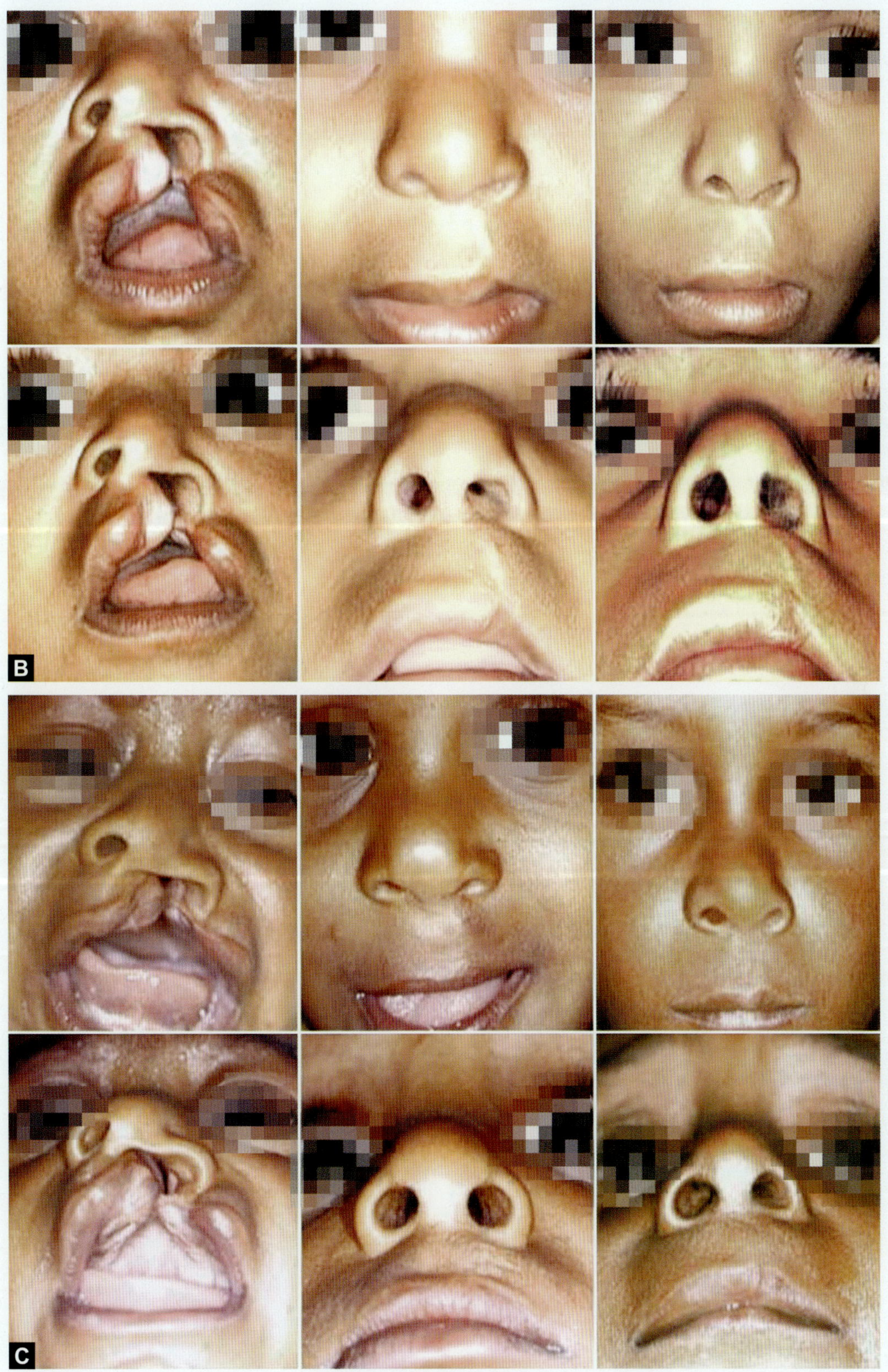

Figs 22B and C

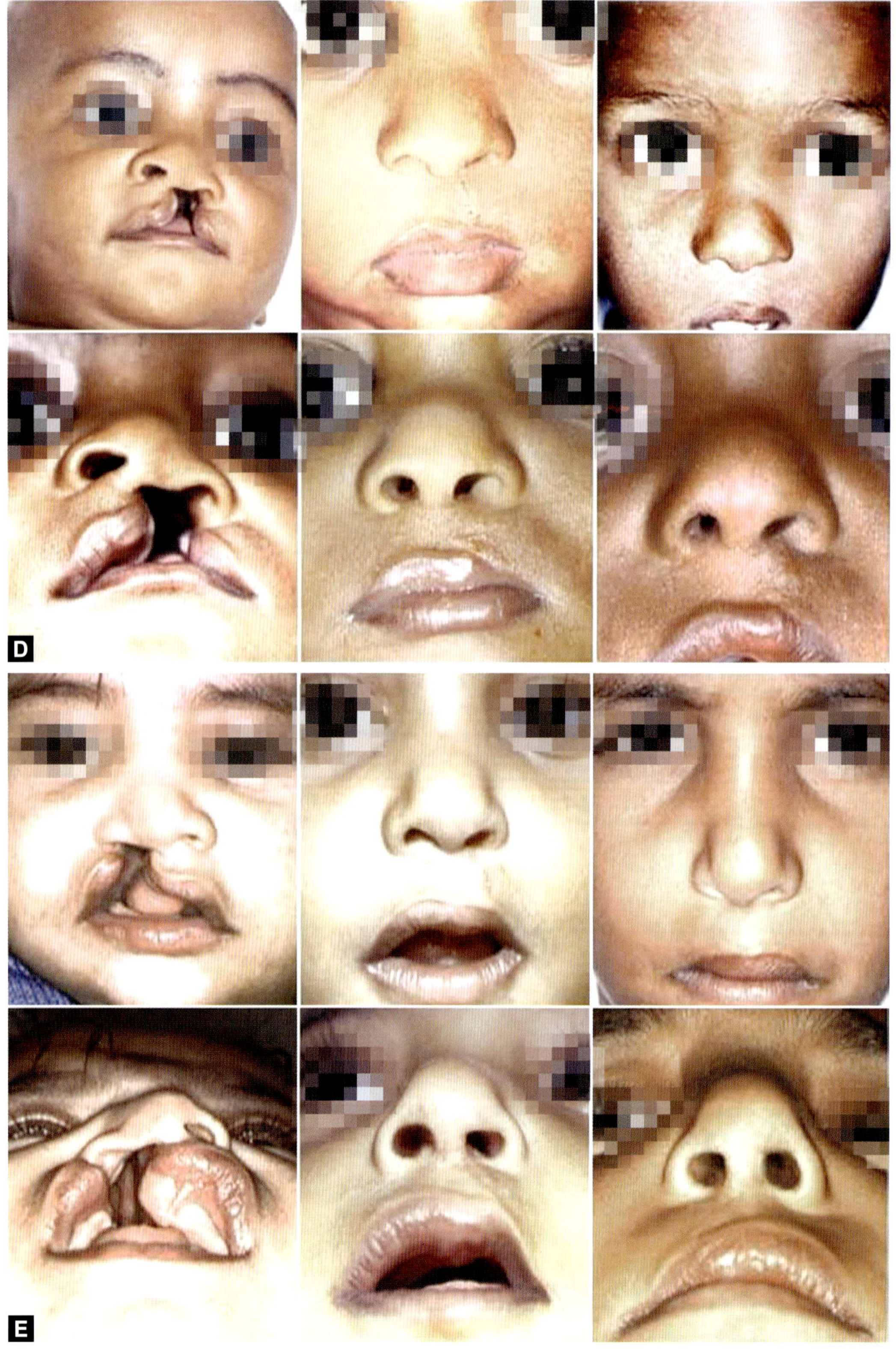

Figs 22D and E

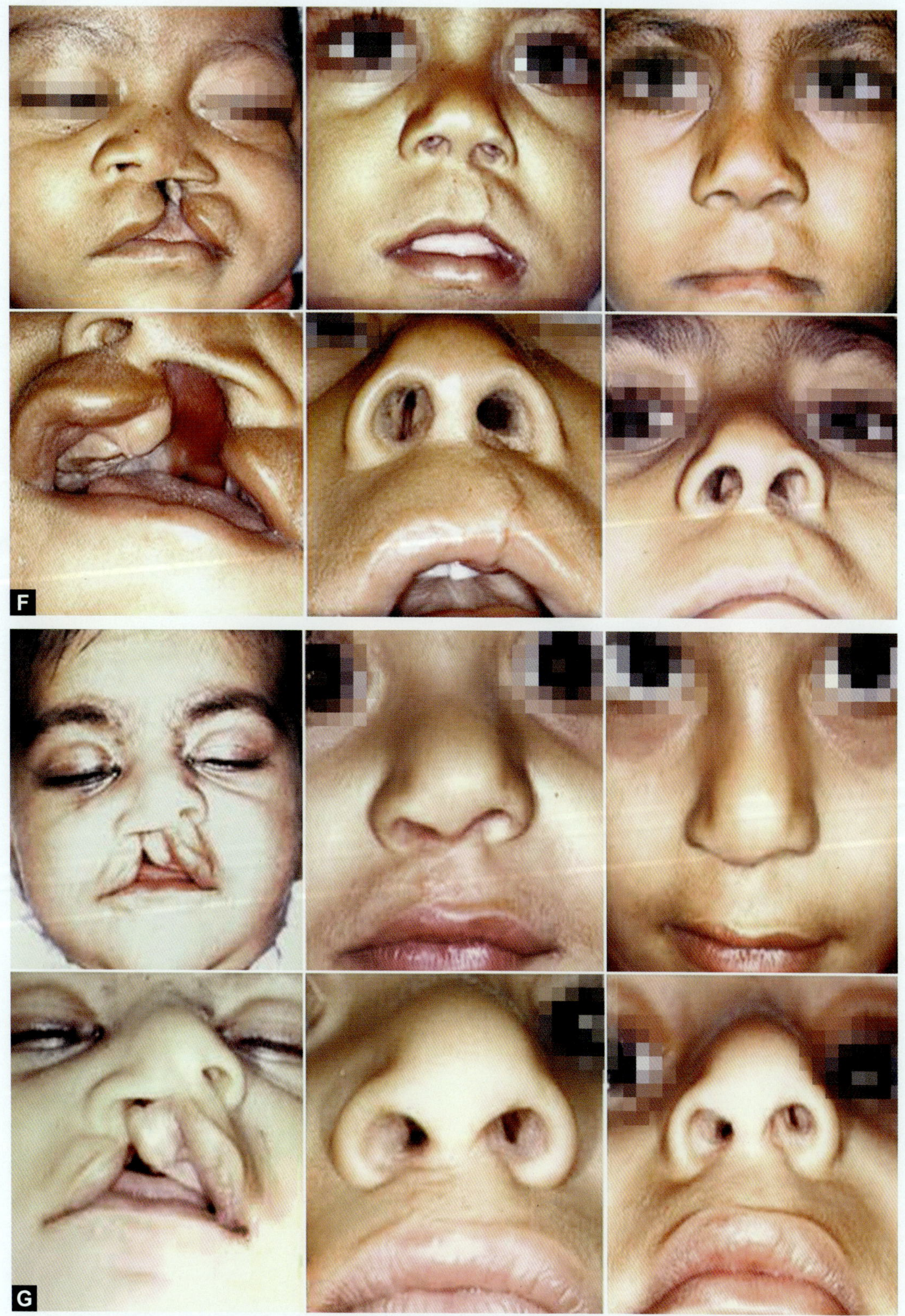

Figs 22A to G: Unilateral complete cleft lip long-term follow-up photographs

Bilateral Complete Cleft Lip (Figs 23A to G)

Directions for Figures

- *First column*: Preoperative anteroposterior and nasal views
- *Middle column*: Postoperative anteroposterior and nasal views with 1 year follow-up of the same patient.
- *Last column*: Postoperative anteroposterior and nasal views over 12 years follow-up of the same patient.

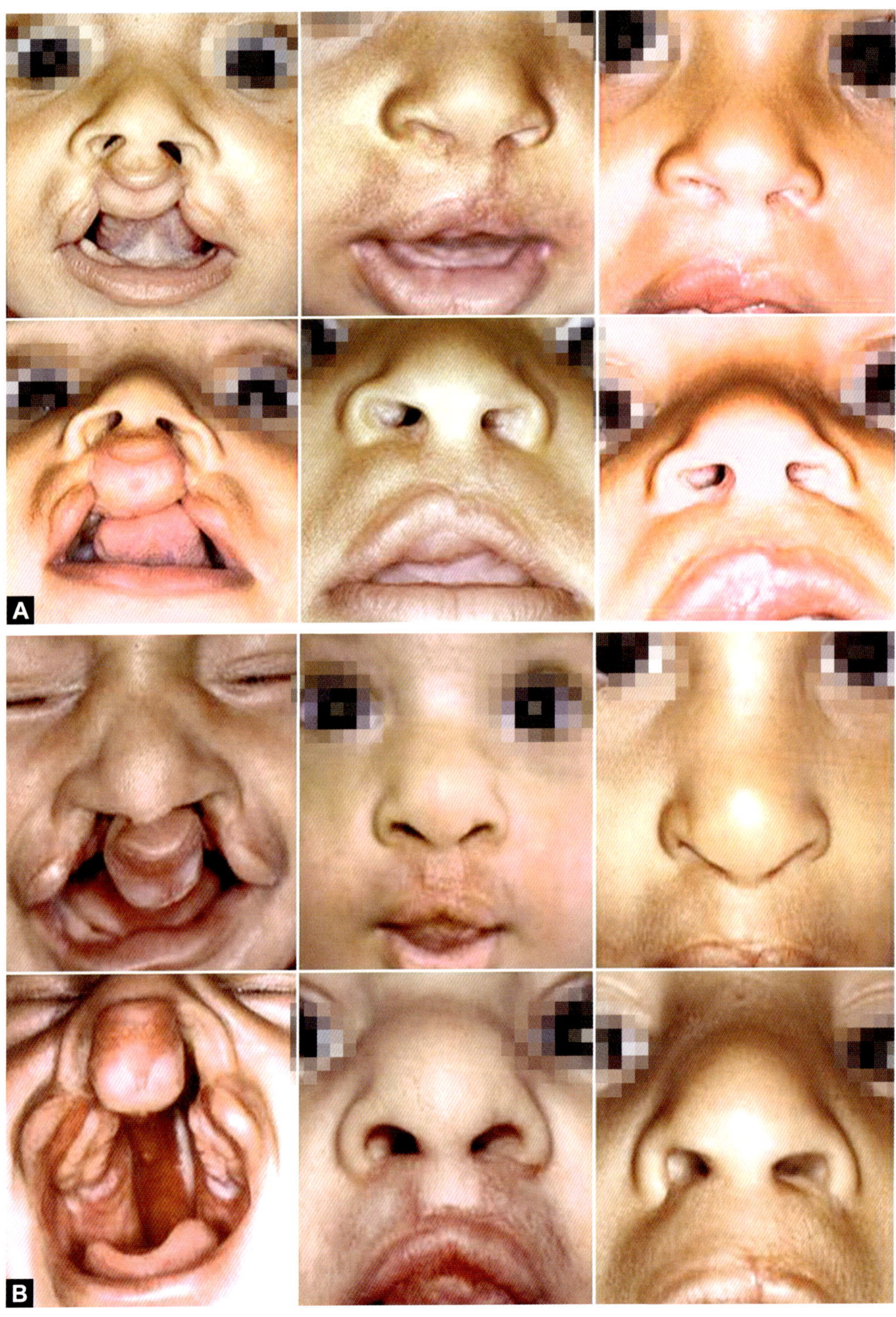

Figs 23A and B

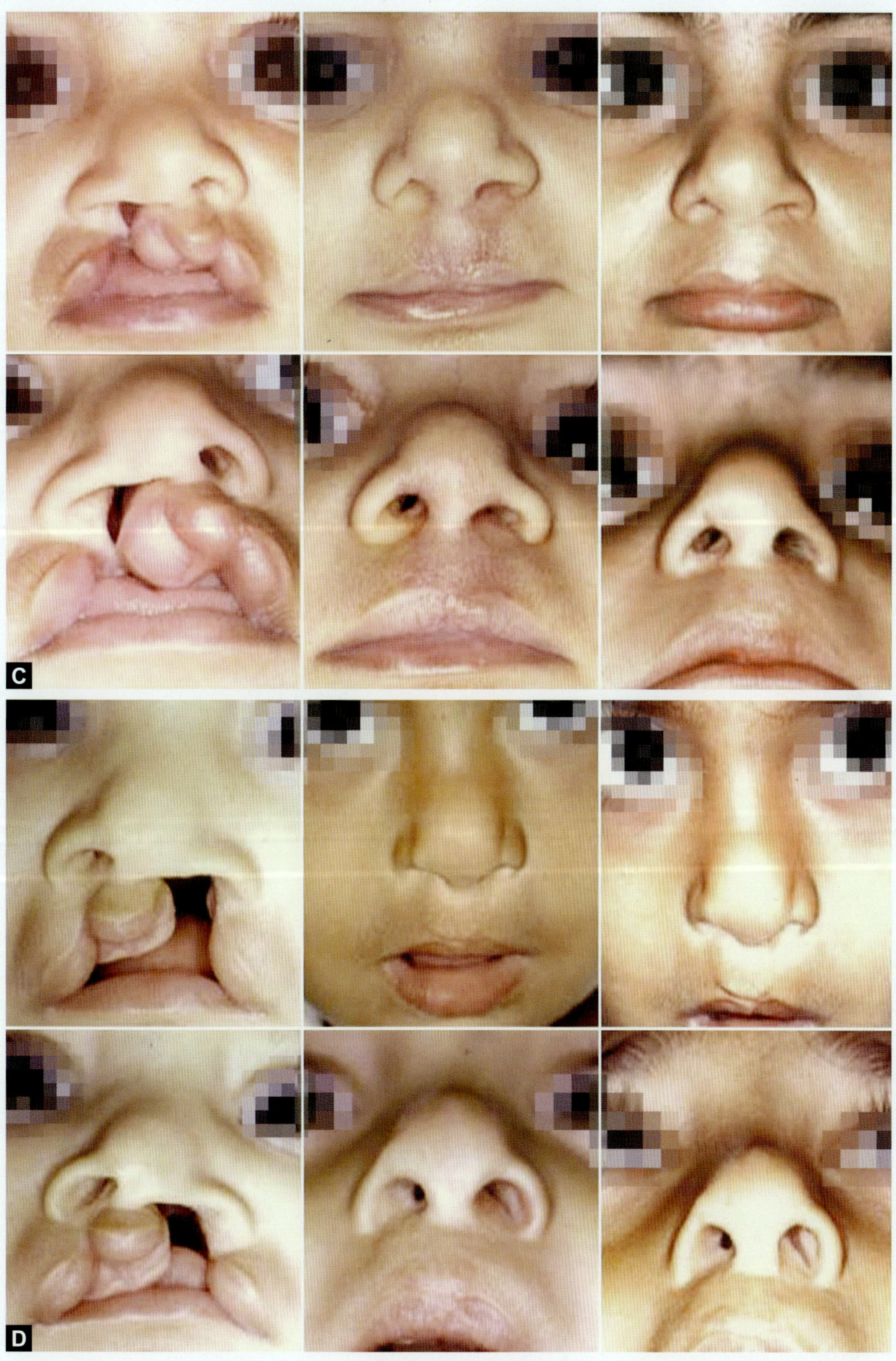

Figs 23C and D

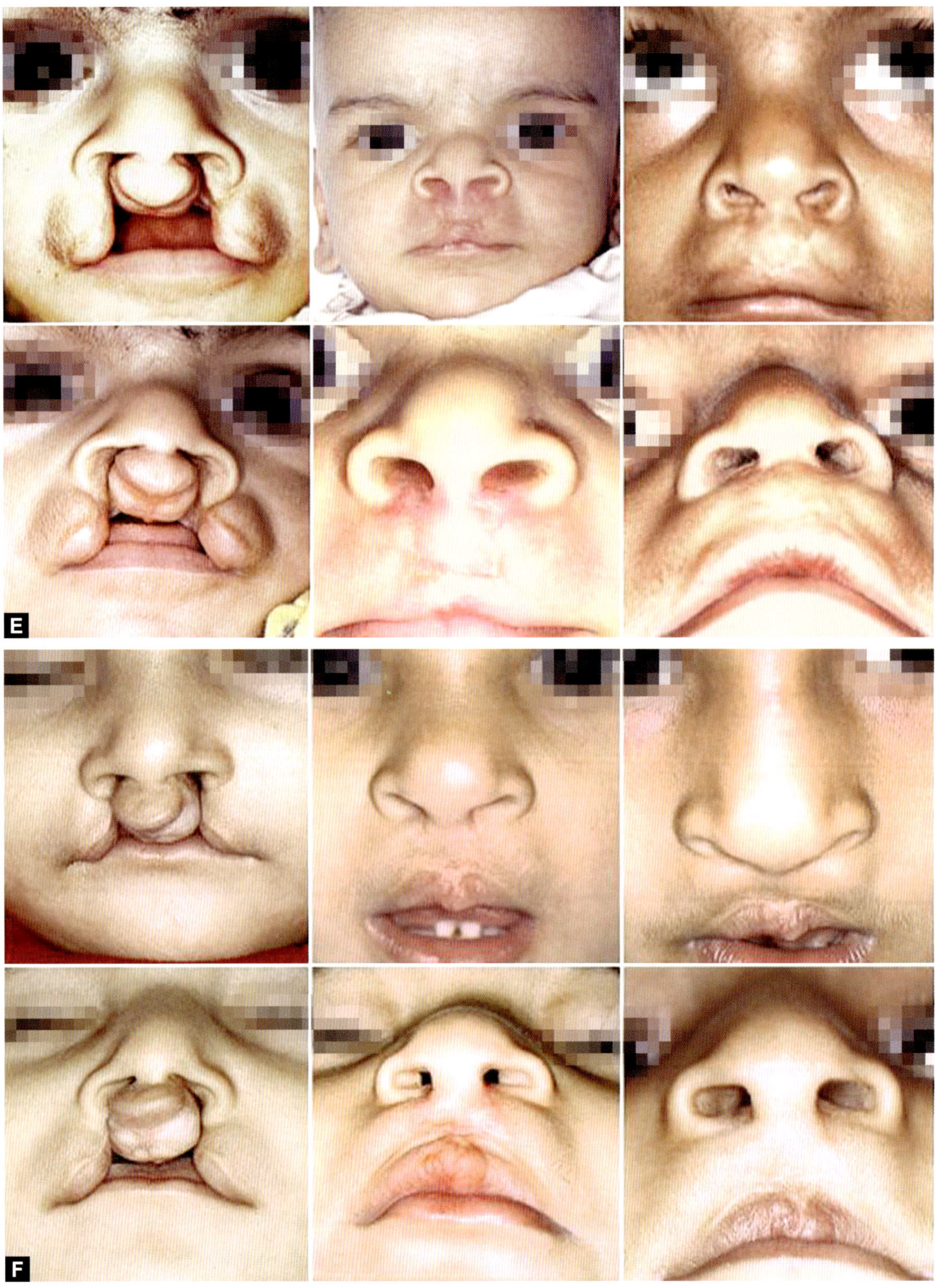

Figs 23E and F

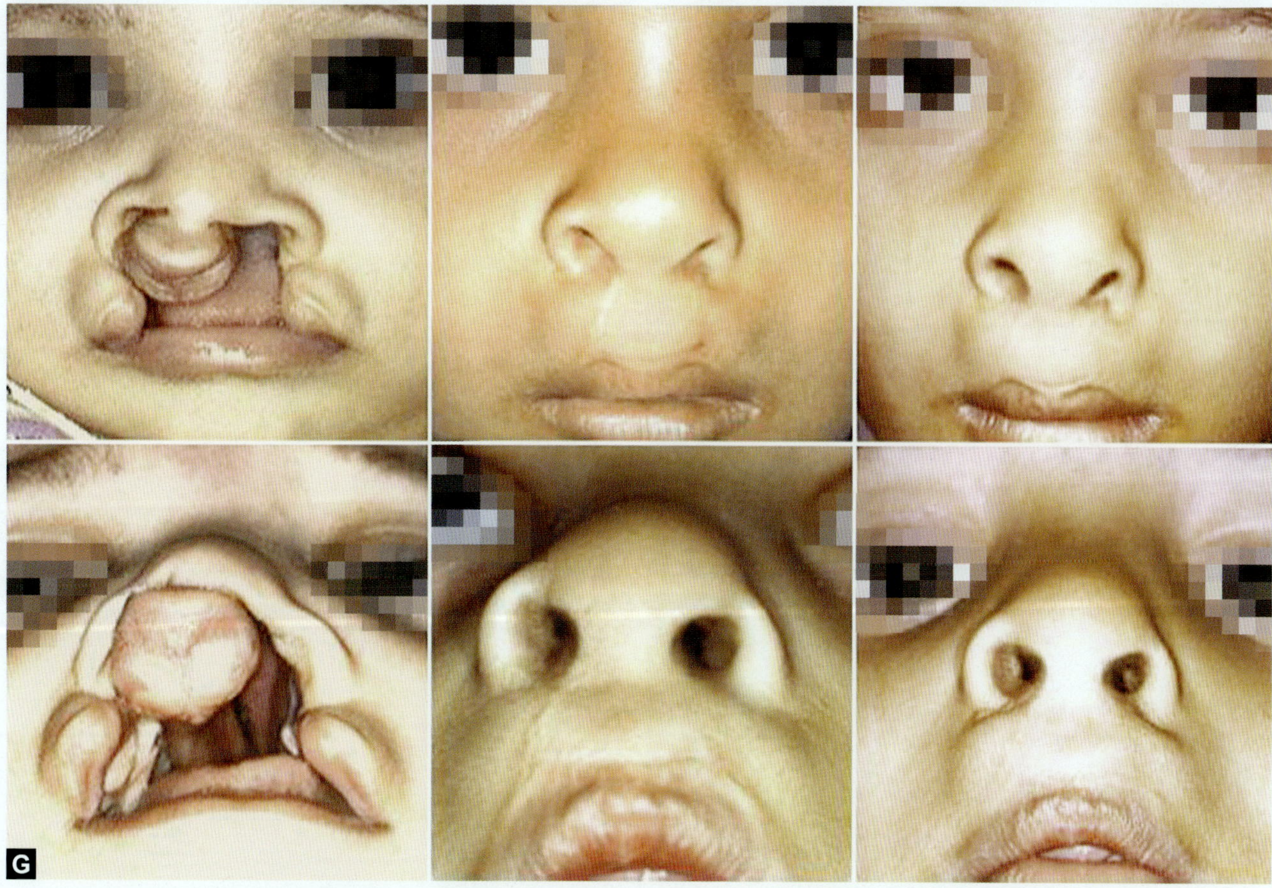

Figs 23A to G: Bilateral complete cleft lip long-term follow-up phtographs

SECONDARY RHINOPLASTY

It should be tailored to suit each patient. It may be soft tissue, cartilage or skeletal corrections.

Soft Tissue Corrections

Soft tissue corrections, such as columellar lengthening by V-Y advancement flaps, fork flap or Cronin flaps, lip reinforcements by Abbe flap from the lower lip, nasal sill narrowing by wedge resections and so on.

Cartilage Corrections

Cartilage dissection, alar repositioning and suspension nasal and columellar augmentation by grafts and tip plasty.

Skeletal Corrections

Skeletal corrections may be as follows according to the deformity and appropriate correction.

- Bone grafting of the alveolar clefts
- Augmentation of the maxilla
- Cantilever bone grafts for nose
- Skeletal base correction by osteotomies
- Correction of malocclusion by orthodontics and orthognathic surgery
- Rhinoplasty.

SECONDARY SEPTORHINOPLASTY IN CLEFT LIP AND PALATE (FIGS 24 TO 29)

Clinical Photographs

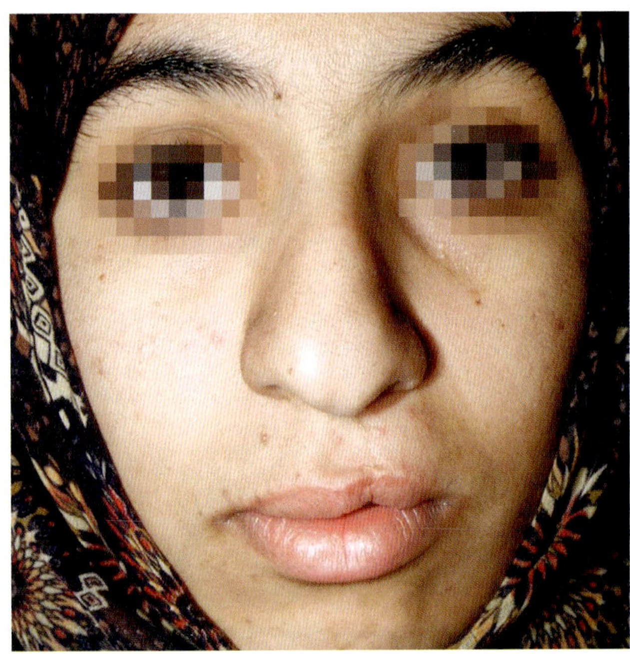

Fig. 24: Frontal view showing the nasal deformity and the vermillion notch

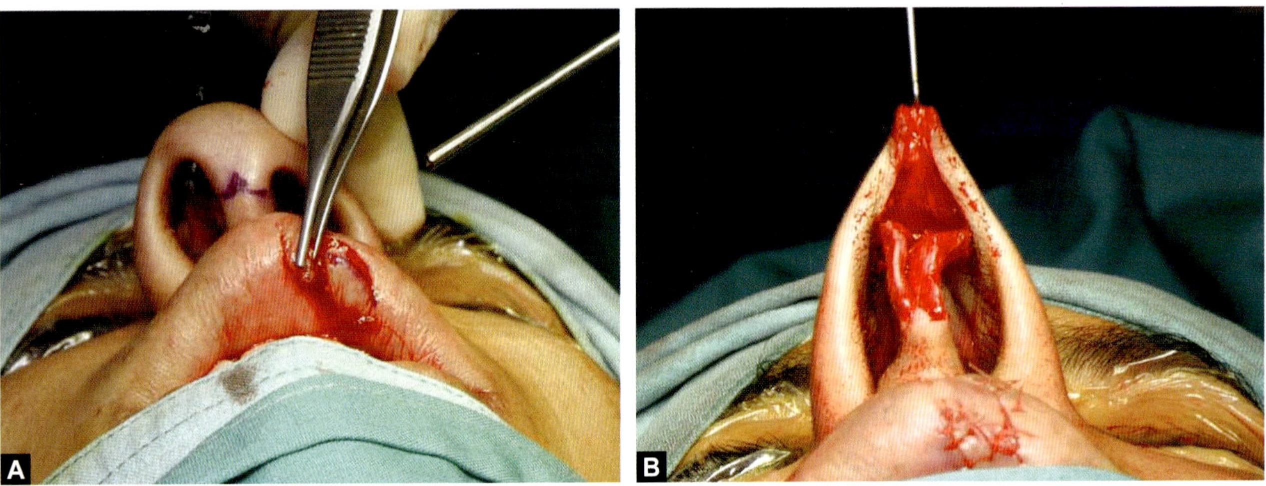

Figs 25A and B: Correction of the vermilion notch by Z-plasty and the septorhinoplasty by open approach

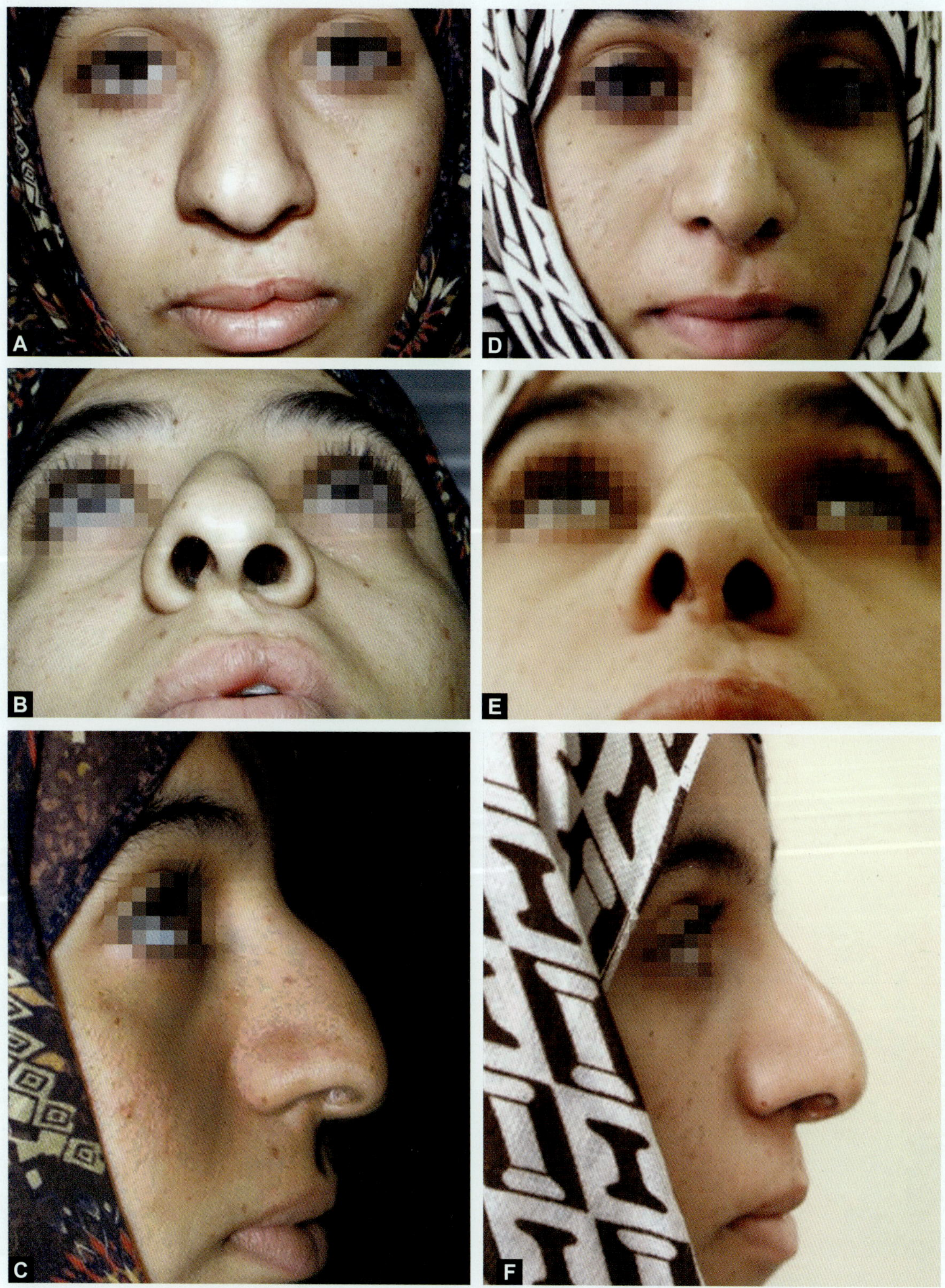

Figs 26A to F: (A to C) Preoperative views; (D to F) Postoperative views

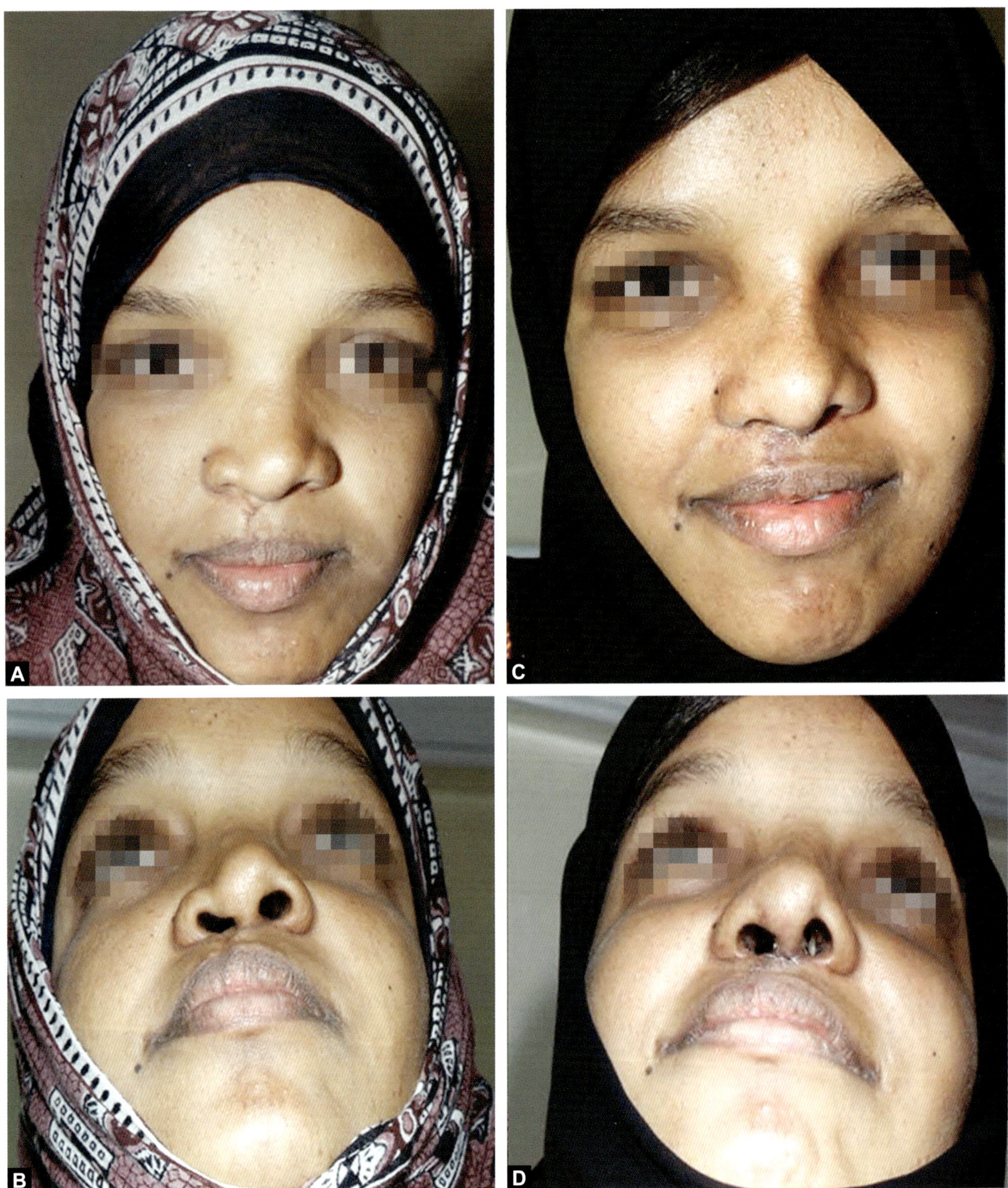

Figs 27A to D: (A and B) Preoperative views; (C and D) Postoperative views

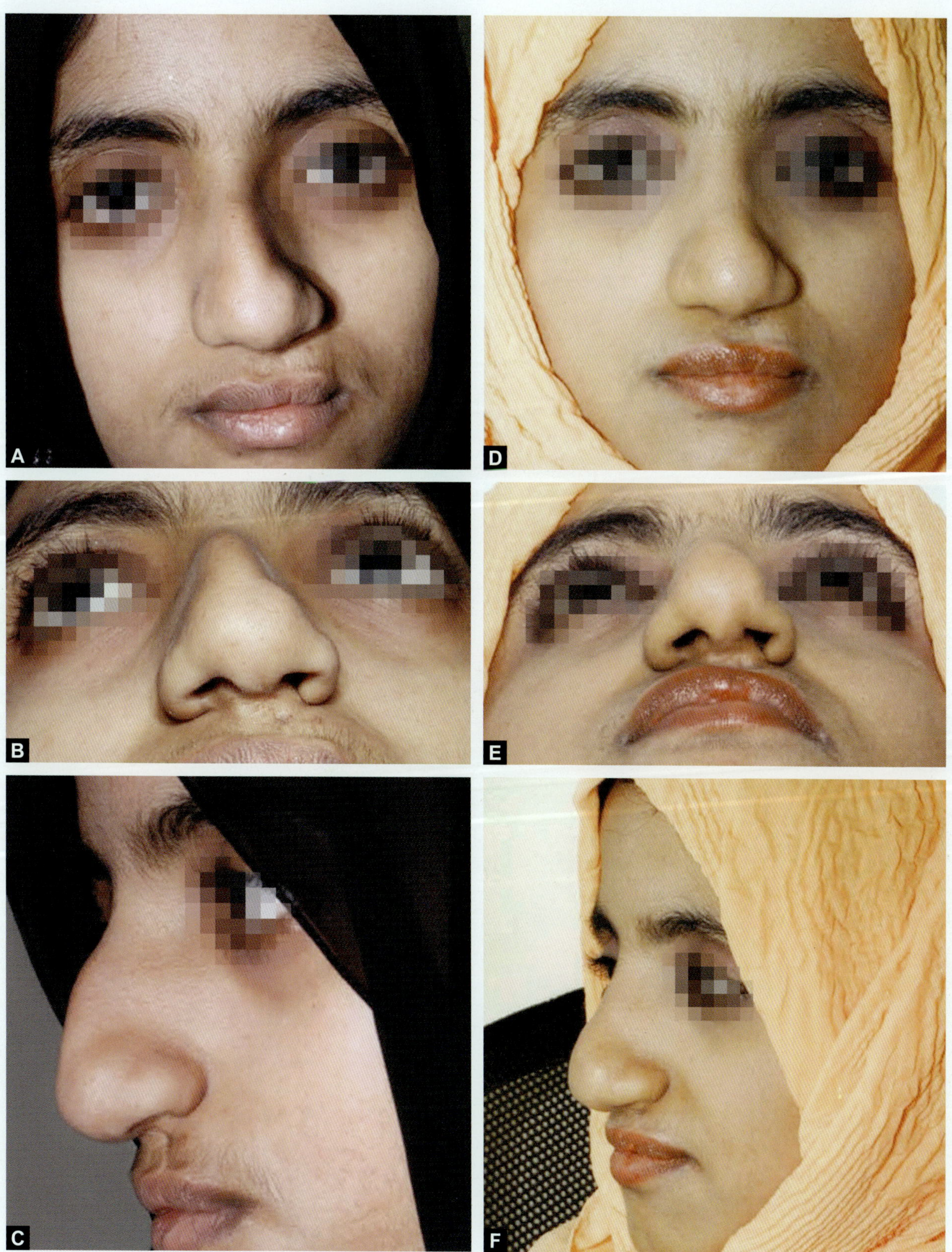

Figs 28A to F: (A to C) Preoperative views; (D to F) Postoperative views

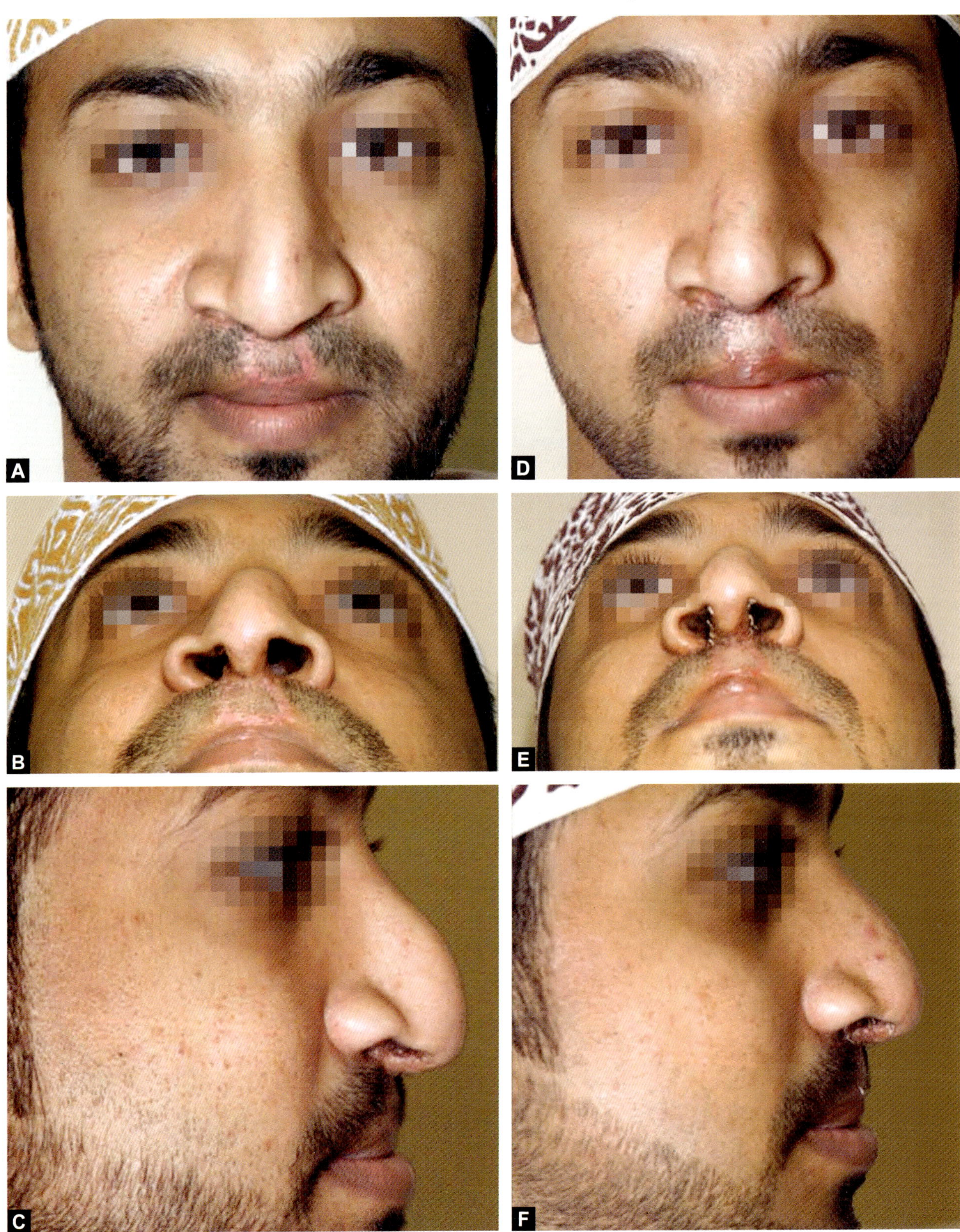

Figs 29A to F: Postoperative bilateral complete cleft lip with septorhinoplasty. (A to C) Preoperative views; (D to F) Postoperative views

BIBLIOGRAPHY

1. Cutting CB. In: Mathes SJ (Ed). Plastic Surgery, 2nd edition. Philadelphia, PA: Saunders; 2006. pp. 217-47.
2. Harashina T. Open reverse-U incision technique for secondary correction of unilateral cleft lip nose deformity. Br J Plast Surg. 1990;43:557-64.
3. Matsuo K, Hirose T. A rotational method of bilateral cleft lip nose repair Plast Reconstr Surg. 1991;87: 1034-40.
4. Millard DR. Refinements in Rotation-Advancement Cleft Lip Technique. Plastic Reconstr Surg. 1964;33:26-38.
5. Tajima S, Maruyama M. Reverse "U" incision for secondary repair of cleft lip nose. Plastic Reconstr Surg. 1977;60: 256-61.
6. Thomas C, Mishra P. Open tip rhinoplasty along with the repair of the cleft lip in cleft lip and palate cases. Br J Plast Surg. 2000;53:1-6.
7. Thomas C. Primary rhinoplasty by open approach with repair of bilateral complete cleft lip. J Craniofacial Surg. 2009;20;1715-18.
8. Thomas C. Primary rhinoplasty by open approach with repair of unilateral complete cleft lip. J Craniofacial Surg. 2009;20;1711-14.
9. Trott JA, Mohan NA. A preliminary report on one stage open tip rhinoplasty at the time of lip repair in bilateral cleft lip and palate: the Alor Setar experience. Br J Plast Surg. 1993; 46:215-22.
10. Trott JA, Mohan NA. A preliminary report on open tip rhinoplasty at the time of lip repair in unilateral cleft lip and palate: The Alor Setar experience. Br J Plast Surg. 1993;46:363-70.

CHAPTER

102 Revision Rhinoplasty: The Lost Tip Support

Hossam MT Foda

INDICATIONS FOR THE SURGERY

Revision rhinoplasty is a very complex and technically demanding procedure. One of the main challenges, in revision cases, is to rebuild the weakened or lost nasal tip support.[1] Loss of tip support results mainly from excessive excisions or resorption of the caudal septum, alar cartilages or anterior nasal spine.

The lost tip support is responsible for most of the functional and aesthetic problems encountered in revision case; this is mainly due to the fact that the loss of support leaves the tip weak and unstable so it can be easily displaced backwards, by the weight of the thick lobular skin and downwards by the constant pull of gravity, leading to loss of tip projection and rotation, resulting in a depressed droopy nasal tip with pollybeak deformity and acute nasolabial angle. Additionally, the weak unsupported tip cartilages can be easily displaced by the contracture forces of healing leading to tip contour irregularities, alar notching or collapse, retracted columella, and shortened nose with an over-rotated tip.[1-3]

A strong caudal septum replacement graft (Fig. 1) is designed to reconstruct the caudal septum and provide good support to the weak buckled medial crura (Fig. 2) in order to correct the functional and aesthetic problems resulting from the lost tip support.

SPECIFIC PREOPERATIVE EVALUATION

The poor tip support can be detected by preoperative examination and confirmed by the intraoperative findings:

I. Digital palpation to evaluate the degree of tip support
   a. Rolling tip skin between index and thumb to detect its relative thickness
   b. Lifting of nasal tip upwards and testing for any improvement in breathing
   c. Pressing on nasal tip to detect amount of cartilage support and degree of recoil
   d. Pressing upwards on the columella to detect any caudal septum deficiency
   e. Pressing inwards on the nasolabial junction to evaluate the premaxilla and anterior nasal spine.

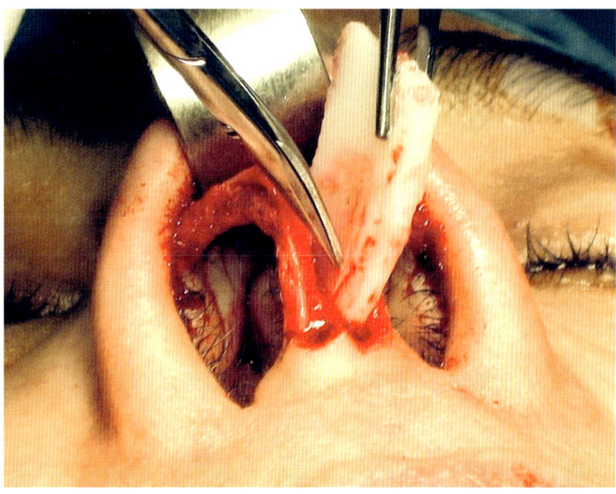

Fig. 1: Intraoperative view of a large caudal septum replacement (CSR) graft

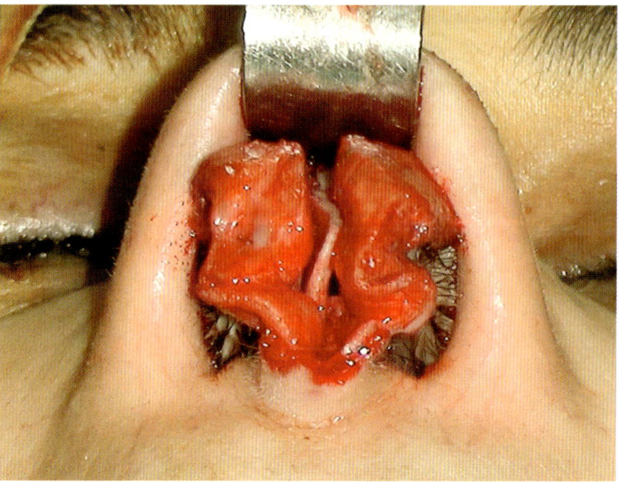

Fig. 2: Intraoperative view of a revision case with total loss of tip support showing weak buckled medial crura and deficient caudal septum due to partial resection and resorption

II. External nasal analysis for signs of loss of tip support (Fig. 3 left, below)
   a. Depressed underprojected nasal tip
   b. Droopy inferiorly rotated nasal tip
   c. Acute nasolabial angle
   d. Retrodisplaced nasolabial junction
   e. Posteriorly inclined upper lip
   f. Retracted columellar base
III. Intraoperative findings in revision cases with lost tip support:
   a. Premaxillary bony deficiency due to previously resected or partially resorped anterior nasal spine
   b. Caudal septal cartilage deficiency from previous excisions or resorption
   c. Medial crura may be weak, fractured, twisted, buckled or partially missing

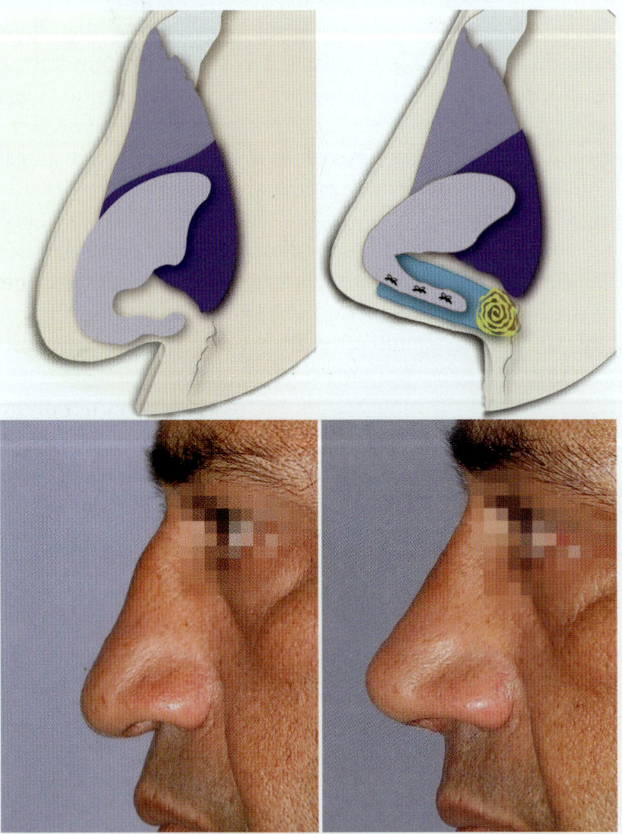

Fig. 3: *Left:* Preoperative schematic illustration and photograph of a patient with caudal septal and premaxillary deficiency showing a depressed droopy tip, acute nasolabial angle, retrodisplaced nasolabial junction and posteriorly inclined upper lip. *Right:* The same patient postoperatively after using a CSR graft and a roll of Mersilene mesh for premaxillary augmentation

SURGICAL STEPS

An external rhinoplasty approach was used to reconstruct the lost support using a cartilaginous caudal septum replacement (CSR) graft combined with premaxillary augmentation using Mersilene mesh.

Premaxillary Augmentation

A pocket is dissected between the footplates of the medial crura till reaching the premaxilla and the anterior nasal spine, which is either previously resected or partially resorped. In such cases, dissection is continued on both sides of the spine to create a pocket for premaxillary augmentation, which is done using Mersilene mesh[4] (Ethicon, Somerville, NJ, USA) after rolling it tightly and marking it, at the midpoint, with a 5/0 silk suture. The roll of mesh is trimmed to an average length of 2 cms (range, 1-3 cms) and its lateral ends tapered. The thickness of the roll depends on the extent of premaxillary deficiency. The prepared roll of mesh is then soaked in Gentamicin solution and introduced into the premaxillary pocket making sure the silk suture rests strictly in the midline to ensure central placement of the implant.

Caudal Septum Replacement Graft

Graft Harvest

Donor cartilage for the CSR graft can be obtained from multiple sources, the first and most preferable choice is autogenous septal cartilage, followed by autogenous conchal cartilage and finally the last choice is autogenous or irradiated costal cartilage homograft. The dimensions of the graft depend mainly on the size of the missing caudal segment and the aesthetic goals of the operation. The length (anteroposterior dimension) of the graft is determined by the amount of tip projection needed, the width (cephalo-caudal dimension) ranged from 7-13 mm depending on the extent of caudal septum deficiency, the thickness of the graft ranged from 2-4 mm for autogenous grafts and from 3-6 mm when irradiated cartilage homograft is used. On using septal cartilage, an inferior mucoperiostium tunnel is elevated off the maxillary crest and the flap elevation is continued upwards to expose the ventral part of the septal cartilage that is attached to the maxillary crest. This is the best part to use for a CSR graft as it is the thickest part of septal cartilage and it is usually found intact even in revision cases with near-total absence of septal cartilage. On using conchal cartilage, it is harvested through an anterior approach using a curved incision parallel to the antihelix but a few millimeters below it to allow the scar to be hidden by the curve of the antihelix and its inferior crus. In order to change the thin concave conchal cartilage into a thick and straight CSR graft; a vertical partial-thickness cut is made on the concave surface of the cartilage, which is then folded on itself in a back-to-back fashion and sutured into a double layer using 6/0 Prolene mattress sutures.

Graft Placement and Fixation

The extent of missing caudal septum is evaluated by instrument palpation. Occasionally, the membranous septum may be found stiff on palpation, giving the impression that some cartilage is present, but on exploration only thick scar tissue is found from the previous surgeries. The medial crura are pulled apart and the thick scar tissue is excised using sharp dissection with No. 15 blade then a fine tenotomy scissors is used to continue the dissection cephalically making sure to stop a few millimeters before reaching the edge of the remaining septal cartilage, thus keeping the created membranous septal pocket isolated from the septum proper. The dissected pocket is then extended posteriorly between the footplates of the medial crura till reaching the premaxillary mesh. The base of the graft is beveled in a concave fashion, to accommodate the roll of Mersilene mesh; the caudal border of the graft is left longer than the cephalic one (Fig. 3 right, above) to prevent any upward displacement of the graft. The graft is then introduced into the membranous septum pocket and pushed downwards till it is tightly pressed against the premaxillary mesh. The graft is fixed, in that position, to the medial crura using 5/0 Prolene sutures in a horizontal mattress fashion. Three sutures are used; the first at the level of the medial crural footplates, the second in the columellar segment of medial crura and the third in the lobular segment of the medial crura (Fig. 3 right, above). Finally, the degree of tip projection is assessed and any excess length of the graft is trimmed to allow approximation of domes to be done above the level of the anterior end of the graft.

TECHNICAL CONSIDERATIONS IN THE SURGERY

In one of our previous studies,[5] it was found that over 75% of cases with caudal septal deficiency were associated with some degree of premaxillary deficiency where the premaxilla and/or the anterior nasal spine were found to be previously resected or partially resorped and the premaxillary fat and soft tissue are atrophied and scarred-down as a result of surgical trauma. In such cases, premaxillary augmentation should be performed before attempting any caudal septal reconstruction, we found Mersilene mesh to be an ideal augmentation material for the premaxilla.[4] It is soft, pliable and its lattice-like structure allows host tissue ingrowth that leads to early fixation of the implant. The presence of the roll of mesh in the premaxilla proved to be very helpful to the CSR graft; it provides a soft cushion on which the base of the CSR graft will rest thus stabilizing the graft and preventing any side-to-side movement, which in absence of the mesh, may cause a "click" against the premaxillary bone. Another advantage of the roll of mesh is that it would guard against any upward displacement of the graft thus avoiding potential overriding between the inserted graft and the septum. Another factor that prevented overriding is that a few millimeters of membranous septum were left undissected thus preventing any direct contact between the graft and the caudal edge of the remaining septum (Fig. 4).

COMPLICATIONS

The CSR graft and premaxillary augmentation with Mersilene mesh was used in over 200 patients with follow-ups for up to 14 years and proved to provide an excellent amount of support to the nasal tip allowing it to maintain its position, over the long-term follow-up period, with no loss in the achieved degree of projection or rotation. Functionally, 85% of the cases with preoperative nasal obstruction reported a significant improvement in breathing (Figs 5 and 6).

No cases of infection, displacement or extrusion of the CSR graft were encountered. However, partial extrusion of the Mersilene mesh occurred in six cases (2%); four of which had associated anterior septal perforations and the remaining two patients had a unilateral cleft-lip nasal deformity. Accordingly, it is better to avoid using Mersilene

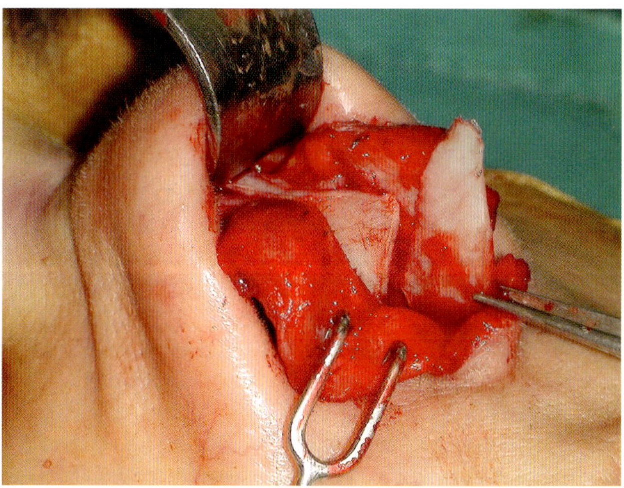

Fig. 4: Intraoperative view showing the minimum distance that should be left undissected between the septum and the CSR graft

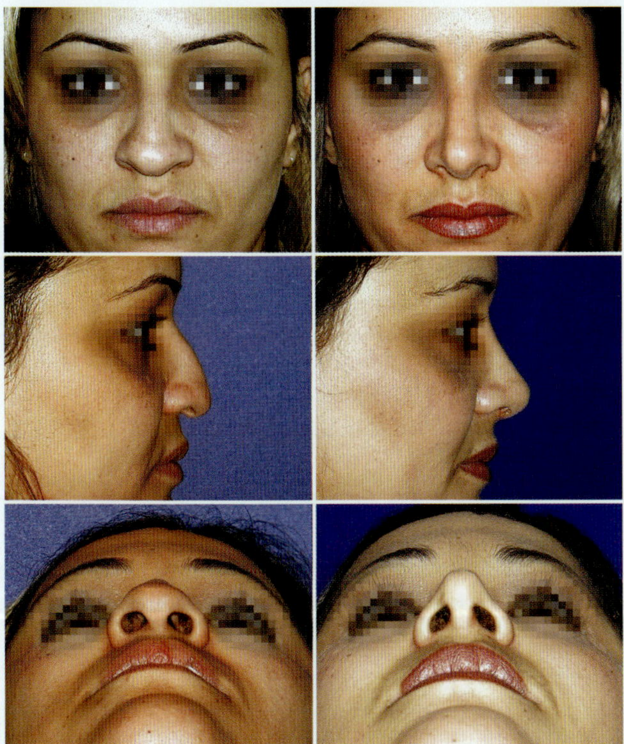

Fig. 5: A revision patient who had a previous septal surgery with resection of caudal septum and anterior nasal spine. *Left:* Preoperative views of the patient. *Right:* Postoperative views of the patient 3 years after reconstruction with an auricular cartilage CSR graft and premaxillary augmentation with Mersilene mesh

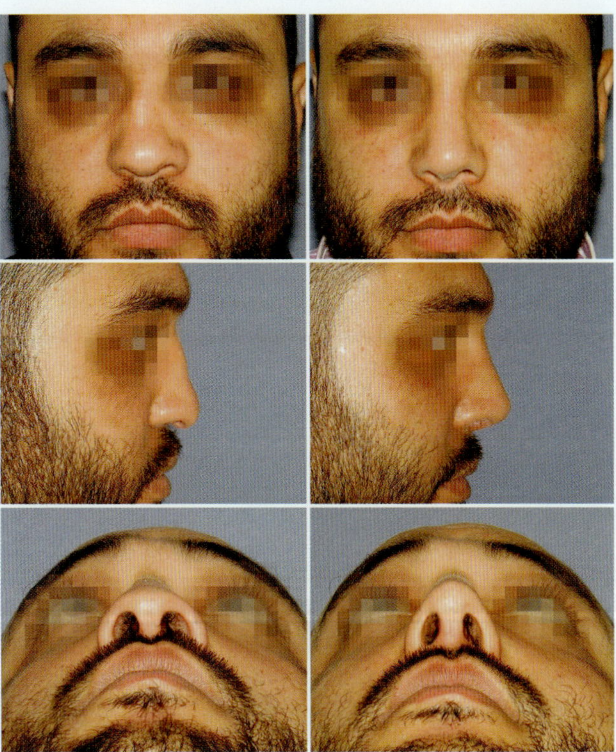

Fig. 6: A revision patient who had a previous septorhinoplasty with an over-resected dorsal and caudal septum. *Left:* Preoperative views. *Right:* Postoperative views of the patient 1 year after reconstruction with a costal cartilage CSR graft and premaxillary augmentation with Mersilene mesh

mesh in the premaxilla in cases with anterior septal perforations. In cleft-lip noses, it is mandatory to exclude the presence of any hidden bony or mucosa fistula that may predispose to contamination and extrusion of the mesh.

OTHER TREATMENT OPTIONS AVAILABLE FOR THE SAME CONDITION

Premaxillary Deficiency

Various kinds of grafts and implants were used to provide premaxillary augmentation; cartilage, which is the most widely used graft material in rhinoplasty, was used successfully in the premaxilla.[8-10] However, as usually a large amount of cartilage is required to provide adequate premaxillary augmentation; the limited thickness of septal and conchal cartilage requires stacking it in layers, which is technically difficult to stabilize. Autogenous bone graft can be used but it is more difficult to shape and carries a significantly higher resorption rate.[11]

Due to the difficulties and limitation associated with the use of autogenous grafts; many types of implants were recommended to provide premaxillary augmentation. Silastic was one of the first implants to be used in the premaxilla,[12,13] however, due to its smooth surface, it does not adhere to the surrounding tissues and is associated with a high incidence of migration and extrusion.[14-16] Unlike Silastic, Proplast[17,18] (Vitek, Houston, TX) and Gore-tex[19] (W.L. Gore & Co., Flagstaff, AZ) are highly porous thus inviting early tissue ingrowth and stabilization, however, they are more difficult to carve and insert and leaves the patient with a rigid unnatural feeling of the solid implant. Mersilene mesh which was used in our technique, shares the advantages of other implants, being readily available in any quantity and not associated with any donor-site morbidity. However, unlike the solid implants, the lattice-like composition of the mesh makes it soft in consistency and easily infiltrated by host tissue thus leading to early fixation and assures a natural feeling of the implant in the lower mobile part of the nose.[4,20,21]

Another major advantage of Mersilene mesh over all other grafts and implants is the pliability of the mesh implant that allows it to be introduced through a small entry opening and to conform well and fill-out the underlying asymmetric areas of bony deficiencies as in cleft-lip noses.[7]

Caudal Septum Deficiency

Many types and shapes of septal extension grafts were used successfully to replace the missing or weak caudal septal cartilage. The major problem of these septal extension grafts is the unnatural rigidity and stiffness of the nasal lobule, which results from fixing the graft to the nasal septum either directly by suturing or via cartilage grafts.[22-28] In our technique, the pocket for the CSR graft is kept separated from the septum by leaving an intact part of the membranous septum to intervene between the septum and the graft,[6] which allowed preserving some of the natural mobility of nasal lobule (Fig. 4).

REFERENCES

1. Foda HM. Rhinoplasty for the multiply revised nose. Am J Otolaryngol. 2005; 26(1): 28-34.
2. Foda HM. External rhinoplasty for the Arabian nose: a columellar scar analysis. Aesthetic Plast Surg. 2004; 28(5):312-6.
3. Foda HM. Management of the droopy tip: a comparison of three alar cartilage-modifying techniques. Plast Reconstr Surg. 2003; 112(5):1408-17.
4. Foda HM. Mersilene mesh in premaxillary augmentation. Aesthetic Plast Surg. 2005; 29(3):169-73.
5. Foda HM. The Caudal Septum Replacement Graft. Arch Facial Plast Surg. 2008;10(3):152-7.
6. Foda HM, Magdy EA. Combining rhinoplasty with septal perforation repair. Facial Plast Surg. 2006; 22(4):281-8.
7. Foda HM, Bassyouni K. Rhinoplasty in unilateral cleftlip nasal deformity. J Laryngol Otol. 2000; 114(3);189-93.
8. Cinelli JA. Correction of combined elongated nose and recessed nasolabial angle. Plast Reconstr Surg. 1958; 21:139-42.
9. Guerrero-Santos J. Cosmetic repair of the acute columellar-lip angle. Plast Reconstr Surg. 1973; 52(3):246-9.
10. Lewis JR. Rhinoplasty and the nasolabial area. Clin Plast Surg. 1988; 15(1):115-24.
11. Adams JS. Grafts and implants in nasal and chin augmentation: A rational approach to material selection. Otolaryngol Clin North Am. 1987; 20(4):913-30.
12. Caronni EP. A new method to correct the nasolabial angle in rhinoplasty. Plast Reconstr Surg. 1972; 50(4):338-40.
13. Fanous N, Yoskovitch A. Premaxillary augmentation: adjunct to rhinoplasty. Plast Reconstr Surg. 2000; 106(3):707-12.
14. Davis PK, Jones SM. The complications of silastic implants. Br J Plast Surg. 1971; 24(4):405-11.
15. Deva AK, Mertin S, Chang L. Silicone in nasal augmentation rhinoplasty: a decade of clinical experience. Plast Reconstr Surg. 1998; 102:1230-7.
16. Proter JP. Grafts in Rhinoplasty: alloplastic vs autogenous. Arch Otolaryngol Head Neck Surg. 2000; 126(4):558-61.
17. Kridel RWH, Kraus WM. Grafts and implants in revision rhinoplasty. Fac Plast Surg Clin N Am. 1995; 3:473-86.
18. Cook TA, Wang TD, Brownrigg PJ, et al. Significant premaxillary augmentation. Arch Otolaryngol Head Neck Surg. 1990; 116(10):1197-201.
19. Schoenrock LD, Reppucci AD. Correction of subcutaneous facial defects using Goretex. Fac Plast Surg Clin North Am. 1994; 2:373-88.
20. Beekhuis GJ. Mersilene mesh to augment the nasal bridge. Am J Cosm Surg. 1986; 3(2):49-53.
21. McCollough EG, Weil C. Augmentation of facial defects using Mersilene mesh implants. Otolaryngol Head Neck Surg. 1979; 87(4):515-21.
22. Slavit DH, Bansberg SF, Facer GW, et al. Reconstruction of caudal end of septum: A case for transplantation. Arch Otolaryngol Head Neck Surg. 1995; 121(10):1091-8.
23. Pirsing W, Kern EB, Verse T. Reconstruction of anterior nasal septum: Back-to-back autogenous ear cartilage graft. Laryngoscope, 2004; 114(4):627-38.
24. Naficy S, Baker SR. Lengthening the short nose. Arch Otolaryngol Head Neck Surg. 1998; 124(7):809-13.
25. Gruber RP. Surgical correction of short nose. Aesthetic Plast Surg. 2002; 26: Suppl 1: S6.
26. Guyuron B, Verghai A. Lengthening the nose with a tongue-and-groove technique. Plast Reconstr Surg. 2003; 111(4):1533-9.
27. Toriumi DM. New concepts in nasal tip contouring. Arch Facial Plast Surg. 2006; 8(3):156-85.
28. Toriumi DM, Pero CD. Asian rhinoplasty. Clin Plast Surg. 2010; 37(2):335-52.

CHAPTER

103 Alar Struts in Rhinoplasty

Patrick T Hennessey, Kofi DO Boahene

INDICATIONS FOR THE SURGERY

Alar rim contour and strength plays an important role in nasal tip esthetics and function. Contour deformities and alar rim collapse may result from congenital weakness or malposition of the lower lateral cartilages (LLCs). In addition, alar pinching and valve collapse may occur as a result of overzealous cephalic trimming of the LLC, when compensatory maneuvers are not performed during rhinoplasty. Alar asymmetries may be noticed in the early postoperative period or as a delayed complication due to scar contracture. More recently, an increased emphasis has been placed on nasal tip grafting and suturing techniques instead of cartilage excision which has allowed for more predictable control of the alar contour. Traditionally, structural and contour deformities of the alar rim have been addressed with batten grafts, strut grafts, composite grafts, and suture techniques.[1-3] A less conventional, but equally effective graft is the alar rim graft placed in a nonanatomic fashion along the alar margin.

In the authors' experience, the two most common indications for placement of alar rim grafts are cephalic malposition of the LLC and correction of alar margin flare. Cephalic malposition of the LLC was first described by Sheen[4] as displacement of the alar cartilage at the midpoint of the alar rim toward the medial canthus instead of laterally toward the lateral canthus. Clinically, the alar rim appears notched and boxy, an appearance classically described as the parenthesis sign (Figs 1A to D). From a series of measurements made in 50 consecutive patients, Daniel[5] noted that the location of the caudal margin of the lateral crus of the LLC, 7 mm or more from the mid-alar margin, highly correlates with malpositioning of the LLC. Cephalic malpositioning of the LLC leaves more of the ala without rigid support. Preoperatively and intraoperatively, it is important to identify this variant of LLC orientation, especially when cephalic trimming is being considered. Injudicious cephalic trimming in a malpositioned LLC has the potential to leave a weakened LLC, which over time will succumb to the forces of scar contracture. Prophylactic placement of alar rim grafts provides additional rim support and corrects the alar notching typically seen.

Alar flaring is a common complaint in patients seeking cosmetic nasal tip rhinoplasty. It can be either congenital or secondary to deprojection of an overprojected nasal tip. Alar flaring has traditionally been addressed with alar wedge resection.[6] The authors have previously shown that alar flaring can be improved by either rim graft alone or in combination with wedge resection without any increased risk of infection or graft loss.[7] The analogy of a collar stay applies here, whereby the placement of a stiff alar rim graft straightens a flared alar or minimizes the degree of secondary flaring resulting from nasal tip deprojection.

Additional indications for alar rim grafting include alar rim collapse, often seen in revision cases when the LLC was overresectioned, and congenital weakness of the LLC. Alar rim grafts may also be used to correct alar margin asymmetries, mild notching, and retraction. The use of alar rim grafts in the correction of alar notching or retraction is a viable option in mild cases (those with approximately 3–4 mm of retraction) when there is adequate lining and skin elasticity to allow stretching and unfurling of the retracted rim.[8] Alar rim grafts can also be used to reduce the relative alar retraction that occurs when septal extension grafts are used to lengthen short noses. For more severe cases of notching or retraction, more aggressive maneuvers, including the use of composite grafts, alar batten grafts, and lateral crural strut grafts, may be needed.

PREOPERATIVE EVALUATION

The ideal alar rim transitions smoothly from the nasal tip defining point to the nasofacial insertion as a gentle line with a slight convexity (Fig. 2). The contour and strength of the alar rim is primarily determined by the semirigid lateral crus of the LLC. As the LLC transitions from the intermediate crus to the lateral crus, it diverges away from the alar margin to a more cephalad position. Thus, the posterior half of the ala is devoid of any rigid support

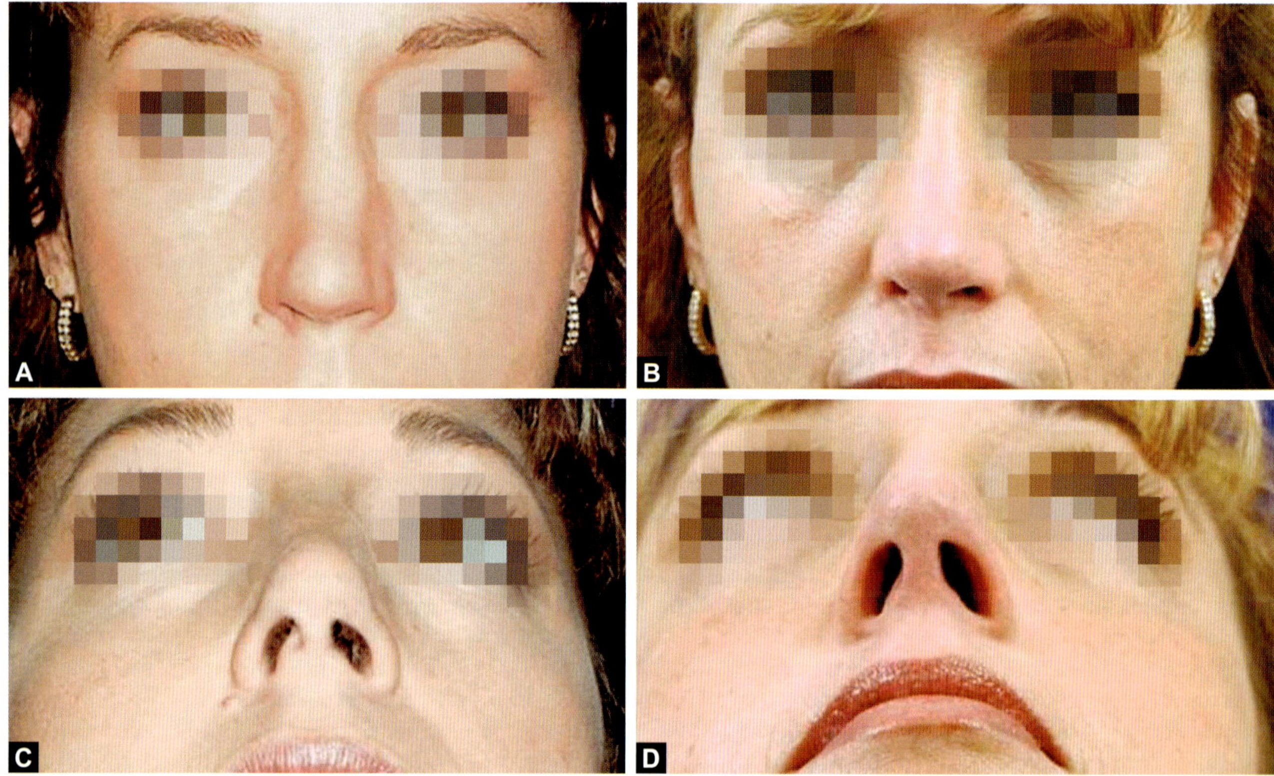

Figs 1A to D: Alar rim grafting for alar margin support and contour correction in a patient with cephalic malpositioned lower lateral cartilages and "boxy" nasaltip. (A) Preoperative front view; (B) Postoperative front view; (C) Preoperative basal view; and (D) Postoperative basal view

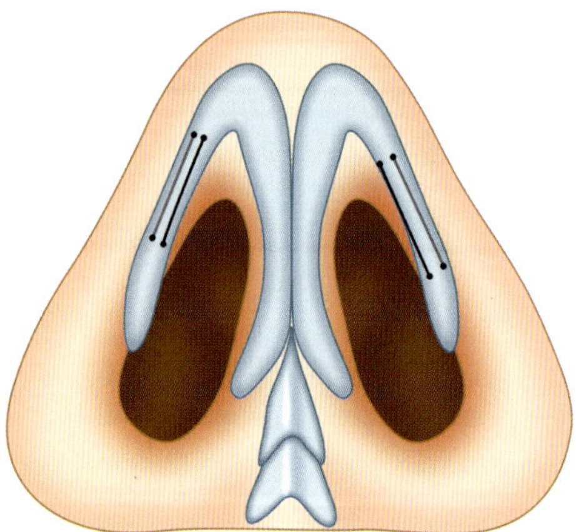

Fig. 2: The ideal alar rim transitions smoothly from the nasal tip defining points to the nasofacial insertion as a gentle curve without a clear demarcation between the nasal tip and alar lobules

(Fig. 3A). The anatomic relationship between the LLC and the alar margin has several structural implications. A greater degree of cephalic rotation of the lateral crus, as seen in congenital LLC malposition, leaves more of the ala without rigid support (Fig. 3B). Overzealous resection of the cephalic margin of the LLC reduces its support of the alar rim. The lack of rigid support along most of the alar rim leaves it vulnerable to inevitable scarring following trauma or rhinoplasty. A weak lateral crus will result in static or dynamic collapse of the alar rim during inspiration. As recently demonstrated,[9] the aesthetically pleasing nasal tip highlights the nasal tip defining points, transitioning smoothly to the alar margin without an interrupting shadow. Dome suturing techniques commonly used in narrowing broad nasal tips often interrupt the alar margin and may result in a pinched nasal tip with an isolated nasal tip lobule. Analogous to a shirt collar stay, the alar rim graft is placed along the alar margin and is capable of directly altering the contour and strength of the alar margin and therefore improving the function and esthetic harmony of the nasal tip (Figs 4A to C).

ANESTHETIC CONSIDERATIONS

As in other rhinoplasty techniques, meticulous injection with local anesthesia containing epinephrine is necessary to ensure hydrodissection and maximal vasoconstriction to allow for excellent visualization during the procedure. This is especially important if performing the procedure in an awake or lightly sedated patient in the clinic setting.

SURGICAL PROCEDURE

After opening the nose in the standard fashion with trans-columellar and marginal incisions, the alar margin is infiltrated with a 1% lidocaine with 1:100,000 epinephrine

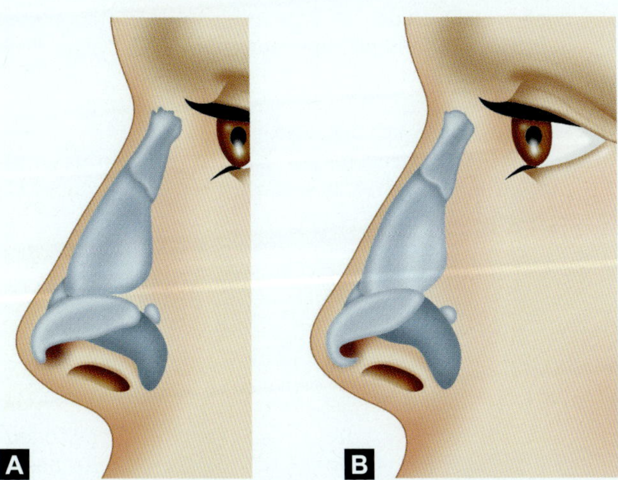

Figs 3A and B: (A) As the lower lateral cartilage transitions from the intermediate crus to the lateral crus, it diverges away from the alar margin to a more cephalad position. Thus, the posterior half of the alar is devoid of any rigid support. (B) With cephalic rotation of the lower lateral crus, a greater portion of the alar is left without rigid support

for hydrodissection and vasoconstriction. The marginal incision and alar margin are then exposed with a wide, double-pronged retractor. With the rim everted, a precise tunnel is dissected along the alar margin beginning from the medial end of the marginal incision to the alar base. Care is taken to avoid penetrating the alar skin. A precise alar tunnel can be safely created with a narrow-tipped scissor and Cottle dissector (Figs 4A to C).

The authors' most commonly fashion alar rim grafts from harvested quadrangular septal cartilage, but other sources of cartilage may be used. The dimensions of the rim graft are first determined by measuring along the alar margin, the region that requires spanning. The rim graft is tailored on a case-by-case basis and measures 2–3 mm wide and 15–25 mm long. The edges of the rim graft should be beveled or contoured to reduce their profile and palpability. The medial edge of the rim graft is softened by gentle crushing with a Brown-Adson forceps or a cartilage morselizer.

Creating a tight and precise pocket minimizes migration of the alar rim graft. To further immobilize the rim graft, a 5.0 fast-absorbing suture is placed around the rim graft, fixing it to adjacent subcutaneous tissue at its medial end. Placing the suture through the thin rim graft often leads to cartilage fracture. After placement, the marginal incisions are closed using 3–4 interrupted 5.0 fast-absorbing sutures.

COMPLICATIONS

Although rare, potential complications include graft extrusion, persistence of external naval valve collapse, infection, and poor cosmetic outcome. Graft extrusion

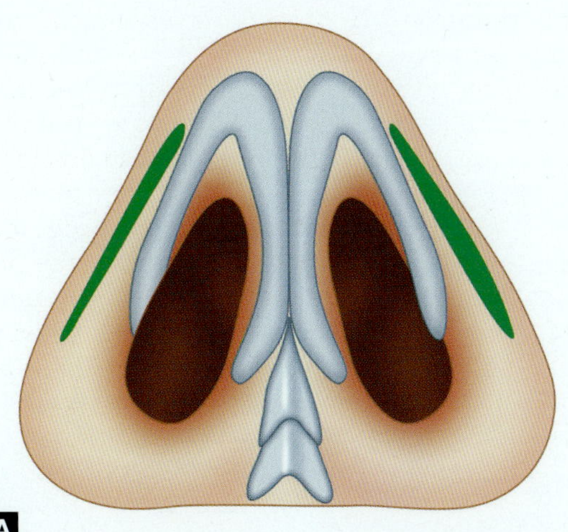

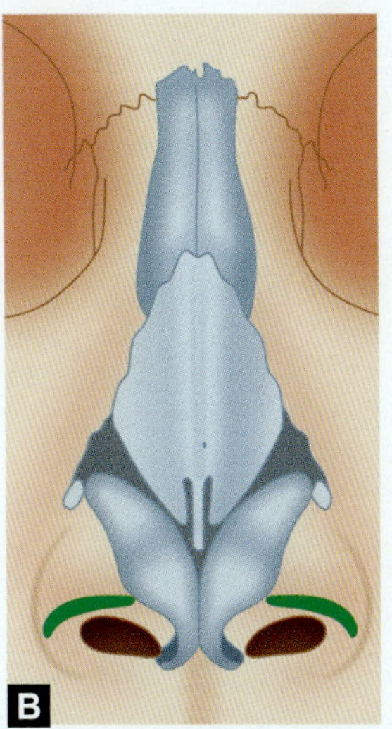

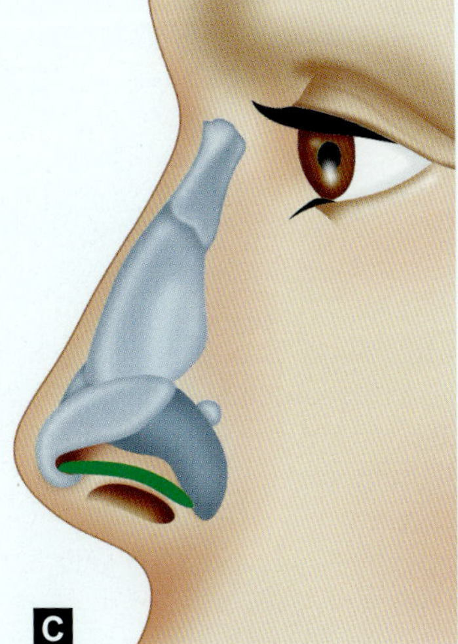

Figs 4A to C: The alar rim graft (green) is placed directly along the alar margin to effect contour changes and provide resilience. (A) Basal view; (B) Front view; and (C) Profile view

can be managed with local wound care and debridement in clinic as needed. Persistence of external nasal valve collapse can occur when an insufficient quantity or poor quality of cartilage is used in grafting. Infection and poor cosmetic outcome can be avoided by proper tissue handling and meticulous skin closure.

SPECIAL INSTRUMENTATION

This procedure can be performed with standard rhinoplasty instrumentation.

REFERENCES

1. Gunter JP, Friedman RM. Lateral crural strut graft: technique and clinical applications in rhinoplasty. Plast Reconstr Surg. 1997;99(4):943-52; discussion 953-5.
2. Kamer FM, McQuown SA. Minicomposite graft for nasal alar revision. Arch Otolaryngol Head Neck Surg. 1987;113(9):943-9.
3. Toriumi DM, Josen J, Weinberger M, et al. Use of alar batten grafts for correction of nasal valve collapse. Arch Otolaryngol Head Neck Surg. 1997;123(8):802-8.
4. Sheen JJ. Aesthetic Rhinoplasty. St. Louis: Mosby; 1978. pp. 264-5.
5. Daniel RK. Discussion: the two essential elements for planning tip surgery in primary and secondary rhinoplasty: observation based on review of 100 consecutive patients. Plastic and Reconstructive Surgery. 2004;114:1582-5.
6. Constantian MB. The two essential elements for planning tip surgery in primary and secondary rhinoplasty: observations based on review of 100 consecutive patients. Plast Reconstr Surg. 2004;114(6):1571-81; discussion 1582-5.
7. Boahene KD, Hilger PA. Alar rim grafting in rhinoplasty: indications, technique, and outcomes. Arch Facial Plast Surg. 2009;11(5):285-9.
8. Brissett AE, Sherris DA. Changing the nostril shape. Facial Plast Surg Clin North Am. 2000;8:433-45.
9. Toriumi DM, Checcone MA. New concepts in nasal tip contouring. Facial Plast Surg Clin North Am. 2009; 17: 55-90, vi.

CHAPTER

104 Augmentation Rhinoplasty

Brajendra Baser, Shenal Kothari

INTRODUCTION

Augmentation is necessary for both esthetic and functional indications, such as the upper or lower lateral cartilages. Traditionally, depressed nose results in diminished social acceptability in India. A prominent nose is considered as a symbol of prestige. Saddle nose is the commonest deformity requesting correction in clinical practice.

Saddle nose deformity results from lack of support to the bony or cartilaginous nasal dorsum. Columellar retraction and collapse of the nasal side walls further worsen the cosmoses. Functional reason for augmentation rhinoplasty includes providing structural support for areas deficient of material weakened cartilaginous support formed in the internal nasal valve area.

Causes for Saddle Nose

- *Congenital*: Nasomaxillary hypoplasia, frontonasal dysplasia, congenital syphilis
- *Traumatic*: Unreduced nasal bone and septal fractures, untreated septal hematoma/abscess
- *Iatrogenic*: Complication of septorhinoplasty and submucous resection (SMR), over reduction of nasal hump (open roof deformity)
- *Secondary*: Granulomatous disorders i.e. leprosy, syphilis, tuberculosis
- Congenital or racial shortness deformity
- Acquired shortness deformity
- Childhood trauma
- *Congenital deformities*: Cleft lip nose, Binder's syndrome
- Dorsal irregularities such as in crooked noses

SPECIFIC PREOPERATIVE EVALUATION

It is true that minor defects meticulously corrected are not as well appreciated as gross defects converted to a less severe deformity. Therefore it is important to be realistic and make the patient understand as to what can be or cannot be achieved postoperatively. The forces applied on septum by the surrounding bones and skin determines its shape and therefore for achieving proper correction of septum, these forces are also to be corrected at the same time. Certain factors that need to be evaluated for best results are as below:

- *Etiological factors*: The etiology of saddle nose plays an important role as in cases of granulomatous disorders. The basic etiological factor should be treated first. For example, in patients with saddle nose due to leprosy, the disease should be under control and not in active phase or in atrophic rhinitis. The nose must be crust-free in atrophic rhinitis. Similarly, for patients requiring a revision rhinoplasty, a period of 6 months to 1 year should have elapsed after primary surgery. Watch for collapsing ala during inspiration. This is because of external valve collapse and is seen in patients who had undergone aggressive reductio rhinoplasty.
- *Degree and site of required augmentation*: The length of the nasal dorsum and its proportion to the rest of the nasal skeleton is important to plan the degree and site of correction. Cases with disproportionately low radix or loss of support in cartilaginous dorsum are difficult to augment and such patients need to be accordingly counseled. Cartilage grafts are the grafts of choice in most situations; septum, concha and rib in order of preference. Occasionally the membranous bones of calvarium are used for nasal augmentation; the last of these procedures is not practiced nowadays. The newer technique for augmentation is diced cartilage in fascia lata. This can be prepared as per the requirement both in respect to size and shape of the recipient area. The nasal bones gain support from the maxilla and the nasal process of the frontal bone. In a bony saddle not only is the dorsum flat but also the side walls which require support.
- *Status of the columella and nasal tip*: Nasal tip augmentation is required for patients with retracted columella and when the tip support is lost. The concept of equilateral rhomboid of nasal tip must be kept in mind for all rhinoplasties.

- *Condition of septal cartilage*: The condition of septal cartilage of nasal septum is assessed. We need to evaluate as to whether it is available for grafting, both in terms of support and availability as a graft material. In conditions like septal abscess or hematoma or following SMR operation there may be complete resorption of septal cartilage whether there is a true septal deviation or it is because of unilateral collapse of cartilage. Pseudodeviation should also be ruled out.
- *Condition of nasal skin*: Nasal cavities must be free of any crust or infection. Nasal skin type varies from individual to individual and varies depending on the racial factors as well. It is important as it has a bearing on the anticipated tissue reaction, wound healing and surgical outcome. This evaluation is important as in a thin-skinned patient the graft outline may be visible. Thick-skinned patient would require more aggressive augmentation. Similarly, connective tissue type becomes significant. It affects skin wrinkling, tissue tension, elasticity and mobility of skin. Post-traumatic scarring; puckered skin following infective conditions or following implant extrusion requires special care.
- *Degree of nasal obstruction*: Evaluation of septal relationship to turbinate is necessary as compensatory turbinate hypertrophy may lead to nasal obstruction. The internal nasal valve is formed by junction of quadrangular cartilage, anterior end of inferior turbinate and floor of nose. This valve should be between 10° and 15°. If the valve is less than 10°, it produces sense of nasal obstruction. Positive Cottle's test is indicative of internal nasal valve collapse. A complete internal nasal examination repeated with aid of topical decongestant and nasal endoscopy allows better visualization of posterior and dorsal septum.
- *Photographic documentation* is important in diagnosis and planning surgery. Postoperative photographs serves to document immediate outcome and function as a historical record to follow surgical changes. The photographs are taken in following standard views viz. frontal, right and left lateral, oblique and basal. The possible outcome is discussed with patient using preoperative photographs. The nose is analyzed in relation to entire face. These photographs help us to understand detailed facial analysis and in diagnosing structural nasal pathology. Facial esthetic units (vertically divided into five equal parts and horizontally into three equal parts) are evaluated separately and in conjunction with nasal dorsum, nasal tip, sidewalls, nasal alae, columella and soft tissue triangle.
- A number of materials are available to the rhinoplastic surgeon to augment the nose. These include alloplasts (synthetic implants), allogenous materials (obtained from cadavers), or autologous implants (harvested from the patient's own tissue). Each has advantages and disadvantages.

Esthetics

The esthetics of the profile must be analyzed critically. No single ideal profile exists, because each individual has his or her own tastes and priorities.

Some considerations for ideal profile are as follows:

- The nasion should be positioned at the level of the supratarsal crease.
- The forehead and glabella must be adequately projected to create an appropriately defined nasofrontal angle.
- A relatively straight dorsum with a slight convexity at the rhinion is most natural and pleasing.
- The tip should project slightly, with the supratip area composing the leading edge of the nasal profile.

ANESTHETIC CONSIDERATION

Although local anesthesia works well especially for small cases, it is preferred to use general anesthesia for majority of the patients. To achieve a clear bloodless field, it is important to inject xylocaine 2% with adrenaline at certain points. A competent anesthetist with controlled hypotensive anesthesia is idle.

CHOICE OF GRAFT MATERIAL

The properties of an ideal graft material for augmentation rhinoplasty includes the following:

- The graft is tolerated by the host without any immunological rejection.
- The shape and size of material should not change with time and forces of healing.
- The material is reasonably malleable to carve or mold into the desired shape.
- The material is easily obtainable and adequate supply of the material is available with minimal donor site morbidity.

Graft Harvesting

- *Septum*: In patients without extensive removal of septal cartilage in the past, abundant quadrangular cartilage is apt to be available for harvest. Maintaining 1.5 cm of the dorsal and caudal septum should be sufficient. An intact L-shaped septal strut is necessary to provide support to the lower two thirds of the nose (Figs 1A to C).
- *Concha*: Auricular cartilage grafts may be harvested from either a posterior incision or an anterior incision.

As long as the anti-helical fold is preserved, the form of the auricle is not significantly altered with removal of the entire cavum conchae and cymba conchae complex. Maintaining the vertical component of the conchal bowl is advised to preserve lateral ear projection. Hydraulic dissection of the subcutaneous plane with the injection of local anesthetic aids in the ease of harvest. The anterior skin is more adherent, although some surgeons prefer to harvest composite grafts from a posterior incision. At times we harvest all the available cartilage from both the ears (Figs 2A and B).

- *Ribs*: The confluence of the 6th and 7th ribs and the confluence of the 9th and 11th ribs have been used successfully for grafting. Care is taken to avoid entrance into the pleural cavity.

Rib cartilages have a strong memory and are very prone to curl. This warping can be limited by taking following steps: (1) remove perichondrium completely, (2) symmetric carving of the costal cartilage from the straightest rib segment, (3) use only the core part of the rib discarding the peripheral pieces, and (4) soak the prepared segment in saline for 10 minutes to identify any acute warping before implantation. The diced rib cartilage is virtually unlimited supply of graft material for most situations.

Allograft

The most commonly used allograft materials include silicone, Medpore and Gortx. Alloplastic materials have numerous advantages. They are readily available with an unlimited supply, they are easy to fashion into the desired shape, they resist warping and resorption, and they have no donor-site morbidity. They are especially popular in southeast Asian countries where nasal augmentation is a very common procedure.

However, alloplastic implants have been noted to have higher rates of infection and extrusion (Figs 3A and B). Infection of the implant may leave the patient with permanent damage to the overlying skin. The use of alloplast in revision cases, septal perforation and the situations where septal support is lacking can be disastrous; the authors prefers to use autologous material only.

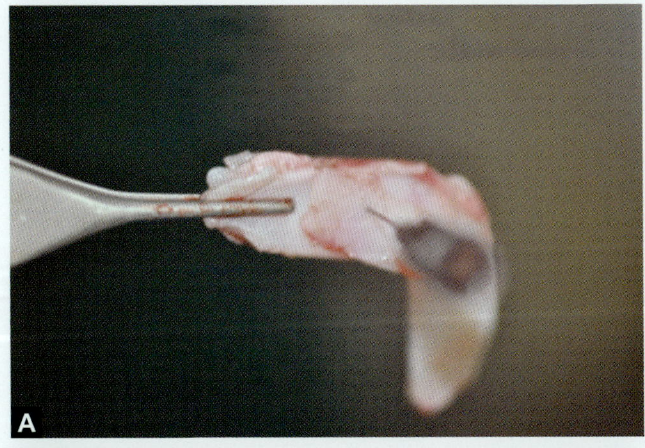

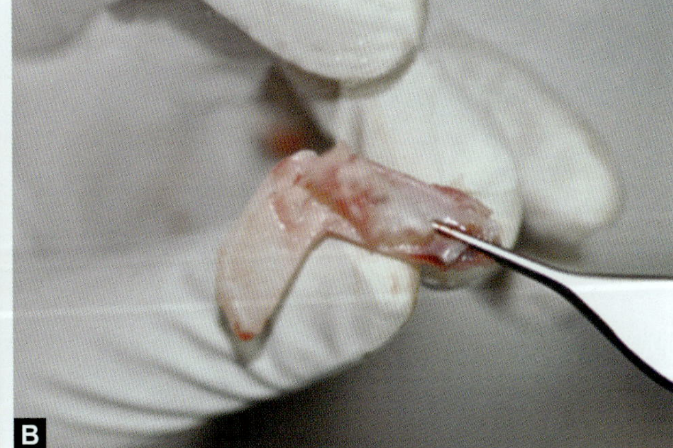

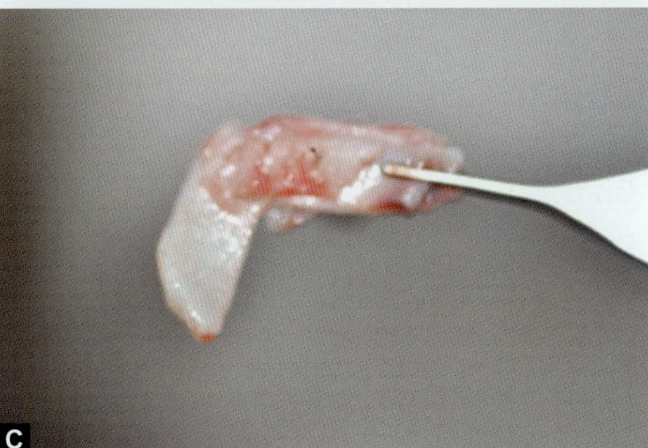

Figs 1A to C: The septal strut support for dorsum. (A) L-shaped strut prepared from septal cartilage (needle is used to fix the two parts); (B) L-shaped strut prepared from septal cartilage, two parts being sutured; (C) L-shaped septal strut ready to use

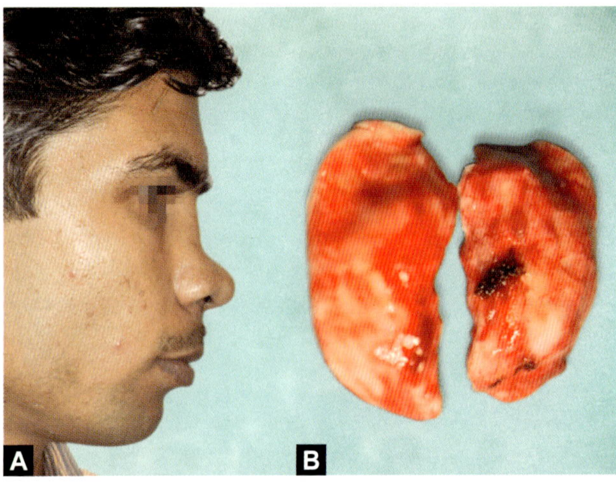

Figs 2A and B: Harvesting cartilage from both conchae for major augmentation. (A) Severe depression; (B) Cartilage harvested from both conchae

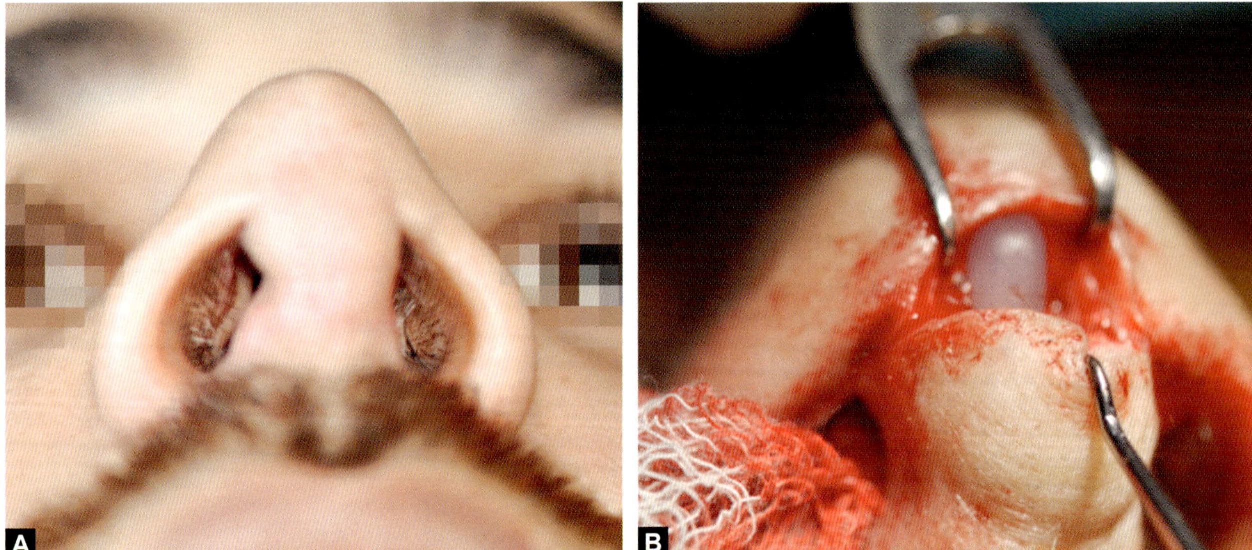

Figs 3A and B: Alloplastic material resulting in extrusion. (A) Infection; (B) Displacement

SURGICAL STEPS

As we describe the steps of rhinoplasty in all such cases, few points must be remembered:

- Open rhinoplasty approach is preferred as it gives a complete view of asymmetry.
- The septum is completely exposed as per the need.
- Care should be taken to avoid perforation of mucoperichondrial flap.
- Osteotomies are done sometime to reduce the width of the nasal dorsum, however, the authors does not recommend it routinely.
- Due importance should be given to the cartilaginous framework and maintain their anatomical position using spreader graft and positioning sutures.

The steps are:

Step 1: Painting and Draping

Like all operations, standard painting and draping technique is adopted. The vibrissae are trimmed to get a better visualization of the operative field.

Step 2: Incision

Various incisions are described to get access to the recipient area like intercartilaginous incision (between upper and lower lateral cartilages), cartilage splitting incision (or intracartilaginous) and the marginal incision (along the lower margin of the ala) for graft insertion. Currently for all minimal or major nasal augmentation we use the Rethi-Goodman external rhinoplasty incision (Fig. 4). This has several distinct advantages: easy access, direct visualization of the operative field to allow creation of symmetrical pockets and elevation of nasal bone periosteum and bone to bone contact is assured. Graft shifting is avoided since the dissected pocket is in mid-line. Lesser risk of extrusion through the incision site is avoided, the incision site being away from the recipient area. Also, augmentation of the side walls is possible through the same incision.

Step 3: Elevation of Dorsal Skin Flap

Now the skin along with the subcutaneous tissue is dissected with the help of a scissors such that the plane of dissection is kept close to the nasal cartilage and bone. However, while we are using a bone graft the dissection is subperiosteal (Fig. 5).

Step 4: Preparation of Recipient Site

A symmetrical pocket of the size slightly larger than the width of the graft to be inserted is dissected in the mid-line to avoid migration of graft and subsequent irregularities. A critical point is the preservation of an adequate soft-tissue envelope during preparation of the pocket for implantation of the graft. The dissection should be performed deep to the subdermal plexus, which not only preserves an adequate thickness of overlying soft tissue but also minimizes subsequent fibrosis and unpredictable healing.

Step 5: Supporting Graft

In post-traumatic and revision cases where septal support to the nasal dorsum is lost, it is important to remake the septal support. A L-shaped frame is made with conchal /septal or rib cartilage (Figs 6 and 7).This frame is fixed with nasal bone and the maxillary spine and the upper lateral cartilage. This is called as the supporting graft. On top of this another esthetic layer of cartilage is placed to give continuity to the dorsum. Figures 8 and 9 demonstrate these procedures in the patients. Figures 10 and 11 show the method of fixing the graft. This supporting frame provides stable foundation and prevents posterior pulling of the dorsal onlay graft, because of the fibrosis in between the septal mucoperichondrial flaps.

Step 6: Diced Cartilage in Facial Tube

This is a very elegant method of nasal augmentation described by Rollin Daniel and is very useful in post-traumatic and revision cases where a large amount of graft material is required or when the skin covering is very tight with scarring.

A fascial tube is prepared (Figs 12A to D) by harvesting temporalis fascia or fascia lata. The sheet of fascia is spread around the tuberculin syringe. The two opposite parallel borders are stitched together and then the base is also sewed to prepare a bag open at one end. Cartilage harvested from concha/septum or rib are made into very small pieces and filled in the tuberculin syringe (Figs 13A to C). The cartilage pieces are pushed inside the facial bag by pushing with the help of the plunger, the syringe is withdrawn while pushing the diced cartilage filled previously in the syringe. Thus a malleable pillow of diced cartilage is formed ready to be used for desired augmentation. Diced cartilage wrapped in facial tube has distinct advantages, like it is simpler procedure, bigger piece of cartilage is available and graft material is autogenous. Grafts can be prepared as per the desired length, shape and size to fit the specific defect as they are highly malleable. Complications like step deformity and extrusion rarely occur and can be easily managed. Over correction and graft visibility are not usually met with.

Step 7: Positioning the Graft in Place

Once the graft is ready, it is pushed into the recipient site and secured in place.

Graft Placement

- *Radix*: The placement of a graft to the radix to correct an overly deep nasofrontal angle can restore a high, strong profile. The graft also produces the appearance of lengthening the nose. A precise pocket is produced deep to the procerus muscle, and the graft is placed. Often, the recipient bed is too large, and the graft should be fixed by placing an absorbable suture through the graft and bringing it out through the skin. It is fixed at this point with a steri-strip for several days. Alternatively, percutaneous K-wires can be placed to secure the graft to the radix and are removed in the office 3 weeks postoperatively. In the authors' experience of utilizing this technique over the last 10 years, all costal bone grafts have had stable bony fusion.
- *Nasal dorsum*: If an endonasal approach is chosen and if the recipient pocket can be created precisely, the graft may be introduced without the need for fixation. Otherwise, fixation is necessary. Multiple options can be used to stabilize the graft. If possible, multiple point fixations are performed. Polydioxanone (PDS) may be used to stabilize the graft to the underlying cartilages. In addition, sutures passed through the skin and left in place for several days are helpful. In addition, suturing of the upper lateral cartilages to the dorsal graft helps support the airway.

Step 8

Finally the skin is closed, nasal packing is done and plaster cast is applied.

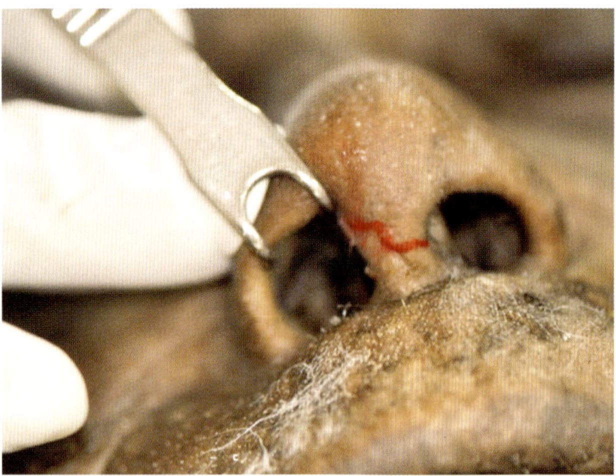

Fig. 4: Columellar incision

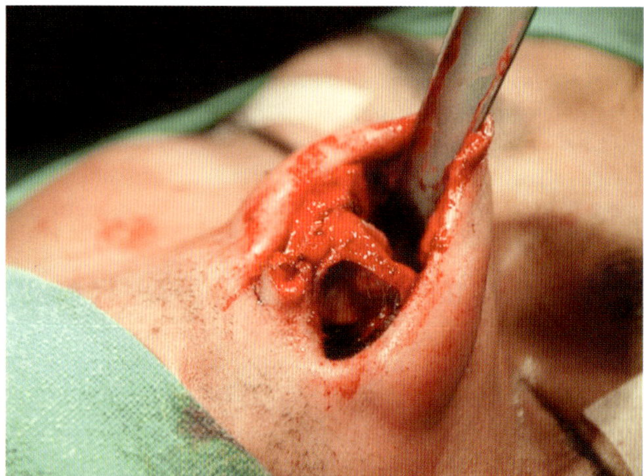

Fig. 5: Creating a symmetrical recipient pocket of the size slightly larger than the width of the graft to be inserted

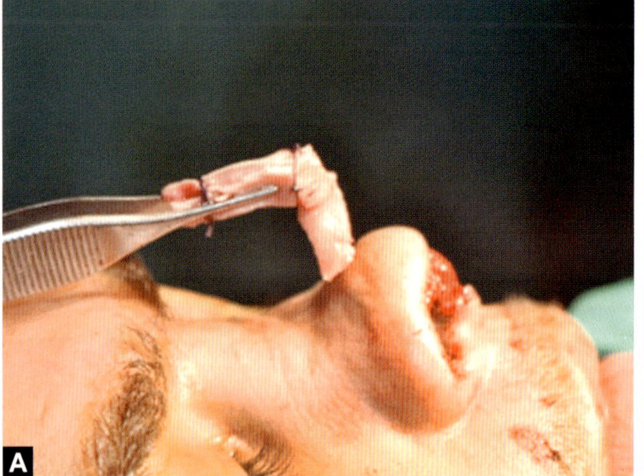

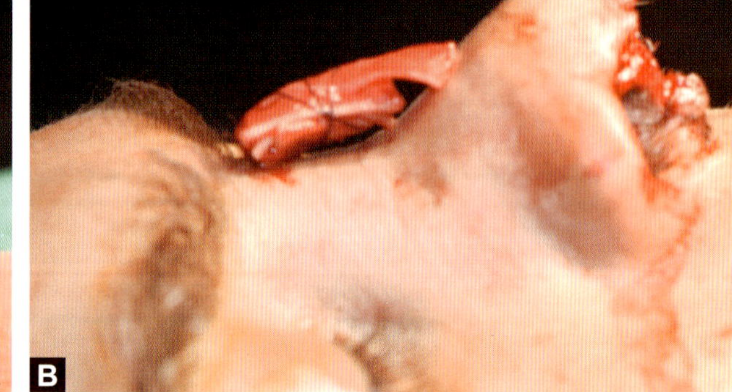

Figs 6A and B: Use of L-shaped support from septal cartilage and bilateral conchal cartilage

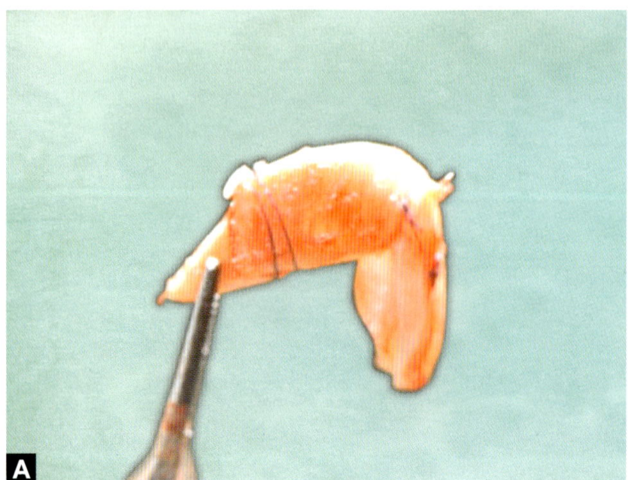

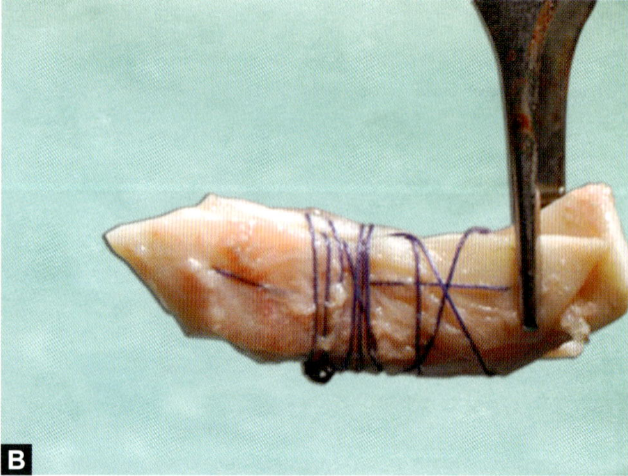

Figs 7A and B: Use of L-shaped support from septal cartilage

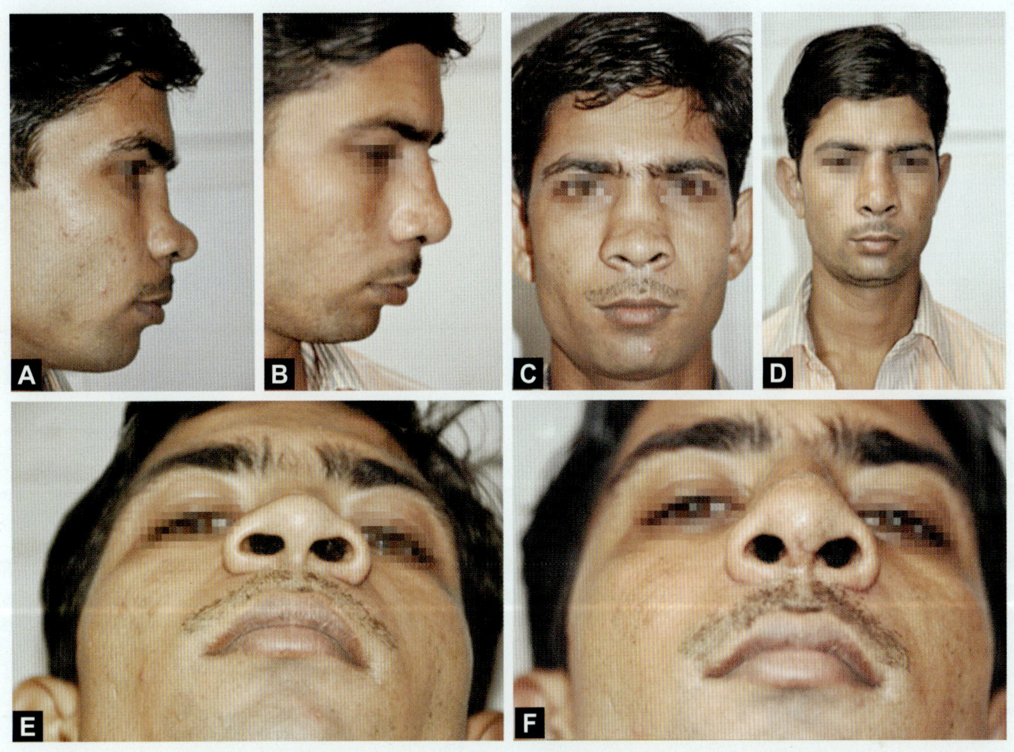

Figs 8A to F: Augmentation using bilateral conchal cartilages

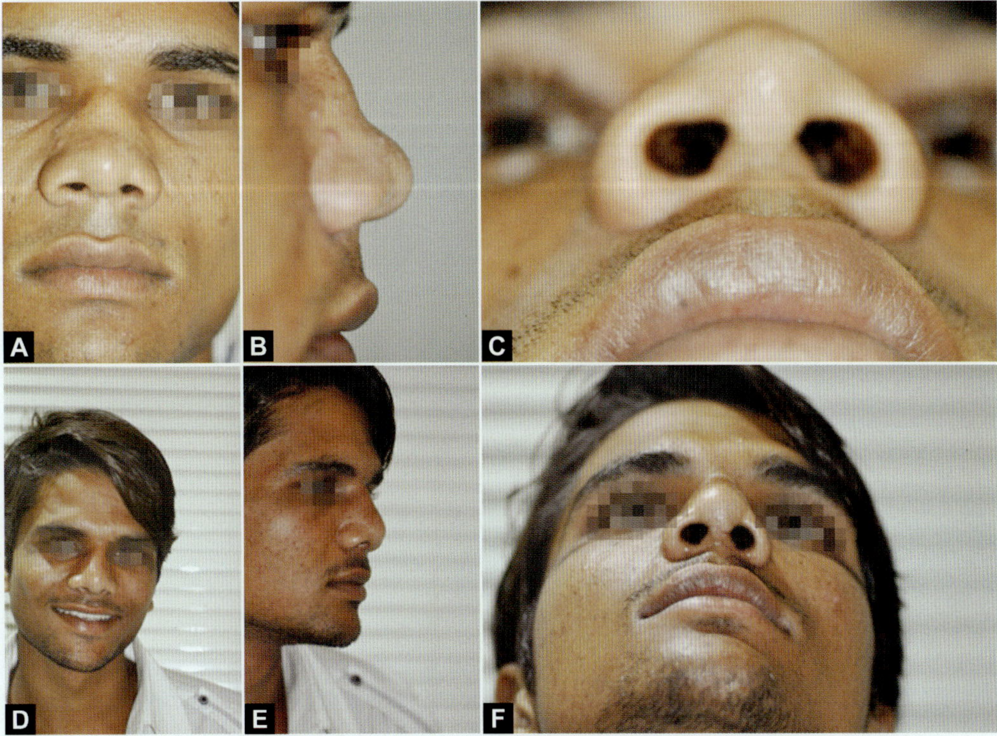

Figs 9A to F: Use of septal cartilage for augmentation

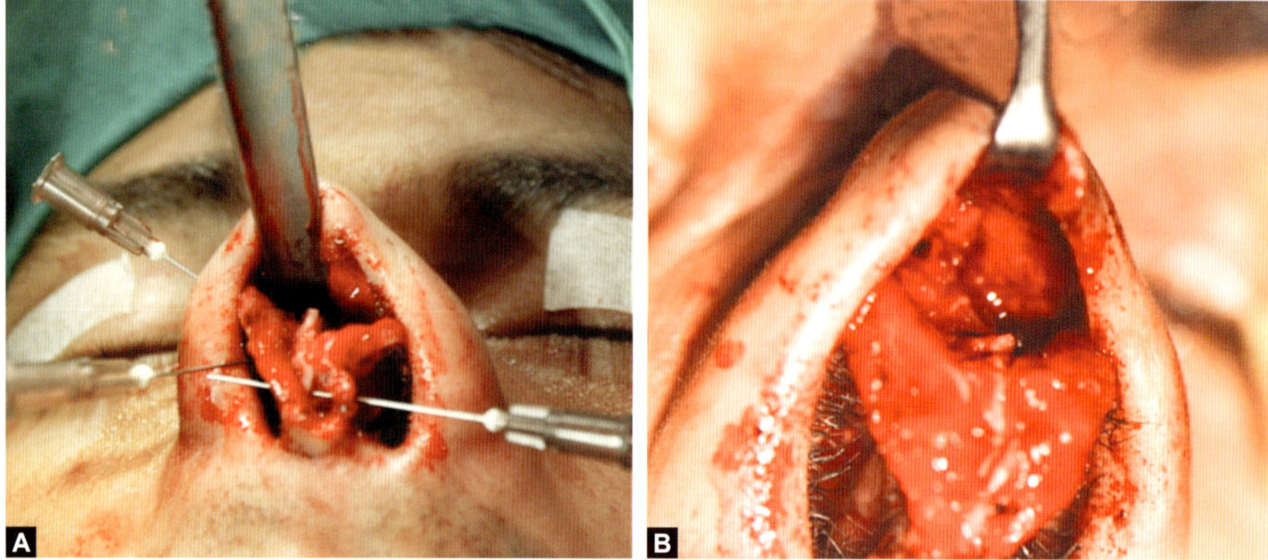

Figs 10A and B: Use of supporting frame to provide stable foundation and placing the dorsal onlay graft. (A) Fixing the supporting frame with nasal bone and the maxillary spine and the upper lateral cartilage; (B) An esthetic layer of cartilage placed on the supporting L-shaped cartilage

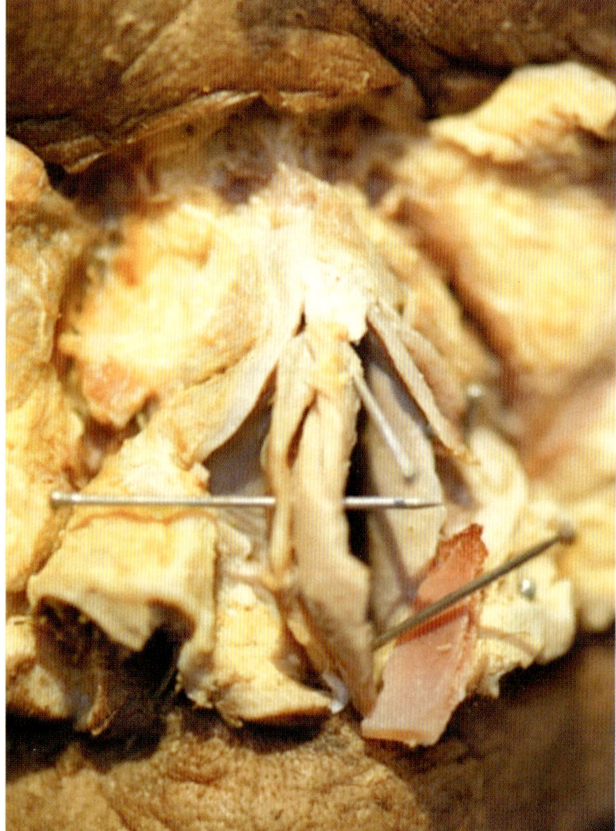

Fig. 11: Fixation of supporting frame with nasal bone and the maxillary spine between the upper lateral cartilage in a cadaver

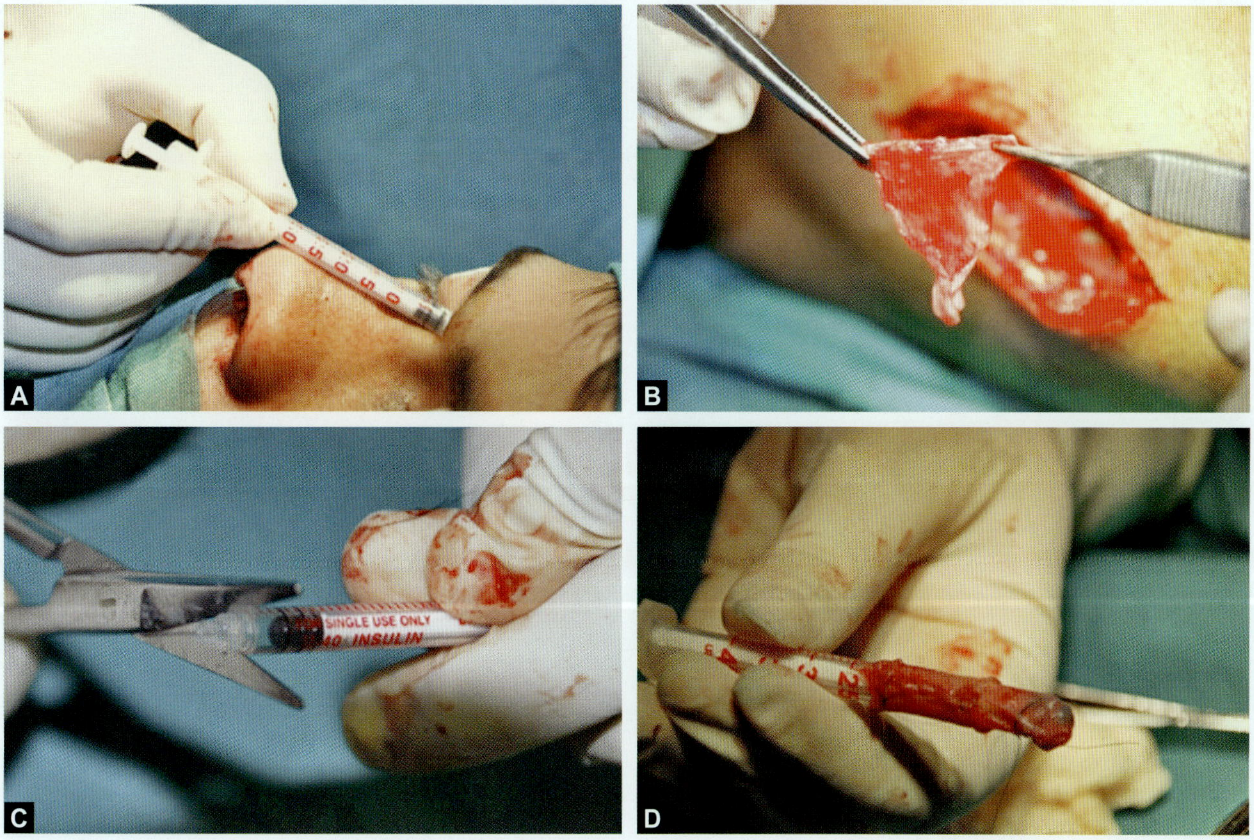

Figs 12A to D: Preparation of fascial tube. (A) Measure the length to be augmented; (B) Harvest the required area of fascia lata; (C) Cut the tip of tuberculin syringe; (D) Prepare the fascial tube

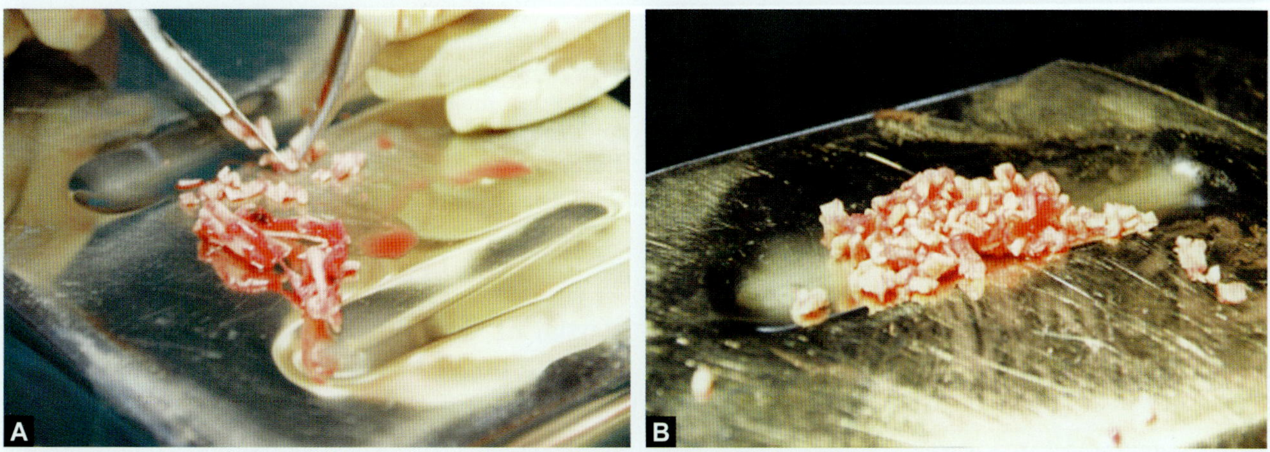

Figs 13A and B

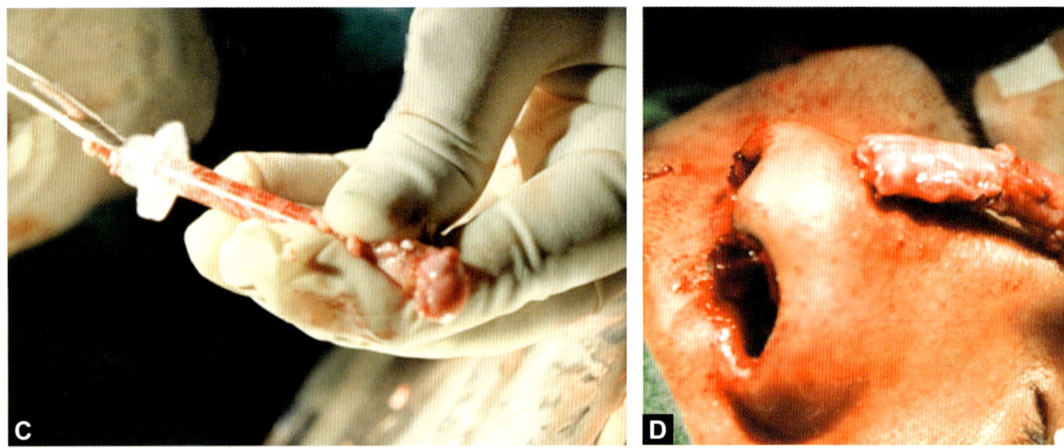

Figs 13A to D: Preparation of diced cartilage graft pillow. (A and B) Cartilage harvested from concha/septum or rib made into very small; (C) Filled in the tuberculin syringe, the cartilage pieces are pushed inside the fascial bag; (D) A malleable pillow of diced cartilage

Step 9

An L-shaped support is created from the septal cartilage remnant and the cartilage bag placed between the two upper lateral cartilages into the desired recipient pocket. In difficult cases where the graft support is inadequate, we use a large L-shaped graft which rests in nasal spine. A columellar strut is used in patients where the caudal septum is deficient. Additional cartilage graft is used for tip augmentation if required.

POSTOPERATIVE DETAILS

The immediate postoperative care is the same as that for primary rhinoplasty. Patients are instructed to leave any splints or tape undisturbed for 1 week. Head elevation is encouraged in the immediate postoperative period. The gentle application of ice on the 1st day minimizes swelling and ecchymosis. The avoidance of strenuous activity is advised for the 1st week. Particular care to avoid any manipulation of the nose, including nose blowing, is stressed for the 1st week. Eyeglasses are not rested on the bridge of the nose but possibly taped to the forehead. The external rhinoplasty sutures are removed on the 7th postoperative day; we recommend use of plaster for 10–15 days.

COMPLICATIONS

Complications and adverse outcomes occur in augmentation rhinoplasties. A certain percentage of patients inevitably require future procedures to achieve a desirable result. This should be clearly explained to the patient before surgery. A particularly relevant adverse outcome of augmentation rhinoplasty is warping and resorption of the grafts, especially with allografts. Asymmetries can occur, despite ideal alignment of the tissues during surgery. These result from asymmetric resorption, warping, and the formation of scar tissue and can occur as long as several months after surgery.

An inadequacy or overabundance of the augmented area may become apparent postoperatively. However, some patients may require revision to achieve a better outcome.

Infection may occur. The infection may cause extrusion of the implant. Removal is then necessary, particularly with alloplasts.

Changes may occur in the skin overlying the graft material. These include persistent erythema, telangiectasias, and contour irregularities due to dermal or subdermal fibrosis. Graft visibility may be a problem in thin-skinned patients.

DIFFICULTIES AND SOLUTIONS

Partial or Complete Absorption of Graft Material

- Whenever possible, prefer cartilage over bone.
- Prefer autologous material over homograft; place the bone grafts subperiosteally to assure a bone to bone contact.
- Proper immobilization of bone grafts. Make the recipient area free of stress

- Remove scar tissue from the recipient site. This can produce contraction and stress over the graft.
- Infection, hematoma and edema in recipient bed should be avoided.
- Make the recipient pocket in midline through external approach.
- Pocket should be made just to accommodate the graft. Avoid extensive skeletalization.

Graft Visibility

Graft outline may be visible in a thin-skinned patient.

- Dissect the pocket close to perichondrial and periosteal plane
- Crushed cartilage may be sutured over the dorsal surface of bone graft or wrapped in fascia.
- Temporalis fascia can be used to cover the dorsal surface of bone graft.

Dorsal Irregularities

Cartilage grafts have tendency to curl, especially the rib cartilage, producing late dorsal irregularities. To minimize recurling of cartilage graft, carve off the graft by trimming the graft in balanced cross section.

Soft Tissue Deficiency

A generous pocket for the implant is essential to prevent graft extrusion and to allow a natural red raping especially in post-traumatic or secondary rhinoplasty cases where the tissue is scarred.

Septum

A deficient septal foundation produces a poor framework and this is taken care by using L-shaped dorsal support.

GRAFT MATERIAL

Historically a wide variety of graft materials has been used to rebuild the nasal dorsum. These include ivory, metals, homograft, allograft, xenograft, bone and cartilage and irradiated rib cartilage. Autografts such as temporalis fascia, denna fat, septal, costal and conchal cartilage, bone from the iliac crest, calvarium, rib, tibia and olecranon.

Choice of Graft Material

The surgeons' choice for selection of graft material in a particular case is as follows:

- *Minor augmentation*: Septal cartilage. If this is not available, conchal cartilage
- *Moderate augmentation*: Septal cartilage or conchal cartilage. Layers of septal and conchal cartilage combined or rib cartilage.
- *Major augmentation*: For severe deformities which require large amount of graft material, calvarial bone graft, rib cartilage or iliac crest bone graft is used. In present day practice, diced cartilage in fascia lata gives the best results.
- *Columellar retraction*: Septal or conchal cartilage strip or tip of 9th rib.

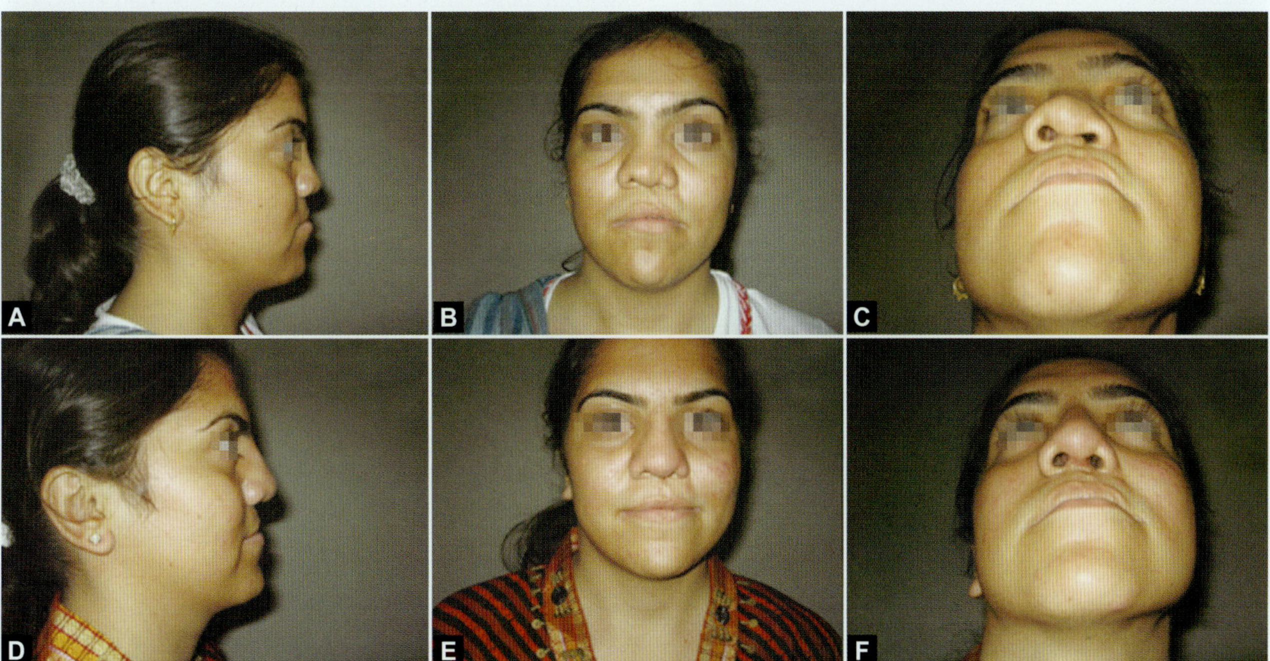

Figs 14A to F: Augmentation rhinoplasty. (A to C) Preoperative images; (D to F) Postoperative images

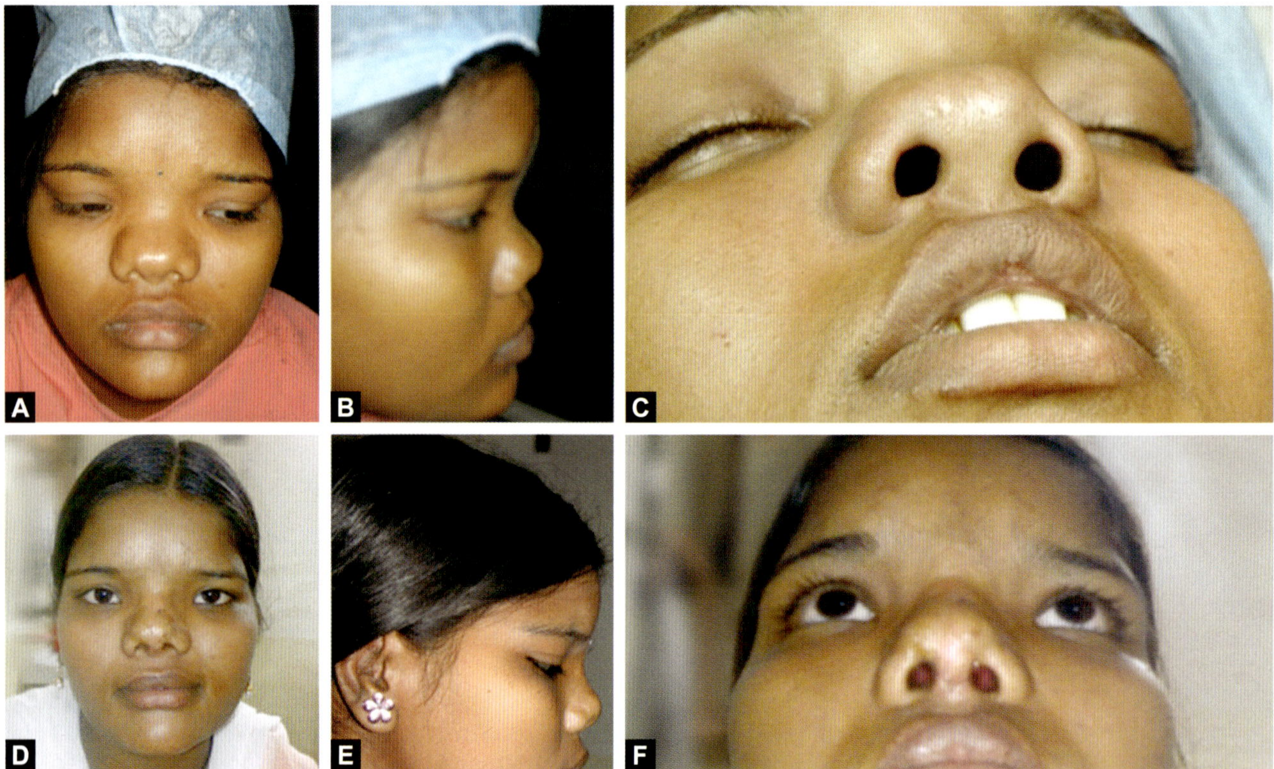

Figs 15A to F: Augmentation using conchal cartilage in a girl with nasomaxillary hypoplasia (Binder's syndrome)

Few preoperative and postoperative pictures of other patients are given in Figures 14 and 15.

BIBLIOGRAPHY

1. Achauer BM, VanderKam VM, Celikoz B, et al. Augmentation of facial soft-tissue defects with Alloderm dermal graft. Ann Plast Surg. 1998;41(5):503-7.
2. Aufright G. Rhinoplasty and face. Plast Reconstr Surg. 1969; 43:219.
3. Baser. B. Aesthetic and Functional Rhinoplasty, 2nd edition. 2004.
4. Bernstein L. Surgical anatomy in rhinoplasty. Otolaryngol Clin North Am. 1975;8:549-58.
5. Fanous N. Unilateral osteotomies for external bony deviation of the nose. Plast Reconstr Surg. 1997; 100 (1):115-23.
6. Gunter JP, Rohrich RJ. Management of the deviated nose. The importance of septal reconstruction. Clin Plast Surg. 1988;15:43-55.
7. Gurlek A, Ersoz-Ozturk A, Celik M, et al. Correction of the crooked nose using custom-made high-density porous polyethylene extended spreader grafts. Aesthetic Plast Surg. 2006;30(2):141-9.
8. Holt GR, Garner EI, McLarey D. Postoperative sequelae and complications of rhinoplasty. Otolaryngol Clin North Am. 1987;20:853-76.
9. Watzinger F, Wutzl A, Wanschitz F, et al. Biodegradable polymer membrane used as septal splint. Int J Oral Maxillofac Surg. 2008;37(5):473-7.
10. Wright MR, Management of patient dissatisfaction with results of cosmetic procedures. Arch Otolaryngol Head Neck Surg. 1980;106:466-71.

CHAPTER

105 Alar Base Reduction

Sara Dickie, Jeremy Warner

INDICATIONS FOR THE SURGERY

The soft tissues of the nasal tip, ala and nostrils are an integral to the success of rhinoplasty surgery and therefore need to be evaluated in every rhinoplasty consult and plan. The primary aims of operating on the alar soft-tissues are to achieve an esthetic balance and natural appearance. This is accomplished by maintaining natural borders, preventing revision surgery and attaining acceptable scars. There are many techniques described in the literature.[1-6] Unfortunately, the most effective or appropriate strategy to achieve superior outcomes can at times remain elusive. The goal of this chapter is to provide the tools necessary to manipulate the alar soft-tissues, including an algorithmic approach to evaluate and treat various anomalies. We will also provide detailed descriptions of the techniques used to alter and improve the appearance of the nasal tip and alar base. Ultimately, these techniques will offer the potential to transform a good result into an exceptional result, ensuring both facial harmony and a satisfied patient.[7]

SPECIFIC PREOPERATIVE EVALUATION

Some alar base irregularities are apparent on preoperative examination. However, many only become apparent after intraoperative manipulation of the nasal tip. Therefore, tip and base assessment should continue throughout the operative course. The surgical planning should not be considered complete without an initial assessment and an intraoperative reassessment of the nasal soft-tissue esthetics. Patients should be evaluated from anterior-posterior, lateral and basal views. If using an open rhinoplasty approach, the analysis of the base width, appreciating both the external and internal components should be performed with the nose completely closed.

The ideal nose parameters on anteroposterior (AP) view are shown in Figure 1. The width of the lower third of the nose should be approximately that of the intercanthal distance. The basal view is shown in Figure 2. From the basal view the nose should be approximately the shape of an equilateral triangle. Alar margins are relatively straight as they travel from the tip of the nose to the alar bases. Nostrils should be ovoid in shape and canted off midline so the inferior aspect is more laterally displaced compared to the superior.

The standard of keeping the width of the nose within the intercanthal distance should be used as a guideline instead of a fixed criterion. The width of the lower third of the nasal tip should be a relative perceptive value depending on the size and shape of the nasal tip rather than an absolute. One must exercise caution to avoid excessive narrowing of the columellar-alar base distance as this may give the appearance of an overly bulky tip. Understanding this concept is necessary to achieve the appropriate balance. Confounding variables such as ethnic differences and patient preference should affect the approach to achieve visual harmony of the face.[8]

Excessive Width of the Lower Third of the Nose

Increased Collumellar-Alar Base Distance and Large or Asymmetric Nostril

There are two surfaces to the ala that affect the width and contour of the alar base.[9] The cutaneous, or the external surface refers to the distance between the columella and the alar base. The vestibular, or the internal surface refers to the nostril diameter. If these are considered independently one can maintain or narrow the width of the alar base and maintain or narrow the nostril size separately.

The first step in planning an alar base reduction is deciding whether to perform an external base reduction, internal base reduction or both. If the columellar-alar base distance (the width of the lower third of the nose) is excessive then typically an external base reduction is warranted (Fig. 3). If the columellar-alar base distance is within the normal range, then a decision needs to be made whether the nostril diameter needs to be decreased to reduce nostril width (Fig. 4). Some patients may require both internal and external base reduction.

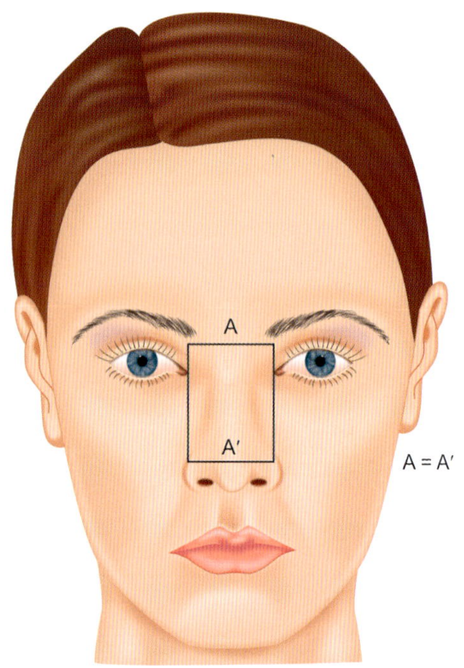

Fig. 1: The ideal nasal proportions as seen from the anteroposterior view. The width of the lower third of the nose is approximately equal to the intercanthal distance

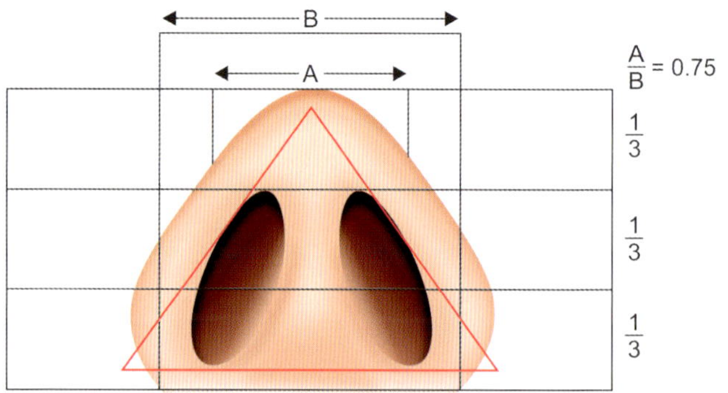

Fig. 2: The ideal nasal proportions as seen from the basal view. The surfaces of the nose approximate an equilateral triangle (shown in red). Alar margins are relatively straight from tip to base. Nostrils should be ovoid in shape and canted off midline

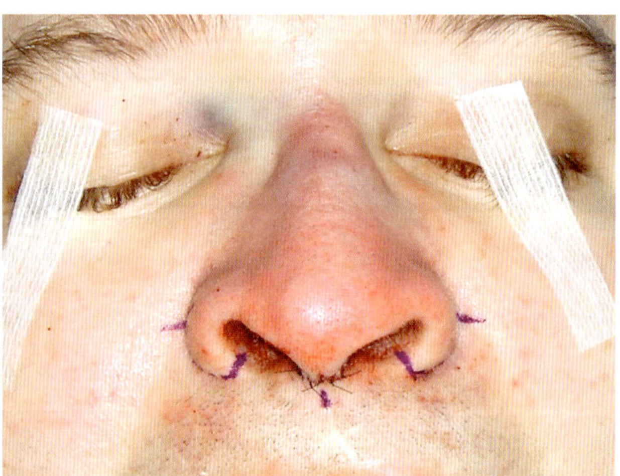

Fig. 3: Intraoperative anteroposterior (AP) view of a patient after open rhinoplasty with columellar incision closed. Note the width of the lower third of the nose is too wide. This is an indication for an external base reduction

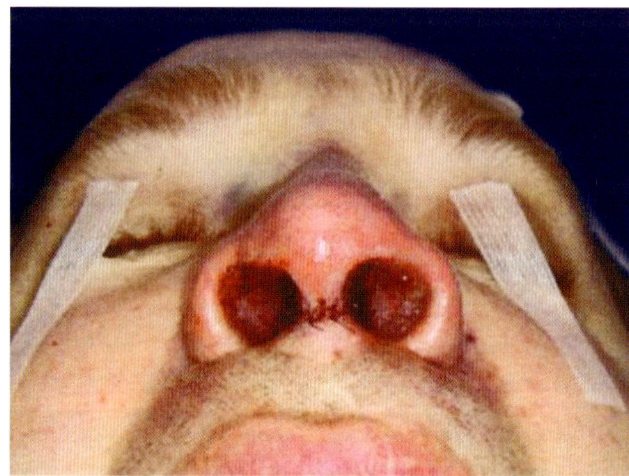

Fig. 4: The same patient from Figure 3 from basal view. Note the nostril diameter is too wide and the nostrils are round. This is an indication for internal base reduction. This patient also exhibits nasal flaring as the lateral wall of the ala bows outward beyond the alar-facial groove

Excessive Alar Flaring

Alar flaring is best evaluated from the basal view (Fig. 4). The alae should be relatively straight as they travel from the tip to the alar base. Flaring is seen when the lateral aspect of the ala extends significantly beyond the alar-facial groove, thus forming a very round nostril. Following the algorithm described below, the sequence of alar flare analysis takes place after alar base reduction. At this point the alar base has been set and the majority of the dissection has already been carried out. It is very common to see flaring when the nose has been deprojected (Fig. 5). Evaluation of nasal flaring should always be performed in this circumstance to address the possible need for flare reduction.

Excessive Alar Hooding

Alar hooding is best evaluated from the lateral view. It is present when the most caudal curve of the ala hangs excessively low. This can occur from either excess alar bulk or from a caudal alar insertion. Hooding obscures the columella from view in the lateral position (Fig. 6). This deformity can be diagnosed using an assessment described by Gunter et al. Looking from the lateral view, a line is drawn through the center of the long axis of the visible nostril.[10] If the alar rim is within 1.5–2.0 mm of this line, then alar position is acceptable. If the distance is less than 1.5 mm or if the nostril is not visible a hanging or hooding ala is present. The amount of hooding can be relative and change depending on columellar show. However, an absolute analysis is more accurate and should be used when deciding whether to reduce bulk of the ala. Intraoperatively, analysis of alar hooding should be performed after the columellar-alar and tip-alar base distances are set.

Algorithm

We have included an algorithm to provide an overview of the aforementioned analysis and the sequence of corrective procedures (Fig. 7). This algorithm should simplify the decision-making process. The rhinoplasty surgeon can sequentially determine the need for each step and then apply the surgical techniques which follow for each indicated procedure.

ANESTHETIC CONSIDERATIONS

Most alar base reductions will be performed simultaneously with rhinoplasty and therefore will likely take place under general or twilight anesthesia. In these cases an oral-ray tube is most effective in maintaining the airway and avoiding interference with the operative field. In cases where alar base reduction is indicated without the need for other surgical procedures of the nose, this can easily be done in the office under local anesthesia alone.

For local anesthetic we prefer 1% lidocaine with 1:100,000 epinepherine. We are not concerned with tissue ischemia of the nasal tip using epinephrine.[11] The duration of vasoconstriction is short lived and the nasal tip has a robust blood supply which will protect these delicate tissues from necrosis. Using a 27 gauge or smaller needle, we infiltrate 2–3 cc at the base of the columella and ala, both internally and externally along the alar margins.

For the anesthetized patient, proper neck and head support is important. One should ensure that the drapes do not prevent free movement of the neck, should turning the head become necessary for access or visualization. Ensure that the endotracheal tube and any other tubing is free from the drapes, so any head movement will not dislodge the tube. In patients who are undergoing alar base reduction under local anesthesia alone, make sure the patient is comfortable and the head well supported before getting started. We prefer to cover the eyes with moist gauze in order to protect the patient from the surgical field and the intensity of the surgical lighting.

SURGICAL STEPS

Alar Base Reduction

External Alar Base Reduction

External alar base reduction decreases the columellar-alar base distance and reduces the apparent width of the lower third of the nose on AP and basal views. It is best performed in the nasal sill. If the goal is to reduce only the columellar-alar width, then an external reduction is planned. In the external reduction the excision is wide at the bottom of the sill and tapered in an "inverted V" pattern (Fig. 8). This allows a narrowing of the base without changing the circumference of the nostril. Patient marking begins with the columellar midline followed by the base of one of the nostril sills (Fig. 9). This distance is measured and used to mark the opposite sill. Using calipers mark the intended area of excision staying medial to the first mark as not to encroach on the ala. The excision is then carried out with a No. 11 blade (Fig. 10). In most cases of alar base reduction, we find it necessary to create a true advancement-rotation flap of the entire alar base to prevent notching. The flap is planned with a 0.5 mm mark above the alar-cheek junction. The incision along the alar base is carried up to a line drawn halfway between the nasal alar base and the alar groove marking the extent of the superior incision in order to prevent blood supply compromise to the nasal tip and superior columellar flap.[12,13] After incision, the alar base is undermined and freed to allow advancement to the medial excisional edge (Fig. 11). The flap allows for a more natural curve and reduces tension along the suture line. It also optimizes scar outcome. In patients with an obtuse alar-cheek junction, patients with a predisposition to poor scarring, and patients with limited isolated internal base reduction we forgo the advancement flap. A single 6-0 nylon suture holds the advancement flap in place to allow assessment of nasal flaring (Figs 12A and B).

When the base reduction is complete the wounds are completely closed with 6-0 nylon sutures. Edges of all incisions should have a well-everted closure which reduces risk of notched scarring in the nasal sill. Rarely, a V-Y closure may become necessary (Fig. 13). No deep sutures are necessary. Most of the cutaneous sutures are removed on postoperative day 4, with the exception of the central sill suture and the more cephalad sutures on the inner portion of the sill, which are left in for 6 days. Sterile skin closure strips (Steri-Strips; 3M, St Paul, Minnesota) are placed for an additional 4 days once the sutures are out.

Internal Alar Base Reduction

For internal alar base reduction one must address only the vestibular alar surface. For this, the sill excision is wide at the top of the sill and tapered in a "V" pattern at the base of the sill (Fig. 14). This allows narrowing of the circumference of the nostril but prevents any change in the columellar-alar base distance. The surgical steps to carry out the internal alar base reduction are the same as for the external alar base reduction (detailed in the preceding section).

Combination

If pre or intraoperative assessment indicates a need for both internal and external alar base reductions, then the appropriate amount of resection is marked at the top of the sill and at the bottom. These marks are connected and define the total area of excision (Fig. 15). The remainder of the surgical steps are identical to those detailed in the external alar base reduction section.

Alar Flare Reduction

If alar flare reduction is indicated, the amount of the lobule to resect is planned and marked (Fig. 16). The planned incision will be from the nasal sill around the alar base. It is important to preserve the natural alar-cheek junction with this incision, so care should be taken to stay just above this line. Also, do not extend the incision outside of the superior alar crease in order to avoid the lateral nasal artery which is just beyond this margin. Excision is performed at the lateral base of the ala, just above the ala-cheek junction. The free edge of the base is grasped with forceps and held taught for wedge-shaped excision using a No. 11 blade (Fig. 17A). This excision simply shortens the tip-alar base distance. If flair reduction is carried out simultaneously with alar base reduction the incision will be continuous with that of the medially located alar base incision along the nasal sill (Fig. 17B). Once the resection is performed, the incisions are completely closed with 6 0 nylon sutures (Fig. 18).

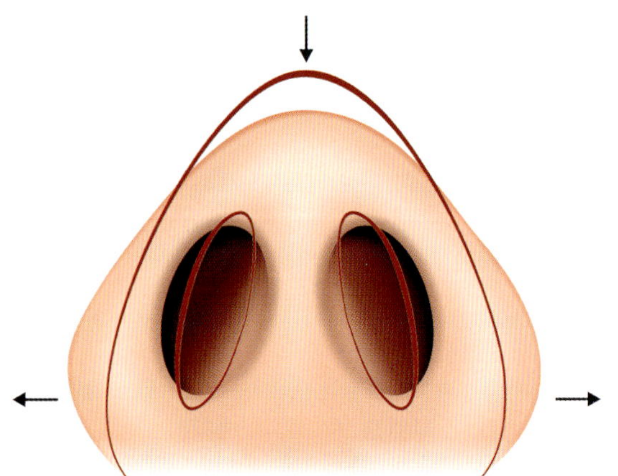

Fig. 5: When the nose is surgically deprojected the alar base widens and alar flaring is increased

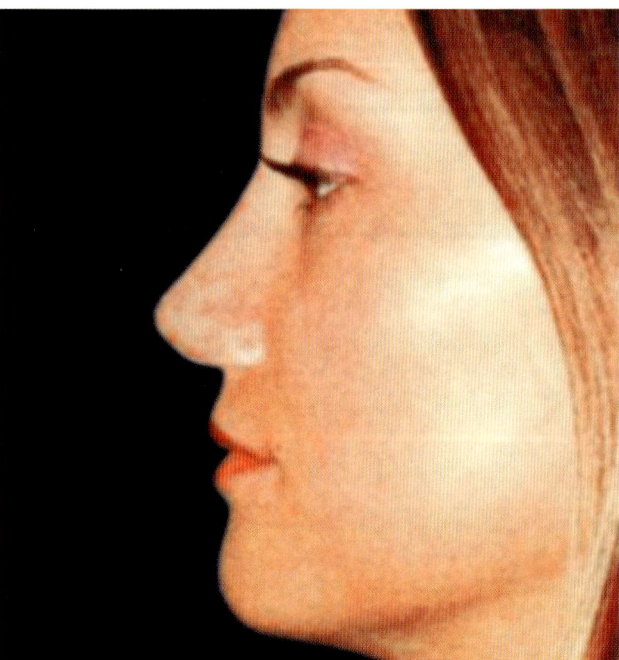

Fig. 6: Direct lateral view showing alar hooding. The caudal curve of the ala obscures the columella

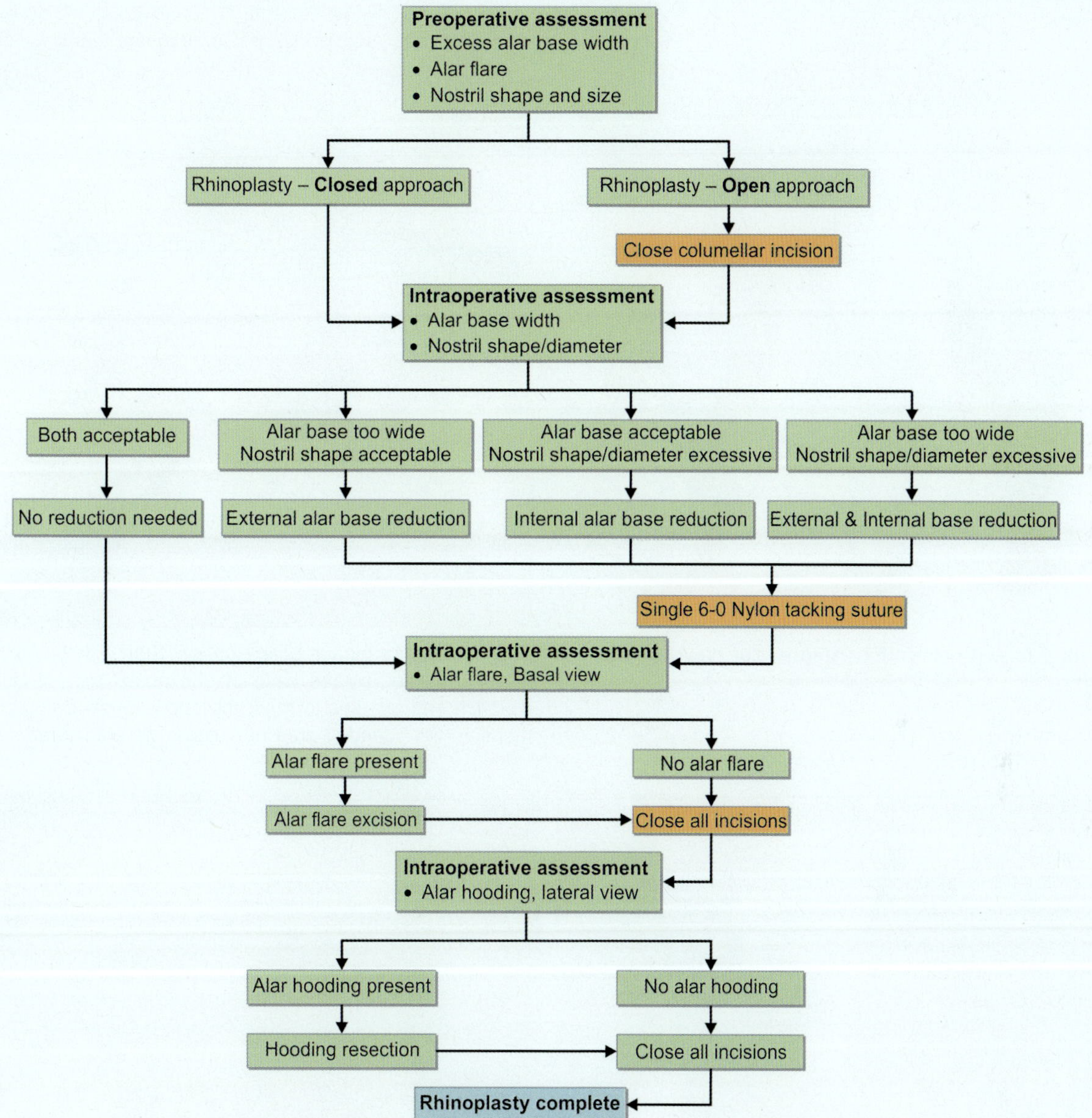

Fig. 7: Algorithm for the analysis and treatment of the alar base

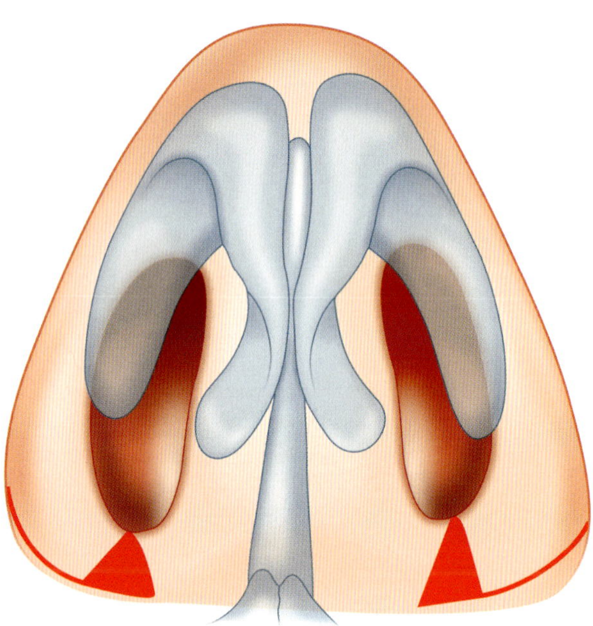

Fig. 8: Excision pattern for external alar base excision

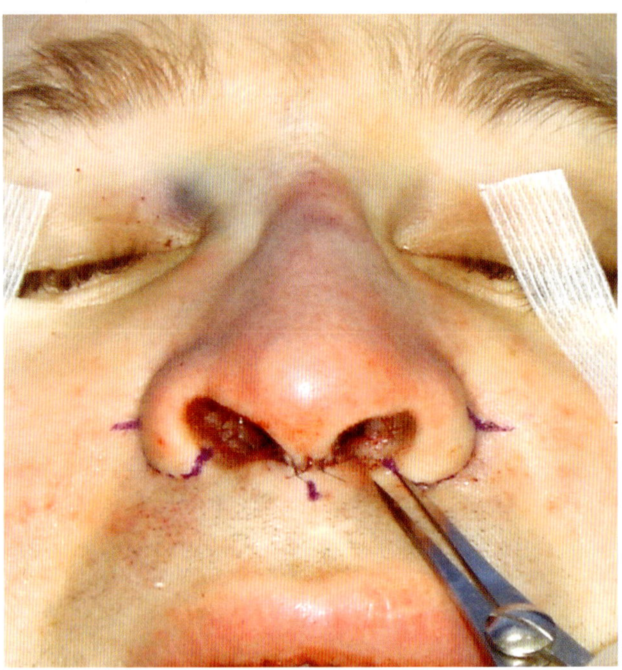

Fig. 9: Markings for alar base excision. Start with the columellar midline followed by the base of one nostril sill. Measure the distance and use this to mark the opposite sill. Using calipers measure the intended area of excision on both sides

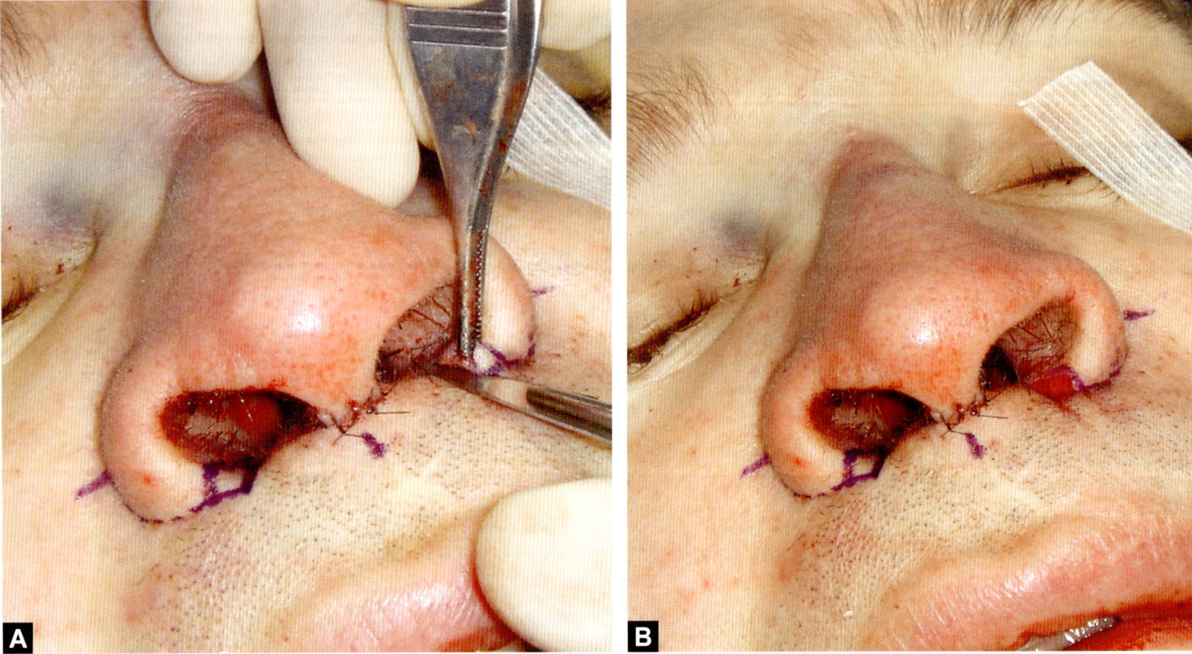

Figs 10A and B: (A) Using a No. 11 blade excise the wedge of tissue at the nasal sill; (B) Shown is a combination of internal and external alar base excision

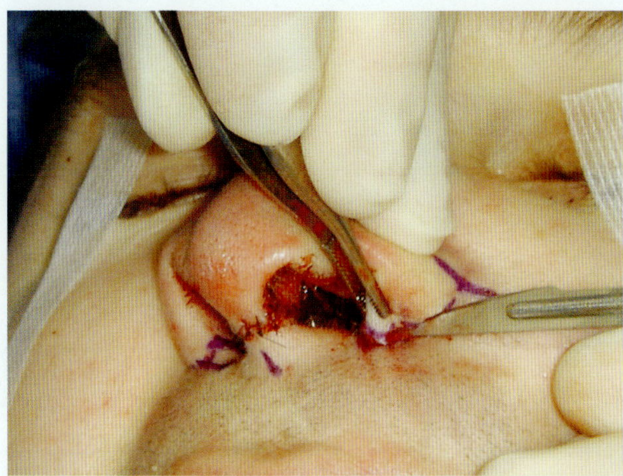

Fig. 11: Advancement-rotation flap to close the alar base excision

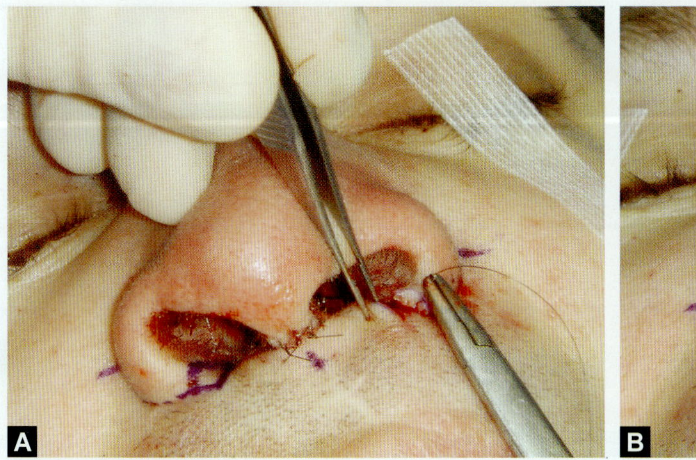

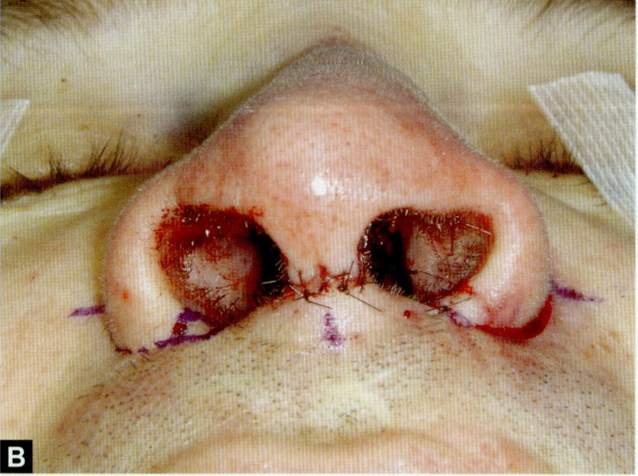

Figs 12A and B: (A) A stay-suture is placed to allow assessment of nasal flaring and contralateral reduction; (B) Note how the base reduction has caused an increase in nasal flaring on the patient's left

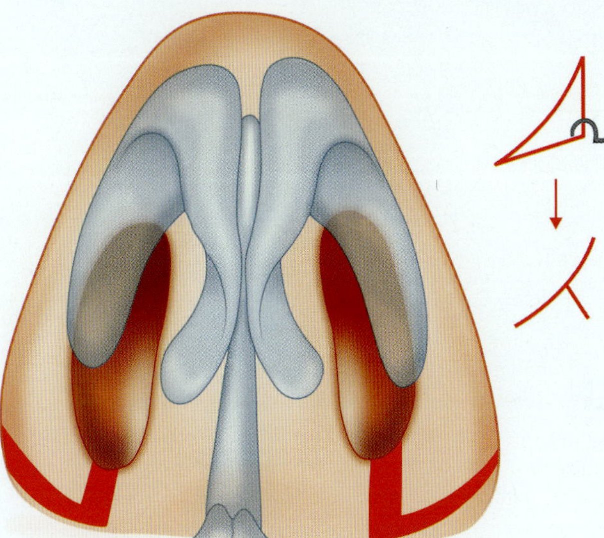

Fig. 13: V-Y closure may be necessary to avoid notching

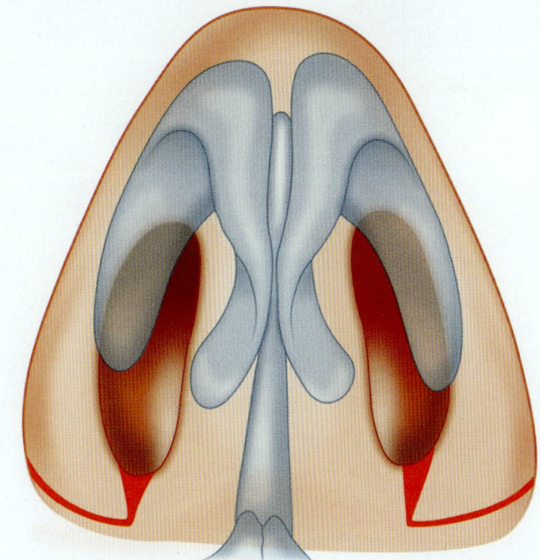

Fig. 14: Excision pattern for internal alar base excision

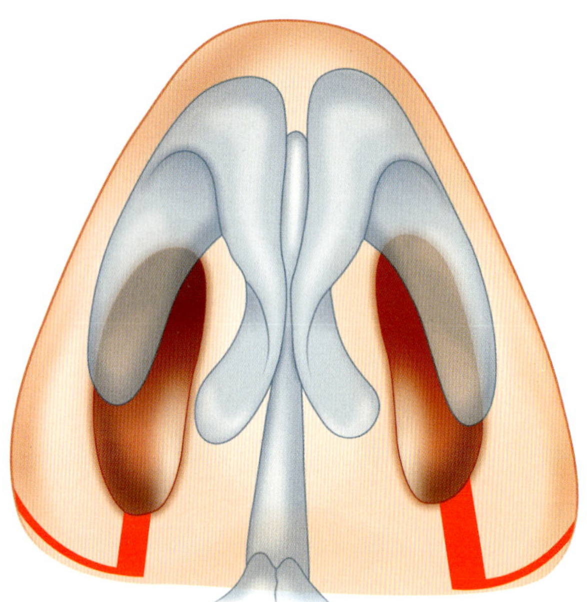

Fig. 15: Excision pattern for combination alar base excision

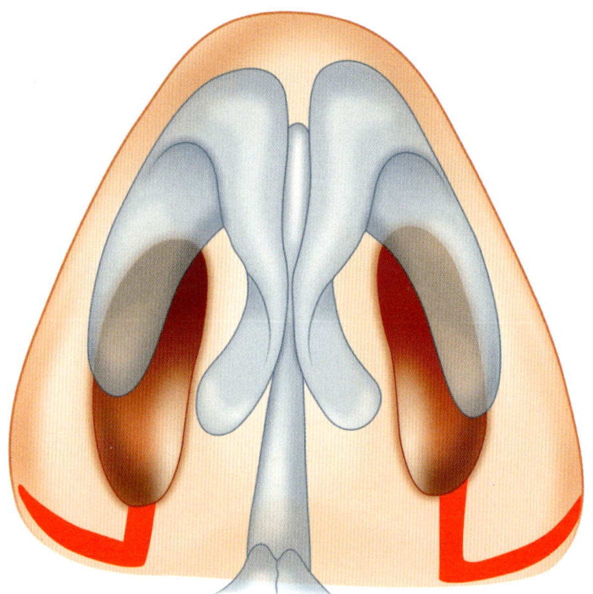

Fig. 16: Excision pattern for alar flare reduction

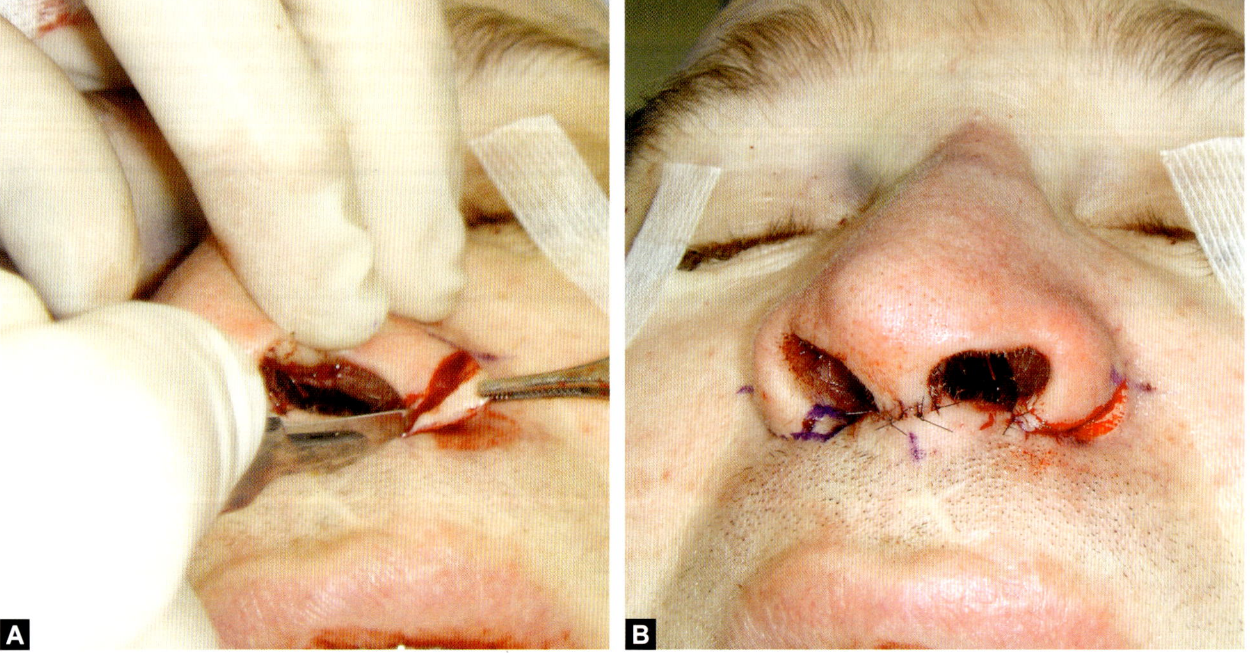

Figs 17A and B: (A) For alar flare reduction a wedge of tissue is resected from the alar base. (B) The wedge resection is continuous with the alar base incision at the nasal sill

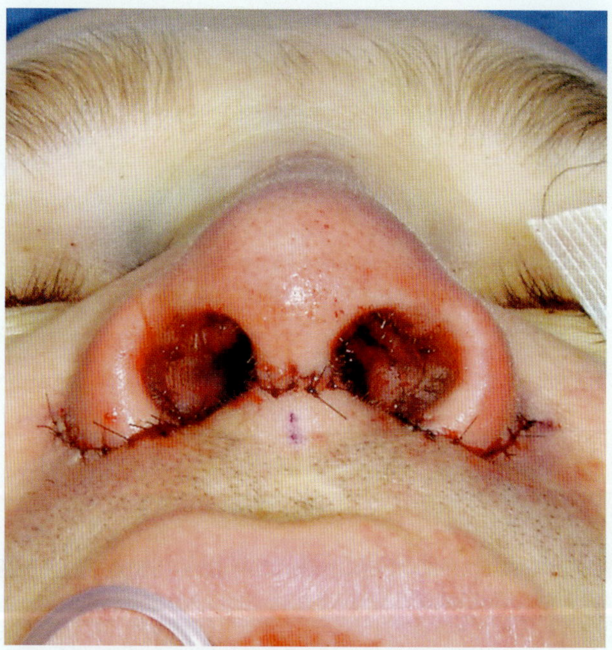

Fig. 18: Completion of alar base and alar flare reduction on both sides of nose

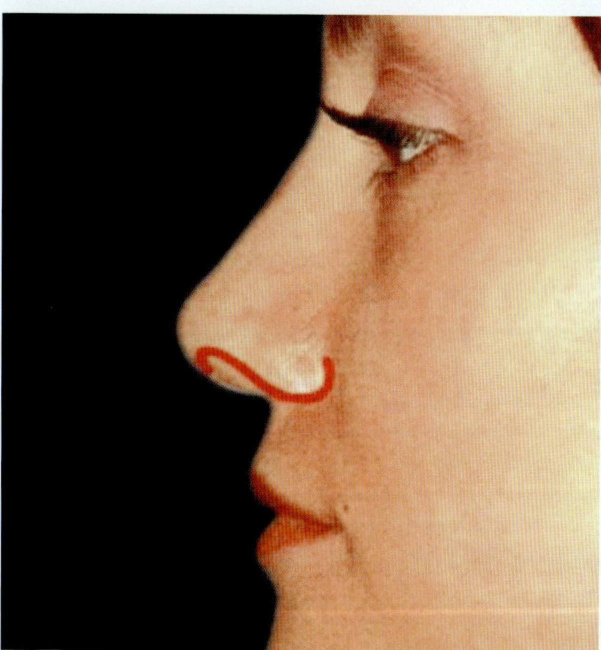

Fig. 19: The ideal visual boarder of the ala is a gentle curve

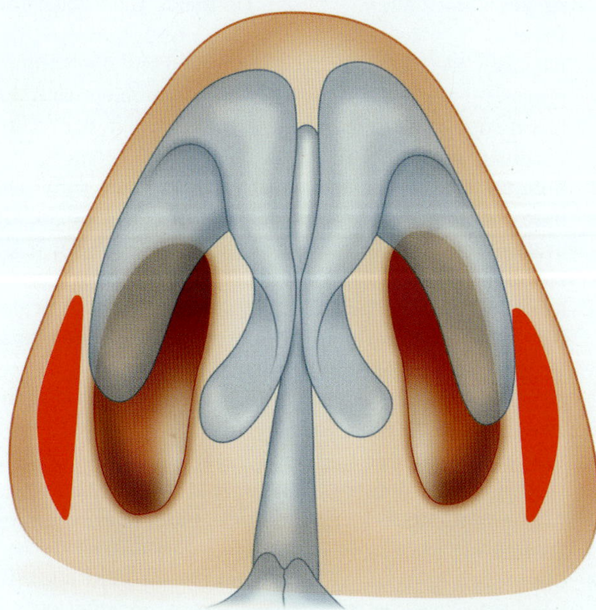

Fig. 20: Excision pattern for alar hooding. Elliptical excisions closed along the natural alar border

Alar Hooding Reduction

This resection is planned using a direct lateral view. The visual border of the ideal alar curve is marked (Fig. 19). An ellipse is drawn on the inner portion of the ala matching the outer visual border. This incision should curve gently to avoid distortion of the nasal ala (Fig. 20).

The wedge of tissue is excised from the inner ala and the wound closed with a running 6-0 nylon suture. The suture line often falls within the visual border of the ala. However, it also occurs in a natural plane, and because of this we have not found healing along this line to be a problem. Sutures are removed on postoperative day 4.

COMPLICATIONS

Scars following the use of these techniques heal exceptionally well. While the possibility of each incision should be discussed with patients preoperatively, reassurance can be given that the scars typically heal well and will result in a more balanced overall rhinoplasty result. Other studies also support low complication rates and good scar outcomes.[14] For alar base excisions requiring an advancement flap, note that excisions carried out too far laterally along the natural curve of the ala may result in an unnatural curve, a notch, or unnatural insertion of the alar base. It is vitally important not to disrupt the natural curve of the alar base.

There is a risk of over correction when resecting the alar base. It is important to recognize that small excisions can make a significant difference, and one should always excise less when there is doubt. Placing a trial stitch allows the surgeon to make decisions regarding further resection (which should only be a millimeter at a time). You can always cut a board sorter, but you cannot cut it longer.

SPECIAL INSTRUMENTS USED FOR THE SURGERY

A rhinoplasty tray containing fine toothed forceps and Castroviejo calipers should be available. We also use a No. 11 blade knife , a fine marking pen, and 6-0 Nylon suture.

A MENTION OF OTHER TREATMENT OPTIONS AVAILABLE FOR THE SAME CONDITION

Excessive alar hooding is a relatively rare problem, and there are multiple ways to correct this deformity surgically. Some authors prefer to keep the elliptical excision inside the nose, bringing the caudal alar border more cephalad. Others have advocated conservative resection of the caudal border of the lateral crus without mucosa, elevating the caudal alar border.[10,15-17] We prefer to use a direct external excision of the caudal border of the ala along the ideal visual border. This approach has been described in cleft nasal surgery. It benefits the surgeon by allowing accurate determination of the visual border and to set it as determined.[18-20] We have found that these scars, even if they are larger, heal just as well as the columellar and alar base incisions and restore and ideal visual border in the ala.

The alar soft-tissue excision techniques presented in this chapter are based on three principles. First, excision of the vestibular sill and rim reduces the outer alar perimeter and narrows the nostril diameter. By angling the excisions in the sill, the surgeon can manipulate the columellar-alar distance and the nostril diameter independently, or use a combination of both. Second, a wedge resection along the rounded caudal margin of the alar lobule decreases the amount of alar flare. Third, in the lateral view there is a natural curve and position of the ala. It should not hang excessively and obscure the view of the columella. Understanding these principles will allow the rhinoplasty surgeon to manipulate these variables and achieve superior esthetic success.

REFERENCES

1. Adamson PA, Oakley S, Tropper GJ, et al. Analysis of alar base narrowing. Am J Cosmetic Surg. 1990;7(4): 239-43.
2. Farkas LG, Hreczko TA, Deutsch CK. Objective assessment of standard nostril types -a morphometric study. Ann Plast Surg. 1983;11(5): 381-98.
3. McKinney PW, Mossie RD, Bailey MH. Calibrated alar base excision: a 20-year experience. Aesthetic Plast Surg. 1988;12(2): 71-5.
4. Gilbert SE. Alar reductions in rhinoplasty. Arch Otolaryngol head Neck Surg. 1996;122(7): 781-4.
5. Becker DG, Weinberger MS, Greene BA, Tardy ME Jr. Clinical study of alar anatomy and surgery of the alar base. Arch Otolaryngol Head Neck Surg. 1997;123(8): 789-95.
6. Guyuron B, Behmand RA. Alar Base abnormalities: classification and correction. Clin Plast surg. 1996;23(2): 263-70.
7. Adamson PA. Alar base reduction. Arch Facial Plast Surg. 2005;7(2):98.
8. Porter JP. The average African American male face: an anthropometric analysis. Arch Facial Plast Surg. 2004:6(2): 78-81.
9. Sheen JH. Alar Resection and Grafting: Dallas Rhinoplasty. 2nd ed. St Louis, MO: Quality Medical Publishing; 2007:553.
10. Gunter JP, Rohrich RJ, Friedman RM. Classification and correction of alar-coumellar discrepancies in rhinoplasty. Plast Reconstr Surg. 1996; 97(3): 643-8
11. Hafner HM, Rocken M, Breuninger H. Epinepherine-supplimented local anesthetics for ear and nose surgery: clinical use without complications in more than 10,000 surgical procedures. J Dtsch Dermatol Ges. 2005;3(3): 195-9.
12. Bafaqeeh SA, Al-Qattan MM. Simultaneous open rhinoplasty and alar base excision: is there a problem with the blood supply of the nasal tip and columellar skin? Plast Reconstr Surg. 2000;105(1): 344-7.
13. Rohrich RJ. Simultaneous open rhinoplasty and alar base excision: is there a problem with the blood supply of the nasal tip and columellar skin? Plast Reconstr Surg. 2000;105(1): 348-9.
14. Kridel RWH, Castellano RD. A simplified approach to alar base reduction: a review of 124 patients over 20 years. Arch Facial Plast Surg. 2005;7(2): 81-93.
15. McKinney PW, Stainecker ML. The hanging ala. Plast reconstr Surg. 1984; 73(3): 247-430.
16. Brown JB, McDowell F. Plastic surgery of the Nose. 2nd ed. Springfield, IL: Charles C Thomas; 1951: 118-9, 134-5.
17. Guyuron B. Alar rim deformities. Plast Reconstr Surg. 2001;107(3): 856-63.
18. Ellenbogen R, Blome DW. Alar rim raising. Plast Reconstr Surg. 1992; 90(1): 28-37.
19. Millard DR Jr. alar margin sculpturing. Plast Reconstr surg. 1967; 40(4): 337-42.
20. Dibbell DG. Cleft lip nasal reconstruction: correcting the classic unilateral defect. Plast reconstr Surg. 1982;69(2): 264-71.

CHAPTER

106 Esthetic Rhinoplasty—Ailed and Ailing Noses

BP Belaldavar

INTRODUCTION

We, the human beings, are in pursuit of beauty from the ancient days of ignorance and illiteracy to the present days of evolved intellectual multimedia. It is true with perceptive of both the subjective and the treating surgeon. The shape and functions of the nose have been dictated with very complex and organized supportive architectural and associated supportive factors. To achieve expected goal these are to be respected and if violated in treatment with overjealous unrealistic expectations, leads to jeopardy and imperfections[1]. Thus patient evaluation and selection for esthetic rhinoplasty goes beyond assessment of anatomical indications. One of the accepted principles of surgeries is greater reliance on established rhinoplasty principles of repair and long term healing concepts.[5]

The human nose is subject to wide array of deformities, abnormalities and anatomical variations. Deformities like congenital, traumatic, postinfections or growth. Abnor malities which cause pathological anatomical change frequently implies functional disturbance. Anatomical variations many of which to a certain extent dependent on race, gender or age and have therefore to be considered within the normal range.[1,3,5,6]

The behavior and outcome of the esthetic results of the nose definitely skeptical and does depend on status and the condition of the nose when the cosmetic or the functional surgery is contemplated. In fact both the end results are complementary to each other. Therefore it is ethical and also sensible in terms of surgical concepts to evaluate clinically and, if needed, with relevant investigations to assess and to know the status and condition of nose in relations to whether is it ailed or ailing nose. The esthetic surgery should be under taken only after proper diagnosis of the ailment, its assessment and appropriate treatment.[2,9]

All the constituents forming the nose, like the skin and its components, fibromuscular envelope bony skeleton and the lining of inside of nasal cavities behave differently to the surgical assault depending on the type and chronicity of ailment[2,3,5,6,9,10,14,17,18] they are being suffered or had suffered. And also nature of outcome of the results depends on the intensity, frequency and duration of the ailment.

Therefore, it is essential to discuss and elaborate different types of ailments and how to account them in relation to philosophy of treating such noses esthetically.

AILED ASSOCIATED NOSES

Ailed noses are the one that have already suffered or had been abused in one or other form and now there is no prevailing active pathology or disease. So for all practical purposes the architectural structures and the covering envelope of the nose are settled well for the surgical exploration and correction. All possible etiological factors can cause the deformities and contribute for the ailed noses (Figs 1 to 28). And this in turn adds up to eccenterated situation in corrective rhinoplasty.[2,3,5,6,9,10,14,17,18]

Congenital Deformities (Figs 1 to 7)

Major congential deformities are often associated with other subtle deformities which need to be identified.

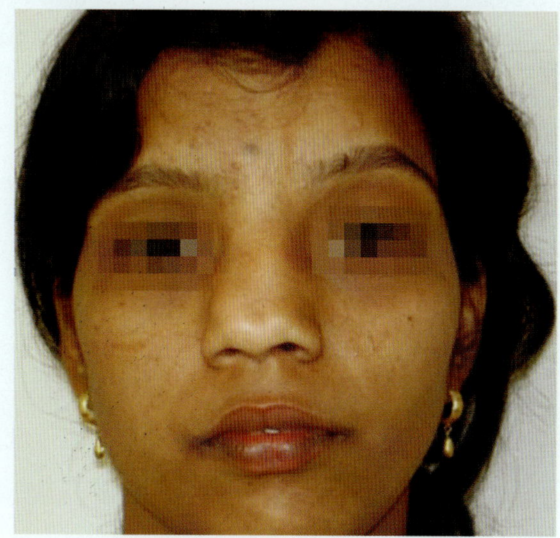

Fig. 1: Poly deformity

Congenital Deformities (Figs 1 to 7)

These are compound poly deformities and such noses are to be evaluated in detail by inspection and palpation so as to identify all deformities for correction.

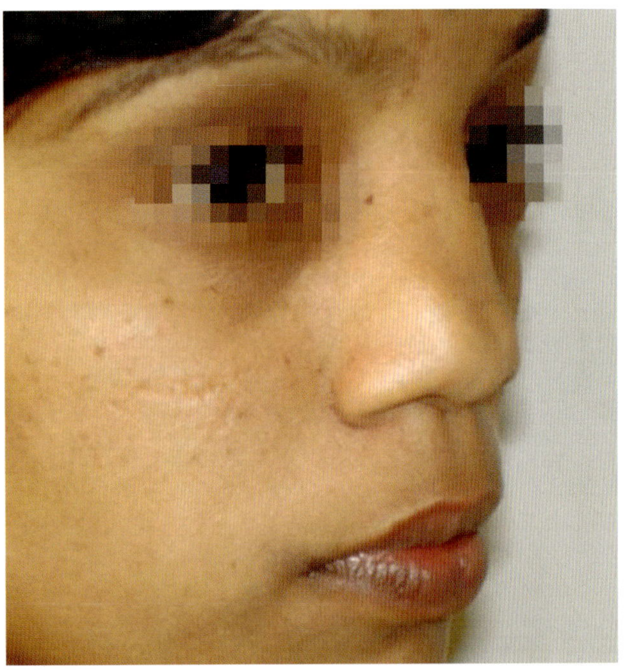

Fig. 2: Congenital Poly deformity

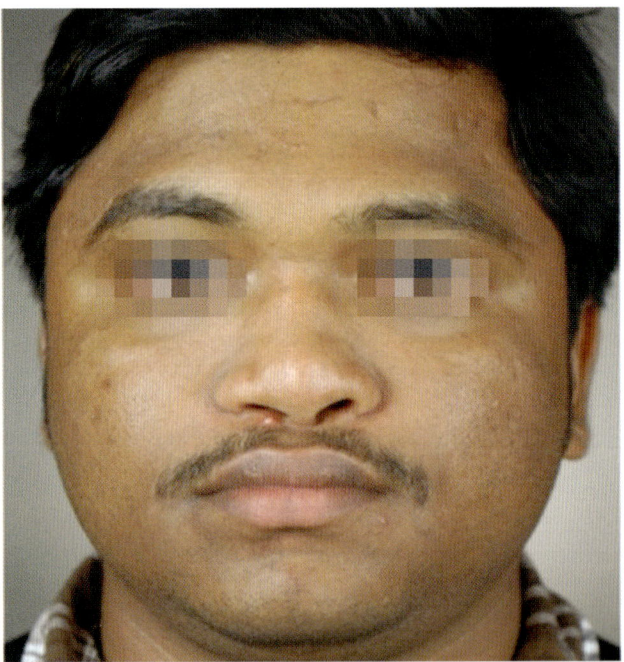

Fig. 3: Small tension nose

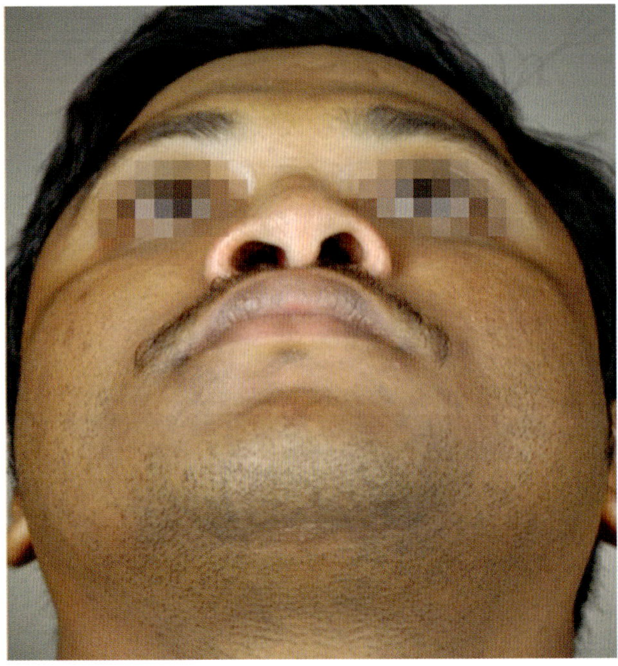

Fig. 4: Short columellar deformity

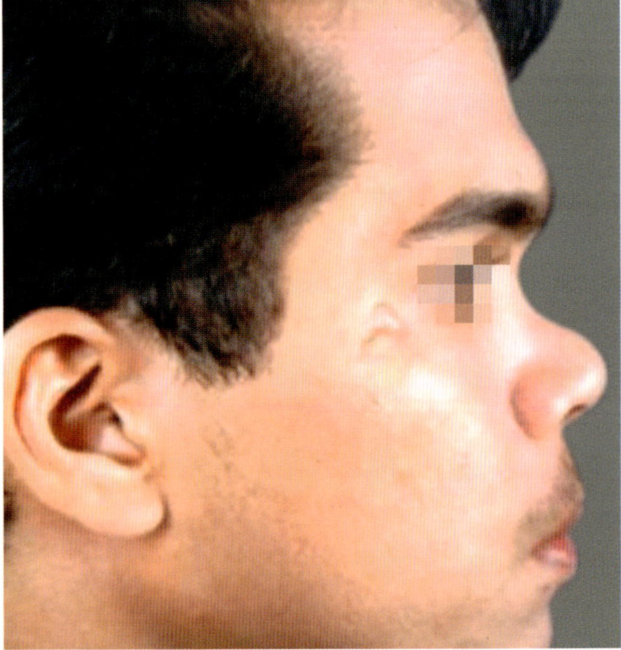

Fig. 5: Small nose with deep NF angle

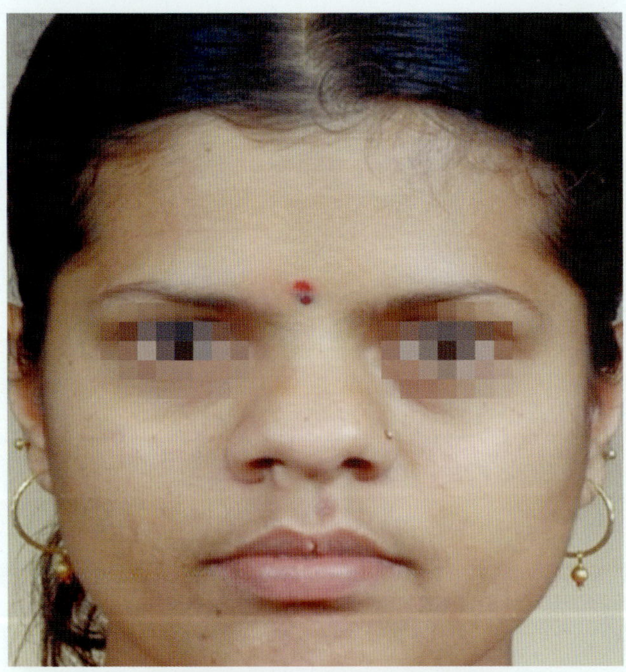

Fig. 6: Big deformed nose with excessive lax and thick skin

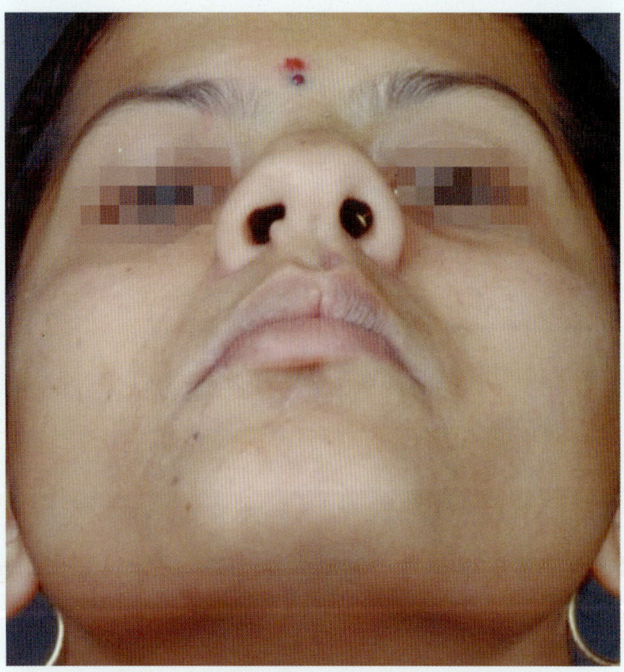

Fig. 7: Thick, short and broad columella

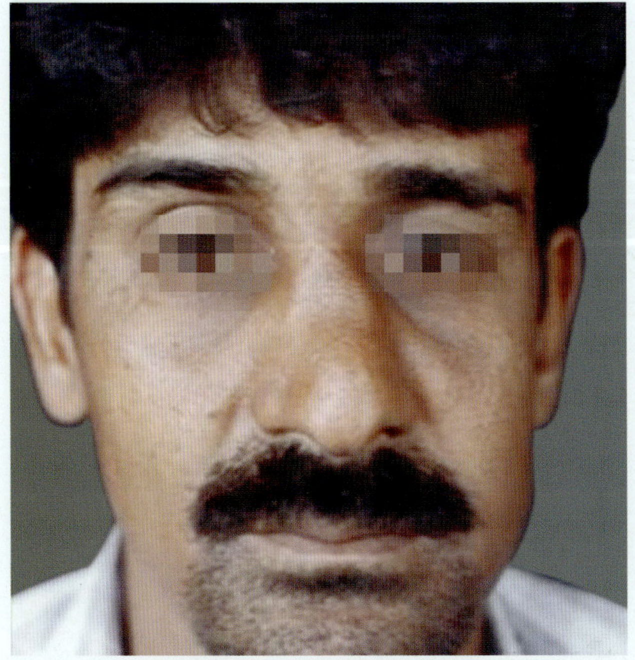

Fig. 8: Large crooked nose

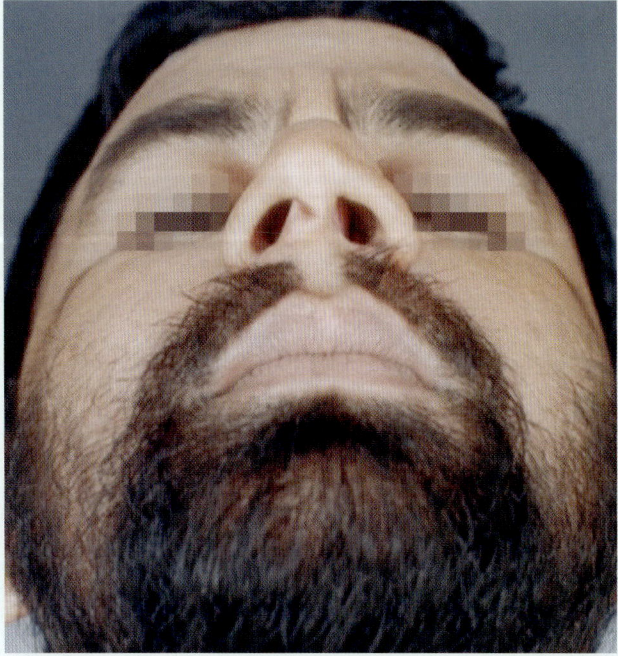

Fig. 9: Skewed nose

Developmental Deformities (Figs 8 to 12)

These types of noses are associated with variant interrelated abnormalities which are due to the continuous influence of some of the factors through the development of the nose. It is ideal to contemplate the surgery after age of of 18 years in males.

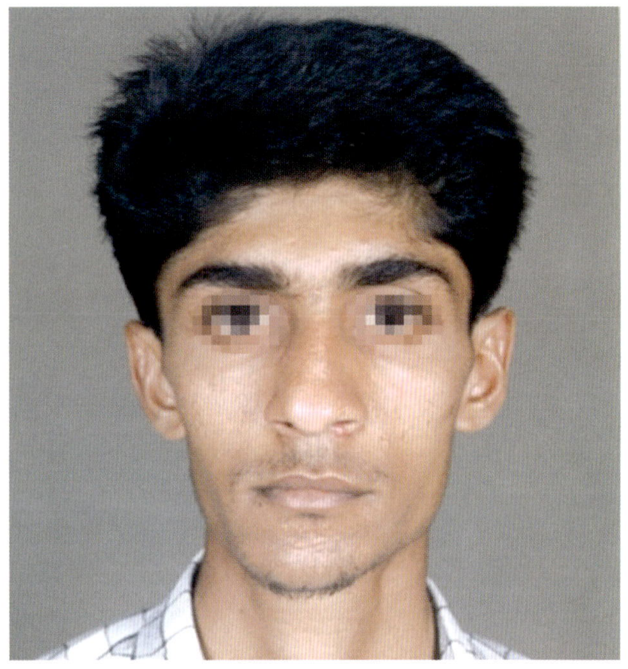

Fig. 10: Long deformed nose

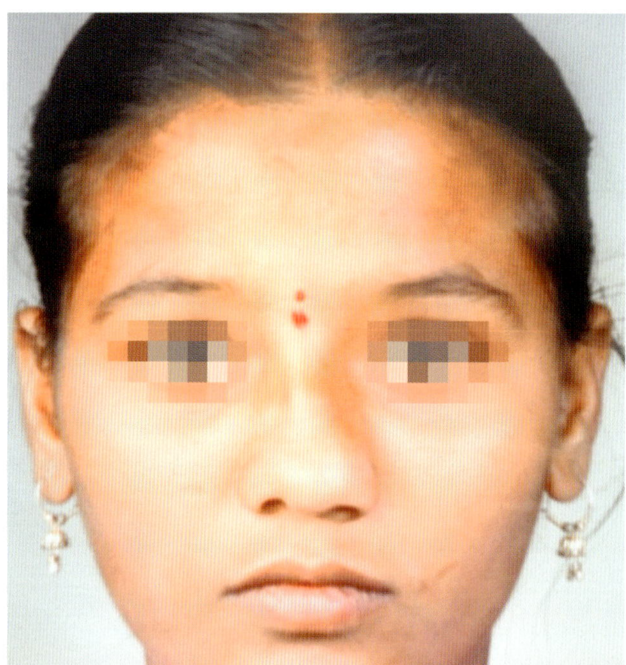

Fig. 11: Broad nose

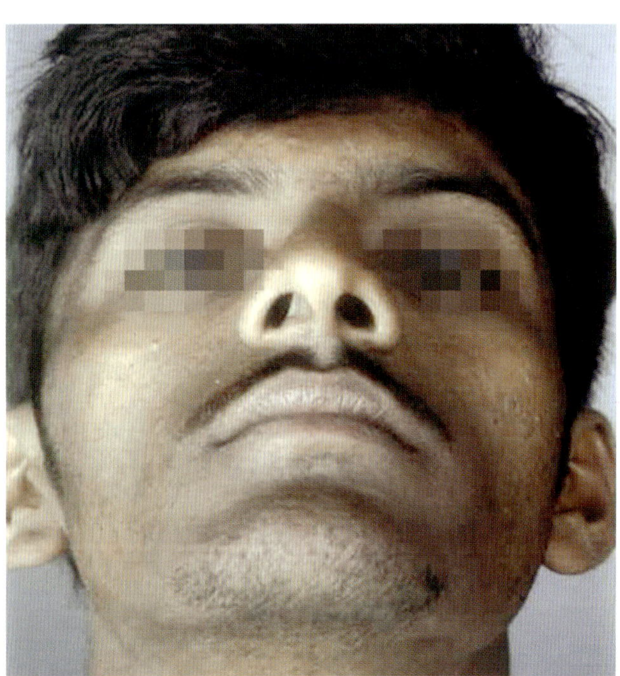

Fig. 12: Septal caudal dislocated nose

Traumatic Deformities (Figs 13 to 17)

It is suggested that the acute traumatic deformities are corrected within 2-3 weeks, if not the correction is done after the optimum period of 6 months.These deformities are difficulty to address

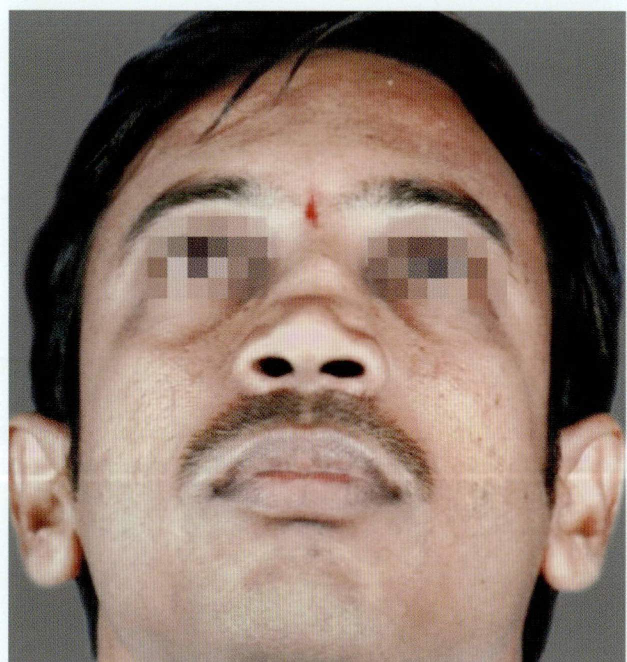

Fig. 13: Saddle nose

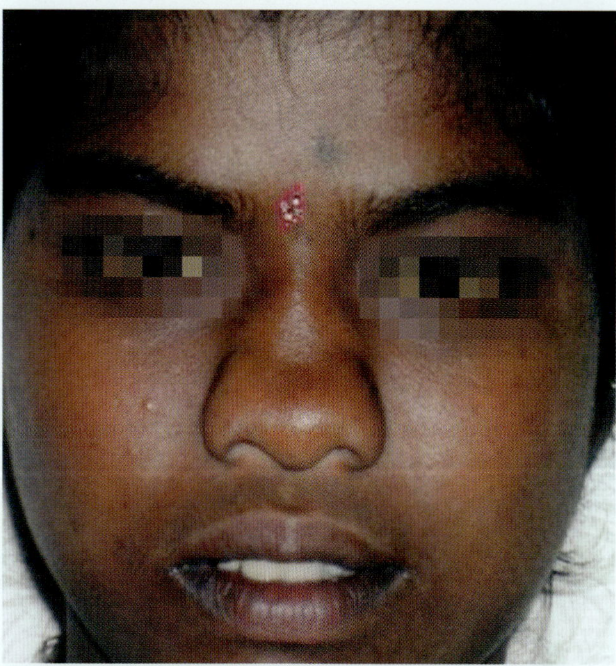

Fig. 14: Broad nose with saddle

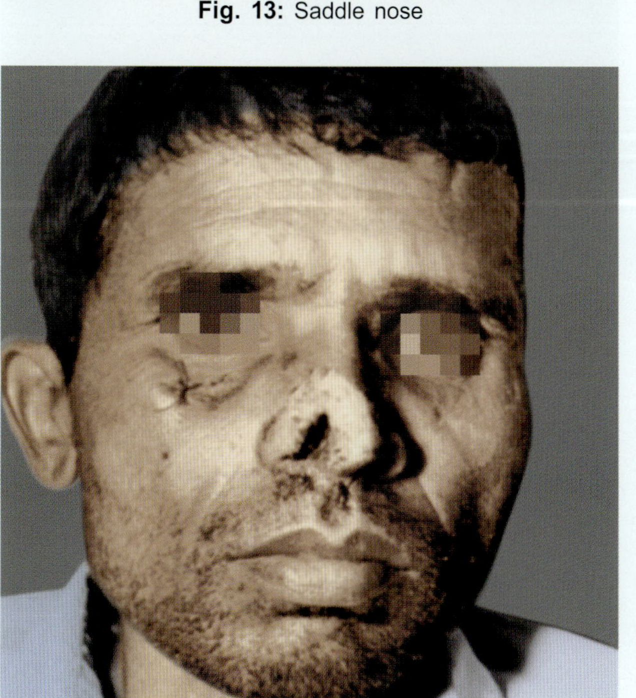

Fig. 15: Chop injury of ala nose

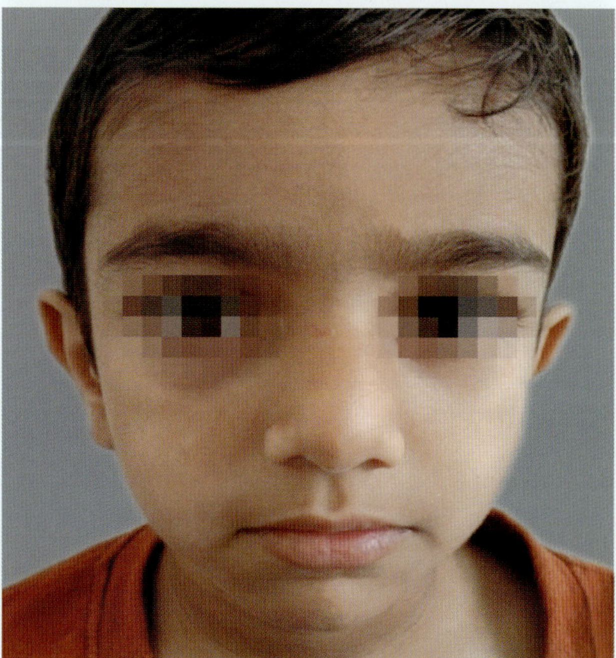

Fig. 16: Big amorphous nose

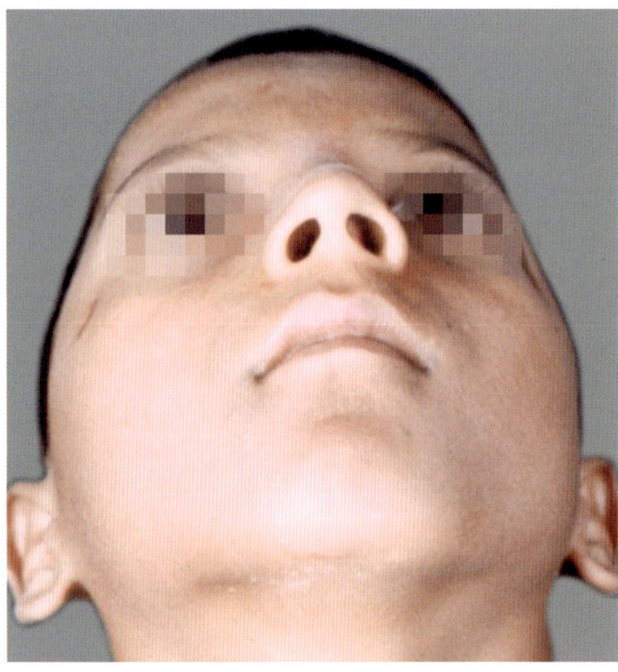

Fig. 17: Caudal dislocated septum in a child

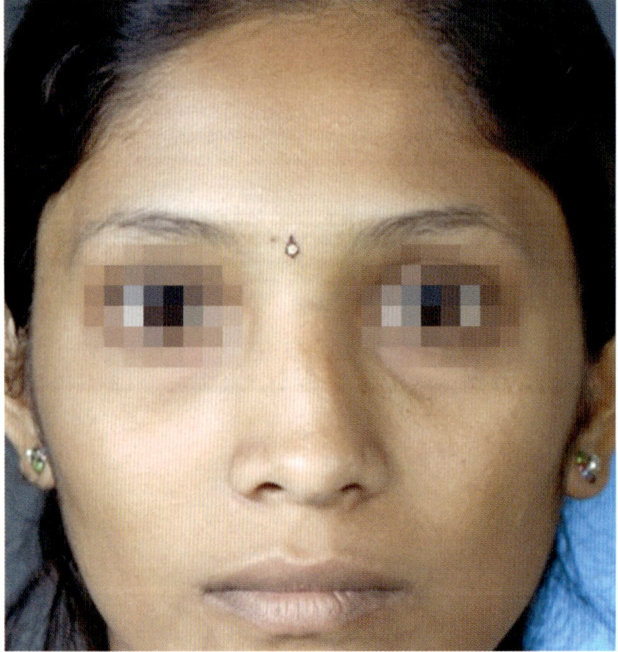

Fig. 18: Post septoplasty

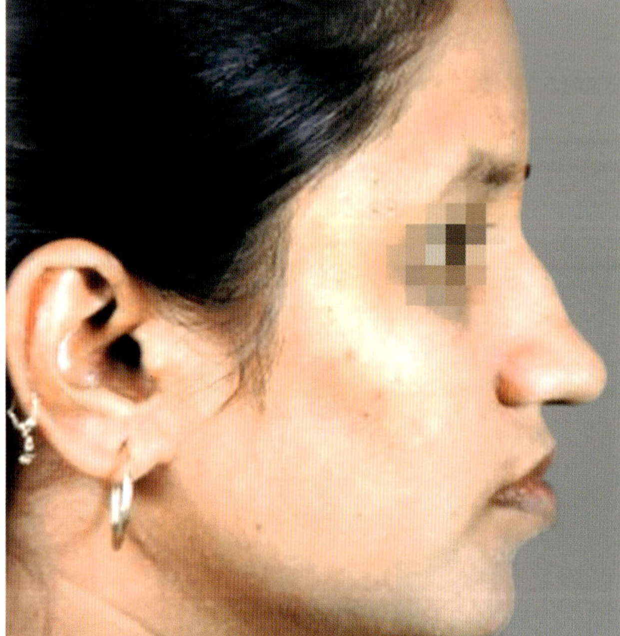

Fig. 19: Post submucosal resection of septum

Iatrogenic Deformities (Figs 18 to 22)

Sometimes nasal deformities do occur because of surgical interventions to correct the nasal disease or the deformities. These could be intentional or non-intentional. Invariably these are unavoidable because of disease process. But, with due care during surgical correction of primary problems the deformities can be reduced to some extent. The revision surgery is done after 6 months to correct the deformities.

Fig. 20: Post septal abscess

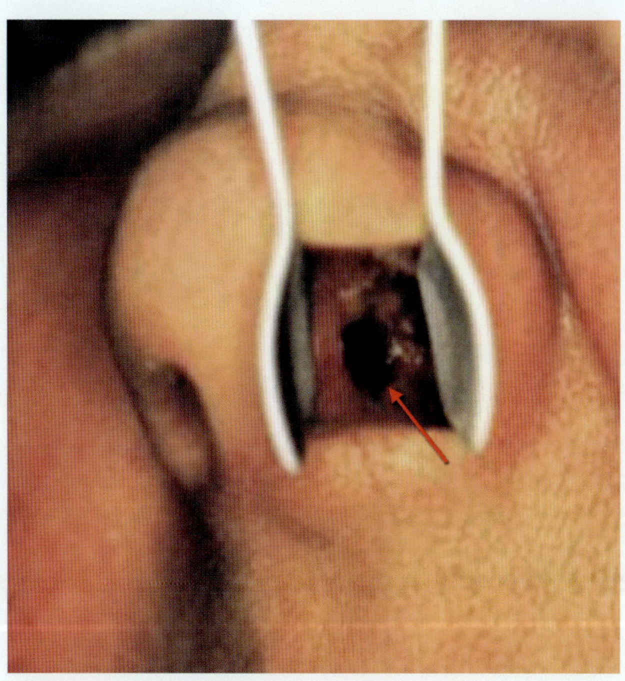

Fig. 21: Post submucosal resection septal perforation

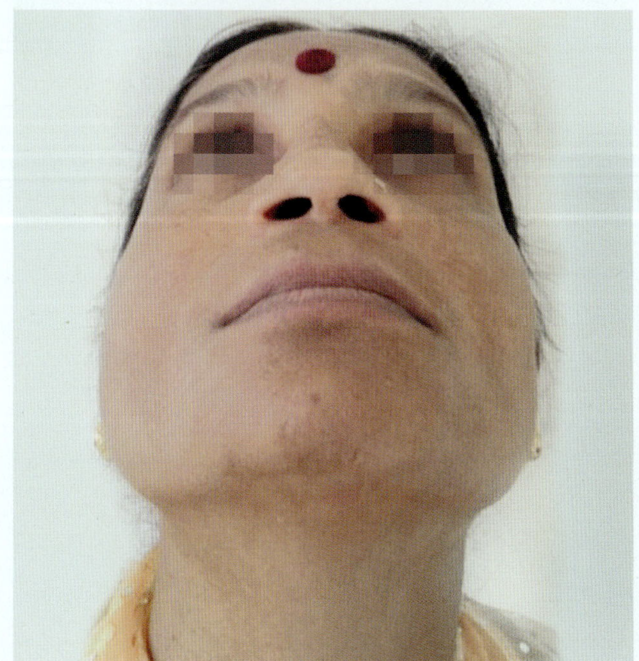

Fig. 22: Post submucosal resection columellar retraction

Skin Conditions (Figs 23 to 25)

Before undertaking corrective surgery of nose it is always wise to diagnose and treat the primary skin diseases especially of the face. It is all the more important in open Rhinoplasty to avoid flaring of the disease and also to prevent the wound infection which may lead to unsightly scars

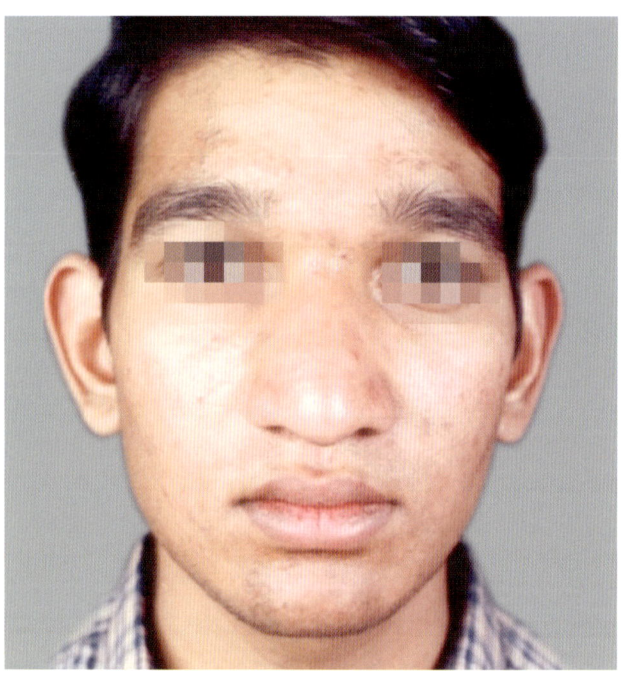

Fig. 23: Acne rosacea

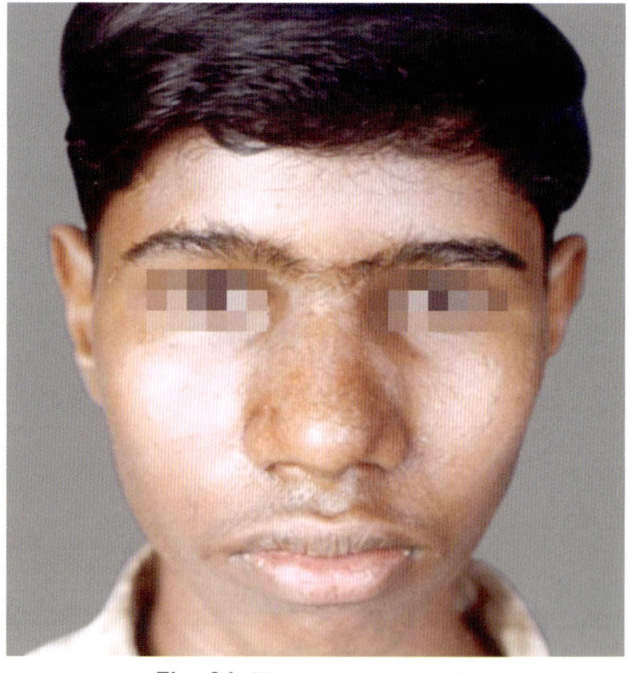

Fig. 24: Thick sebaceous skin

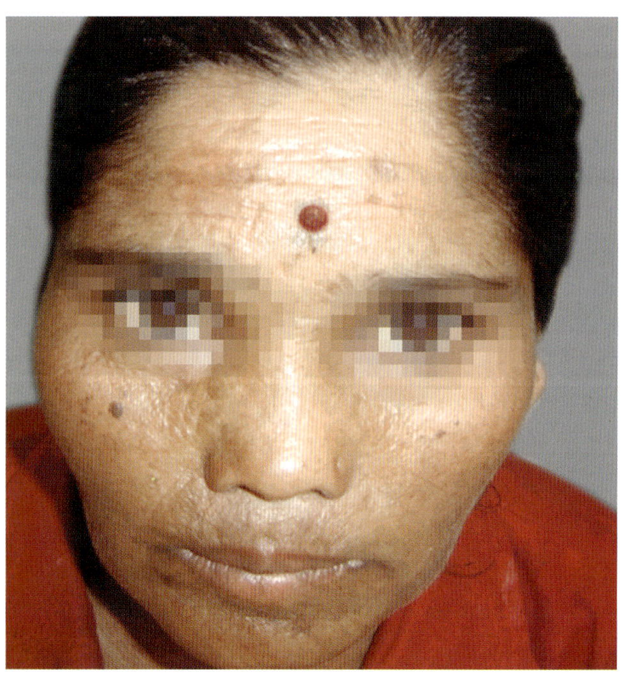

Fig. 25: Lipoid proteinosis—Fine shining yellowish nodules

Chronic Diseases (Figs 26 and 27)

Because of long lasting disease process it takes quite a long time to make the chronic disease to heal and it is worth to cure the chronic disease before undertaking the corrective surgery of nose to achieve acceptable, reliable and sustainable results.

Fig. 26: Atrophic rhinitis – causing Saddle and Broad nose

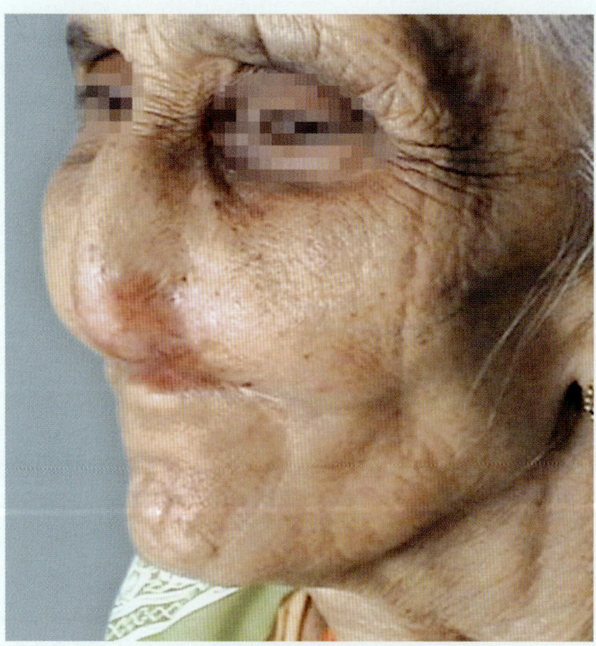

Fig. 27: Burnt out rhinoscleroma – Conjoint l lip Columella and nasal lobule

Associated Deformities

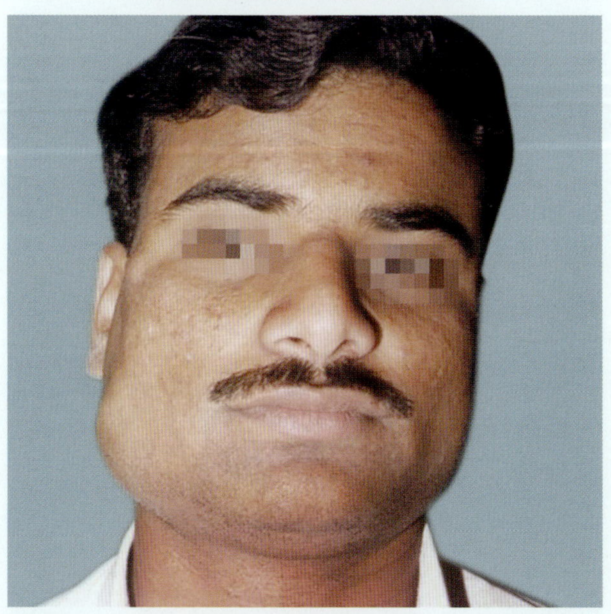

Fig. 28: Hypertrophied masseter muscle – Dysharmonic esthetic face

So the satisfactory outcome of surgical results is possible only after thorough evaluation and understanding of the exact nature of the tissue healing and associated problems and addressing the same with extra care during corrective surgery of the nose.

Rhinoplasty in the aging nose is distinctly different entity, whose unique characterization must be appreciated by the rhinoplasty surgeon to optimize the functional and esthetic results.[11]

Early surgeries before patients have reached puberty when properly performed will not alter nasal development and normal nasal growth, even after medial and lateral osteotomies, cartilage repositioning and conservative septoplasty.[14]

Fractures of the nasal complex are the most common facial fractures. This is because it is most prominent, made up of composite structures and less force is required. It is always a rule and mandatory to allow minimum of 6 months time before the definitive corrective surgery on such noses to allow all the tissues to settle and edema to subside completely.[3,4,12,14]

AILING ASSOCIATED NOSES

Many of the time noses get affected by active disease or diseases (ailing nose) (Figs 28 to 41). In such noses, the tissues forming the nose are edematous, fragile and render the nose more ugly looking. Therefore the esthetic surgeries on such noses are definitely not undertaken for the obvious known reasons. By operating on such actively ailing noses one will end up with most disastroussituation, as the tissue healing process will be bizarre and unpredictable. Infact, operating on such noses is unphilosophical, unethical and unwarranted[3,4,6,8,15,20]

Infections (Figs 29 to 36)

Acute infections whether mild or fulminant are to be treated energetically then only patient is operated for esthetic correction of nose.

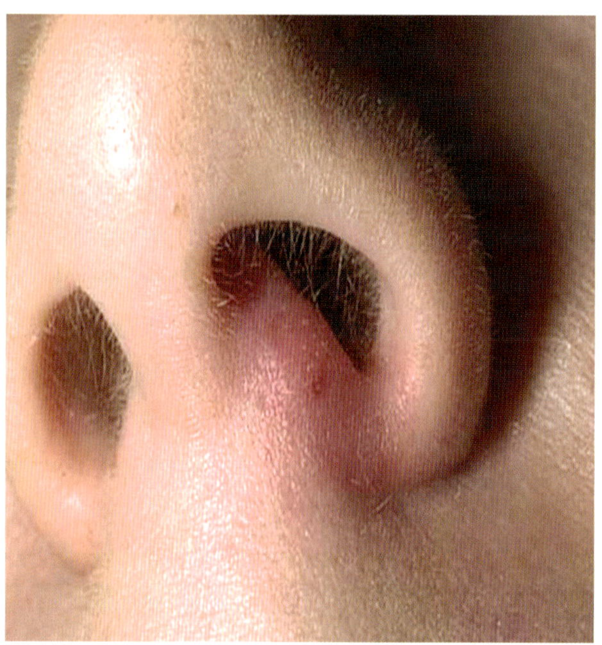

Fig. 29: Nasal vestibulitis—Farunculosis

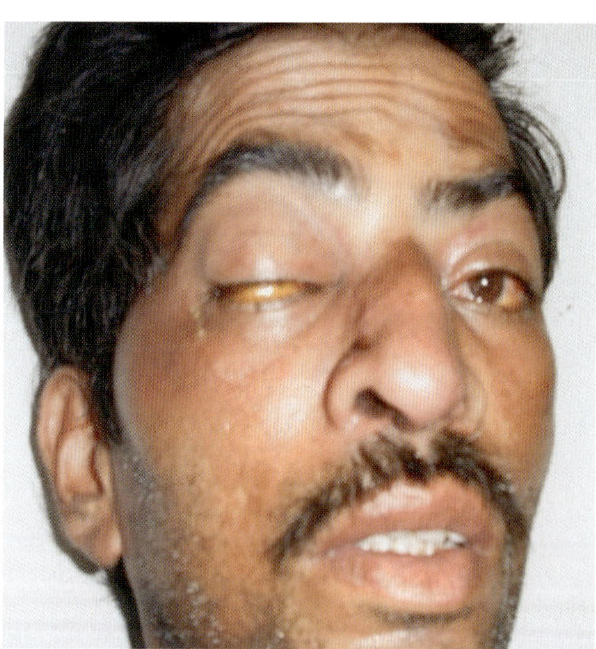

Fig. 30: Cavernous sinus thrombophlebitis

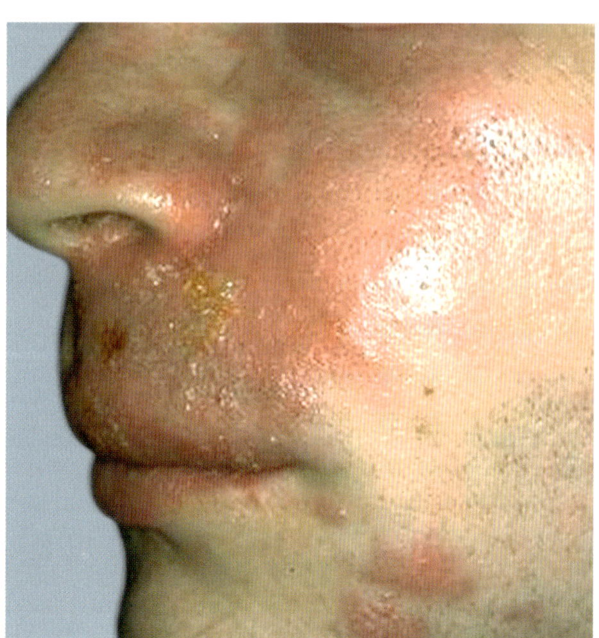

Fig. 31: Erysipelas

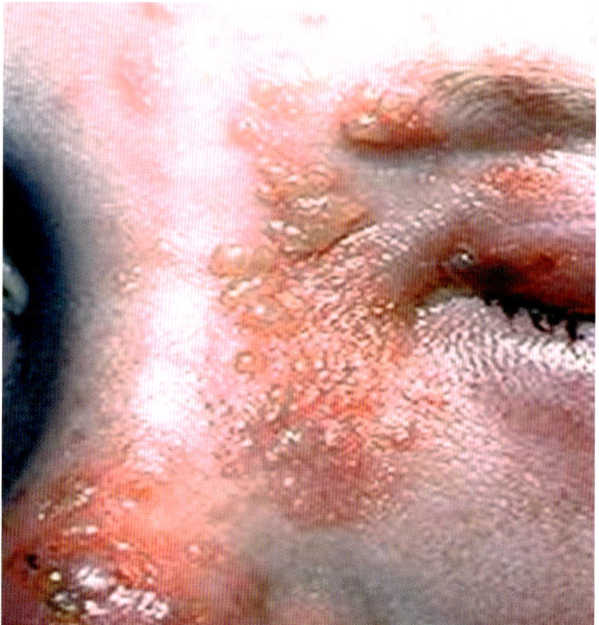

Fig. 32: Herpes zoster—vesicles

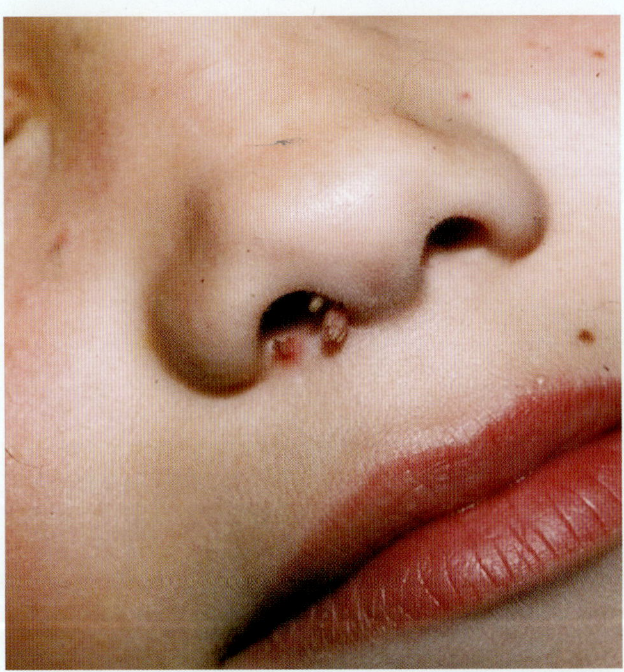

Fig. 33: The wart—lesions

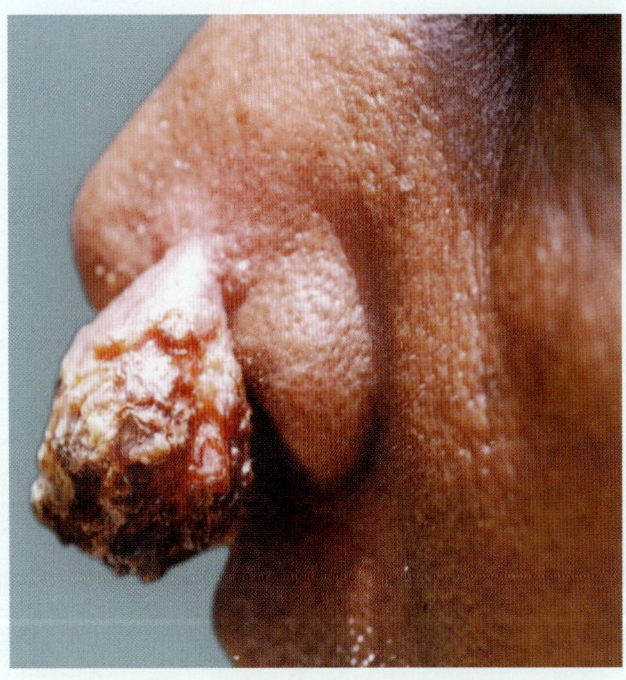

Fig. 34: Rhinosporidiosis—mass

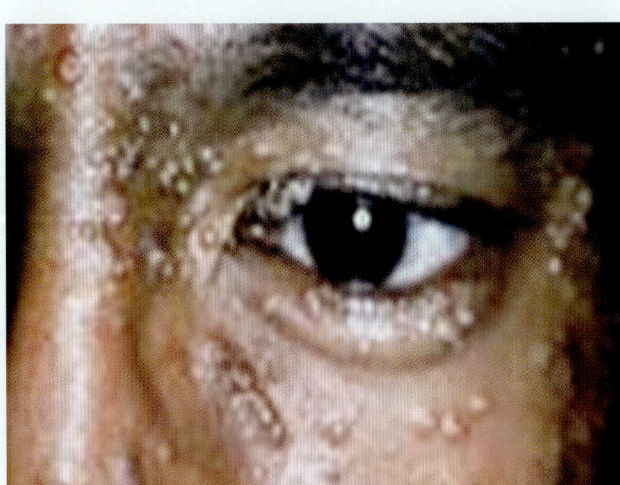

Fig. 35: Molluscum contagiosum lesions

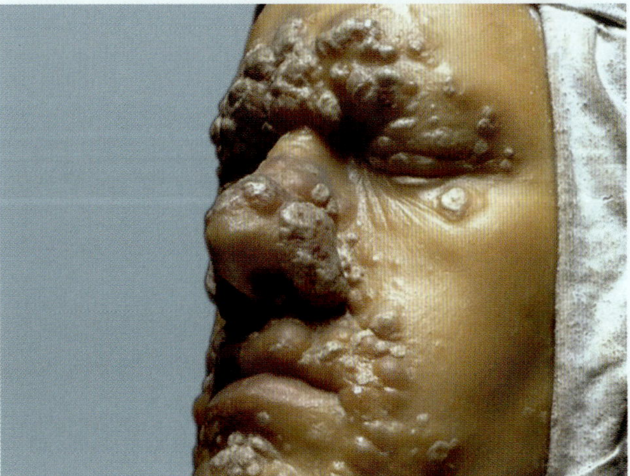

Fig. 36: Syphilis lesions

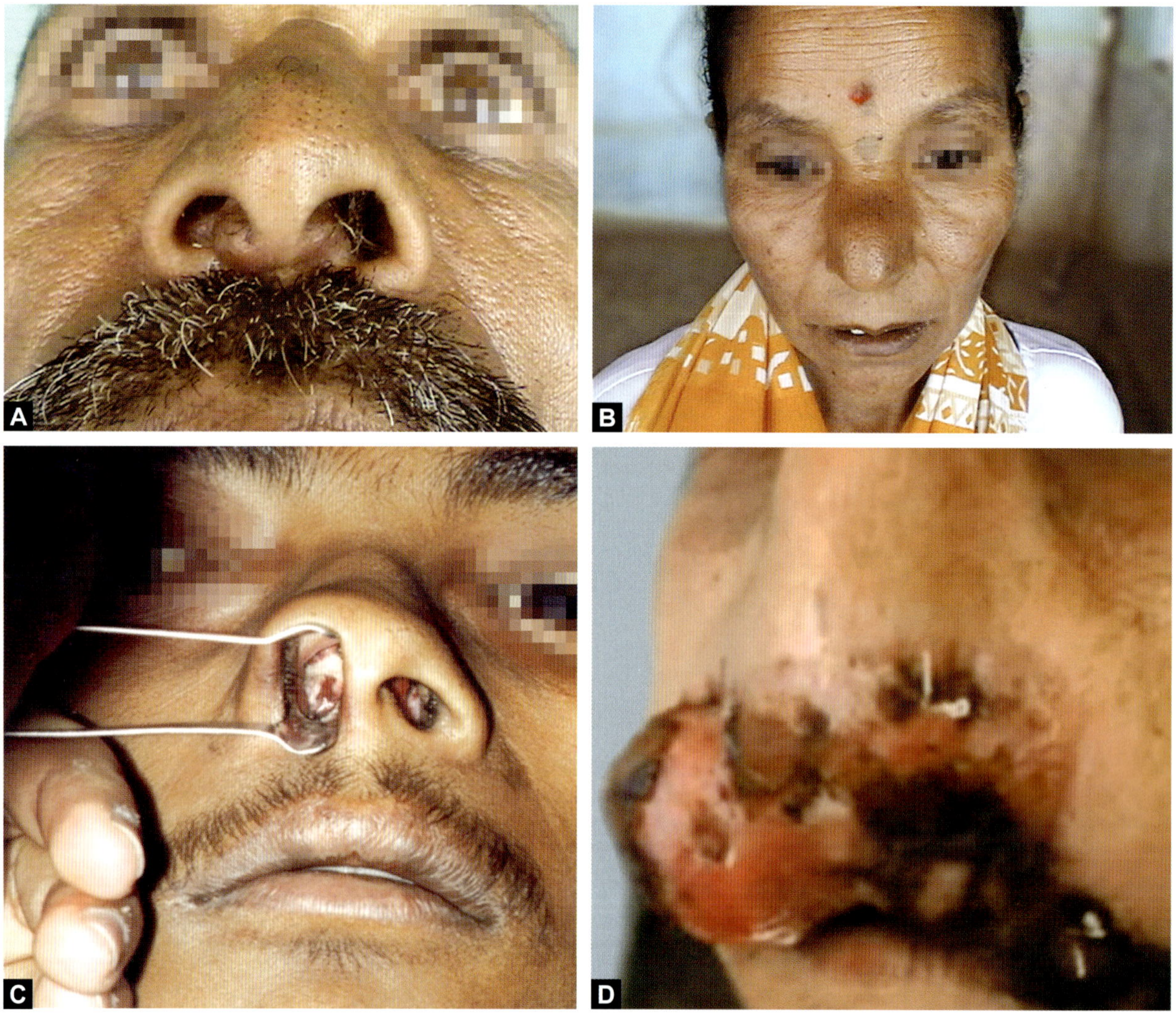

Figs 37A to D: Rhinoscleroma noses—mild to florid lesions

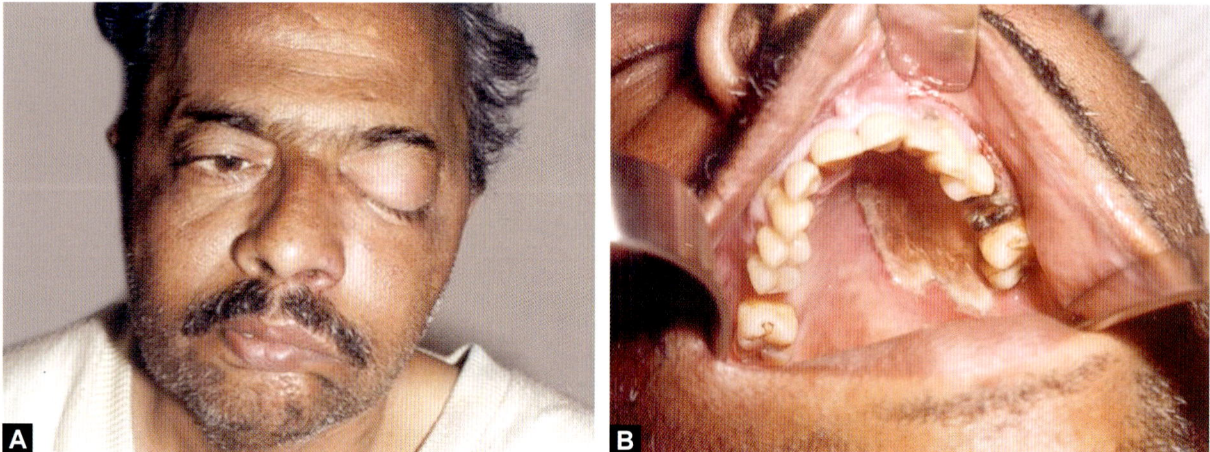

Figs 38A and B: Fungal diseases—involving the sinus and adjacent structures

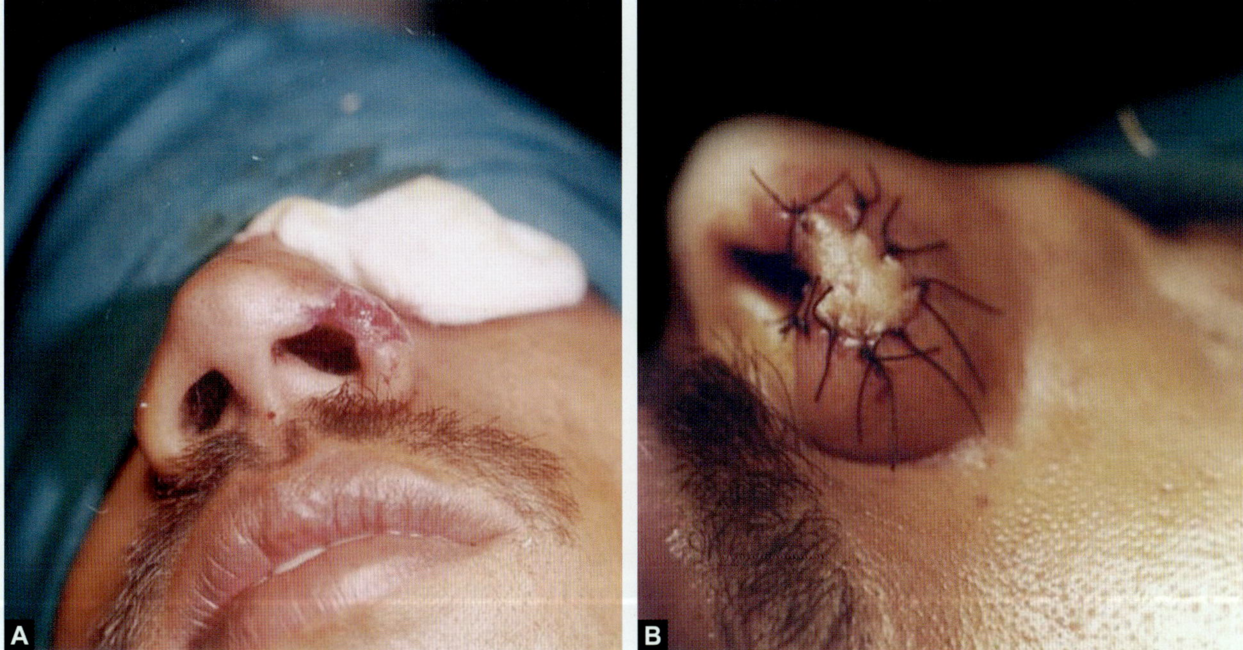

Figs 39A and B: Human bite and its correction with auricular graft

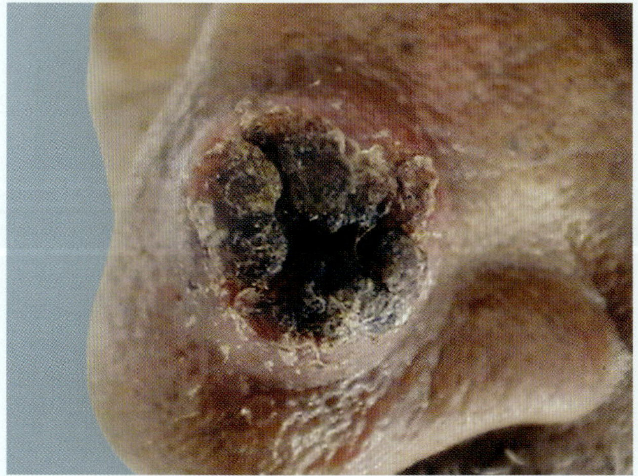

Fig. 40: Acanthoma

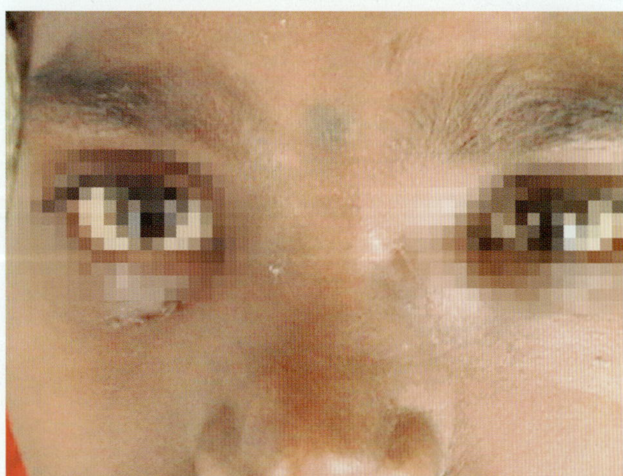

Fig. 41: Dacryocystitis

The primary modality of managing such ailing noses is proper accurate diagnosis of the disease, investigating the same and treating it appropriately. The esthetic surgery is contemplated only after the primary disease is completely cured and sufficient time is allowed for complete healing of the tissues. Otherwise it leads to inefficient local anesthesia, excessive oozing peroperatively and loss of tissue planes. And postoperatively exaggerated tissue edema, delayed healing, more pain and sometimes may get infected and leading to unexpected results of the surgery and permanent morbidity.

ASSOCIATION-EVALUATION (FIGS 42 TO 47)[3,6,8,13,16]

Whether the nose is ailed or ailing the proper evalua tion is done with paramount care and precision, in relation to nasal skeleton and its envelope. The sensitivity of the skin is examined for the easy bruising and ecchymosis. The condition of the nasal mucosa and skin along with the status of the septal cartilage is noted. The degree of deformity and the site of correction or rectification are also appreciated. The optimum timing for surgery is 6 months to 1 year in chronic and traumatic noses.

Special conditions, like atrophic rhinitis, rhinoscle roma, fungal diseases and skin conditions, are to be taken care of and are to be addressed. Diagnostic, and if needed functional endoscopy is done either concurrently or at different interval depending on the need of the same.

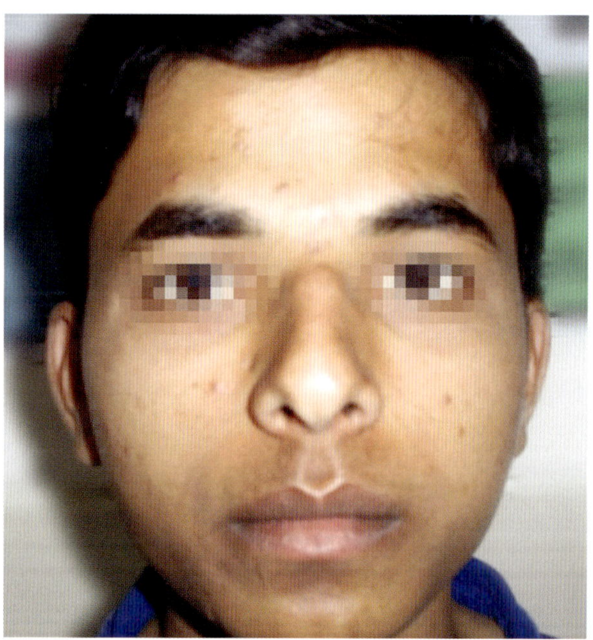

Fig. 42: Acnetic skin and sensitive skin

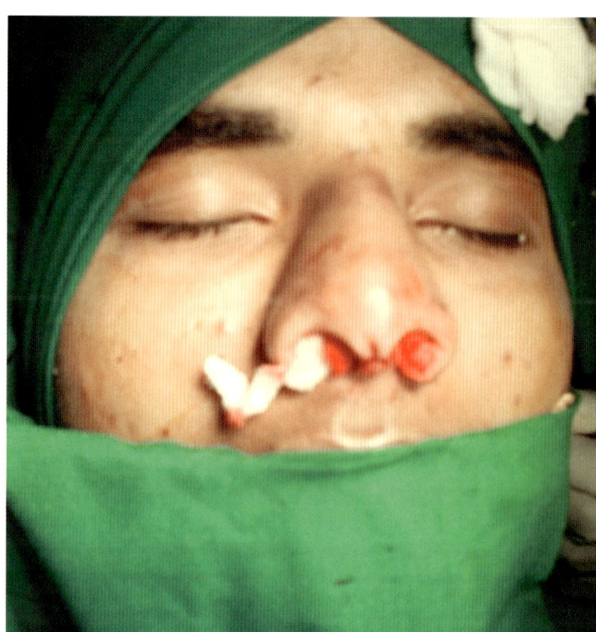

Fig. 43: Peroperative ecchymosis of skin

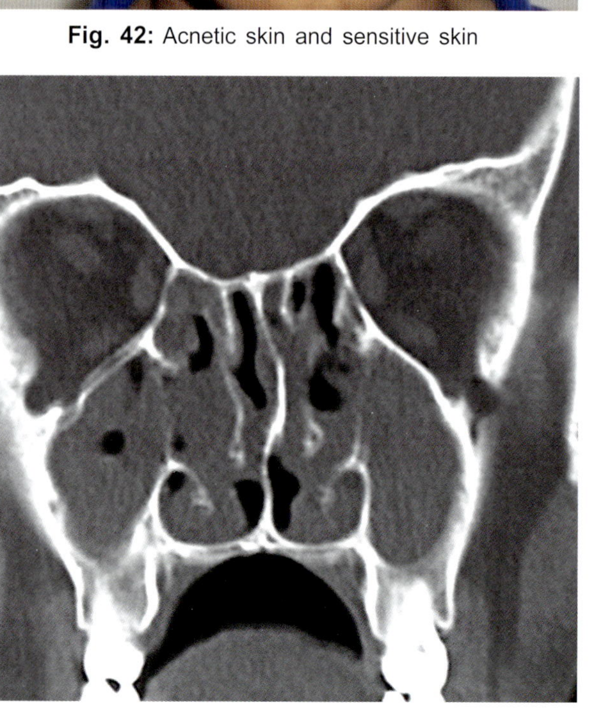

Fig. 44: CT scan evaluation—Chronic sinus disease

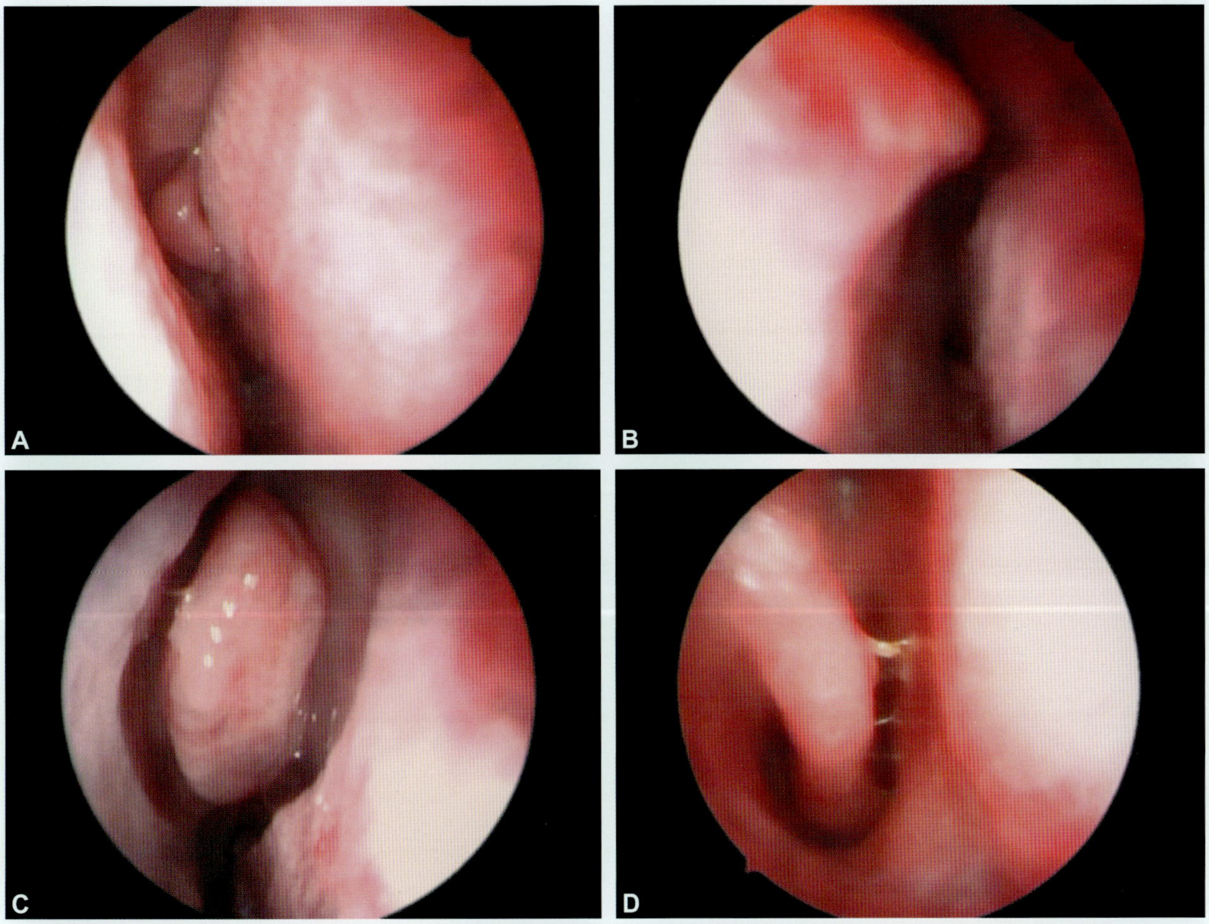

Figs 45A to D: Nasal endoscopy-showing DNS, Spur, Hypertrophied turbinate and Secretions respectively

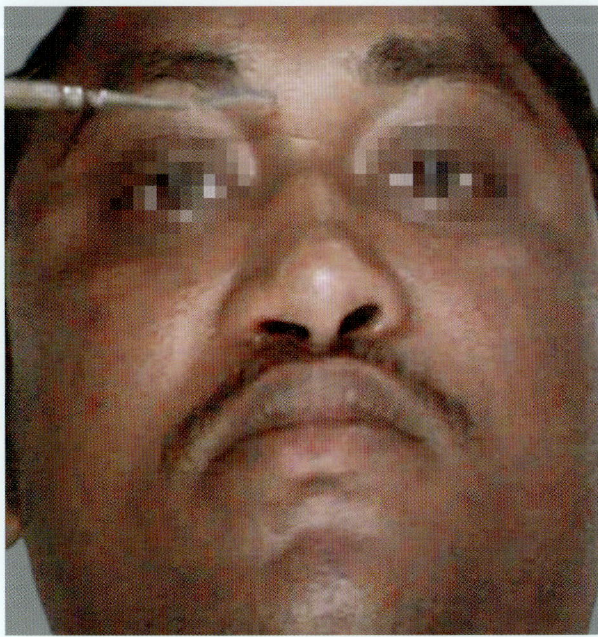

Fig. 46: Inspection and palpation of obvious and subtle structures

Apart from routine, patients are subjected for special investigations like nasal endoscopy and, if needed, some times CT scan as well. The manual palpation for subtle details, even for minimum tissue details, is quite useful for proper planned surgery to avoid unexpected situations peroperatively and for the good results.

HOW TO RECTIFY[2,3,6,8,9,11,14,15,18]

As it is appreciated, the basic challenge in esthetic surgery in ailed and ailing noses is the influence of the disease process directly or indirectly on the architectural and skin soft tissue envelope of the nose. This effects the diagnosis, management, surgical evaluation, procedure, healing process and thus directly on the result and the morbidity. If this entity is not taken into consideration and compromised, it leads to cosmetic as well as functional morbidity and many a time it leads to psychosomatic disorder.

The architectural balance between tension and compression get affected in such ailments leading to deformities. Restoration of this balance is necessary for stable reconstruction. The corrective rhinoplasty is done with basic concepts with permutation and combinations of various complimentary procedures and grafts in the form of fillers, spreaders, suspensors, plums, battens, shields, umbrellas and various modified sutures (Figs 48A and B).

SOME OF THE EXAMPLES OF AILED AND AILING NOSES BEFORE AND AFTER ESTHETIC SURGERY

Some of the examples of ailed and ailing noses before and after esthetic surgery are depicted in Figure 49 (two columns).

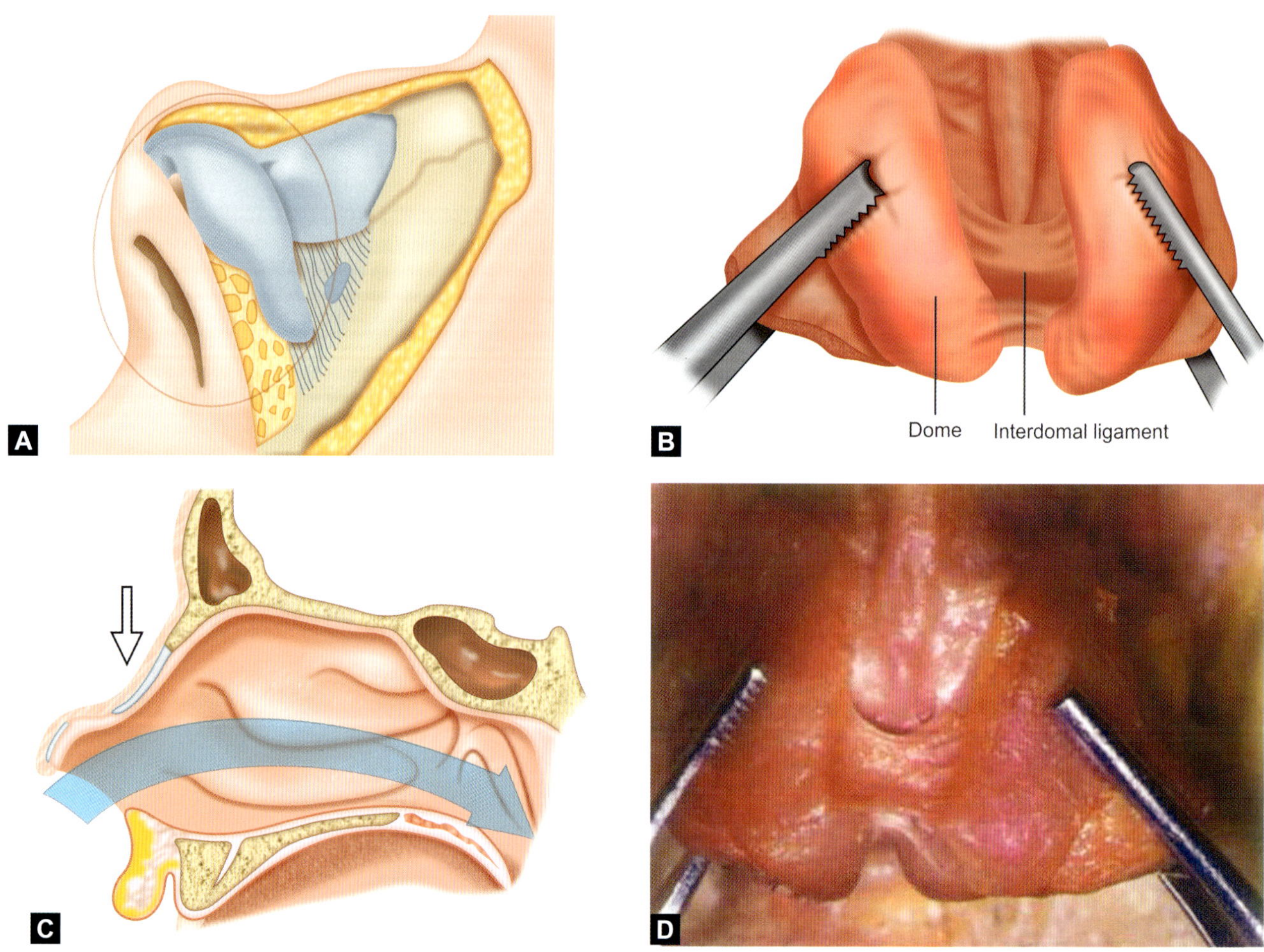

Figs 47A to D: (A and B) Showing the tip and dome configuration; (C and D) Showing the dedirected inspired air currents in saddle nose and anterior septal angle respectively

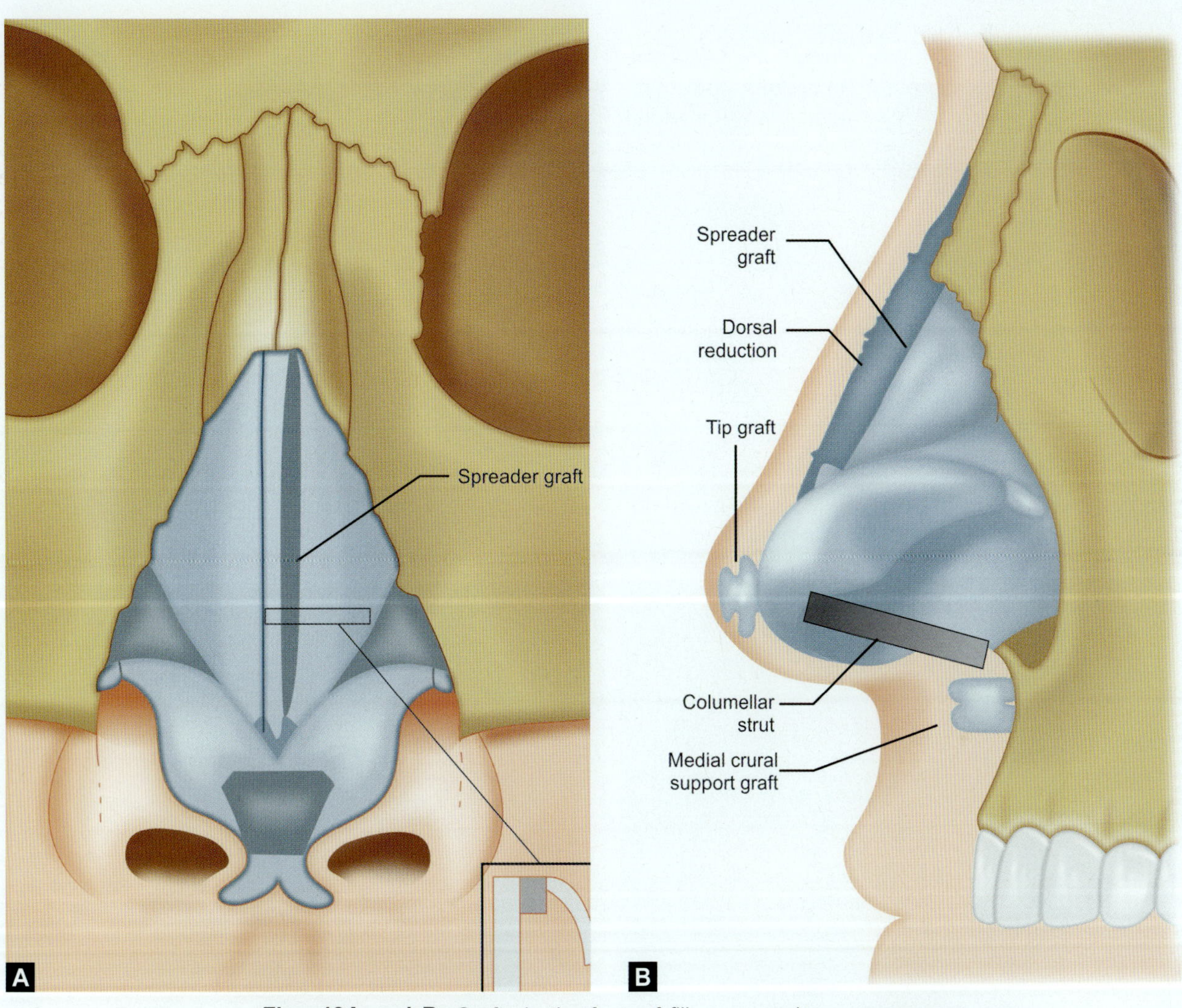

Figs 48A and B: Grafts in the form of fillers, spreaders, suspensors, plums, battens, shields, umbrellas and various modified sutures

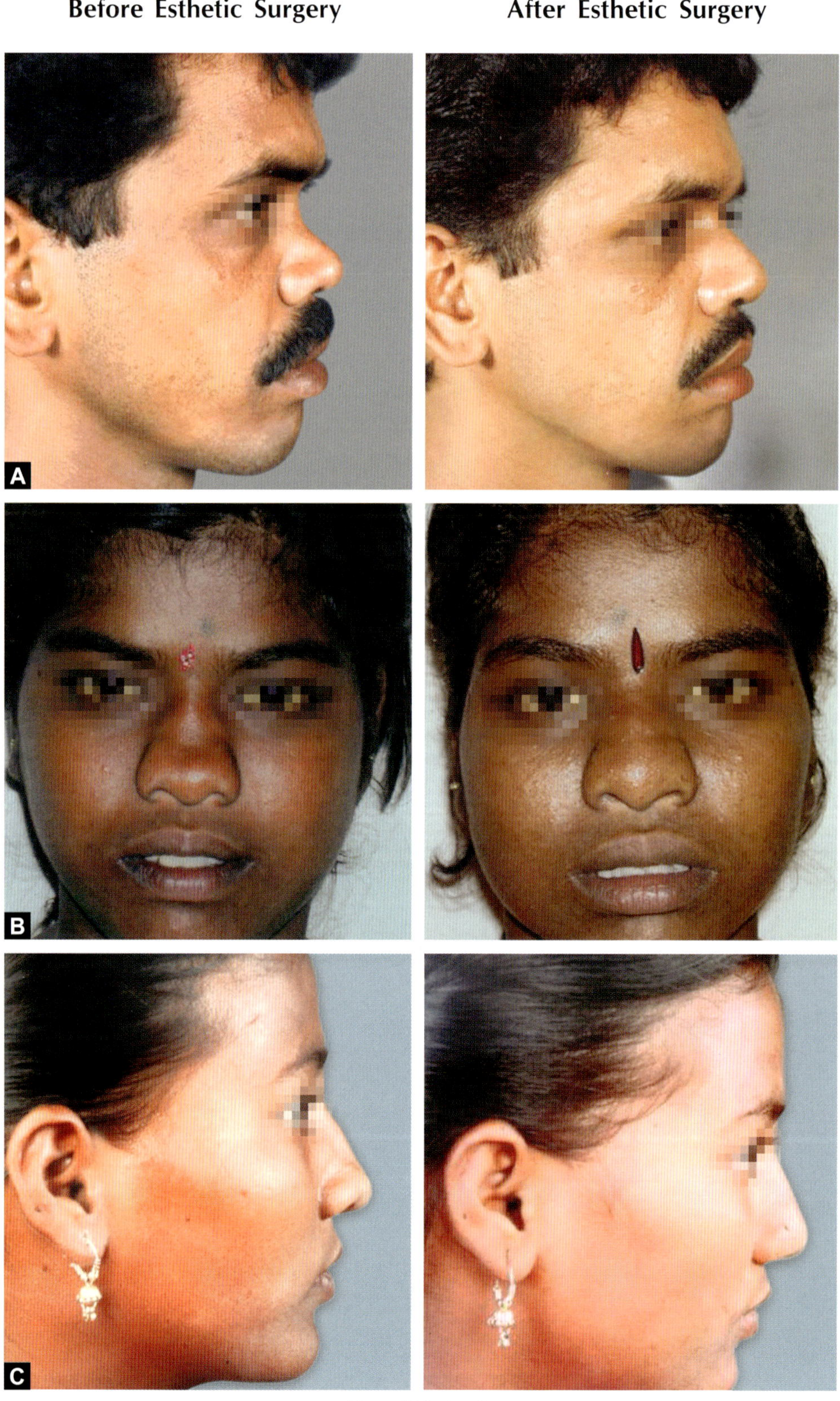

Figs 49A to C

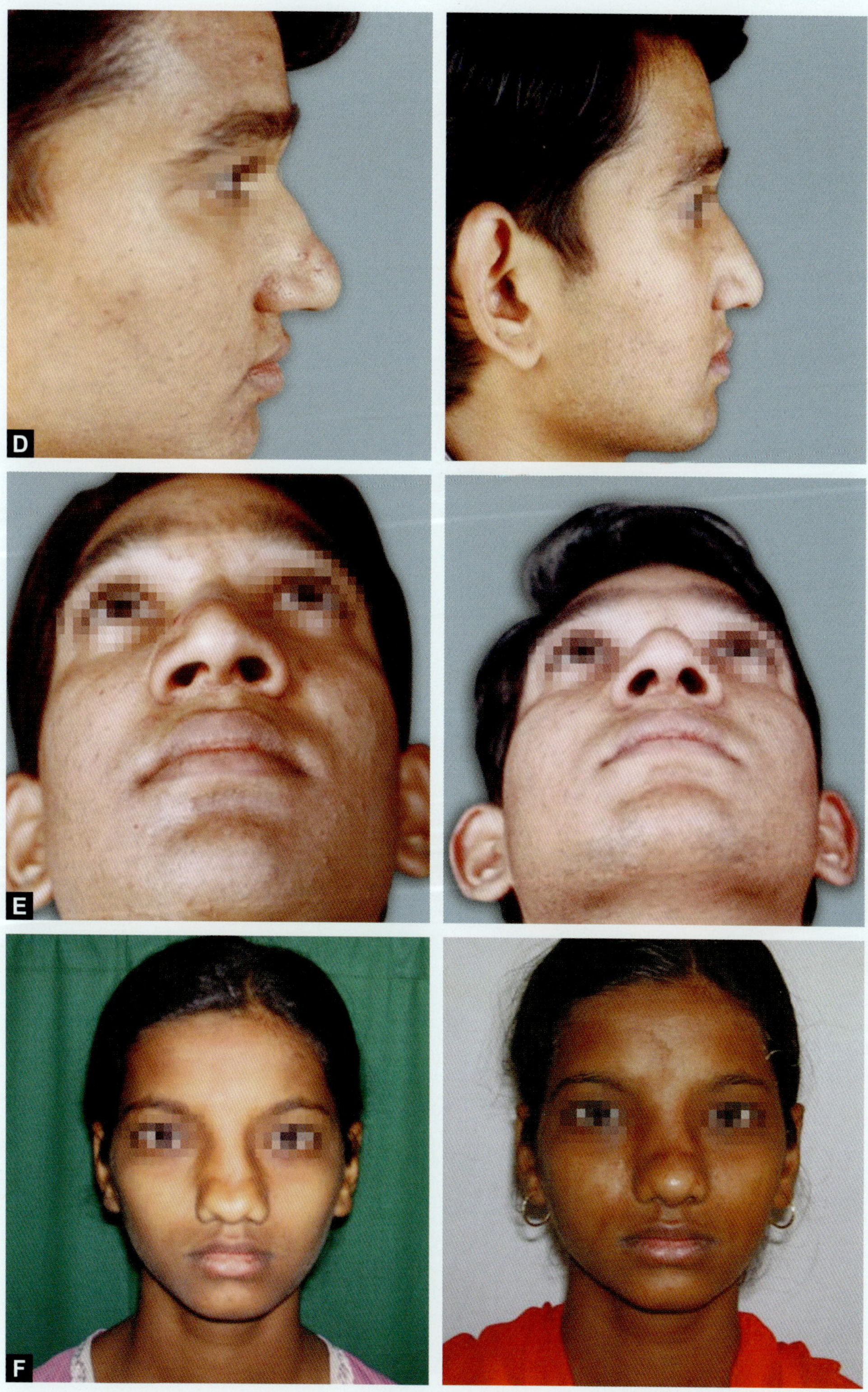

Figs 49D to F

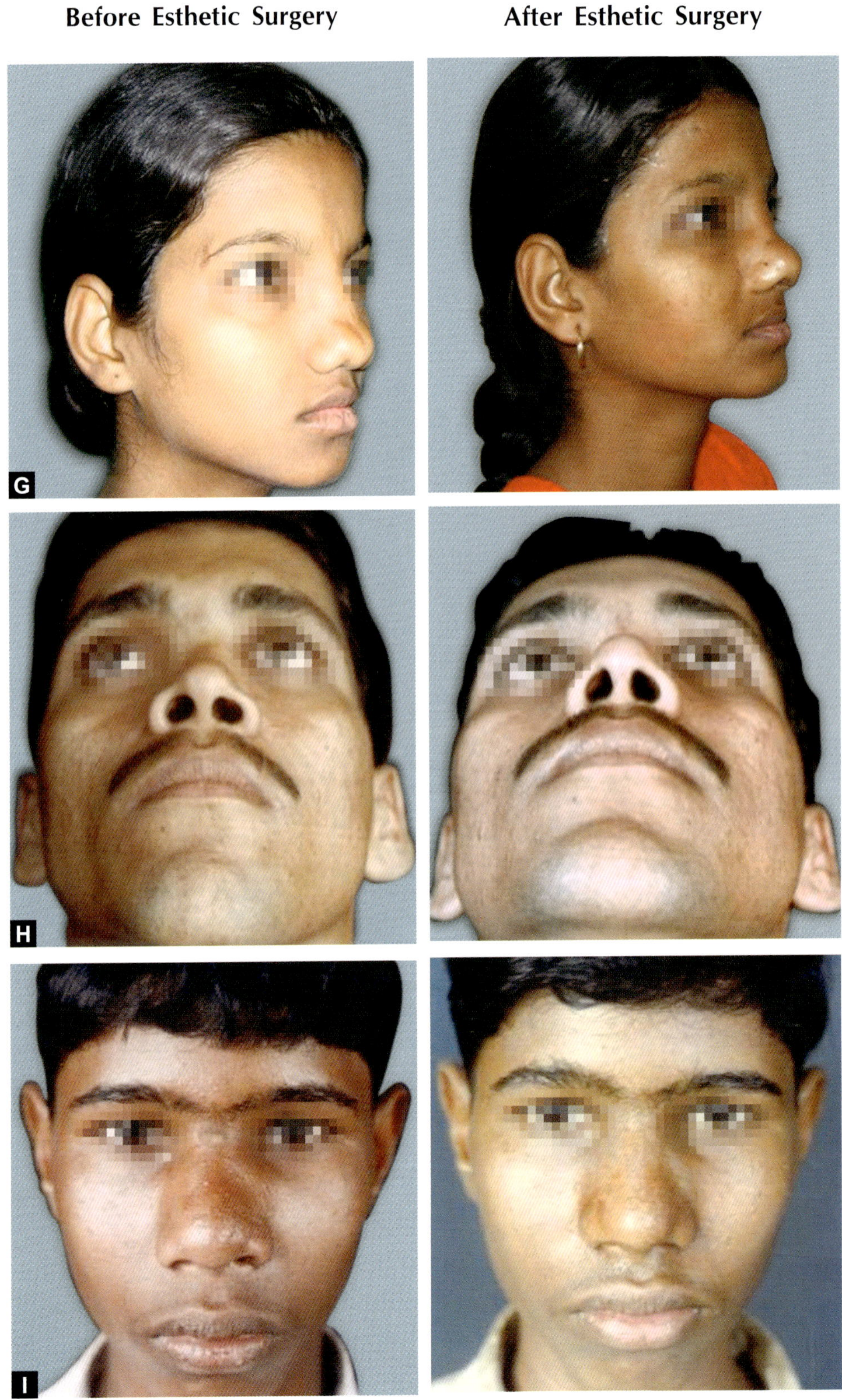

Figs 49G to I

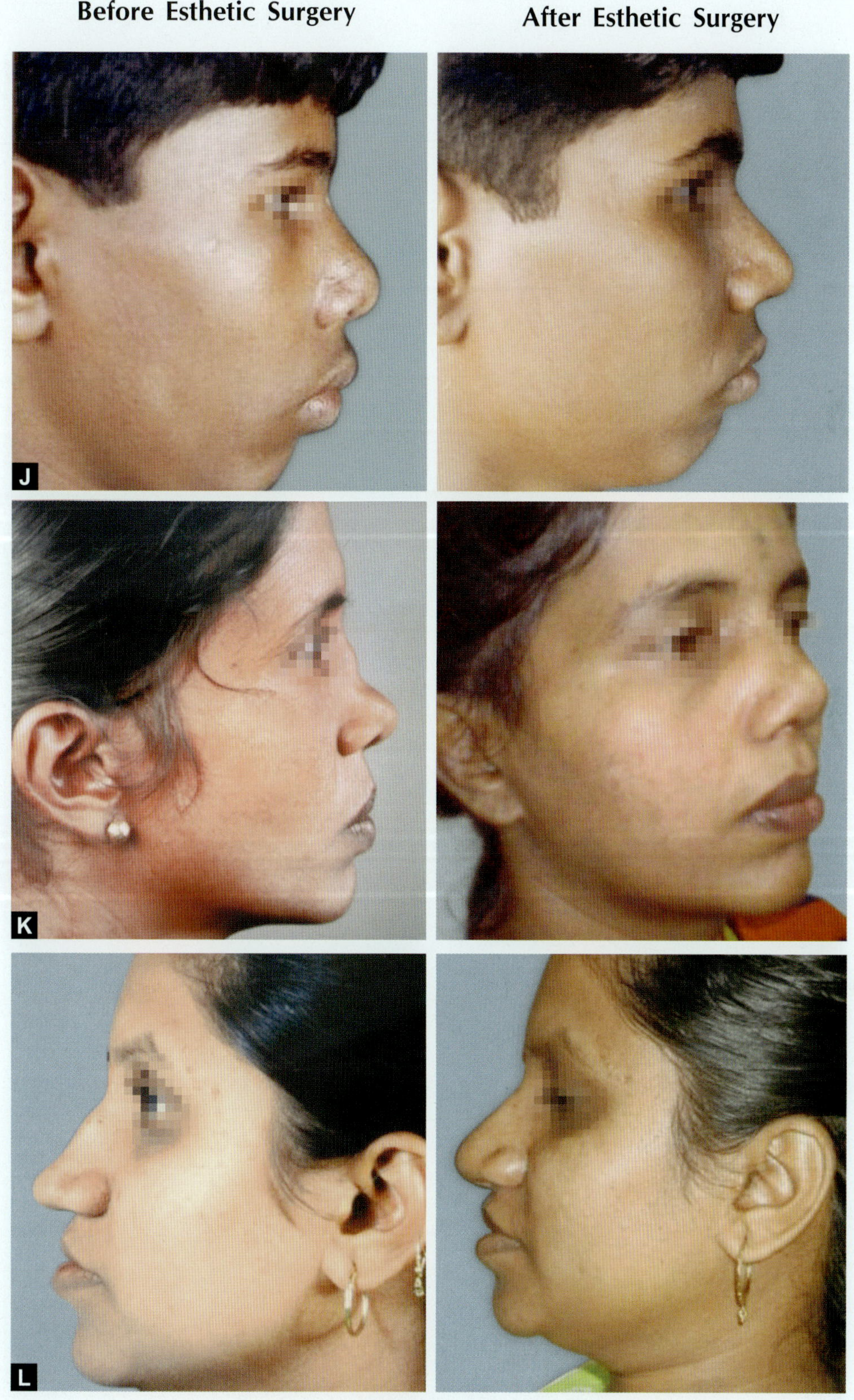

Figs 49J to L

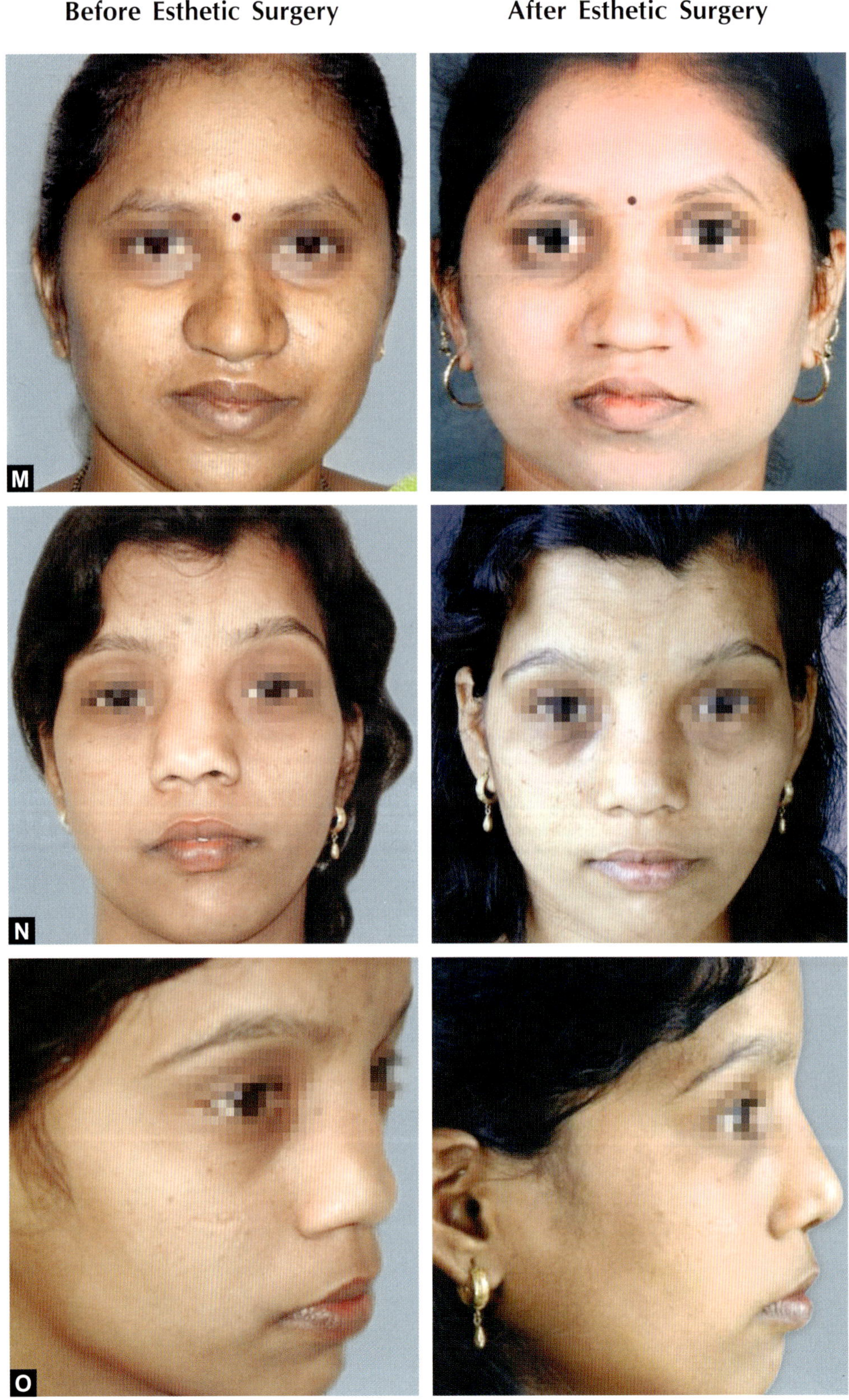

Figs 49M to O

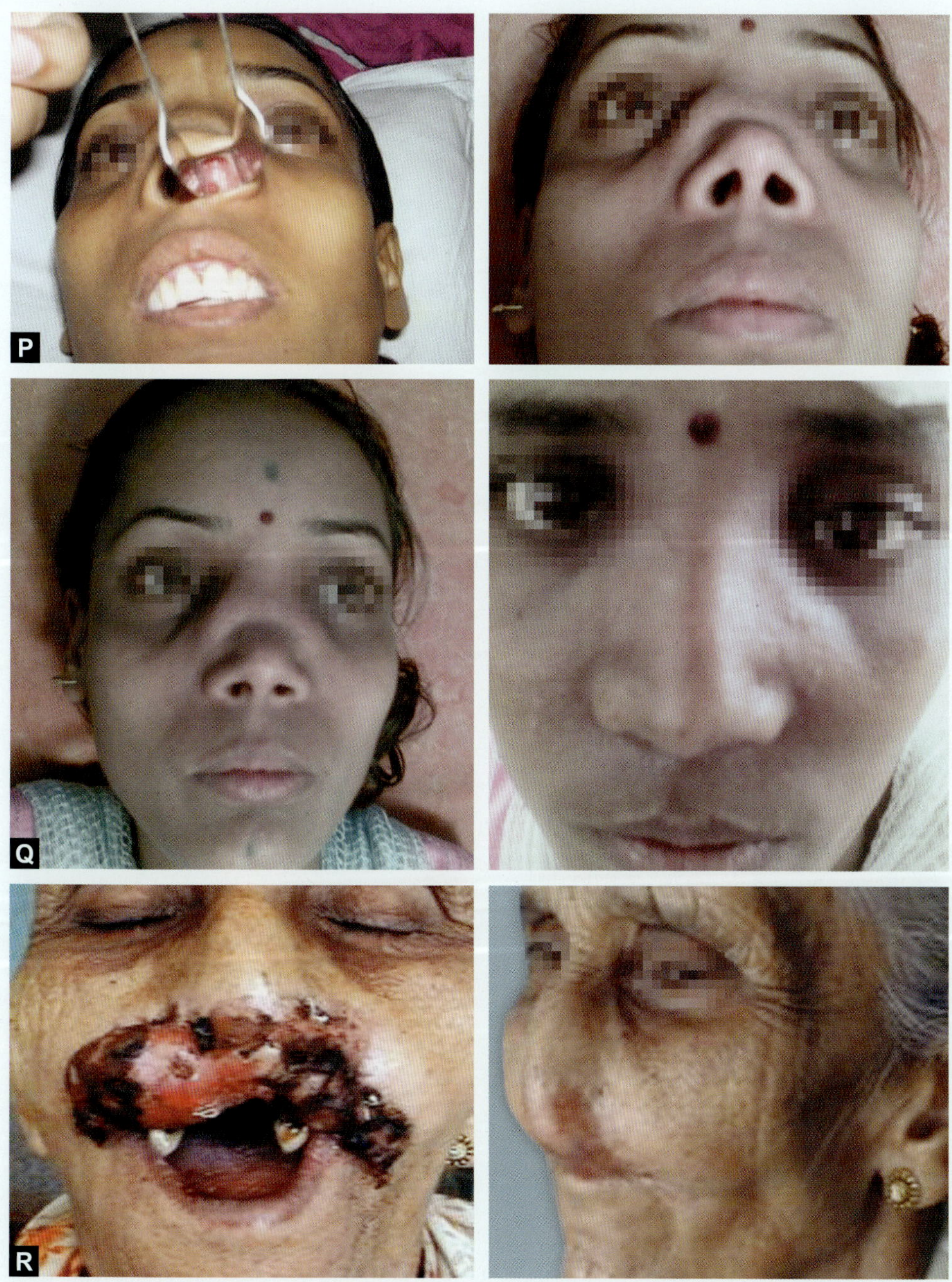

Figs 49P to R

Before Esthetic Surgery

After Esthetic Surgery

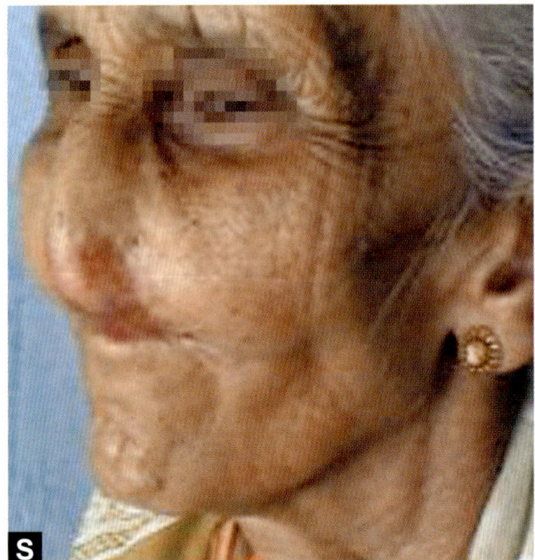

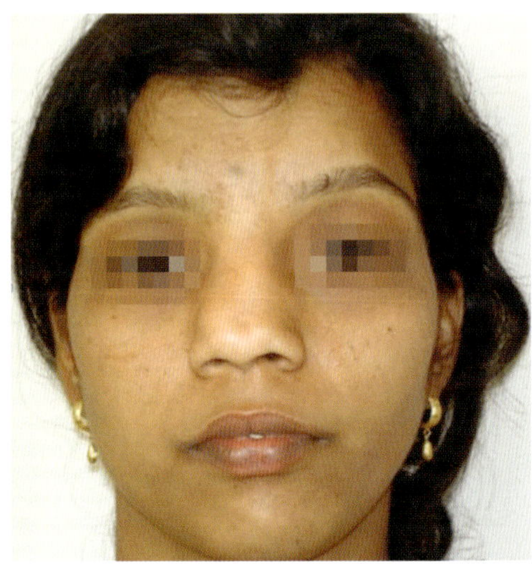

Figs 49A to S: Some of the samples of ailed and ailing noses before and after esthetic surgery

So, the acute and subacute afflictions are to be treated first and primarily. Decision of precision to address the conspicuous or subtle and expressed or unexpressed features is necessary. One has to keep in mind the innate idiosyncrasy of the healing tissues. It is comforting to confirm that the rules are not cut and dried and still there is plenty of room for individual differences of opinion. Whatever it may be the result should produce reliable stable reconstitution of deformity with minimum complications. With more control and predictability it should reduce reoperation rate and improve esthetic and functional problems. The soft tissue envelope of the nose get relaxed over time. Maintaining an open attitude, proper evaluation and listening to the patient help the surgeon to have fair judgment in the management of ailed and ailing noses appropriately in esthetic rhinoplasty.

REFERENCES

1. Tardy Jr. ME, Denneny 3rd. J, Fritsch MH. The versatile cartilage autograft in reconstruction of the nose and face. Laryngoscope. 1985; 95: 523-33.
2. Congdon D, Sherris D, Specks U, McDonald T. Long-term follow up of repair of external nasal deformities in patients with Wegener's granulomatosis. Laryngoscope. 2002;112: 731-7.
3. Trenite GN. Rhinoplasty: A practical guide to functional and aesthetic surgery of nose. Kugler Publications Hague. 2005.
4. Disant F, Bessède JP. [Guidelines for the clinical practice: aesthetic and functional rhinoplasty].; Societe Francaise d'Oto-Rhino-Laryngologie et de Chirurgie de la Face et Cou; Societe Francaise de Stomatologie et Chirurgie Maxillo Faciale. Rev Laryngol Otol Rhinol (Bord). 2007;128(4):203-30.
5. Sood VP. Corrective Rhinoplasty. CBS Publishers New Delhi (India), 2008.
6. Browning GG. Burton MJ, Clarke R, Hibbert J, et al. 2008. Scott-Brown's otolaryngology (7th ed., Hodder Arnold international ed.). London.
7. Belaldavar B.P. Lipoid Proteinosis—Aspect of Otorhinolaryngologist: A rare case report. Journal of Scientific Society. 2008;35(1):73-6.
8. Fuchs HA, Tanner SB. Granulomatous disorders of the nose and paranasal sinuses. Curr Opin Otolaryngol Head Neck Surg. 2009;17(1):23-7. doi: 10.1097/MOO.0b013e32831b9e58.
9. Shah AR, Zeitler D, Wise JB. Nasal reconstruction of the leprosy nose using costal cartilage. Otolaryngol Clin North Am. 2009;42(3):547-55. doi: 10.1016/j.otc.2009.03.009.
10. Pribitkin EA, Ezzat WH. Classification and treatment of the saddle nose deformity. Otolaryngol Clin North Am. 2009; 42(3):437-61. doi: 10.1016/j.otc.2009.03.004.
11. Rainsbury JW. The place of rhinoplasty in the ageing face. J Laryngol Otol. 2010;124(2):115-8. doi: 10.1017 S0022215109990892. Epub 2009 Sep 18.
12. Bremke M, Gedeon H, Windfuhr JP, Werner JA, Sesterhenn AM. Nasal bone fracture: etiology, diagnostics, treatment and complications. Laryngorhinootologie. 2009;88(11): 711-6. doi: 10.1055/s-0029-1224106. Epub 2009 Jun 26.
13. Sachse F, Stoll W. Nasal surgery in patients with systemic disorders. Laryngorhinootologie. 2010;89 Suppl 1:S103-15. doi: 10.1055/s-0029-1246127. Epub 2010 Mar 29.
14. Wright RJ, Murakami CS, Ambro BT. Pediatric nasal injuries and management. Facial Plast Surg. 2011;27(5):483-90. doi: 10.1055/s-0031-1288931. Epub 2011 Oct 25.
15. Larson K, Gosain AK. Cosmetic surgery in the adolescent patient. Plast Reconstr Surg. 2012;129(1):135e-141e. doi: 10.1097/PRS.0b013e3182362bb8.
16. Ghosh SK. Rhinoplasty in atrophic rhinitis. J Indian Med Assoc. 2012;110(4):246-7.

17. Anghel I, Anghel AG. Reconstructive rhinoplasty in cases with basal cell carcinoma of the nose. Chirurgia (Bucur). 2012;107(3):373-8.
18. Pisera P, Antoszewski B, Fijałkowska M, Kasielska A, Iljin A. Long-term aesthetic results of rhinoplasty in congenital nose deformities—comparison of surgeon's and patient's evaluation. Otolaryngol Pol. 2012;66(4):280-4. Epub 2012 May 4.
19. Lawrence R. Pediatric septoplasy: A review of the literature. Int J Pediatr Otorhinolaryngol. 2012;76(8):1078-81. doi: 10.1016/j.ijporl.2012.04.020. Epub 2012 May 15.
20. Picavet VA, Grietens J, Jorissen M, Hellings PW. Rhinoplasty from a rhinologist's perspective: Need for recognition of associated sinonasal conditions. Am J Rhinol Allergy. 2012; 26(6):493-6. doi: 10.2500/ajra.2012.26.3816.

CHAPTER

107

Cleft Lip and Palate

G Spinelli, G Carnevali, D Lazzeri, L Autelitano

OVERVIEW

Cleft lip and palate (CLP) are congenital facial malformations related to abnormal development of the cephalic structures (upper lip, hard and soft palate) during gestation. Because of the rarity of these conditions and the lack of standardization of methods of storage, the exact incidence of this pathology is still unknown, and estimates vary widely. The frequency at birth is approximately 1-700, with greater variability in different ethnic groups:[1]

- *Caucasian*: 0.69–2.35/1,000
- *Chinese*: 1.31–3.18/1,000
- *Japanese*: 1.65–2.71/1,000
- *Native Americans*: 0.55–2.50/1,000
- *Africans*: 0.32–0.82/1,000

European Collaboration on Cranial Facial Anomalies (EUROCRAN) estimated that there are about 876 new cases per year in Italy. Two-thirds of the cases involve the lip with or without palate deformities (more frequent in males), and the remaining one-third occur as isolated deformities of the palate (especially in females). In unilateral forms, left side is the most affected. In most cases, the cleft is sporadic and has a multifactorial etiology. The incidence increases with the age of parents and in multiparae.

According to the hypothesis that the condition occurs through the interaction of multiple factors, the malformation depends on genetic predisposition and various teratogenic agents. The importance of the genetic contribution in orofacial clefts is evidenced by the concordance in monozygotic twins (40% for CLP, 35% for isolated cleft palate). Using "linkage" analysis and allelic association, several potentially involved genes and cytokines, such as MSX1 and transforming growth factor ß3 (TGFß3), have been identified.

Many human teratogens are associated with an increased risk of sporadic clefts, including ethanol, diphenylhydantoin, trimethadione, aminopterin, methotrexate, retinoids and hyperthermia. Cigarette smoking during pregnancy, especially in combination with TGFa and folic acid deficiency appears to be related to an increased probability of facial deformities and abnormalities in neural tube closure. Five percent of all cleft cases are syndromic; syndromes occur more frequently with isolated cleft palate. From 1990 to the present, about 340 syndromes that present with an orofacial cleft have been identified. Most of these syndromes are genetically based (Tables 1 and 2).[2]

Table 1: Syndromic clefts with relative mutated genes

Cleft lip, cleft lip and palate			
Autosomal-dominant developmental malformations, deafness and dystonia	ACTB	Gorlin	PTCH1
Familiar gastric cancer and CLP	CDH1	CLP, ectodermal dysplasia	PVRL1
Craniofrontonasal	EFNB	Holoprosencephaly	SHH
Roberts	ESCO2	Holoprosencephaly	SIX3
Holoprosencephaly	GLI2	Branchio-oculo-facial	TFAP2A
"Oro-facial-digital"	GLI3	Holoprosencephaly	TGIF1
Hydrolethalus	HYLS1	Ectrodactyly-ectodermal dysplasia-clefting	TP63
Van der Woude/popliteal pterygium	IRF6	Ankyloblepharon-ectodermal dysplasia-clefting	TP63
X-linked mental retardation and CLP	PHF8	Tetra-amelia with CLP	WNT3

Contd...

Contd...

Cleft palate			
Oculofaciocardiodental	BCOR	"Oro-facial-digital"	GLI3
CHARGE	CHD7	Van der Woude/popliteal pterygium	IRF6
Lethal and Escobar multiple pterygium	CHRNG	Andersen	KCNJ2
Stickler type 1	COL2A1	Kabuki	MLL2
Stickler type 2	COL11A1	Cornelia de Lange	NIPBL
Stickler type 3	COL11A2	X-linked mental retardation	PQBP1
Desmosterolosis	DHCR24	Isolated cleft palate	SATB2
Smith-Lemli-Opitz	DHCR7	Diastrophic dysplasia	SLC26A2
Miller	DHODH	Campomelic dysplasia	SOX9
Craniofrontonasal	EFNB1	Pierre Robin	SOX9
Kallmann	FGFR1	DiGeorge	TBX1
Crouzon	FGFR2	X-linked cleft palate and ankyloglossia	TBX22
Apert	FGFR2	Treacher-Collins	TCOF1
Otopalatodigital types 1 and 2	FLNA	Loeys-Dietz	TGFBR1
Larsen syndrome; atelosteogenesis	FLNB	Loeys-Dietz	TGFBR2
Hereditary lymphedema-distichiasis	FOXC2	Saethre-Chotzen	TWIST1
Bamforth-Lazarus	FOXE1		

Source: Modified from Dixon MJ, Marazita ML, Beaty TH et al. Cleft lip and palate: understanding genetic and environmental influences. Nat Rev Genet. 2011;12(3):167-78.

Table 2: Nonsyndromic cleft associated genes

Confirmed	*Likely*	*Intensively studied*
IRF6	ABCA4 locus	CRISPLD2
VAX1	BMP4	FGF8
8q24 locus	FGFR2	GSTT1
	FOXE1	MTHFR
	MAFB	PDGFC
	MSX1	PVRL1
	MYH9	SUMO1
	17q22 locus	TGFA
		TGFB

Source: Modified from Dixon MJ, Marazita ML, Beaty TH, Murray JC. Cleft lip and palate: understanding genetic and environmental influences. Nat Rev Genet. 2011;12(3):167-78.

EMBRYOLOGY

The heterogeneity of facial deformities is attributable to the extreme embryogenetic and anatomical complexity of this region. During embryogenesis, there are several phases in which the fusion of various processes creates the continuity and shape of the lip, nose and palate. Any alteration at these points may cause a facial cleft.

Each process consists of ectodermal tissue, derived from the hindbrain and midbrain neural crest, and mesodermal tissue.

The fate of these cells and tissues is determined by several genes and cytokines that control migration, development, apoptosis and therefore, the formation of the face (Fig. 1).[3]

During the sixth week of embryonic life, the medial and lateral nasal processes fuse with the maxillary processes, generating the base of the nose, nostrils, upper lip and primary palate (Fig. 2).[3] During the eighth week, the palatal processes become horizontal and fuse with the septum to form the secondary palate (Figs 3 and 4).[3] The marginal ectodermal components undergo apoptosis and the mesenchyme unifies the structure.

The anterior primary palate fuses with the secondary one and then ossifies. Facial clefts occur in case of failure of fusion of processes in one or more of these different stages of development. The cleft may be complete or incomplete, depending on the nature of the fusion failure. When the defect concerns the fusion of the medial nasal processes

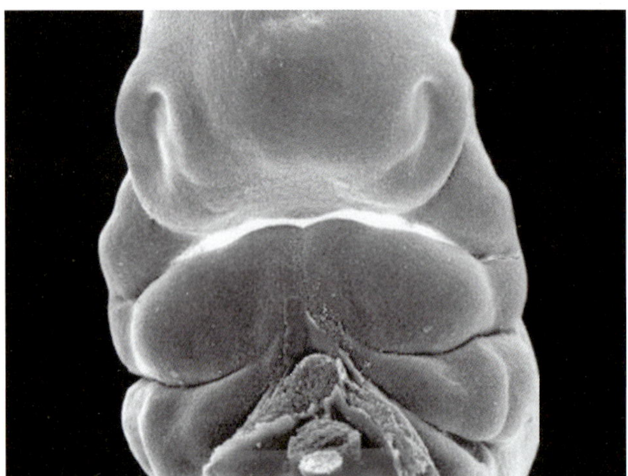

Fig. 1: Facial scanning by electronic microscope of a 5-week old embryo

Source: Cohen MM. Malformations of the craniofacial region: evolutionary, embryonic, genetic, and clinical perspectives. Am J Med Genet. 2002;115(4):245-68.

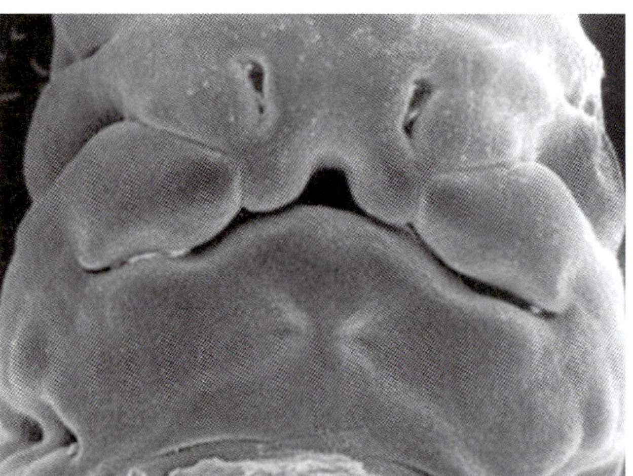

Fig. 2: A 6-week old embryo by electronic microscopy. During the sixth and seventh week of gestation, the maxillary and the nasal processes fuse. The upper lip is still incomplete

Source: Cohen MM. Malformations of the craniofacial region: evolutionary, embryonic, genetic, and clinical perspectives. Am J Med Genet. 2002;115(4):245-68.

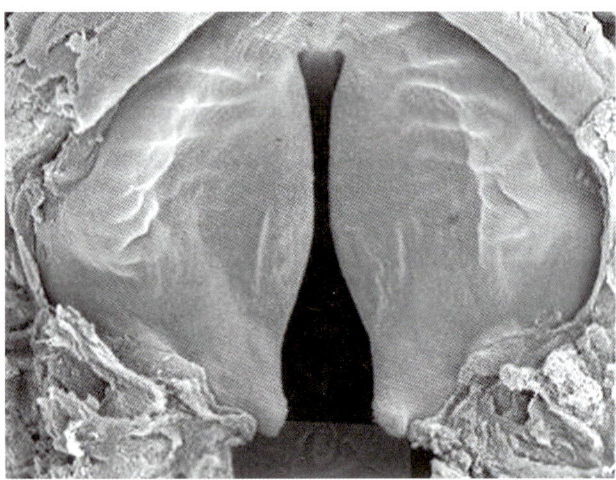

Fig. 3: Secondary palate in a 53-day old embryo, after the fusion with the primary palate

Source: Cohen MM. Malformations of the craniofacial region: evolutionary, embryonic, genetic, and clinical perspectives. Am J Med Genet. 2002;115(4):245-68.

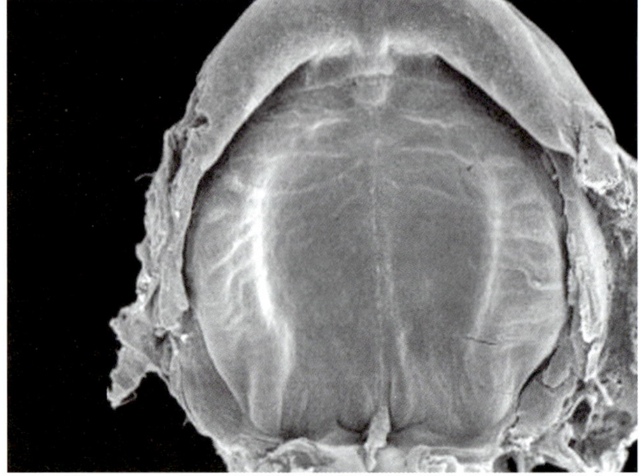

Fig. 4: After 59 days of gestation, the fusion of the secondary palate is complete

Source: Cohen MM. Malformations of the craniofacial region: evolutionary, embryonic, genetic, and clinical perspectives. Am J Med Genet. 2002;115(4):245-68.

with the maxillary and the lateral nasal processes, there is the development of a cleft lip and/or a maxillary cleft. If the defect concerns the rotation/fusion of one or both palatal processes, a mono- or bilateral cleft of the secondary palate will be developed, respectively.

FUNCTIONAL ANATOMY

To understand the functional defect and the classification and grading of surgical treatment of a cleft of the lip and palate, the muscular and neurovascular anatomical

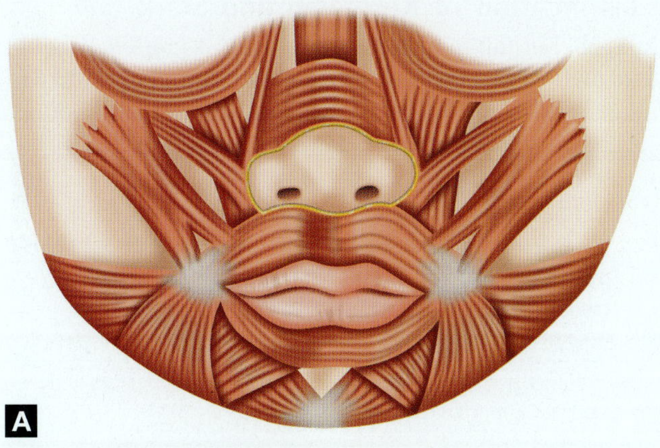

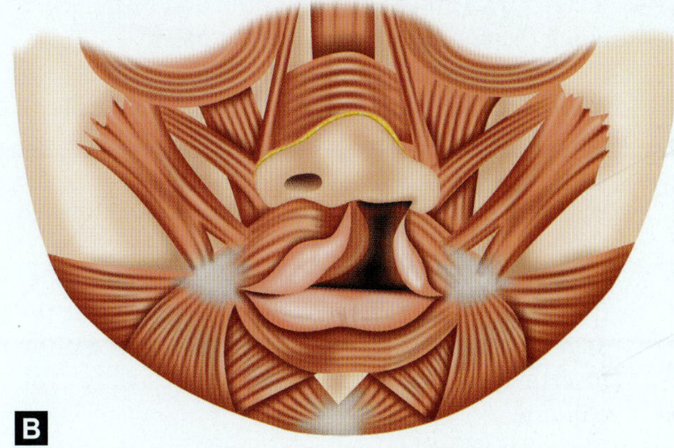

Figs 5A and B: Musculature of the normal lip and in cleft lip: note the insertion on both sides of the cleft to the wing of the nose and the columella

characteristics must be understood. The cleft-related anatomical abnormalities correspond to an equal number of defects developed during the embryonic formation of the muscular structures, particularly when the fusion of each process with its counterpart fails. The non-union of the orofacial muscles during gestation results in abnormal and non-functional insertions, with subsequent hypoplasia.

- *Muscles of the lip*: The orbicularis oris. This is a single and median muscle that surrounds the oral rim. It is composed of:
  - A superficial (external) portion composed of bundles from other mimic muscles of the face (such as the canine, buccinators, triangular, incisors). It is divided into two semicircles that meet in the midline. It inserts in the deep skin of the lip, nose and membranous septum.
  - A deep (internal) portion that is located close to the free edge of the lips. This is composed of an upper and lower ring that cross at the labial commissures and insert on the deep surface of the skin and mucosa. It works exclusively as a constrictor of the mouth.

The labial muscular fibers (compressor labii, musculus cutaneomucosus, rectus labii) are obliquely interspersed between the skin and the mucous membrane, and they contribute to the act of sucking. These fibers typically disappear after breast-feeding.

In the complete CLP, the fibers of the orbicularis muscle rotate upward from the lateral zone to the medial zone, along the edge of the cleft. These fibers then stop on the base of the nasal wing and the columella (Figs 5A and B), where they fit one over the other, or fade in subcutaneous tissues.

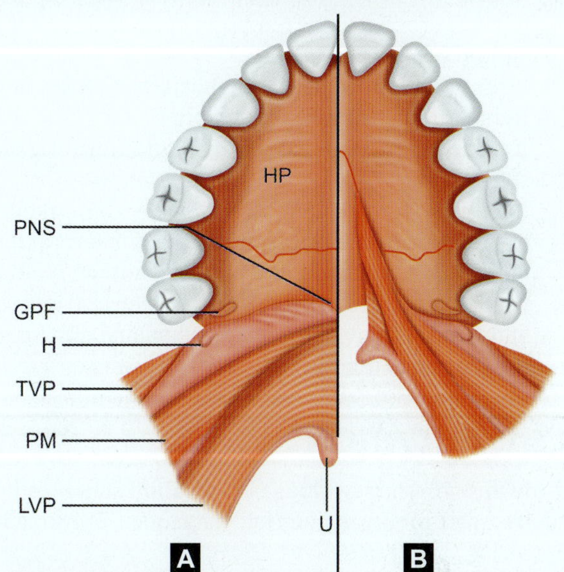

Figs 6A and B: (A) Normal palatal muscles and (B) Cleft palate muscles

(HP: Hard palate; PNS: Posterior nasal spine; GPF: Greater palatine foramen; H: Hamulus; TVP: The tensor veli palatini; PM: Pharyngopalatine muscle; LVP: Levator veli palatini; U: Uvula; →: Aponeurosis of the veil)

Source: Modified from Maue-Dickson W, Dickson DR. Anatomy and physiology related to cleft palate: current research and clinical implications. Plast Reconstr Surg. 1980;65(1):83-90.

- *Muscles of the palate*: Tensor veli palatini (TVP) and levator veli palatini (Figs 6A and B).[4]
  - The TVP originates from the pterygoid process, the sphenoidal angular horn and the anterolateral portion of the Eustachian tube.

- It runs in an anteriorinferior direction by inserting along the anterior third of the soft palate.
- Its contraction lengthens and elevates the soft palate near the hamulus and enlarges the orifice of the Eustachian tube.
- Depending on the circumstances, it may act synergistically or antagonistically with the levator veli palatini.
- In children with CLP, this muscle appears thinner than normal, and its insertion is located at the edge of the cleft palate as a single beam or tendon inserting in the thickness of the levator veli palatini.
- A smaller part of the muscle inserts into the posterior nasal spine (PNS) or the posterior edge of the palatine bone.
- The levator veli palatini is an equal cylindrical muscle which originates from the apex of the petrous process of the temporal bone and from the carotid canal.
- It runs in a groove below the Eustachian tube, and its insertion is located at the raphe.
- Its action consists of moving back and elevating the soft palate.
- In children with CLP, this muscle is markedly hypoplastic. Its posterolateral portion inserts at the palatal arch and the basis of uvula, and its medial portion is located at the edge of the cleft and inserts at the nasal spine, the edge of the palatal bone and the tendon of the TVP.

CLASSIFICATION

Over the past 70 years, various classification schemes for CLP have been proposed, but few have been universally accepted.

Classification of the International Confederation of Plastic and Reconstructive Surgery

Based on embryology, three different groups are recognized. The groups are further subdivided if the defect is unilateral or bilateral.

- *Group 1*: Defects involving lip and alveolus
- *Group 2*: Cleft of secondary palate [hard palate (HP), soft palate or both]
- *Group 3*: Any cleft involving the primary or/and secondary palate.

Spina reviewed this classification and proposed by adding a fourth group to include all of the rare and atypical facial clefts.

Classification of Kernahan and Stark

In 1958, Kernahan and Stark proposed a graphic scheme that divides the region of the potential malformation in nine areas, according to the anatomical and embryological characteristics of the incisive foramen (Figs 7 to 9).[5,6]

- *Areas 1 and 4*: Lip
- *Areas 2 and 5*: Alveolus
- *Areas 3 and 6*: Palate between alveolus and incisive foramen
- *Areas 7 and 8*: Hard palate
- *Area 9*: Soft palate.

PRENATAL DIAGNOSIS

Prenatal diagnosis is essential to minimize the impact on parents. Ultrasonography in pregnancy has become a routine, noninvasive, inexpensive and well-accepted technique of investigation. In most cases, the diagnosis is made incidentally during routine ultrasonography or during ultrasonographic investigation of concerns unrelated to the cleft. The sensitivity of this instrumental examination (the so-called detection rate) varies widely in different centers. The detection rate has increased recently, as ultrasound techniques and the therapeutic protocols have improved. Every effort is made to define the nature and the etiology of the defect and to exclude any syndromic deformities. A geneticist consult may be critical, especially in the cases of inherited syndromes.

There is no consensus in the scientific community about the probability that a prenatally diagnosed cleft is part of unrecognized syndromic spectrum. Based on the reliable studies, the risk is around 10–12%. It is important to educate the parents about the nature of defects, the functional consequences, prospectives and expectation of treatment efficacy. This information includes the psychological consequences of decision making regarding the defect, including the possible voluntary termination of pregnancy after communication of the diagnosis. It is essential that the mother receive care in a dedicated center, where several specialists including the surgeon can discuss the primary and secondary problems associated with the available surgical strategies (Fig. 10).

PRESURGICAL ORTHOPEDICS

Unilateral Cleft Lip and Palate

Since the 1970s, a passive plate made with hard and soft resin[7] is used to:

- Separate the oral and nasal cavity (allowing adequate force for sucking and swallowing)

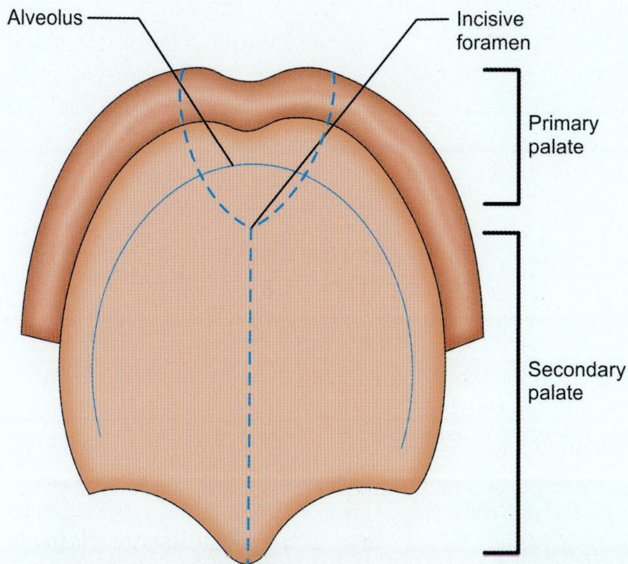

Fig. 7: Embryology and anatomy of the incisive foramen

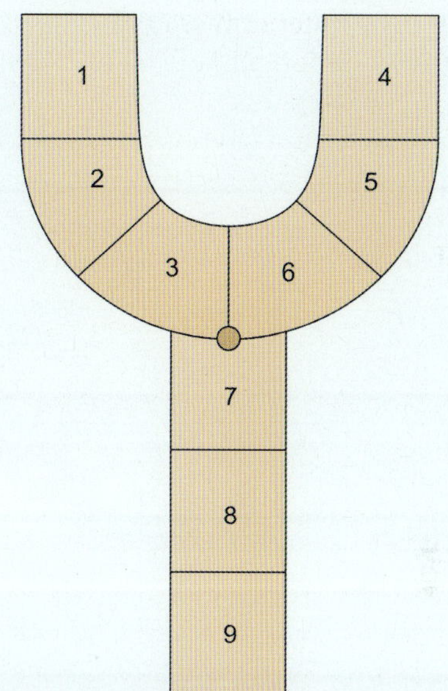

Fig. 8: The nine areas of Kernahan and Stark Classification
Source: Modified from Kirschner RE, LaRossa D. Cleft lip and palate. Otolaryngol Clin North Am. 2000;33(6):1191-215, v–vi.

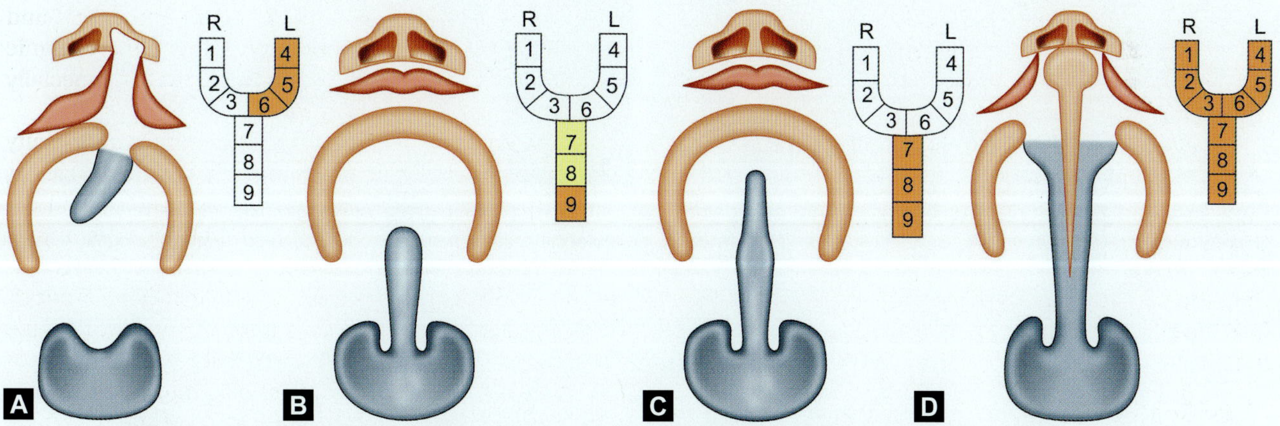

Figs 9A to D: Classification chart of some cleft, according to the classification of Kernahan and Stark
Source: Modified from Kernahan DA, Stark RB. A new classification for cleft lip and cleft palate. Plast Reconstr Surg Transplant Bull. 1958;22(5):435-41

- Facilitate breathing through the correct positioning of the tongue
- Direct growth vectors
- Guide the development of the two maxillary abutments (using progressive selective attachments applied on the plate itself) (Figs 11 and 12).[8]

Bilateral Cleft Lip and Palate

The need for presurgical orthopedics in bilateral clefts to retract the premaxilla (which is typically protruded) is universally accepted. Several methods have been proposed, but the most simple and widely used method provides for the use of a passive plate in association with a tape to push back the premaxilla. Since 1996[9] an orthopedic plaque has been used to remodel the nasal and alveolar processes. This procedure allows the gradual reversal of the premaxilla and the simultaneous elongation of the columella, which otherwise remains short and flattened (a typical stigmata of a BCLP) (Figs 13A and B).

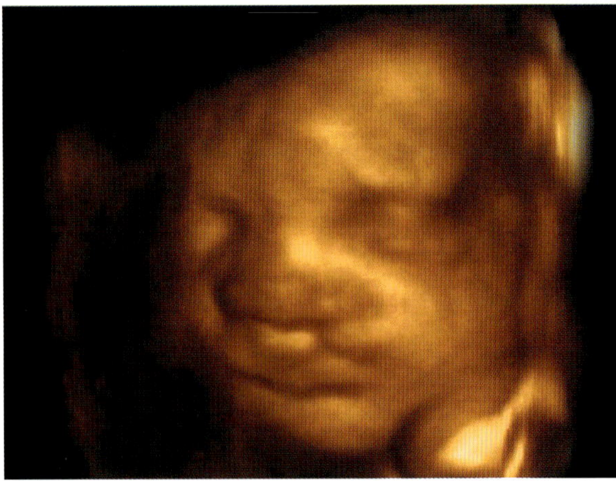

Fig. 10: Ultrasound scan with three-dimensional (3-D) reconstructions of cleft palate; the malformation is visible as a deep and central recess below the nose

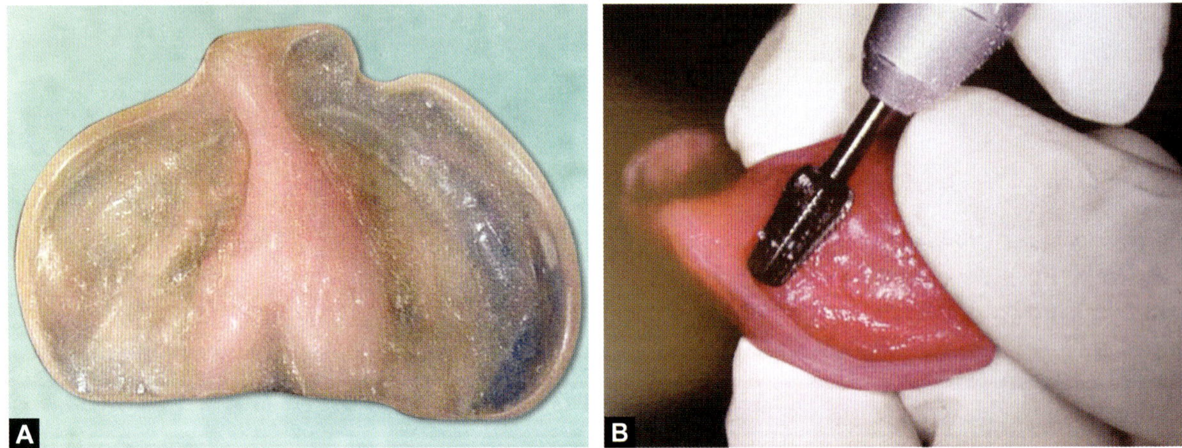

Figs 11A and B: Complete unilateral cleft lip and palate (UCLP), Hotz passive plate and selective grinding
Source: Meazzini MC, Brusati R, Bozzetti A, et al. Malformazioni craniofacciali: coordinamento ortodontico-chirurgico. *Bologna*: edizioni Martina; 2011.

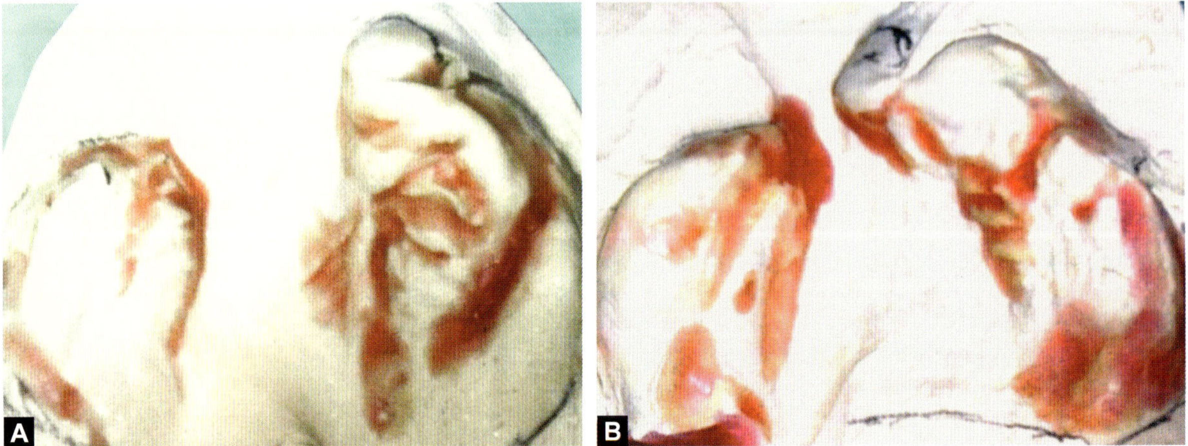

Figs 12A and B: Plaster models of complete unilateral cleft lip and palate (UCLP), note the distance of the stumps after the use of the plate of Hotz
Source: Meazzini MC, Brusati R, Bozzetti A, et al. Malformazioni craniofacciali: coordinamento ortodontico-chirurgico. *Bologna*: edizioni Martina; 2011.

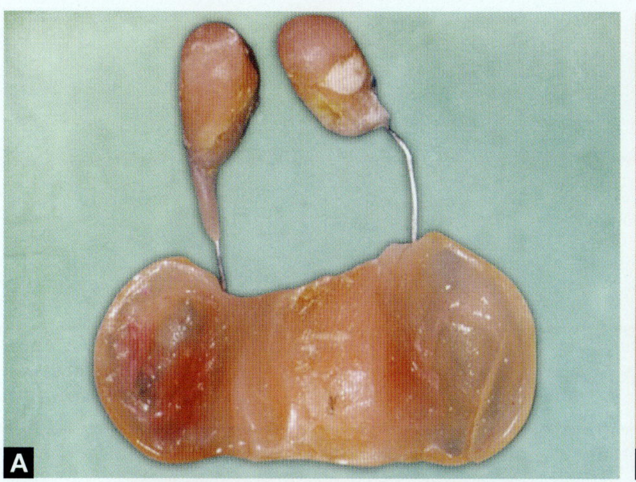

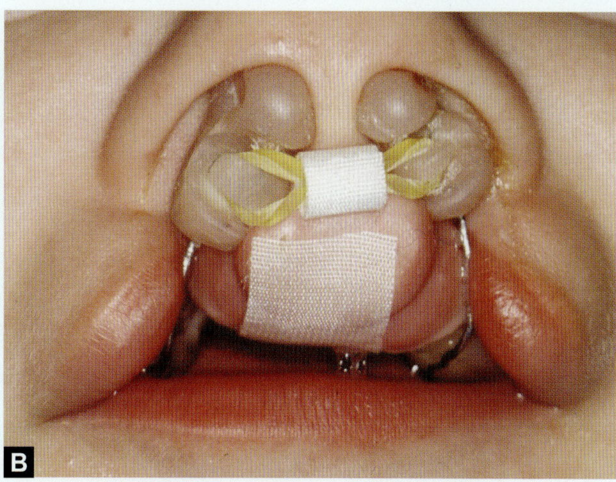

Figs 13A and B: Bilateral cleft lip and palate (BCLP), orthopedic nasoalveolar remodeling plate

SURGICAL TREATMENT

Surgery remains the mainstay of treatment for the CLP.

The principles underlying the repair proposed in the 1930s by the anatomical studies of Veau remain fundamental:

- All tissues are present, retracted or displaced.
- The correct remodeling of the displaced structures is essential for proper repair.
- The defect in facial growth or facial function is primarily a consequence of a poor anatomic reconstruction.

Although the essence of treatment has remained unchanged, several protocols and surgical techniques are currently followed (EUROCLEFT found 194 different therapeutic protocols in 201 European Centers).

The basics of the surgical treatment is influenced by both surgical indications and surgeon's experience, are shown below.

Cheilorhinoplasty of a Unilateral Cleft in Two Steps

First Step

At 4–6 months of age; often after an orthopedic treatment with passive plate to guide the maxillary growth.

- *Palatoplasty*: An incision is made along the margins of the soft palate cleft from the uvula to the posterior third of the HP. The dissection highlights the palatine aponeurosis and the tendon of TVP, and a tenotomy is performed (Figs 14A and B). A nasal mucoperiosteal flap from the pterygoid process and the palatine lamina on both sides is prepared, and a suture of the nasal plane from the HP to the tip of the uvula is performed. With the aid of a microscope, the surgeon isolates and prepares the palatine muscles, which are rotated from the nasal plane toward the midline (Figs 15A and B). After superimposition, this site is carefully sutured. After the release of the mucoperiosteal flaps, with or without lateral incisions, the oral plane is sutured to cover the previously repaired nasal floor (Figs 16A and B).
- *Cheilorhinoplasty*: The landmarks for reconstruction, including the top of the Cupid's bow of the healthy side, the top of the Cupid's bow of the pathological side, the base of columella and the base of the nasal ala on the pathological side, are identified (Fig. 17). Skin marks and incisions are made according to Millard's approach (Figs 18 and 19).[10] The region of the nasal spine is exposed through a mucosal incision. A subperichondrial dissection with a dislocation of the foot of the septum is performed to reposition it along the median plane (Figs 20A and B). Then, the buccal mucosa, transverse nasal muscle, external orbicularis, anterior nasal floor and finally, the skin undergo reconstruction (Figs 21 and 22). If it is necessary to obtain a better symmetry of the Cupid's bow, a small Z-plasty (Figs 23A and B) in the lower part of the lip is performed to obtain vertical elongation of the pathological side.
- At the end of surgery, nasal conformers, if necessary, are applied.

Second Step

At 18–24 months of age, the residual alveolar and HP cleft is corrected. The action of the labial and palatal musculature generally significantly reduces the gap between the two stumps (Figs 24 to 26).

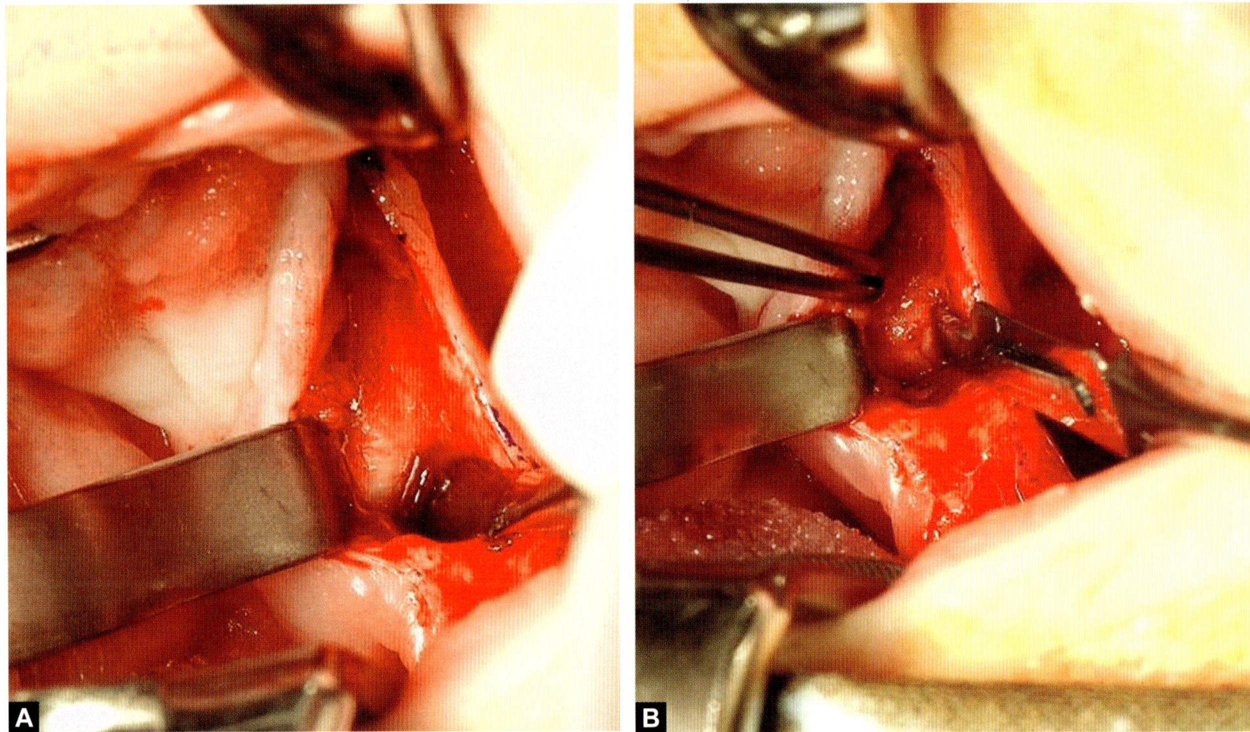

Figs 14A and B: Palatoplasty, retrieval and tenotomy of the tensor veli palatini (TVP)

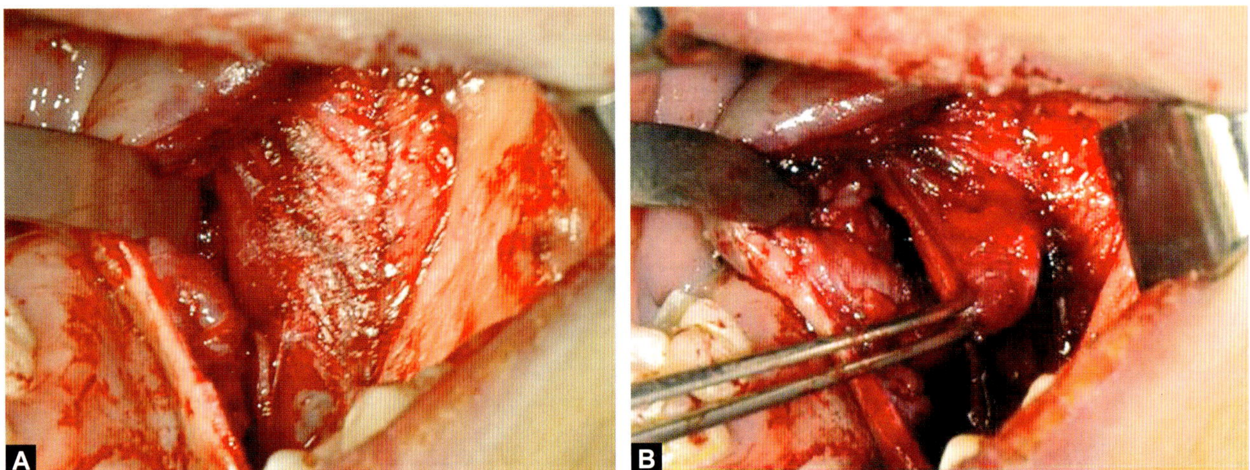

Figs 15A and B: Palatoplasty, preparation and rotation on the midline of the palatine musculature

- *Gingivoalveoloplasty and repair of the hard palate*: The repair begins with an intrasulcular incision on the smaller stump, and then lifting of a vestibular mucoperiosteal flap following distal vertical release incision. The same procedure is then repeated on the larger stump. After a palatine incision is made along the margins of the cleft, a mucoperiosteal dissection of the oral and nasal sides is performed. Then the nasal, oral, palatine and buccal planes are sutured, restoring the continuity of the fibromucosal flaps in the cleft area. This alveolar space is covered on all sides by mucoperiosteal tissues, which allows the formation of new bone tissue without any need for secondary bone grafting.

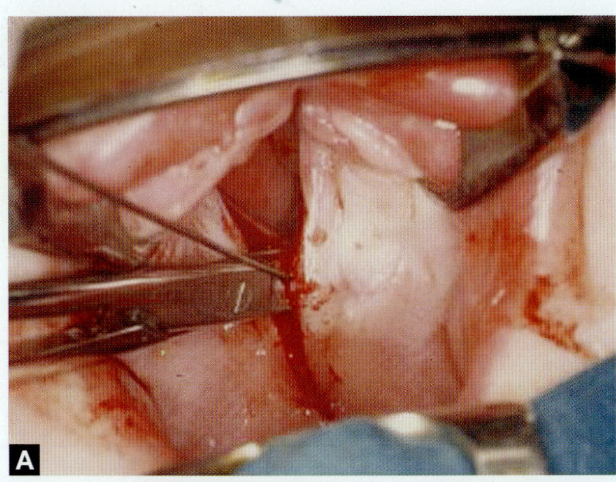

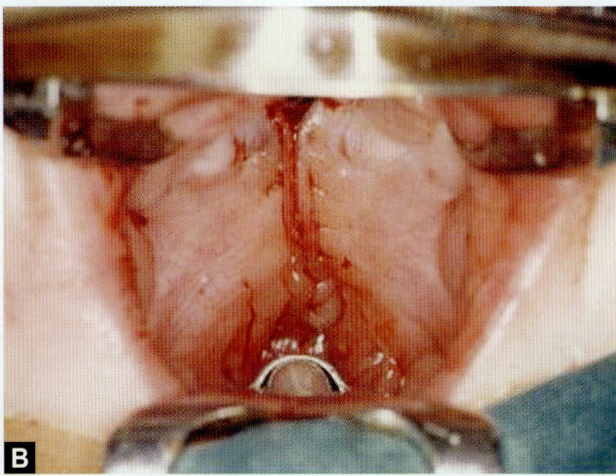

Figs 16A and B: Palatoplasty, reconstruction of the oral side without releasing incisions

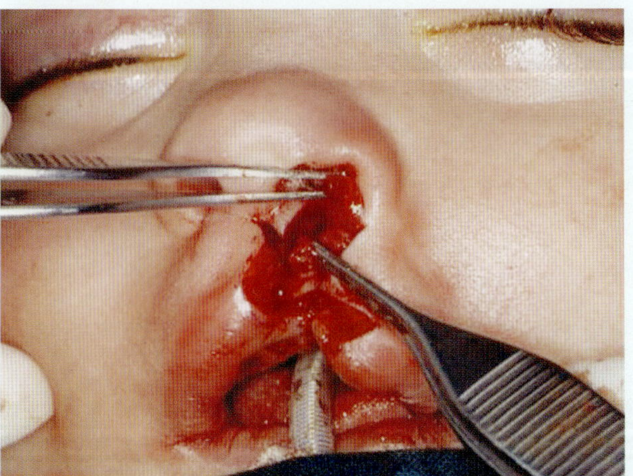

Fig. 17: Cheilorhinoplasty, identification and preparation of nasolabial muscles

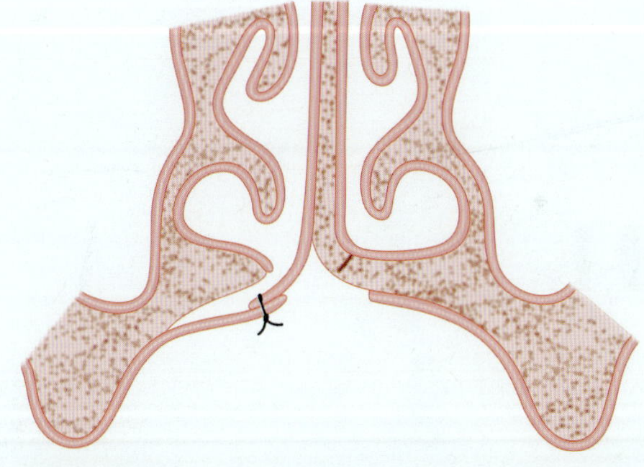

Fig. 18: "All in one" cheilorhinoplasty, preparation of the Pichler flap

Source: Modified from Furlow LT. Cleft palate repair by double opposing Z-plasty. Plast Reconstr Surg. 1986;78(6):724-38.

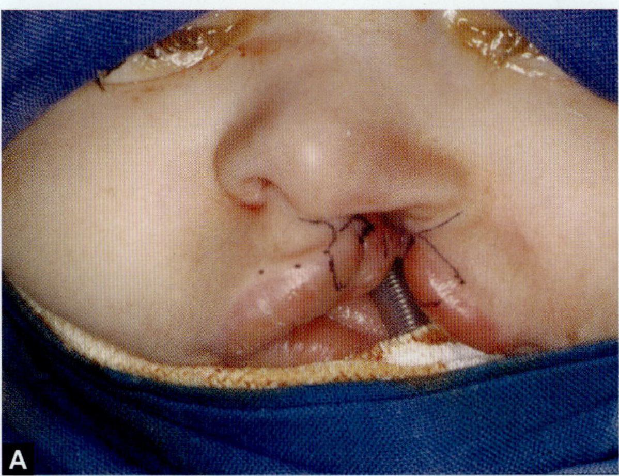

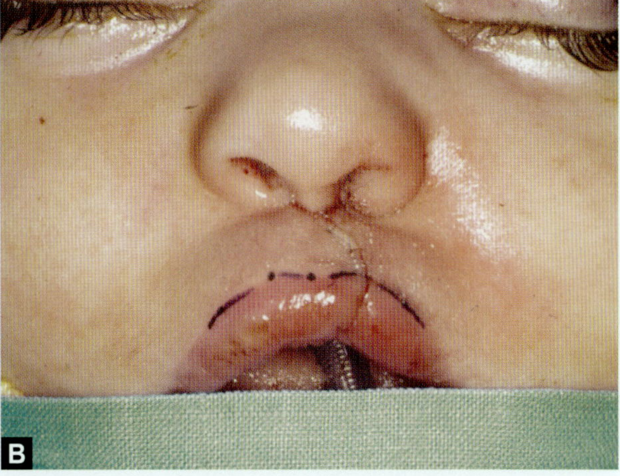

Figs 19A and B: Cheilorhinoplasty, skin incision and reconstruction of the lip with the Millard's technique

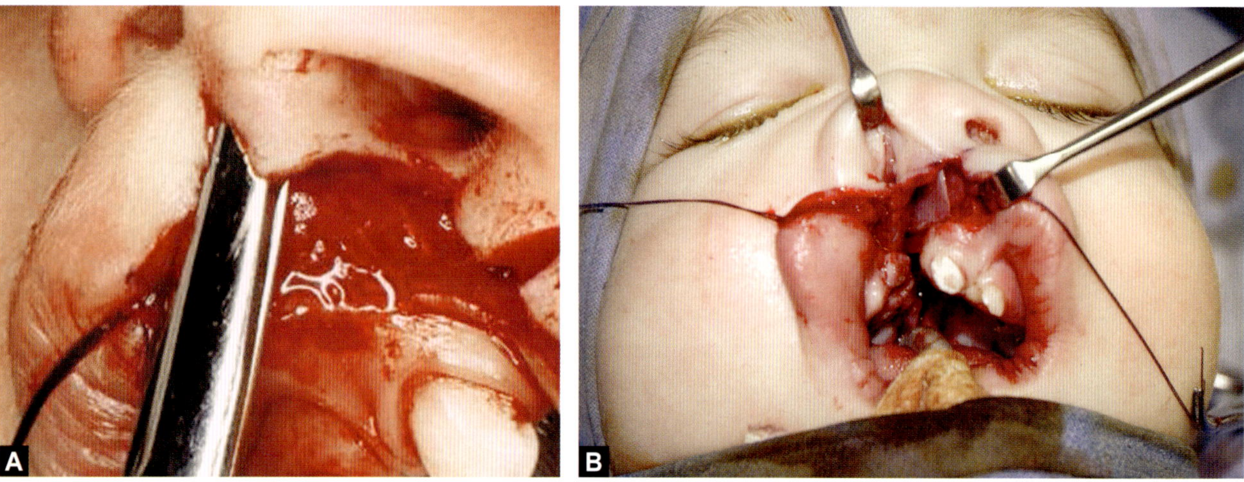

Figs 20A and B: Cheilorhinoplasty, dissection of intercrural cartilage and dislocation of the nasal septum

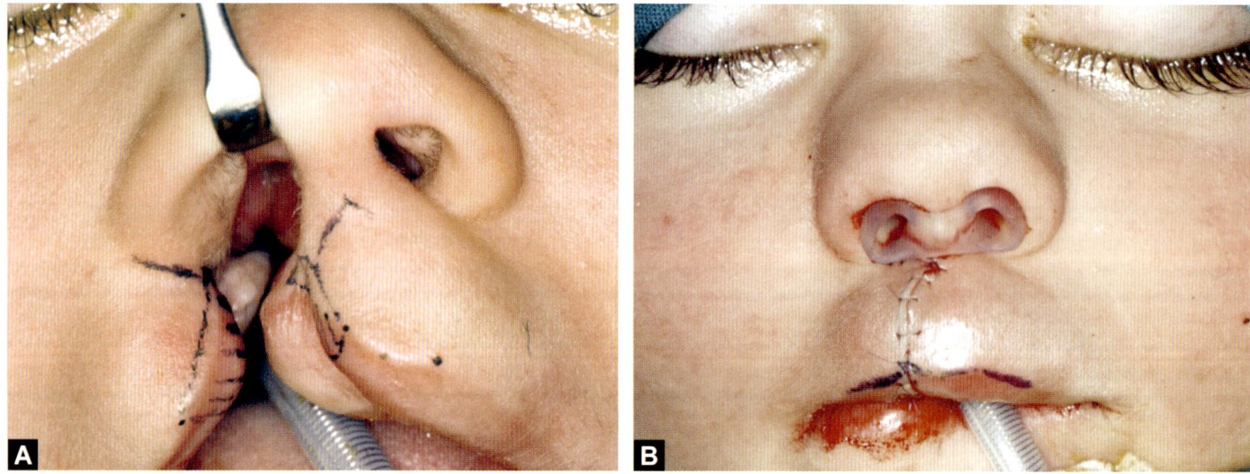

Figs 21A and B: Cheilorhinoplasty, skin incision and reconstruction with the Mohler's technique

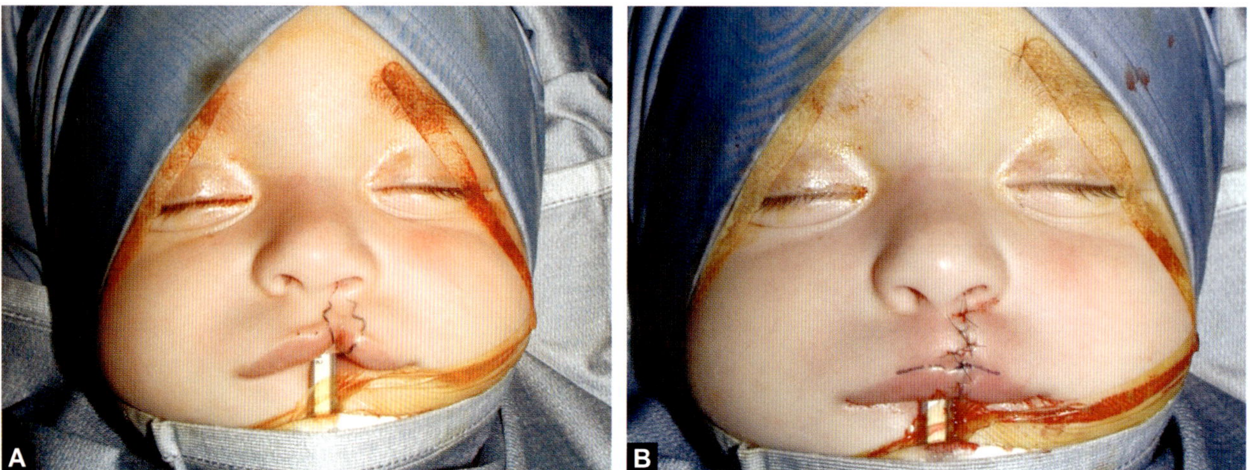

Figs 22A and B: Cheilorhinoplasty, skin incision and lip reconstruction with the Wave technique

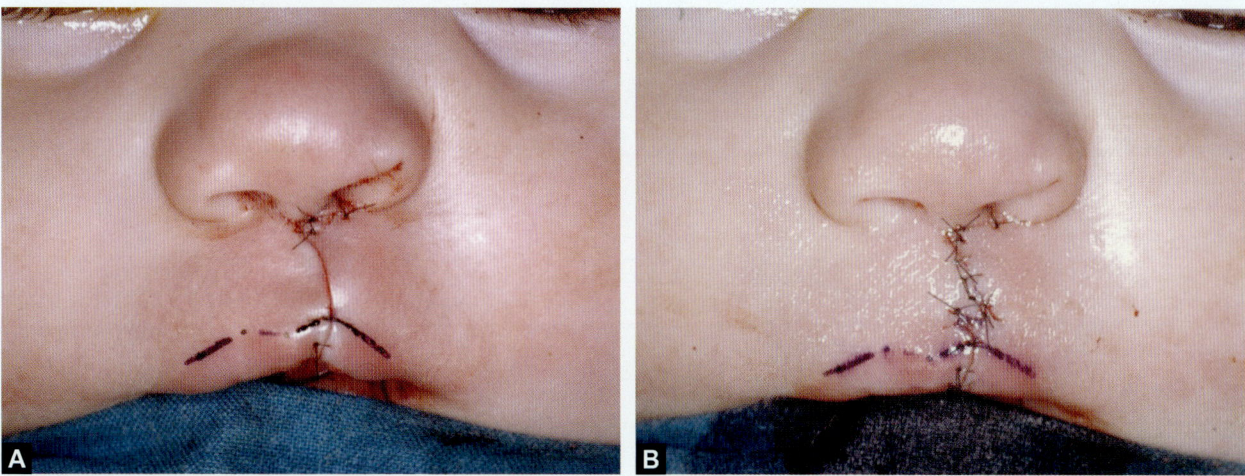

Figs 23A and B: Cheilorhinoplasty, reconstruction of the lip with the Millard's technique and small elongating Z-plasty

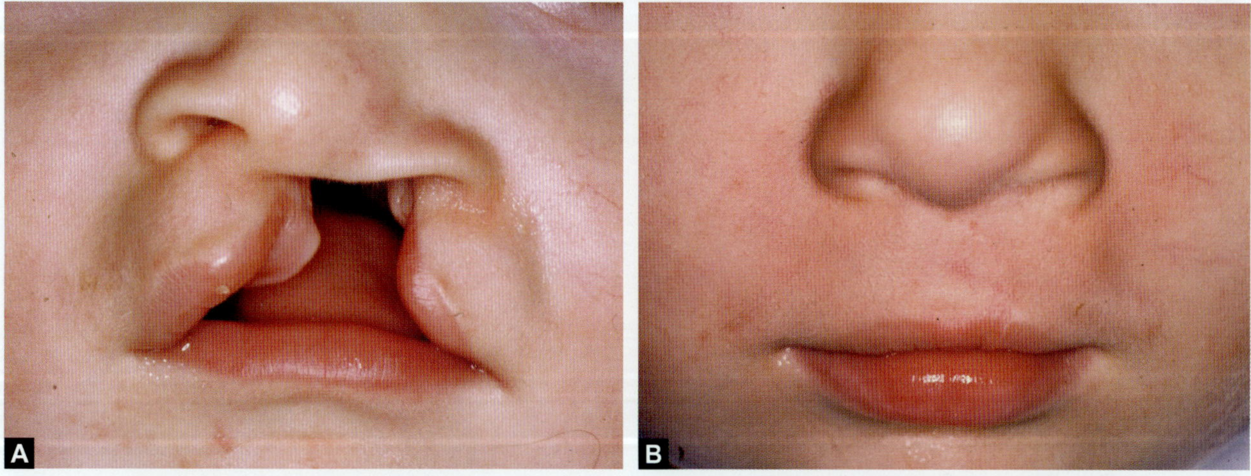

Figs 24A and B: Unilateral cleft lip and palate (UCLP), before and after primary reconstruction

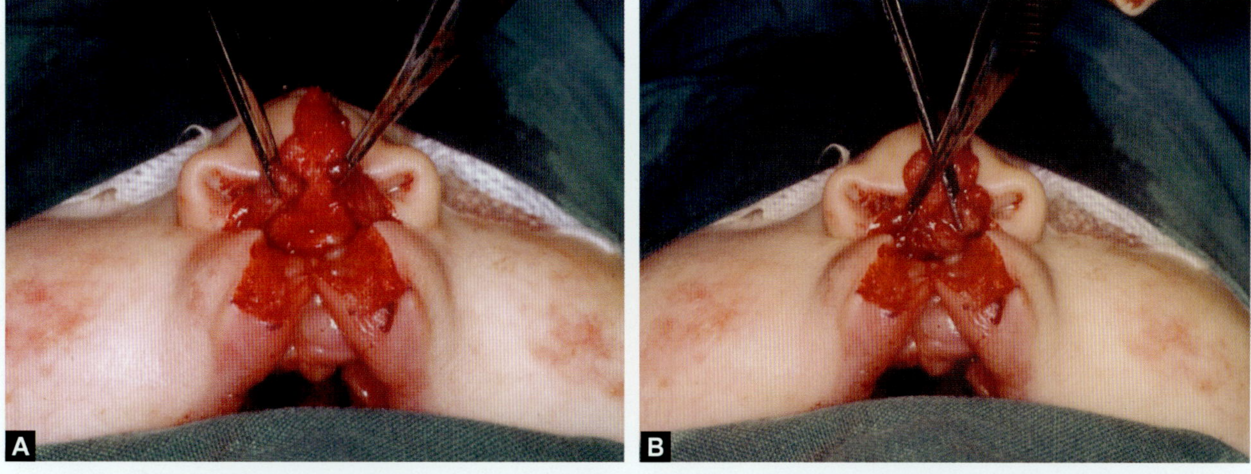

Figs 25A and B: Bilateral cleft lip and palate (BCLP), Delaire cheiloplasty and Delaire modified cheiloplasty

Cheilorhinoplasty of a Unilateral Cleft with an "All in One" Technique

This technique can be applied if the palate cleft does not exceed 10–12 mm.

When the alveolar processes of the cleft are near each other or in contact, the repair of the defect can be performed following the same two-step surgical protocol, but in a single operation. Otherwise, it is necessary to perform an alveolar bone graft at about 6 years of age.

Cheilorhinoplasty of a Bilateral Cleft in Two Steps

The basic principles are those that regulate the two-step treatment of the unilateral cleft. The role of the preoperative orthopedics is extremely important in these cases.

First Step

The operation starts with the reconstruction of the soft palate according to the surgical steps described above. The lip correction is performed in a manner similar to that described above, after a careful orthopedic preparation to obtain sufficient elongation of the columella and an adequate approximation of the stumps (Figs 27A to D).

If the protrusion of the premaxilla is extreme, it is preferable to carry out the so-called lip adhesion intervention, which consists of the suture of the skin and mucosa of the upper two-thirds of the cleft lip. This technique creates a partial cleft in order to retract the premaxilla in a few months, creating a favorable situation for the repair.

Incisions according to Mulliken approach are performed (Figs 28A and B).[11] The alar cartilages are

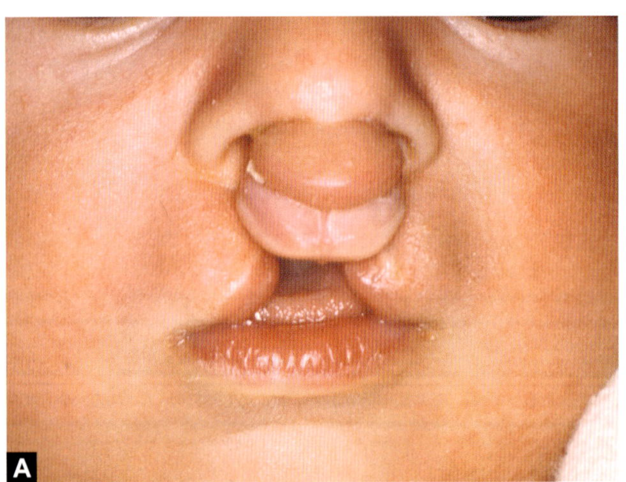

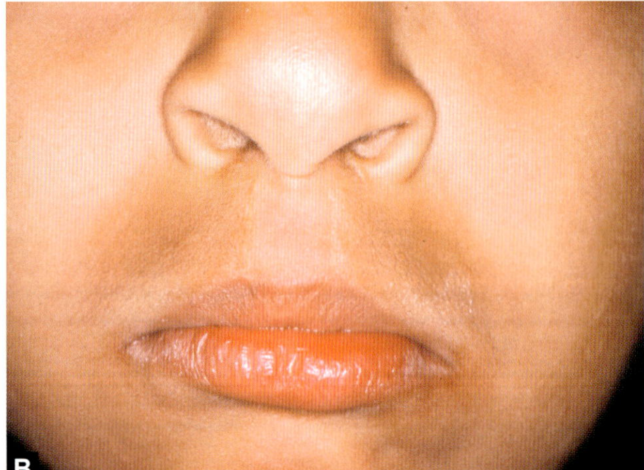

Figs 26A and B: Bilateral cleft lip and palate (BCLP), before and after primary reconstruction

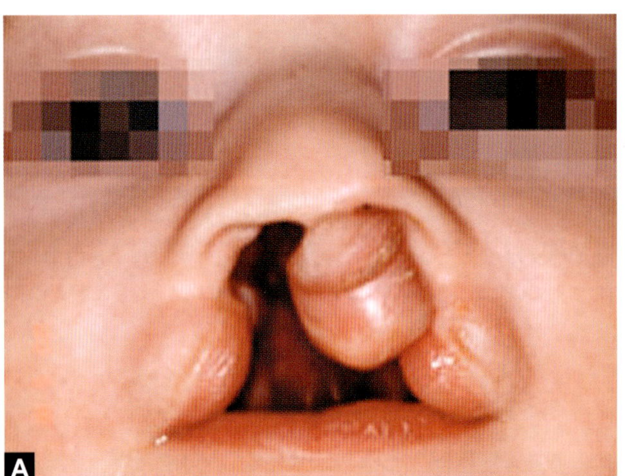

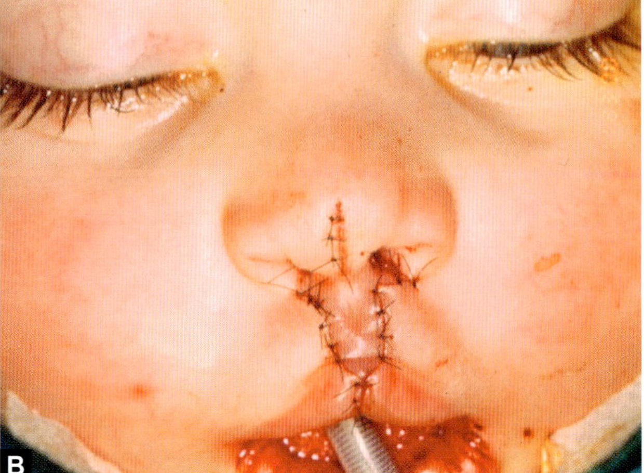

Figs 27A and B

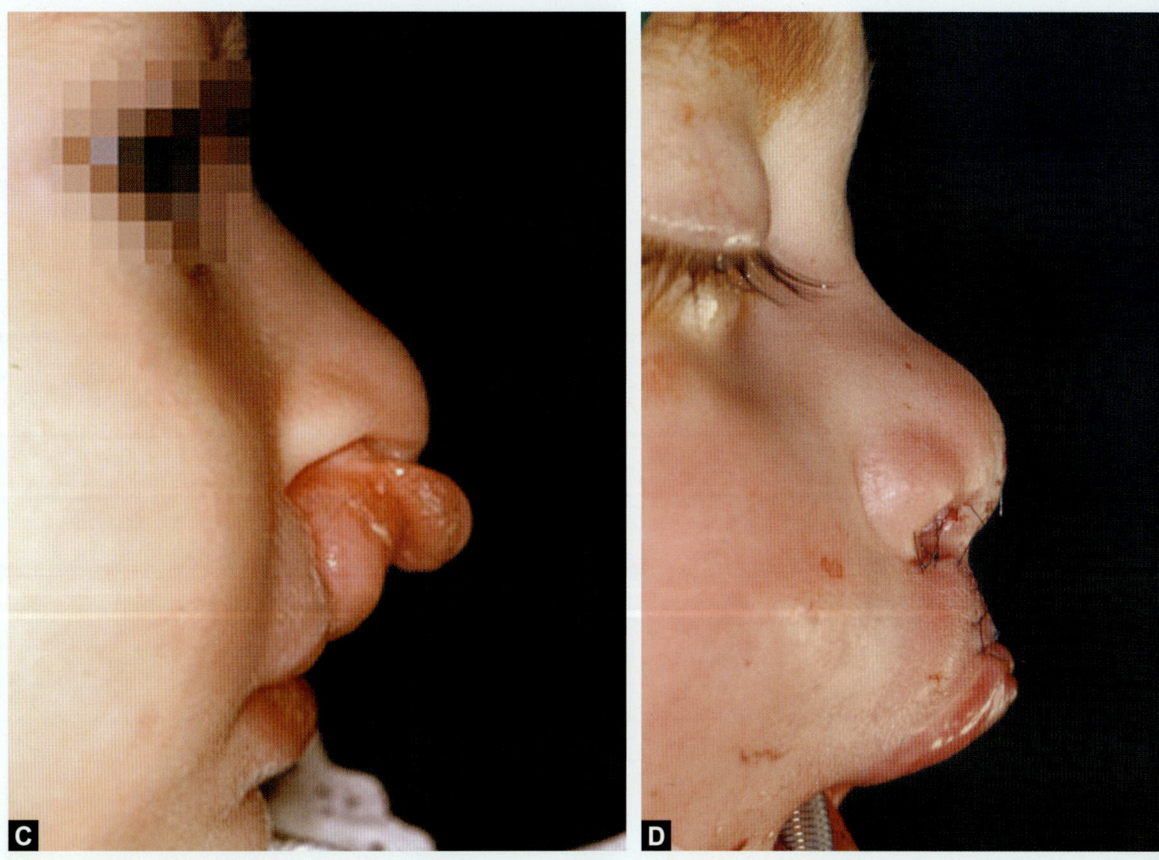

Figs 27A to D: Bilateral cleft lip and palate (BCLP), cheilorhinoplasty with primary columellar elongation

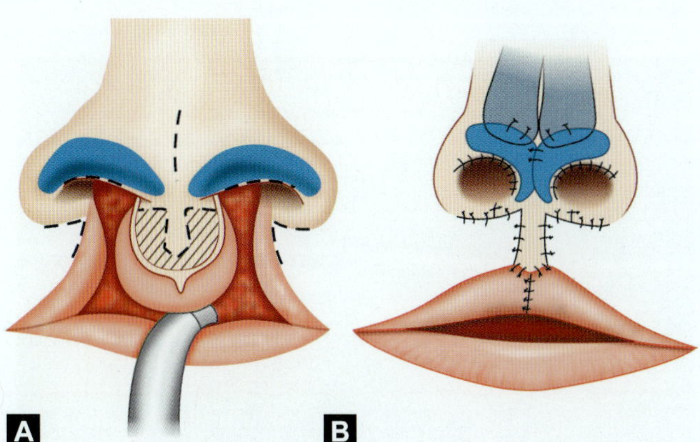

Figs 28A and B: Bilateral cleft lip and palate (BCLP), cheilorhinoplasty with primary columellar elongation
Source: Modified from Mulliken JB. Bilateral complete cleft lip and nasal deformity: an anthropometric analysis of staged to synchronous repair. Plast Reconstr Surg. 1995;96(1):9-23; discussion 24-6.

undermined from skin through marginal endonasal incisions and are brought towards the midline and sutured together.

The surgeon then sutures the transverse nasal and orbicularis oris muscles to rebuild the muscular plane of the lip. The labial skin is reconstructed and the nasal conformers are applied.

Second Step

At 18–24 months of age, the residual alveolar/HP cleft undergo repair following the same surgical procedures described for the unilateral cleft. It is important to pay particular attention to the preparation of the premaxillary flaps to avoid compromising the blood supply. This depends exclusively on the vestibular side, and therefore, the dissection should be minimal.

SURGICAL OUTCOMES

Nasal Fistulae

This complication occurs with frequency ranging from 2% to 30%, depending on the number of cases and the surgical techniques. These occur at the transition point between the hard plate and soft palate or more rarely, behind the premaxilla in bilateral clefts. The defect is repaired using local pedicle flaps, dissected and positioned without tension. In severe cases, due to the large size of the fistula or the poor quality of tissues resulting from past failures, the surgeon may use pedicle flaps obtained from the tongue or cheeks.

Velopharyngeal Insufficiency

In the case of failure in rehabilitative speech therapy, secondary surgery may be considered. Several techniques can be applied, including microscope-aided muscular repair, the Furlow technique of rotational Z-flaps, and sphincterial pharyngoplasty with rotation and suture of the posterior wall of pharynx and posterior palatine pillars. In extreme cases the superior pedicle velopharyngoplasty may be used, although this technique has potential side effects, including closed rhinolalia, sleep apnea and difficulty in blowing the nose (Figs 29 to 31).

Maxillary Hypoplasia

Depending on the series, the incidence in CLP patients is 15–45% and varies in relation to the surgical techniques used (Figs 32A and B), the timing of the operation and the operator's skill. As for the other jaw deformities, the optimal time for the osteotomy is after skeletal maturation. The intervention consists of a high Le Fort I osteotomy with mobilization of the bone segment and stabilization with plates and screws. The bony gaps are filled with autologous or bank bone grafts and stem cells (Figs 33 and 34). If large advancements are required due to the opposition offered by the existing scars, osteodistraction (Figs 35A to D) should be combined with the osteotomy using internal or external distractors. In selected cases, this technique can be performed before skeletal maturity occurs.

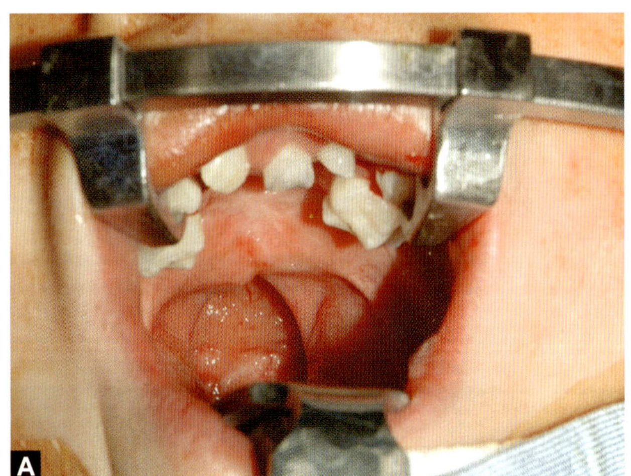

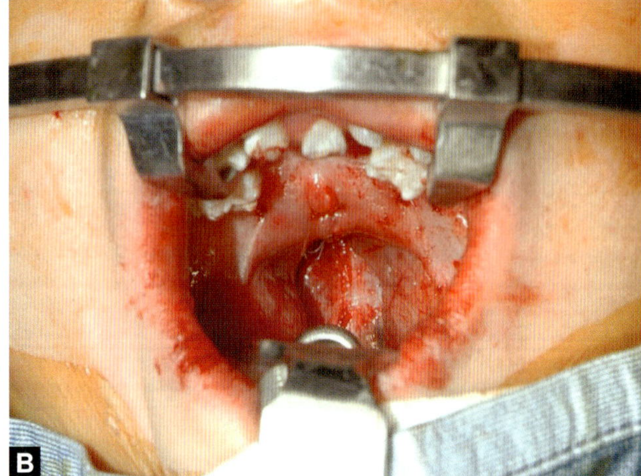

Figs 29A and B: Surgical outcomes, Sanvenero-Rosselli velopharyngoplasty

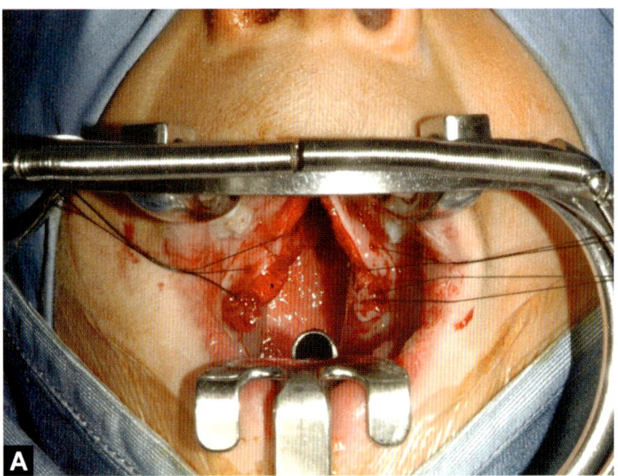

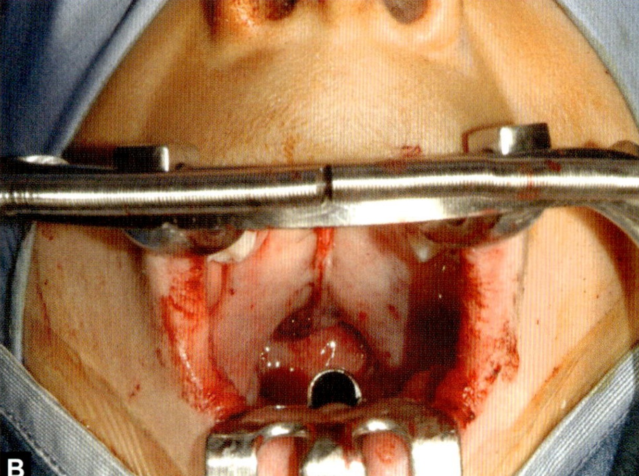

Figs 30A and B: Surgical outcomes, Hynes velopharyngoplasty

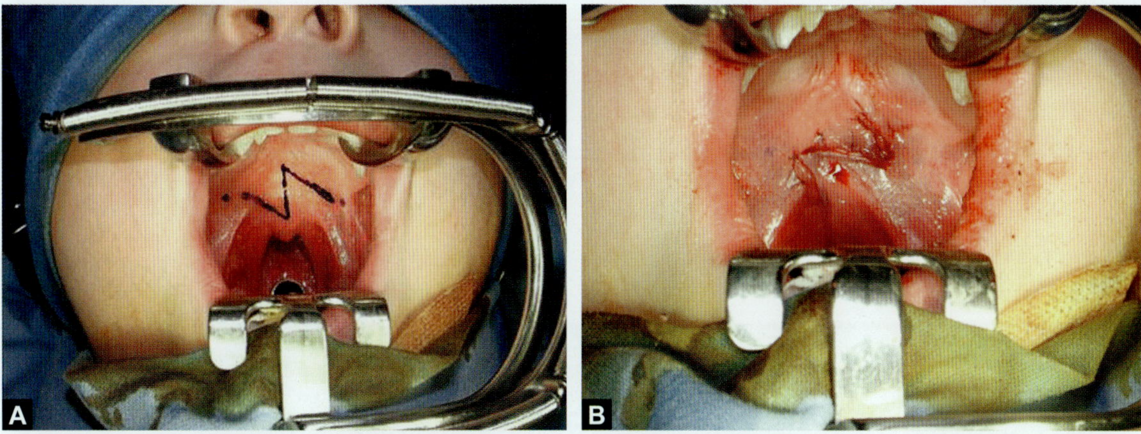

Figs 31A and B: Surgical outcomes, Furlow velopharyngoplasty

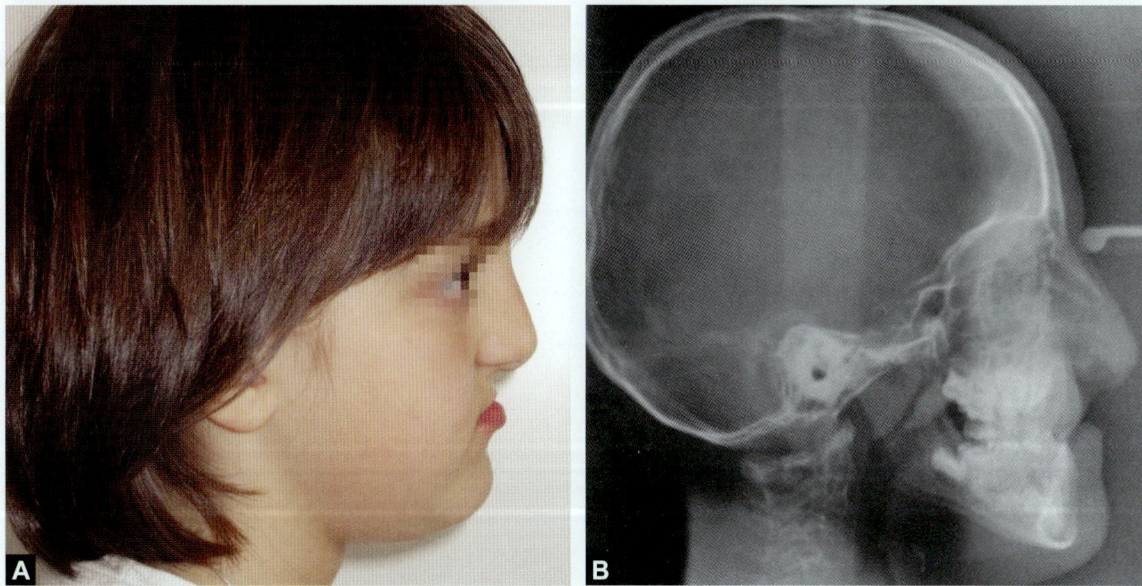

Figs 32A and B: Cleft lip and palate (CLP) outcomes, maxillary hypoplasia

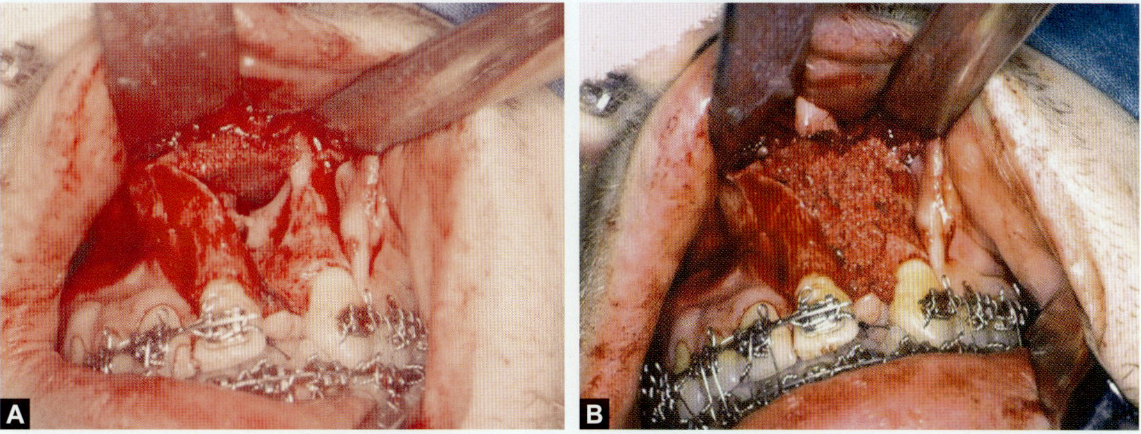

Figs 33A and B: Surgical outcomes, bone graft

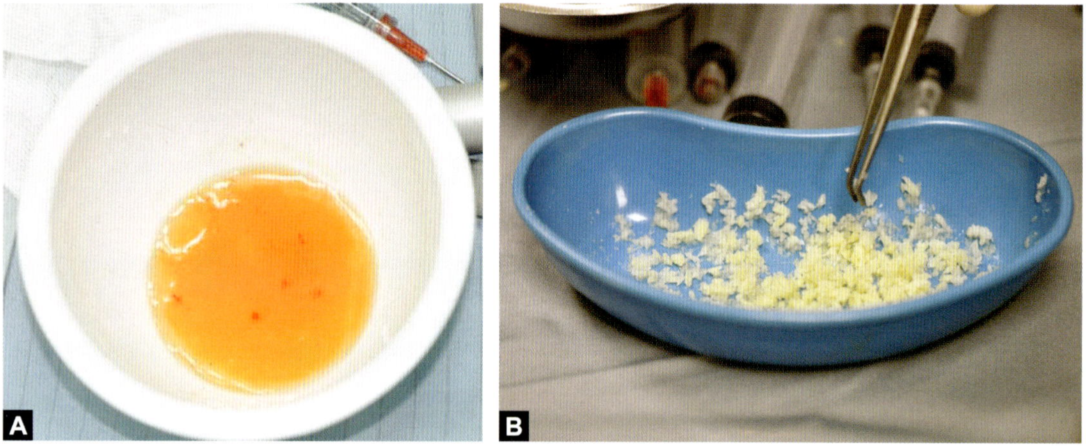

Figs 34A and B: Surgical outcomes, bone graft using homologous bone chips and stem cells

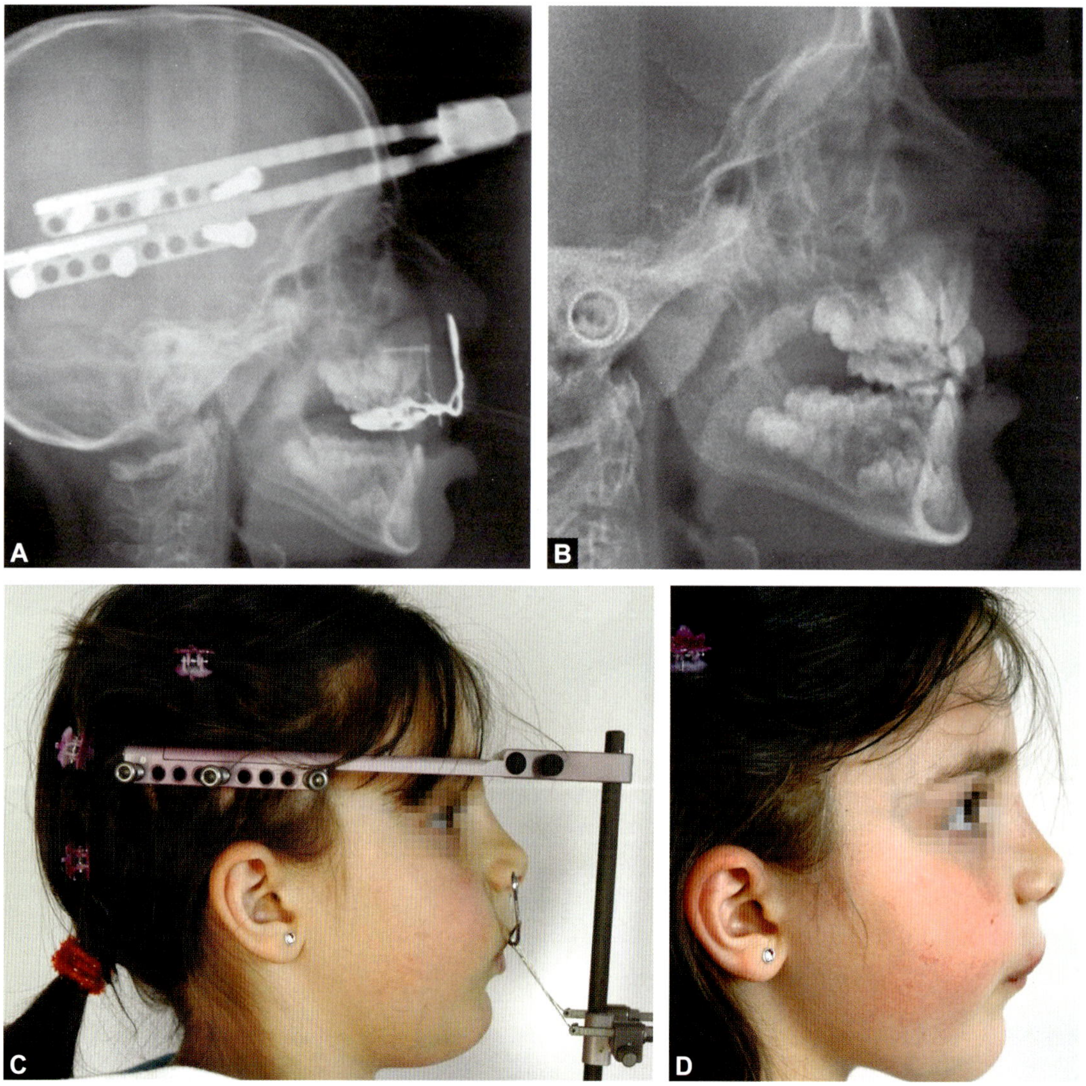

Figs 35A to D: Surgical outcomes, maxillary osteodistraction

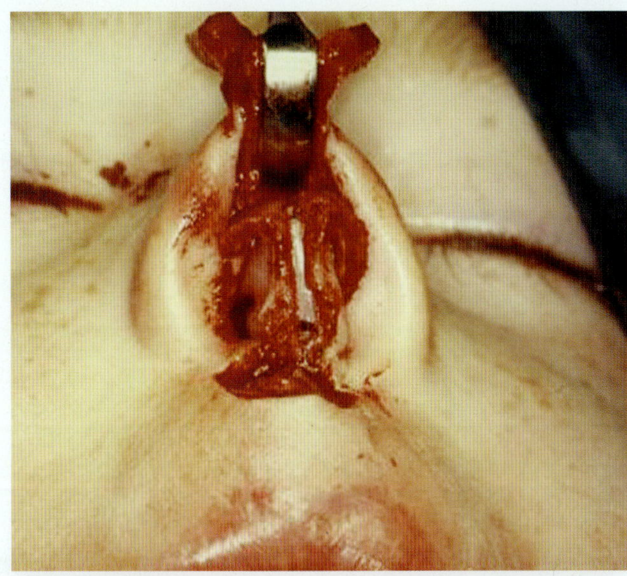

Fig. 36: Surgical outcomes, open rhinoseptoplasty

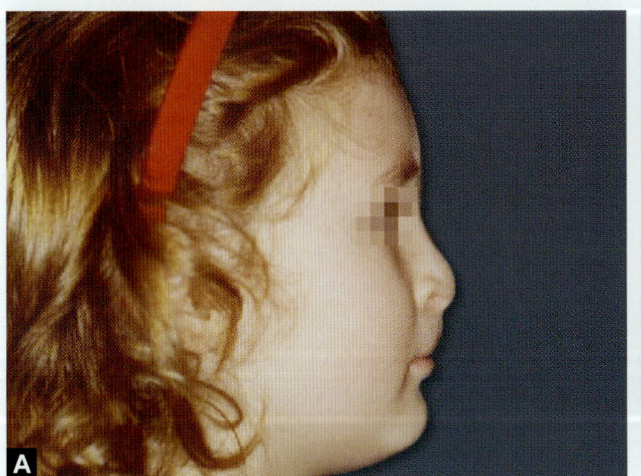

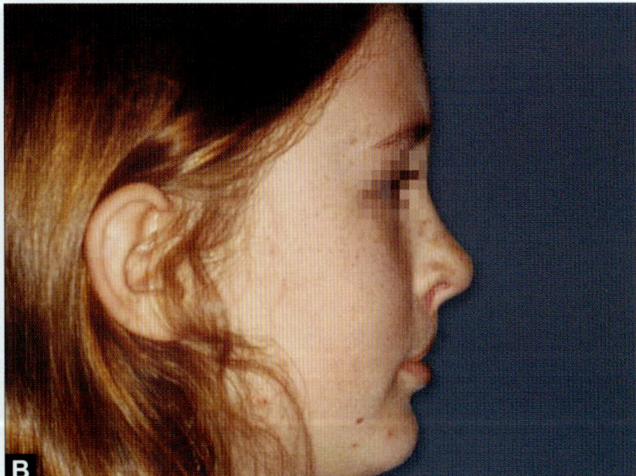

Figs 37A and B: Surgical outcomes, before and after open rhinoseptoplasty

Nasolabial Outcomes

These deformities and asymmetries are frequent and widely variable depending on the type of the cleft and the skill of the surgeon.

The most common nasolabial deformities and asymmetries, along with related treatment options include:

- *Cupid's bow asymmetry*: Lengthening with a Z-plasty or shortening through excision
- *Uneven mucocutaneous border*: Excision and realignment
- *Insufficient/inadequate muscle reconstruction*: Reopening of the scar, muscle-periosteal release, realignment and closure
- *Asymmetry of the free edge of the lip and/or insufficient thickness*: V-Y plasty, vestibular mucosal advancement and/or lipofilling
- *Nasal asymmetries associated with dystopia of the alar cartilage*: Open rhinoplasty (Figs 36 and 37) with reduction of the triangular cartilages, removal of the Gibbus and basal osteotomies. It is important to remember that a good rhinoplasty is not possible without a proper reconstruction of the nasolabial muscles
- *Shortness of the columella and alar cartilages diastasis*: Columellar lengthening is performed through preparation of two skin flaps carved along the previous scars. The alar cartilages are approximated. Bone grafts from the septal cartilage may be performed to support the tip.

REFERENCES

1. Gundlach KKH, Maus C. Epidemiological studies on the frequency of clefts in Europe and world-wide. J Craniomaxillofac Surg. 2006;34(2):1-2.
2. Dixon MJ, Marazita ML, Beaty TH, et al. Cleft lip and palate: understanding genetic and environmental influences. Nat Rev Genet. 2011;12(3):167-78.
3. Cohen MM. Malformations of the craniofacial region: evolutionary, embryonic, genetic, and clinical perspectives. Am J Med Genet. 2002;115(4):245-68.
4. Maue-Dickson W, Dickson DR. Anatomy and physiology related to cleft palate: current research and clinical implications. Plast Reconstr Surg. 1980;65(1):83-90.
5. Kirschner RE, LaRossa D. Cleft lip and palate. Otolaryngol Clin North Am. 2000;33(6):1191-215, v-vi.
6. Kernahan DA, Stark RB. A new classification for cleft lip and cleft palate. Plast Reconstr Surg Transplant Bull. 1958;22(5):435-41
7. Hotz M, Gnoinski W. Comprehensive care of cleft lip and palate children at Zürich university: a preliminary report. Am J Orthod. 1976;70(5):481-504.
8. Meazzini MC, Brusati R, Bozzetti A, et al. Craiofacial anamalies: Surgical-orthodontic management. Bologna: edizioni Martina; 2011.
9. Cutting C, Grayson B, Brecht L, et al. Presurgical columellar elongation and primary retrograde nasal reconstruction in one-stage bilateral cleft lip and nose repair. Plast Reconstr Surg. 1998;101(3):630-9.
10. Furlow LT. Cleft palate repair by double opposing Z-plasty. Plast Reconstr Surg. 1986;78(6):724-38.
11. Mulliken JB. Bilateral complete cleft lip and nasal deformity: an anthropometric analysis of staged to synchronous repair. Plast Reconstr Surg. 1995;96(1):9-23; discussion 24-6.

BIBLIOGRAPHY

1 Al-Omari F, Al-Omari IK. Cleft lip and palate in Jordan: birth prevalence rate. Cleft Palate Craniofac J. 2004;41(6):609-12.
2 Balboni GC. Anatomia umana. (terza edizione). Milano: edi-ermes; 1990.
3 Burd RS, Mellender SJ, Tobias JD. Neonatal and childhood perioperative considerations. Surg Clin North Am. 2006;86(2): 227-47, vii.
4 Campbell A, Costello BJ, Ruiz RL. Cleft lip and palate surgery: an update of clinical outcomes for primary repair. Oral Maxillofac Surg Clin North Am. 2010;22(1):43-58.
5 Cheng LR. Asian-American cultural perspectives on birth defects: focus on cleft palate. Cleft Palate J. 1990;27(3): 294-300.
6 Croen LA, Shaw GM, Wasserman CR, et al. Racial and ethnic variations in the prevalence of orofacial clefts in California, 1983-1992. Am J Med Genet. 1998;79(1):42-7.
7 Cutting C, Grayson B. The prolabial unwinding flap method for one-stage repair of bilateral cleft lip, nose, and alveolus. Plast Reconstr Surg. 1993;91(1):37-47.
8 Davies D. The one-stage repair of unilateral cleft lip and palate: a preliminary report. Plast Reconstr Surg. 1966;38(2):129-36.
9 De Mey A, Swennen G, Malevez C, et al. Long-term follow-up of UCLP at the Reine Fabiola Children's Hospital. B-ENT. 2006;2(Suppl 4):44-50.
10 Delaire J, Talmant JC, Billet J. [Evolution of techniques in cheiloplasty for cleft-lip (and study of a few complementary measures)]. Rev Stomatol Chir Maxillofac.
11 Dion K, Berscheid E, Walster E. What is beautiful is good. J Pers Soc Psychol. 1972;24(3):285-90.
12 Elahi MM, Jackson IT, Elahi O, et al. Epidemiology of cleft lip and cleft palate in Pakistan. Plast Reconstr Surg. 2004;113(6):1548-55.
13 Fara M. The musculature of cleft lip and palate. In: McCarthy JG (Ed). Plastic Surgery, 2nd edition. Philadelphia, PA: WB Saunders; 1990. pp. 2598-626.
14 Farina R. [Total unilateral harelip: correction of severe deformity of the palate & lips in a single operation; Le Mesurier's cheiloplasty & Veau-Ernst's gnatho-urano-staphyloplasty]. Ann Chir Plast. 1958;3(3):199-205.
15 Forrester MB, Merz RD. Descriptive epidemiology of oral clefts in a multiethnic population, Hawaii, 1986-2000. Cleft Palate Craniofac J. 2004;41(6):622-8.
16 Fudalej PS. One-stage repair of complete unilateral cleft lip and palate dentofacial treatment outcome. Wijchen: Benda Drukkers; 2011.
17 Grollemund B, Guedeney A, Vazquez MP, et al. Relational development in children with cleft lip and palate: influence of the waiting period prior to the first surgical intervention and parental psychological perceptions of the abnormality. BMC Pediatr. 2012;12:65. Doi: 10.1186/1471-2431-12-65.
18 Honigmann K. One-stage closure of uni- and bilateral cleft lip and palate. Br J Oral Maxillofac Surg. 1996;34(3):214-9.
19 Hunt O, Burden D, Hepper P, et al. The psychosocial effects of cleft lip and palate: a systematic review. Eur J Orthod. 2005;27(3):274-85.
20 Jones MC. The risk than an apparently isolated cleft lip with or without cleft palate will be associated with anomalies that impact outcome: follow-up of 32 cases ascertained through prenatal diagnosis. Proc Greenwood Genetic Center. 2000;19:122-3.
21 Kaplan I, Ben-Bassat M, Taube E, et al. Ten-year follow-up of simultaneous repair of cleft lip and palate in infancy. Ann Plast Surg. 1982;8(3):227-8.
22 Kaplan I, Dresner J, Gorodischer C, et al. The simultaneous repair of cleft lip and palate in early infancy. Br J Plast Surg. 1974;27(2):134-8.
23 Kaplan I, Taube E, Ben-Bassat M, et al. Further experience in the early simultaneous repair of cleft lip and palate. Br J Plast Surg. 1980;33(2):299-300.
24 Kim S, Kim WJ, Oh C, et al. Cleft lip and palate incidence among the live births in the Republic of Korea. J Korean Med Sci. 2002;17(1):49-52.
25 Kirby R, Petrini J, Alter C. Collecting and interpreting birth defects surveillance data by hispanic ethnicity: a comparative study. The Hispanic Ethnicity Birth Defects Workgroup. Teratology. 2000;61(1-2):21-7.
26 Landheer JA, Breugem CC, van der Molen AB. Fistula incidence and predictors of fistula occurrence after cleft palate repair: two-stage closure versus one-stage closure. Cleft Palate Craniofac J. 2010;47(6):623-30.

27 McLeod NM, Urioste ML, Saeed NR. Birth prevalence of cleft lip and palate in Sucre, Bolivia. Cleft Palate Craniofac J. 2004;41(2):195-8.

28 Meyerson MD. Cultural considerations in the treatment of Latinos with craniofacial malformations. Cleft Palate Craniofac J. 1990;27(3):279-88.

29 Millard DR. Nasal and labial flaps for alveolar and hard palate closure. In: Millard DR (Ed). Cleft Craft: The Evolution of Its Surgery. Alveolar and Palatal Deformities, Volume 3. Boston, USA: Little Brown and Company; 1980. pp. 249-62.

30 Millard DR Jr. Rotation-advancement principle in cleft lip closure. Cleft Palate J. 1964;12:246-52.

31 Mohler LR. Unilateral cleft lip repair. Plast Reconstr Surg. 1987;80(4):511-7.

32 Msamati BC, Igbigbi PS, Chisi JE. The incidence of cleft lip. cleft palate, hydrocephalus, and spina bifida at Queen Elizabeth Central Hospital, Blantyre, Malawi. Cent Afr J Med. 2000;46(11):292-6.

33 Mulliken JB. Correction of the bilateral cleft lip nasal deformity: evolution of a surgical concept. Cleft Palate Craniofac J. 1992;29(6):540-5.

34 Peterson-Falzone SJ, Hardin-Jones MA, Karnell MP. Cleft Palate Speech, 3rd edition. St Louis: Mosby; 2000.

35 Pfeiffer P. [Adhesive bridges for care of patients with cleft lip and palate after maxillofacial surgery and orthodontic treatment]. Quintessenz. 1987;38(6):1015-24.

36 Sanvenero-Rosselli G. [Cleft palate plastic surgery using a pharyngeal flap]. Langenbecks Arch Klin Chir Ver Dtsch Z Chir. 1960;295:895-900.

37 Shaw WC, Semb G, Nelson P, et al. The Eurocleft project 1996-2000: overview. J Craniomaxillofac Surg. 2001;29(3):131-40; discussion 141-2.

38 Strauss RP. Culture, health care, and birth defects in the United States: an introduction. Cleft Palate J. 1990;27(3): 275-8.

39 Suleiman AM, Hamzah ST, Abusalab MA, et al. Prevalence of cleft lip and palate in a hospital-based population in the Sudan. Int J Paediatr Dentist. 2005;15(3):185-9.

40 United States Census Bureau. Population by Age, Sex, Race, and Hispanic or Latino Origin for the United States: 2000 (PHC-T-9). [online]. Available from: www.census.gov/population/cen2000/phc-t9/tab01.pdf. [Accessed November 2012].

CHAPTER

108 Lip Reconstruction

Jagadish Tubachi, Karthikeyan Balasubramanian, Sumeet Pahwa, Sultan Pradhan

INTRODUCTION

The lips are important in both an esthetic and functional sense. Tumor ablative surgery of lip results in considerable cosmetic and functional morbidity. So, optimal reconstruction of the lip is important to minimize the esthetic and functional morbidity.[1] Choice of surgical reconstruction of lip defects depends on the location and extent of the defect. A number of methods have been described, but only few are a practically simple and reliable. The ultimate goal of lip reconstruction is to achieve oral competence and good aesthesis, which is socially acceptable.

ANATOMY

The lips comprise of two mobile structures that represent the anterior boundaries of the oral cavity. The lips function dynamically in deglutition, speech and facial expression. The normal lip is at about 5–6 cm long. The orbicularis oris muscle forms the main bulk of the lip and maintenance of it's continuity is important for oral competence. This muscle has no bony attachments. A second group of dilator muscles are attached in radial manner around the orbicularis oris, consisting of the mentalis, depressor anguli oris, depressor labii inferioris, risorius, zygomaticus major and minor, levator anguli oris and levator labii superioris. In opening and closing of the mouth, the orbicularis works synergistically with a group of dilator muscles arranged in a radial fashion around the mouth.

Blood supply is from the paired superior and inferior labial branches of the facial artery. The labial arteries run submucosally on the intraoral side of the lips, meeting in the midline (Fig. 1).

Superior labial artery branches from facial artery deep to zygomaticus major. It gives off angular artery and then enters orbicularis oris. It runs along the upper lip and anastomoses with opposite side (see Figs 2A to D).

The average distance of the superior labial artery from the labial commissure is about 12.1 mm. This is important in planning of axial flaps. To preserve the arterial integrity during raising of axial flap, the point of rotation should have minimum of 13–15 mm of tissue preserved near the oral commissure.[2]

Inferior labial artery branches from facial artery near the commissure. It traverses deep to depressor angularis oris to enter orbicularis oris and runs along lower lip to anastomose with opposite side.

Inferior labial artery is located at an depth ranging from 5 mm to 10 mm from the free border of lip.[3] Thus, it can be said that during harvesting of Abbe-Estlander flap, a 10 mm pedicle thickness is enough to preserve the arterial integrity.

Motor supply to the lip muscles is from the facial nerve, primarily the buccal and marginal mandibular branches.

The vermilion is dry due to a lack of mucous glands and has exposed position outside the oral cavity, whereas the "wet" portion of the lip is well supplied with mucous by minor salivary glands. The red color is due to the rich blood supply to the region. A thin pale junctional zone of skin (known as the "white line") demarcates the junction between vermilion and skin. This white line should be aligned correctly during lip repair for optimal esthetic outcome (Fig. 1).

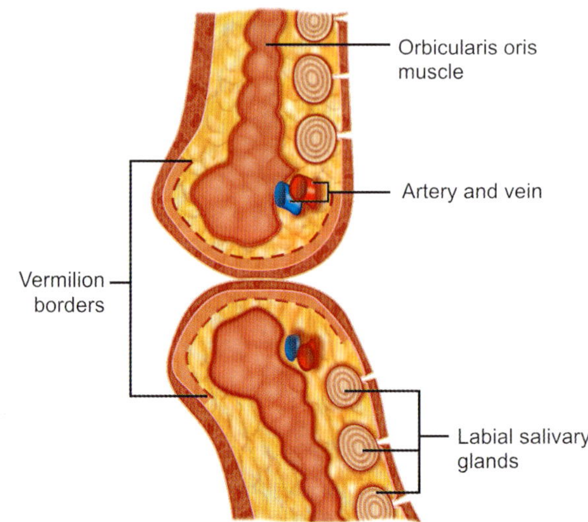

Fig. 1: Schematic representation of cross-section of lip: The labial arteries run submucosal on the intraoral side of the lips

RECONSTRUCTION OF LIP DEFECTS

Reconstruction of Vermilion Defect: Vermilion Advancement

Very superficial carcinoma of the lip is treated by lip shave. Primary closure of wound is ideal for small defects[4] (Figs 2A to D). A large defect is reconstructed by the vermilion advancement. After resection, assistant stretches the lip with skin hooks and only the mucosa is lifted from the underlying orbicularis oris. As the elevation is continued toward the labial sulcus, a layer of minor salivary glands is encountered (Fig. 1). Flap elevation is continued between orbicularis oris and the layer of minor salivary glands into gingivolabial sulcus and above the periosteum of lower alveolus (Fig. 2E). During

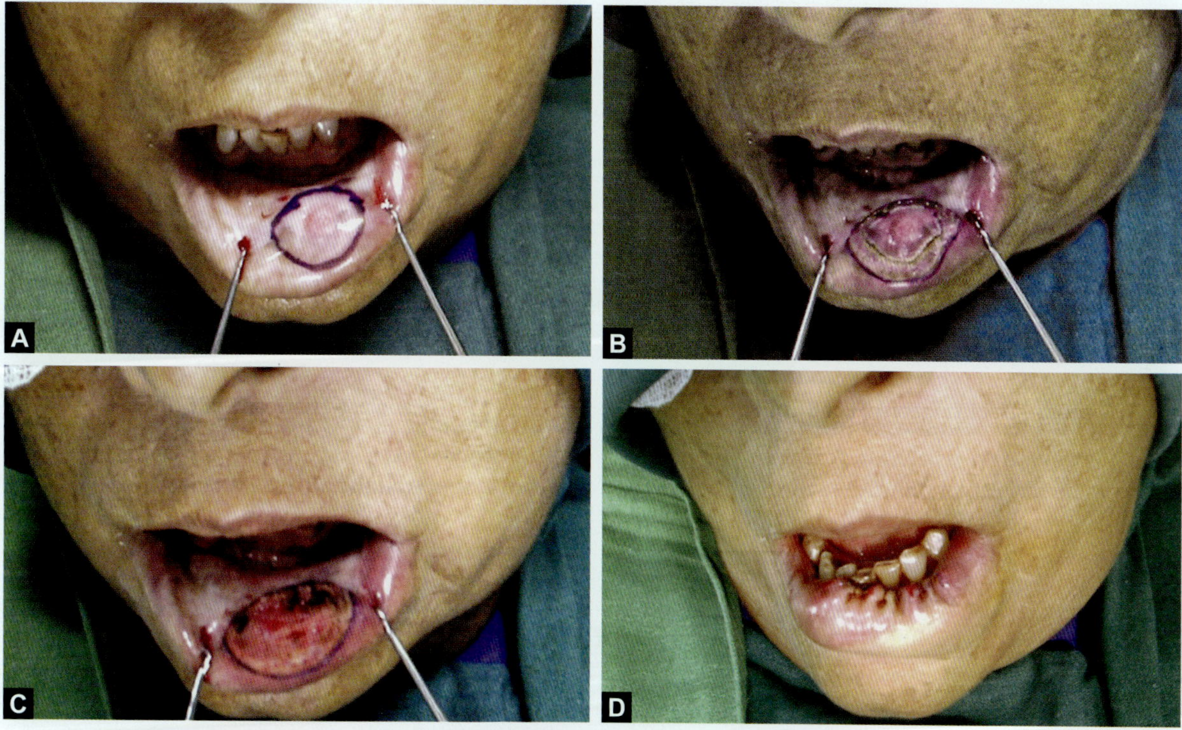

Figs 2A to D: Very superficial carcinoma of lip is treated by lip shave. A resultant small defect was primarily closed

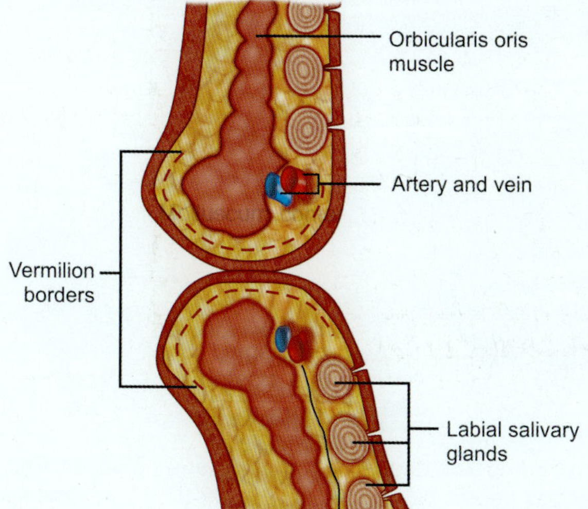

Fig. 2E: Plane of dissection for vermillion advancement

the flap elevation, "button holing" is avoided. Adequacy of flap is assessed. If the flap is short, release incision is made in the gingival sulcus.[4] The flap is draped over the defect in a tension less manner and sutured with non-absorbable material of surgeon's choice.

RECONSTRUCTION OF LIP DEFECTS: LESS THAN ONE-THIRD OF LIP DEFECT

Small lesion involving full thickness of lip can be excised in V-shaped manner. The resultant defect is primarily closed. Larger lesion can be excised in a rectangular fashion. The defect is closed by advancing the lip through release incision in the lip-chin crease (Figs 3A and B).[5]

RECONSTRUCTION OF LIP DEFECTS: ONE-HALF TO TWO-THIRDS OF LOWER LIP

Primary closure of defects larger than one-half of the lip is difficult. So, the defect is reconstructed by borrowing "like" tissue from the opposite lip.

ABBE CROSS-LIP FLAP

Abbe cross-lip flap is based on the principle of creating a labial artery based full thickness lip flap, which includes skin, muscle and mucosa. This flap is switched from donor lip to defect in the opposite lip. This flap is based on the labial artery—either superior or inferior. This is an ideal for lesions involving from one-third to two-thirds of the lip (Figs 4 and 5).[5,6]

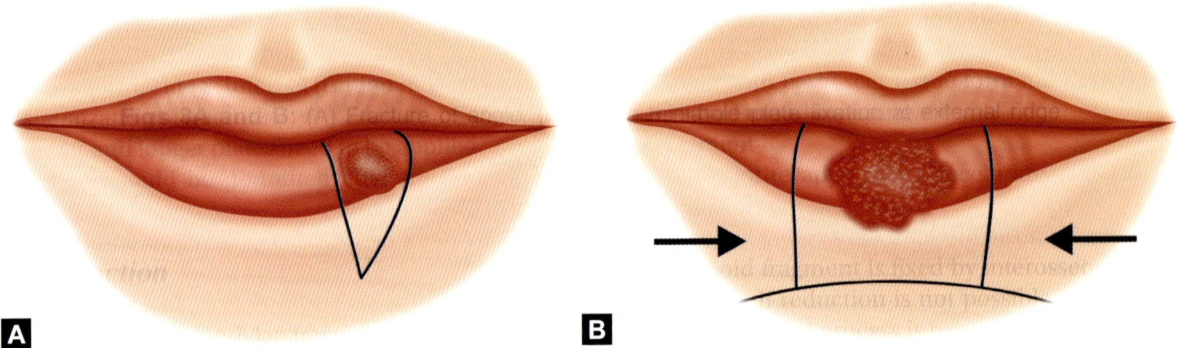

Figs 3A and B: Direct excision and repair of lower lip lesions. Defect less than one-half can be repaired primarily. Small lesions can be excised using the "V" excision and the defect is closed in three layers. The larger lesions can be excised as a rectangle and incisions made in the lip-chin crease to allow advancement of lateral lip tissue for closure

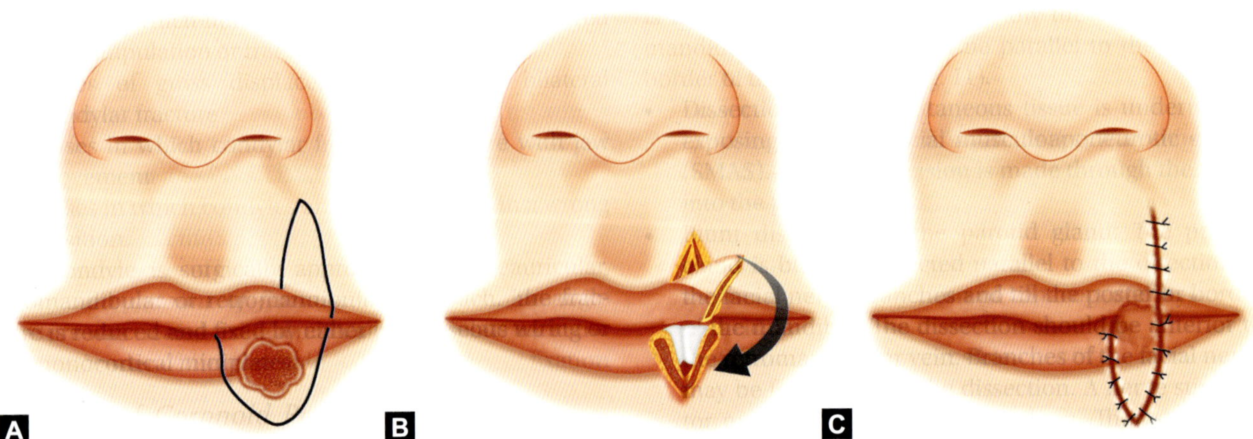

Figs 4A to C: Abbe cross-lip flap: (A) V-shaped excision is planned around the lower lip lesion and proposed flap from upper lip; (B) Lesion is excised. Flap is designed with same height as defect, but only 50% of width; (C) Flap is transposed and sutured into defect

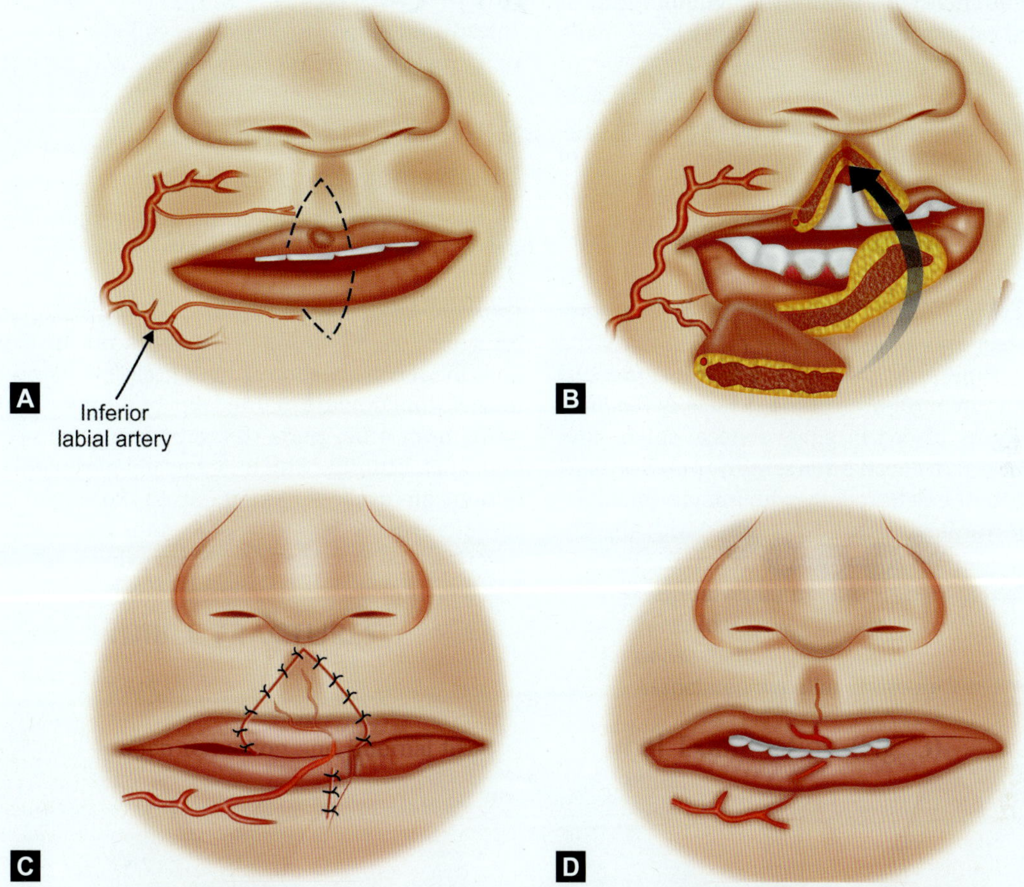

Figs 5A to D: Schematic representation of vascular pedicle of Abbe cross lip flap

Flap Design

The flap width should be approximately one-half of the width of the defect so that width of both the upper and the lower lips is reduced by the same amount. Two centimeter is the maximum recommended width of the flap.

Surgical Steps

The surgical steps of Abbe cross lip flap are as follows:

- Measure the lip defect.
- Design the flap on the opposite lip to be half the width and same height as that of the defect.
- Incise skin with knife. Incision is deepened through subcutaneous tissue, orbicularis oris and mucosa. Incision stops just short of white line to protect underlying vascular pedicle.
- Rotate the flap into the defect.
- Flap is sutured in three layers.
- The pedicle is divided after 3 weeks and necessary esthetic adjustments are made.

Postoperative Care

There is a risk of damage to the vascular pedicle either by dental trauma or by opening mouth widely. So patient is advised liquid and pureed diet till the vascularity is established.

Advantage

- Technically easy to raise the flap.

Disadvantages

- This is a two-staged procedure.
- There is risk of damage to the pedicle by dental trauma or by opening mouth is wide.
- Relative microstomia, which depends on the size of defect.

THE ESTLANDER FLAP

The Estlander flap is quite similar to the Abbe flap. It is ideal for reconstruction of defect involving the oral commissure. The flap is raised similar to Abbe flap. The key difference is that the rotation occurs around the commissure. It provides a good esthetic outcome(Figs 6A to F).[5]

Karapandzic Flap

This flap involves reconstruction of central lip defect (30 to 80%) with intact commissure by medial mobilization of skin, muscle and mucosa of nasolabial region. While doing so, blood and nerve supply of orbicularis is preserved.[9]

Flap Design (Figs 7A to C)

The key surgical steps begin with drawing the incision around the defect and continuing the incisions into the nasolabial fold superiorly. Only skin and subcutaneous tissue is incised down till orbicularis muscle is reached. Mucosal incision is placed in gingivobuccal sulcus and sufficient mucosa is advanced. Then skin and mucosal flaps are advanced into the defect along with intact orbicularis oris. Mucosa and orbicularis oris are sutured with absorbable suture material. Vermilion edges of both the cut end are approximated to achieve optimal esthetic appearance.

Advantages

The advantages of this flap are as follows:

- It preserves perioral sensation and function of the orbicularis oris.
- It provides good cosmoses.

Disadvantage

- Microstomia, which is directly proportional to the size of defect.

Reconstruction of Total Lip Defect

After total resection of lip, there is no lip tissue available for reconstruction. In such case, it is not possible to give functional lip. The aim of surgery is to import tissue from other parts of the body to give near normal appearance of lip, which is socially acceptable. Various options are available ranging from nasolabial flap (NLF) to microvascular free tissue transfer.[7] Here, authors describe few reliable local flaps, which are technically less demanding.

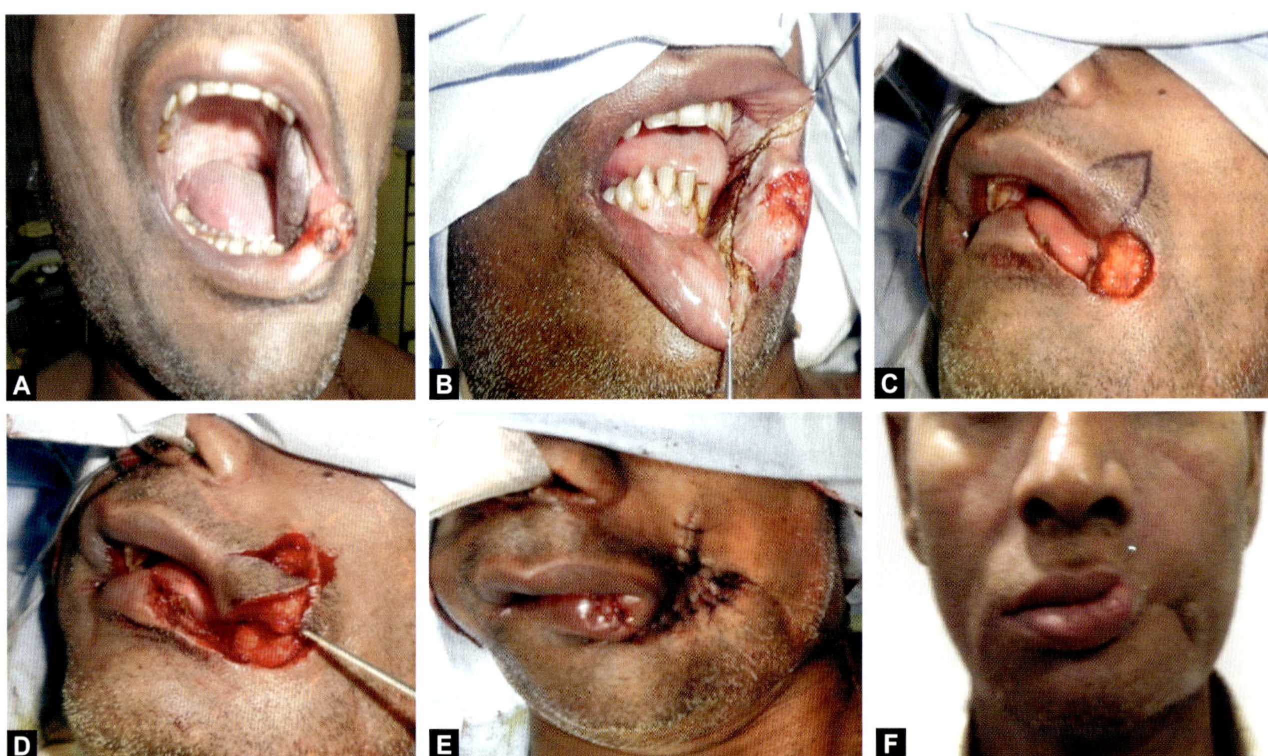

Figs 6A to F: Abbe-Estlander flap: A 45-year-old patient with second primary over left one-third of the lower lip and angle of mouth. Full thickness excision of lateral third of lower lip with angle of mouth was done. The proposed Estlander flap is outlined. Flap is raised, rotated and sutured into defect. Postoperative view 6 months later

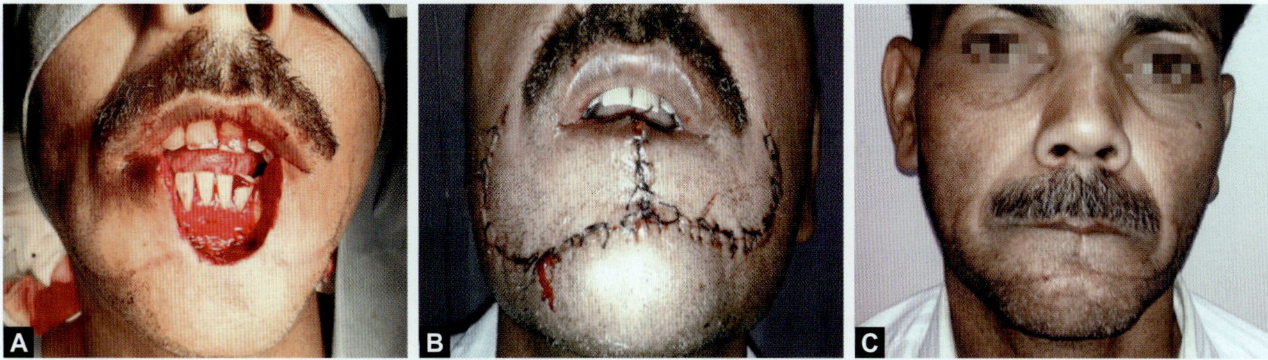

Figs 7A to C: Karapandzic flap reconstruction: Carcinoma of middle third lower lip (Figs A to C) is represented. Full thickness resection was done. Incision for Karapandzic flap is outlined. Flap is raised and sutured in place. Meticulous approximation of vermilion border is done for good esthetic appearance. Postoperative appearance after 2 years

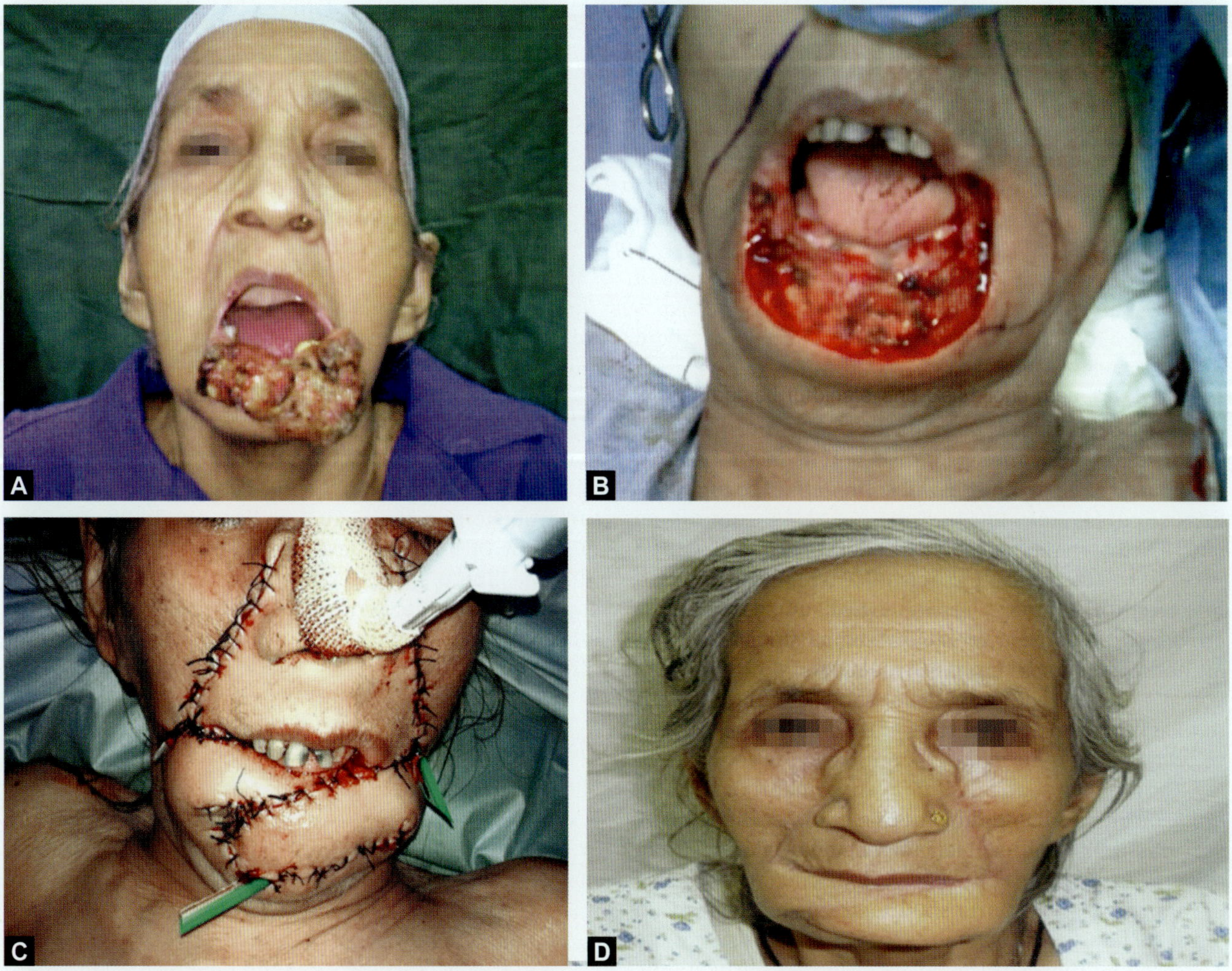

Figs 8A to D: Elderly female presenting with carcinoma of lower lip. Full thickness total lower lip resection was done. The defect was reconstructed with bilateral NLF. Postoperative appearance after 3 years

Bilateral Nasolabial Flap

A total lower lip resection is a difficult situation for reconstruction. Author prefers bilateral NLF for reconstruction of total lower lip defects (Figs 8A to D).

Flap Design

The length of NLF should be approximately same as the length of the excised lower lip. The height of defect corresponds to the width of NLF. This flap is based on subcutaneous and dermal plexus.[7] In case of thin skin of patient, flap can be harvested to include underlying musculature to increase the bulk of flap.

Surgical Steps

The surgical steps of this flap are as follows:

- Full thickness excision of lower lip defect is carried out.
- *Marking for the flap*: The flap is outlined such that the length of NLF should be approximately same as the width of the excised lower lip. The height of defect corresponds to the width of NLF. The suture line of flap donor site should follow natural nasolabial fold to minimize esthetic morbidity.
- Incise the skin and subcutaneous tissue. Depending on the situation, thickness of the flap can be modified by including sufficient subcutaneous tissue. Nasolabial flap is elevated on both sides.
- Both the flaps are mobilized. One of the flaps is sutured to remaining labial alveolar mucosa, and other flap is sutured to skin at outer resection margin. Then, both flaps are sutured together.

Reconstruction of Upper Lip Forehead Visor Flap

Visor flap is very useful in reconstruction of entire upper lip (Figs 9A to D).[10]

Flap Design

The forehead visor flap is based on bilateral superficial temporal (ST) vessels. So, this is a bipedicled flap. Superficial temporal artery divides approximately 2 cm above the zygomatic arch into anterior and posterior branches, which then sends perforators to the overlying subdermal layer.[8]

Procedure

- Bilateral ST vessels are traced using doppler ultrasonography. Flap is designed around the ST vessels. The height of flap should be twice the height of defect, so when folded, it forms both mucosal and skin lining
- Skin is incised with scalpel till the level of pericranium. Flap is raised above the pericranium. One should be careful not to violate pericranium, which forms the bed for skin grafting.

Advantages

- Technically less demanding.
- Flap has excellent vascularity, so chances of flap necrosis are minimal.

Disadvantages

- The donor site needs skin grafting and the resultant cosmosis is poor. The donor site morbidity is minimized by the use of a tissue expander.
- This is a two-staged procedure, which requires flap division.

RECONSTRUCTION OF LIP COMPOSITE DEFECT

Advanced carcinoma of lower lip involves paramandibular soft tissues. Curative surgery involves full thickness lip resection with segmental mandibulectomy. Reconstruction mandible and surrounding soft tissue is essential to provide adequate oral competence and appearance.[4]

Reconstruction of Lip Composite Defect with Pectoralis Major Myocutaneous Flap[11]

It has an axial blood supply. It is based on the pectoral branch of the acromiothoracic artery.

Positioning, Prepping and Draping

The patient is placed in a supine position with the chest exposed. Entire chest and ipsilateral axilla are scrubbed and chest is draped as shown in Figure 10.

Surface Markings of the Vascular Pedicle

The surface markings of the vascular pedicle are determined by drawing a line from the shoulder to the xiphisternum and another line, vertically from the midpoint of the sternoclavicular notch to intersect the first line. The point, 2–3 cm medial to corocoid process, approximately represents surface marking of vascular hilum. From this point the pedicle runs in a curved direction towards the point of bisection which is already described (Fig. 10).

Flap Design (Fig. 10)

The flap is employed as musculocutaneous island flap. It is based on the pectoral branch of the acromiothoracic artery. The skin paddle is designed at the level of nipple so that the flap reaches till the site of defect. In order to ensure that the flap is of adequate length, the distance between the superior edge of the skin paddle and the clavicle should be equal to the distance between the inferior margin recipient site and the clavicle. Size of the flap should be slightly bigger than the size of defect to compensate for the shrinkage of skin paddle.

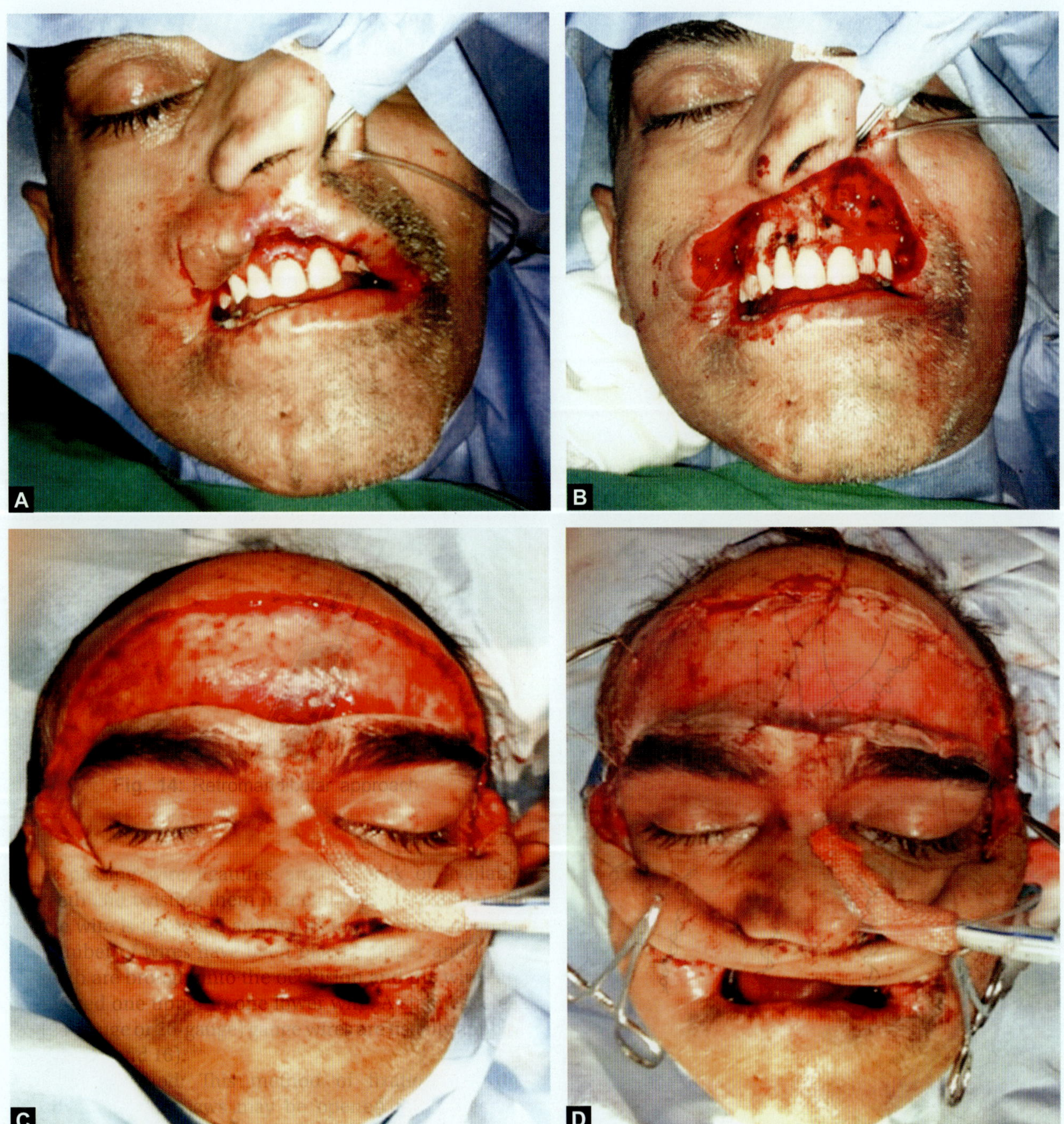

Figs 9A to D: Recurrent carcinoma upper lip involving entire lip (Figs A to D). Full thickness excision with premaxillectomy was done. Superficial temporal vessels are traced by using doppler ultrasonography. Flap is designed on bilateral ST vessels. Bipedicled forehead flap is raised and sutured to the margins of defect. Rest of the flap is tubed. Donor site is covered with split thickness skin graft

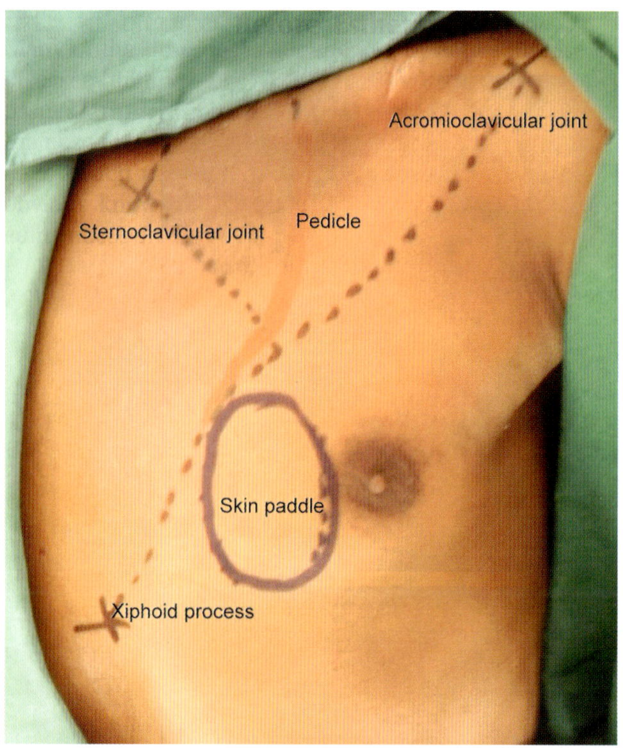

Fig. 10: Surface markings of pectoral branch of acromiothoracic artery

Procedure

- Skin incision is made with scalpel. Incision is further deepened with electrocautery to minimize blood loss. An incision is extended laterally from the peripheral margin of the skin paddle along the anterior axillary fold, which corresponds with the lateral margin of the pectoralis major muscle. Incision is carried through subcutaneous tissue to the level of pectoralis muscle. Superior flap is developed till the level of clavicle. At this stage, lateral edge of pectoralis major muscle is identified. A plane is created through the loose areolar tissue present between pectoralis major and minor muscle, until the vascular pedicle is identified. The pectoralis major muscle is divided lateral to the pedicle. While doing so, the pedicle is always kept in view. At this stage, muscle is rotated medially and attachment of muscle from the rib is released with electrocautery. Medial end of the muscle is divided such that perforators of internal mammary vessels are preserved. Pectoral nerves are encountered during mobilization of flap are divided.
- *Skin tunnel over clavicle*: The flap is generally passed into the neck, superficial to the clavicle through a wide subcutaneous tunnel, which is created at the level of clavicle (Fig. 10). The tunnel should be large enough to permit easy delivery of the flap into the neck without

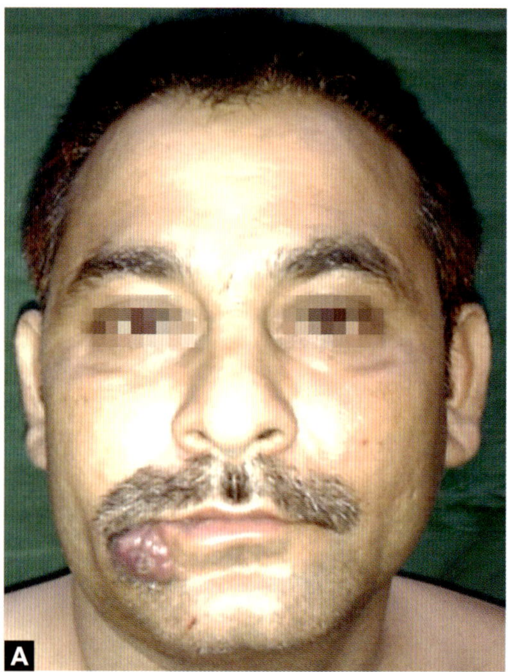

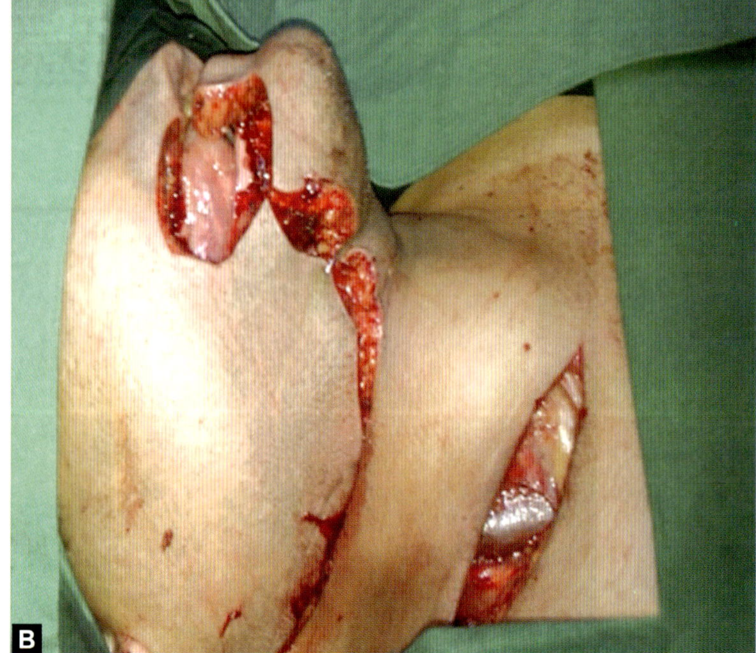

Figs 11A and B

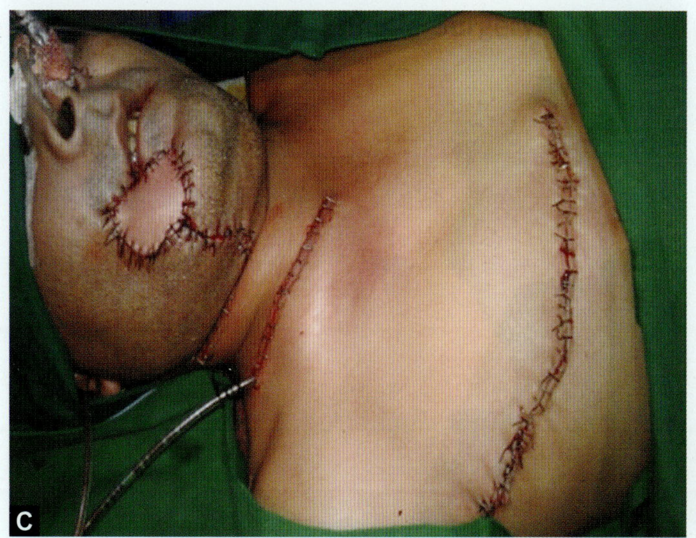

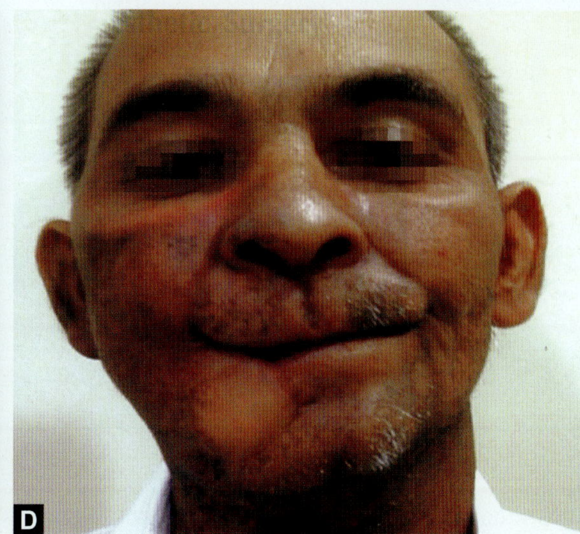

Figs 11A to D: Reconstruction of lip composite defect with pectoralis major myocutaneous flap. Carcinoma of right lower gingivolabial sulcus with involvement of lateral third of lower lip is represented (Figs 11A to D). Full thickness lip composite resection was done. Defect was reconstructed with bipaddled pectoralis myocutaneous (PMMC) flap. Postoperative appearance after 6 months

shearing the musculocutaneous perforators supplying the skin paddle and to avoid strangulating the vascular pedicle. The flap is passed through the subcutaneous tunnel and fed into the recipient area.

Closure of Donor Site Defect

The donor site is closed primarily by mobilization of the surrounding skin.

REFERENCES

1. Moretti M, Vitullo, et al. Surgical management of lip cancer. ACTA otorhinolaryngologica italica. 2011;3:5-10
2. Schutle DL, David A, et al. The anatomical basis of the Abbé flap. The Laryngoscope. HYPERLINK "http://onlinelibrary.wiley.com/doi/10.1002/lary.v111:3/issuetoc." 2001;111(3): 382-6.
3. HYPERLINK "http://www.ncbi.nlm.nih.gov pubmed?term=Edizer%20M%5BAuthor%5D&cauthor=tre&cauthor_uid=12794457" Edizer M, HYPERLINK "http:/www.ncbinlm.nih.gov/pubmed?term=Ma%C4%9Fden%2O%5BAuthor%5D&cauthor=true&cauthor_uid=12794457" Maden O etal.Arterial anatomy of the lower lip: a cada eric study. HYPERLINK "http://www.ncbi.nlm.nih gov/pubmed/12794457"\o"Plastic and reconstructive surgery." Plast Reconstr Surg. 2003;111(7):2176-81.
4. Ramon M, Micheal A. Lip Cancer. Head & Neck Surgery: Otolaryngology, p. 1541.
5. Alzacko SM. Surgical treatment of squamous cell carcinoma (SCC) of the lip in northern Iraq. The Iraqui Postgraduate Medical Journal. 2010; 9(2).
6. Papel I, et al. Facial plastic and reconstructive surgery. Chapter 51: Lip Reconstruction. Thieme Publishing, New York, NY; 2002; 634-45.
7. Eckardt, et al. Reconstruction of oral mucosal defects using the nasolabial flap: clinical experience with 22 patients. Head & Neck Oncology. 2011, 3:28.
8. Kleintjes WG. The vascular anatomy the forehead and related forehead flaps and it's application in plastic and reconstructive surgery. Dissertation for the degree of PhD at the University of Stellenbosch; 2007. p. 37.
9. Karapandzic M. Reconstruction of lip defects by local arterial flaps. Br J Plast Surg. 1974;27:93-7.
10. Nthumba P, Carter L. Visor flap for total upper and lower lip reconstruction: a case report. Journal of Medical Case Reports. 2009;3:7312.
11. Gregor RT. The use of the myocutaneous reconstruction after major head and neck surgery SAMEDIESE TYDSKRIF. 1982; pp. 788-92.

CHAPTER

109 Operative Techniques in Mandible Fractures

Rajesh R Yadav, PV Dhond

INTRODUCTION

In the modern era of rapid life, vehicular accidents and violence are a common occurrence. Fractures of the mandible are gaining attention due to the upward trend of accidents of two wheelers and other motor vehicles. The fracture treatment consists of reduction and immobilization. Type of reduction depends upon type of fracture.

REDUCTION

Reduction of fracture means bringing two fractured segments in original anatomical position. In the dentate mandible, reduction must be anatomically precise.

IMMOBILIZATION

Following accurate reduction of fragments, the fracture site needs to be immobilized to allow the bone-healing to occur.

TYPES OF REDUCTION

- Closed reduction
- Open reduction.

INDICATIONS FOR THE SURGERY

Closed Reduction

- Fractures which are favorable (undisplaced) with minimal disturbance of occlusion
- Fractures in children involving developing dentition
- Simple coronoid fractures
- Most of the condylar fractures.

Open Reduction

- All unfavorable fractures with change in occlusion
- Displaced bilateral condylar fractures
- Malunited fractures
- Nonunion of fractures
- If associated with complex facial fractures
- Cases in which closed reduction is contraindicated
- All complex and comminuted fractures
- Cases of severely atrophic edentulous mandible with displacement.

SPECIFIC PREOPERATIVE EVALUATION

Before taking patient on table, the following things should be evaluated:

- Head injuries should be ruled out.
- Spine injuries should be ruled out.
- Patient should be hemodynamically stable.
- A brief history should be taken. Previous convulsion and psychiatric disorder should be ruled out as these may be contraindications for intermaxillary fixation.
- Thorough examination should be done. Associated fracture of face and mandible should be ruled out, trauma to temporomandibular joint (TMJ) should be ruled out
- Occlusion of patient should be evaluated. In case of malocclusion, previous occlusion should be judged by looking at wear facet, previous dental treatment papers or patient's photograph.
- X-ray of left and right mandible, in oblique lateral view, is a must.
- Panoramic film is desirable, as it gives single overall view of the mandible.
- CT scan should be done, in case of:
  - Multiple facial injuries
  - Comminuted fractures
  - Missile injuries
  - Infected malunion, nonunion fractures
  - Vertical splint fractures.

ANESTHETIC CONSIDERATIONS

Preoperative

- Explain the patient about postoperative events, like brief mouth closure.
- Assess nostril patency

- Check for evidence of basal skull fracture and cerebrospinal fluid (CSF) leak, which makes nasal intubation contraindicated
- In a case of severe trismus, where postoperative edema may be anticipated, tracheostomy should be considered
- Submental intubation should be considered in case of a panfacial trauma.

Perioperative

- Trismus make intubation look potentially difficult preoperatively as the mouth opening is markedly limited due to the muscle spasm, hematoma, pain, but these tend to relax following induction.
- Nose should be packed with 4% lidocaine with adrenaline or Otrivin nasal drop should be used.
- A rapid sequence induction with suxamethonium is appropriate.
- A marked swelling may make intubation difficult and awake fiberoptic intubation may be required.
- Gas induction, while applying the face mask, is often difficult due to pain.
- Make sure that the patient, when comes out from anesthesia, should not be sedated and should be completely awake from the anesthesia.
- If throat pack is placed around, the tube should be removed before the application of wires.

Postoperative

- Observe the patient for some time in recovery before sending it to the ward.
- Start humidified oxygen.
- Always keep a wire cutter and a suction machine beside the patient's bed (to cut the wires in case of emergency).
- Shift the patient with nasopharyngeal airway to the ward.

SURGICAL STEPS

- Closed reduction and immobilization
- Open reduction and immobilization.

Closed Reduction and Immobilization

This means fracture segment is reduced manually without any incision, followed by immobilization. There are many methods of immobilization. Most commonly used method is arch bar fixation.

Steps in arch bar fixation:

- Selection of appropriate length and contouring of Erich arch bar according to arch of teeth (Fig. 1A).
- Arch bar to be placed around the teeth for a proper measurement. Extra length of the arch bar needs to be trimmed and the posterior edge of the bar needs to be bent to prevent soft tissue injury (Fig. 1B).
- After giving local block (using 2% lidocaine and adrenaline with one and half inch needle—26 #), wire is passed above and below the arch bar and tightened so that it does not obstruct the lug. It is important to make sure that these wires have been tightly applied. This is done by checking whether any vertical movement of arch bar is possible. The wires used are normally of 26 gauge (Figs 1C and D).
- Intermaxillary fixation can be established by either wires or by elastic (Fig. 1E).

General Considerations

There are important points to consider before starting.

- The occlusion must be checked. In the case of jaw malformations, like a deep bite deformity, it may be impossible to use arch bars.
- One pitfall, while using arch bars, is the risk of acquisition of blood-borne infection from patients.
- Passing the wires to secure the arch bar can result in a puncture or tear in the surgeon's glove and thereby, possibility of infection.

Open Reduction and Immobilization

Generally, open reduction is done under general anesthesia. Depending on the site and type of fracture, three approaches are used:

1. Extraoral approach
2. Intraoral approach
3. Use of existing wound.

Extraoral Approach

Submandibular approach: In 1934, Risdon described this technique. This is the same incision used for excision of the submandibular gland.

- Indications: This approach is used for fractures of the mandibular body and angle regions. Generally, this is used in complex and comminuted fractures, where intraoral reduction, exposure and reconstruction plate placement would be difficult.
- Incision: The incision can either be parallel to the inferior border of the mandible, at least 2 cm below the angle of the mandible or be placed in an existing skin crease for maximum cosmetic benefit (Fig. 2). Incision is performed after infiltrating the area with 2% lidocaine with adrenaline.
- Elevation of flap: Subplatysmal flap elevated up to the mandible with help of cautery.
- Preservation of marginal mandibular nerve: The main neural structure is the marginal mandibular branch of the facial nerve (cranial nerve VII). The facial artery and vein are also encountered during this dissection.

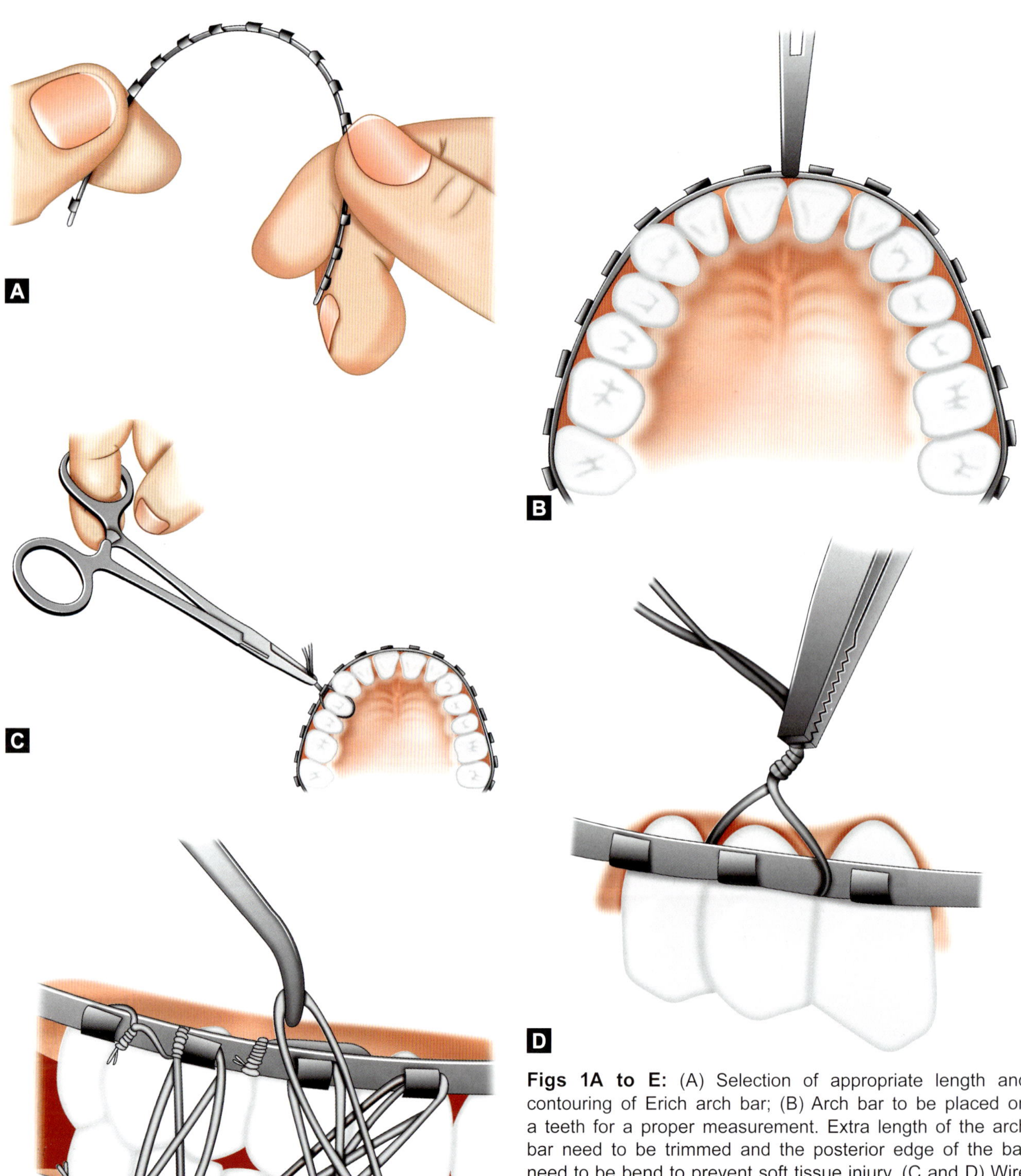

Figs 1A to E: (A) Selection of appropriate length and contouring of Erich arch bar; (B) Arch bar to be placed on a teeth for a proper measurement. Extra length of the arch bar need to be trimmed and the posterior edge of the bar need to be bend to prevent soft tissue injury. (C and D) Wire is passed above and below the arch bar and tightened so as not to obstruct the lug. It is important to make sure that this wires have been tightly applied by checking whether any vertical movement of arch bar is possible. The wire used are of normally of 26 gauge; (E) Intermaxillary fixation can be established by either wires or by elastic

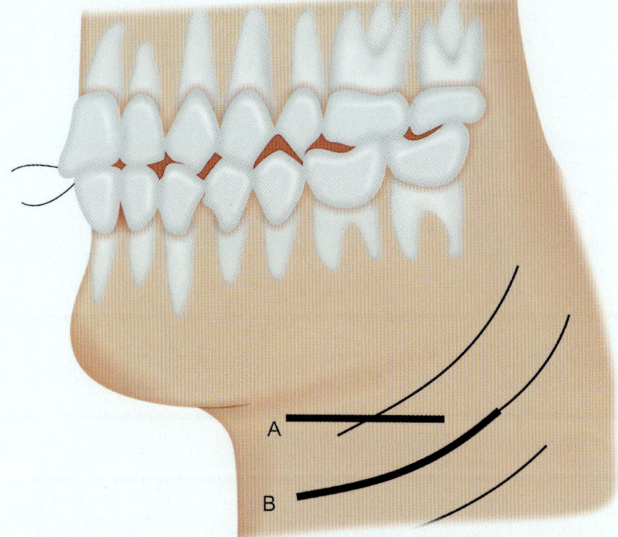

Fig. 2: Various submandibular incision

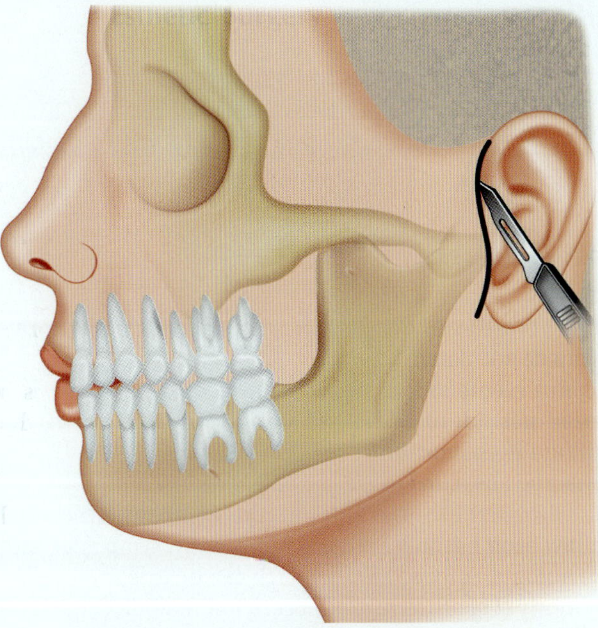

Fig. 3: Face lift incision(preauricle incision)

They are commonly located 1 cm below the angle of the mandible. This neurovascular structure is identified by Holder Martin's method in which facial vessels are identified and they are retracted, so that they are safe in the flap. The dissection is carried out through the deep cervical fascia.

- Muscle dissection: The muscle and periosteum are cut with the help of cautery, and retracted upward. Mucoperiosteum is incised and elevated to expose the fracture segment.
- Wound closure: Wound is sutured in layers; first the muscle layer, then platysma layer and then the skin layer is sutured keeping the drain in the wound.

Preauricular approach: The preauricular approach can be used to access and treat fractures in the mandibular condylar head and neck region.

- Preservation of important neurovascular structure: Branches of the facial nerve may be involved in this incision and dissection. The superficial temporal artery and vein are commonly encountered in this surgical approach. The vessels should be conserved if possible.
- Incision: Dingman described this incision. The incision is made in a preauricular skin crease. This incision is called face lift incision. Incision is not extended below the lower end of tragus (Fig. 3).
- Identification of temporal fascia
  - Carry the incision through the skin and subcutaneous tissues to the depth of the temporal fascia. The temporal fascia is a glistening white tissue layer that is best appreciated in the superior portion of the incision.
  - The superficial temporal vessels may be retracted anteriorly with the skin flap, or left in place.
  - Then, palpate for zygomatic arch. Ask the assistant to move the jaw so that you can palpate mandibular condyle.
- Incising temporal fascia parallel to frontal branch of facial nerve
  - An oblique incision through the superficial layer of the temporal fascia above the zygomatic arch is performed, ensuring that it is parallel to frontal branch of the facial nerve.
  - Strip the periosteum off the lateral zygomatic arch by inserting the periosteal elevator beneath the superficial layer of the temporal fascia.
  - Dissection will be carried inferiorly to expose the capsule of the TMJ.
  - The frontal branch of the facial nerve is protected within the superficial layer of the deep temporal fascia.
  - Dissection can be carried out inferiorly—dissection is proceeded furthur in a subperiosteal plane to reach the neck of the mandibular condyle.

  A disadvantage of this approach is that the surgeon can reach only a limited portion of the condylar neck region.
- Wound closure: If the TMJ capsule has been incised to access the condylar head, it must be closed as the first step. The temporal fascia is closed as the next step. Skin and subcutaneous sutures are placed.

Intraoral Approach

This approach is used for:

- Fracture of symphysis and body
- Fracture of condylar process and ramus.
  In practice, intraoral approach is more commonly used.
- Advantages
  - Intraoral approach is more rapid than extraoral approach
  - No external scar
  - More exposure for horizontal mandible anteriorly.
- Disadvantage
  - Only labial cortex is visualized. Thus, there is a possibility of significant gap remaining in the lingual cortex.

Intraoral approach to the symphysis and body

- Vestibular incisions: The intraoral approach is the usual access for simple fractures of the body, symphysis, and angular regions. The approach can be extended posteriorly (Fig. 4) for better access to the body, angle and ramus regions. In complex fractures, including comminuted, edentulous and infected fractures requiring the placement of load-bearing reconstruction plates, an extraoral approach may provide better access.
- Incision: Infiltrate the area with a local anesthetic (2% lidocaine with adrenaline) and wait for a while. Make an incision through the mucosa in the vestibule. Between the canines, the incision is made 10–15 mm away from the attached gingiva in a curvilinear fashion. Posterior to the canine, the incision is only 5 mm away from the attached gingiva, staying superior to the mental nerve.

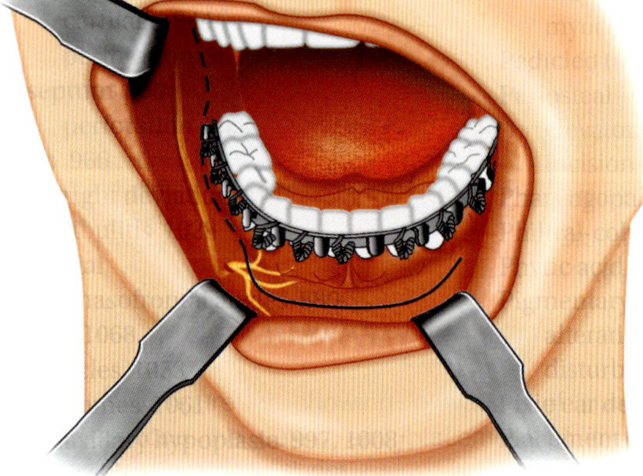

Fig. 4: Intraoral incision for symphysis and body fracture

- Protection of mental nerve: The mental nerve is an important structure which needs to be preserved; if it is severed, there will be paresthesia, numbness at the lips, chin and vestibule.
- Precautions: When the incision is extended posterior to the canine teeth, the mental nerve can be damaged; this should be kept in mind and then dissect. Keep the incision superior to the mental nerve in the body region that can be done by making incision 5 mm away from attached gingiva posterior to canine.
- Dissection: Below the mucosa, lies the mentalis muscle. Saving the mental nerve, incision on mentalis muscle is performed with the help of cautery. Keep adequate stump attached to mandible so that mentalis muscle can be resutured back.
- Exposure of fracture site: Mucoperiosteal flap is incised and elevated to expose the fracture.
- Wound closure: After thoroughly irrigating the wound and checking for hemostasis, the incision is closed. Anteriorly, the mentalis muscle is reapproximated to prevent drooping of the chin tissues. The mucosa is closed with interrupted or running resorbable sutures. A crep bandage is applied on the chin region to prevent hematoma formation and to support soft tissue.

Intraoral approach to the angle

- Vestibular incisions: The intraoral approach is used for the majority of simple angle fractures.
- Mark the incision: Where there is no third molar present, or where one is present but has to be left in place, a purely vestibular incision approximately 5 mm away from the attached gingiva is made (Fig. 5A). When an erupted third molar is to be removed, the incision must incorporate the attached gingiva around the buccal side of the tooth (combination of vestibular and envelope incision) (Fig. 5B).
- Infiltration: Inject 2% lidocaine with adrenaline at the marked site.
- Preservation of sensory buccal nerve: The sensory buccal nerve crosses the upper anterior rim of the mandibular, ascending ramus in the region of the coronoid notch. It is usually below the mucosa running above the temporalis muscle fibers. When the posterior vestibular incision is taken sharply along the bony rim, the buccal nerve is at risk of transsection, followed by numbness in the buccal mucosal region. Therefore, to protect the nerve, the posterior dissection is to be extended bluntly as soon as the lower coronoid notch is reached.
- Buccinator muscle: On performing the incision, lower attachment of buccinator muscle is transected—After incision taken, buccinator muscle is transected. With the help of cautery, mucoperiosteum is elevated and fracture segment is identified.

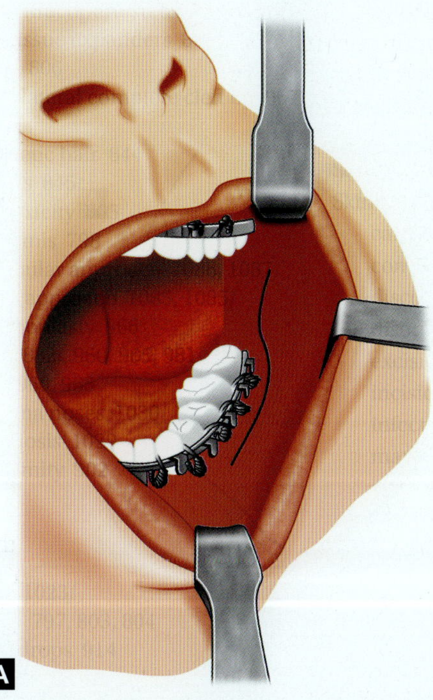
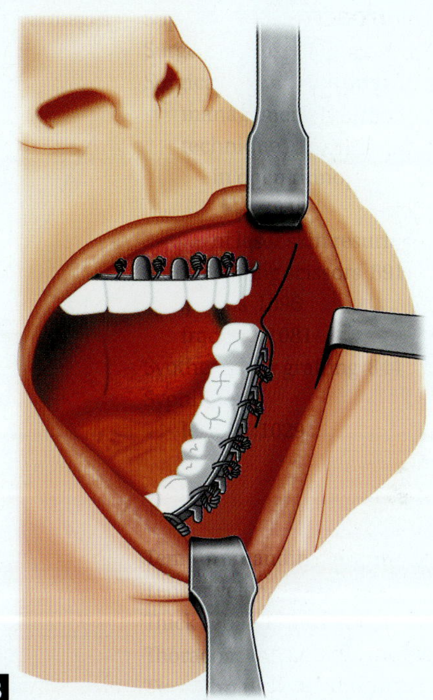

Figs 5A and B: (A) Mucosal incision for angle fracture; (B) Mucosal incision for angle fracture when erupted third molar have to be removed

- Wound closure of the vestibular incision: To reattach the muscle, the sutures in the lateral vestibular region should not only be superficial. The suture should catch all layers (mucosa and muscle) to ensure muscle reattachment. After thoroughly irrigating the wound and checking for hemostasis, the surgeon can close the incision.

An elastic pressure dressing covering the angle region helps support the soft tissues, and prevent hematoma formation. Wound closure is done using envelope flap.

The envelope portion of the flap is undermined with scissors to facilitate tension-free advancement over extraction site. Generally, resorbable sutures are used for this closure. The flap is advanced and closed over the extraction site.

The Use of Existing Lacerations

Frequently, patients with facial fractures also have lacerations. Very often, these existing soft-tissue injuries can be used to directly access the facial bones for management of the fractures.

The surgeon may elect to extend the laceration to provide adequate access to the fractured area, following the relaxed natural skin creases.

Wound closure: Wound closure for this incision is the primary closure of the laceration. Proper cleansing, debridement, and hemostasis should be accomplished prior to closure. The laceration is closed in layers with resorbable interrupted sutures, realigning the anatomic structures and eliminating dead space.

Steps After Exposure of Fracture Fragment

Reduction of Fracture Fragment

After exposure, fracture fragment is reduced to normal alignment. Teeth occlusion alignment is more important than bone alignment. The occlusion of patient is brought to pre-existing alignment with manipulation, and an intermaxillary fixation is put.

Fixation

Although many methods of osteosynthesis have been described, but most practiced, easy and reliable method of osteosynthesis is miniplate osteosynthesis.

Champy's Lines of Osteosynthesis

Champy and coworkers, after careful consideration of the biomechanics of mandible, have described osteosynthesis line for placing the miniplate in the mandible (Figs 6A and B).

- A line drawn at the base of the alveolar process corresponds to the line of tension. A miniplate and a screw can be fixed along this line. In the parasymphysis region, another line is drawn to neutralize the tension force.

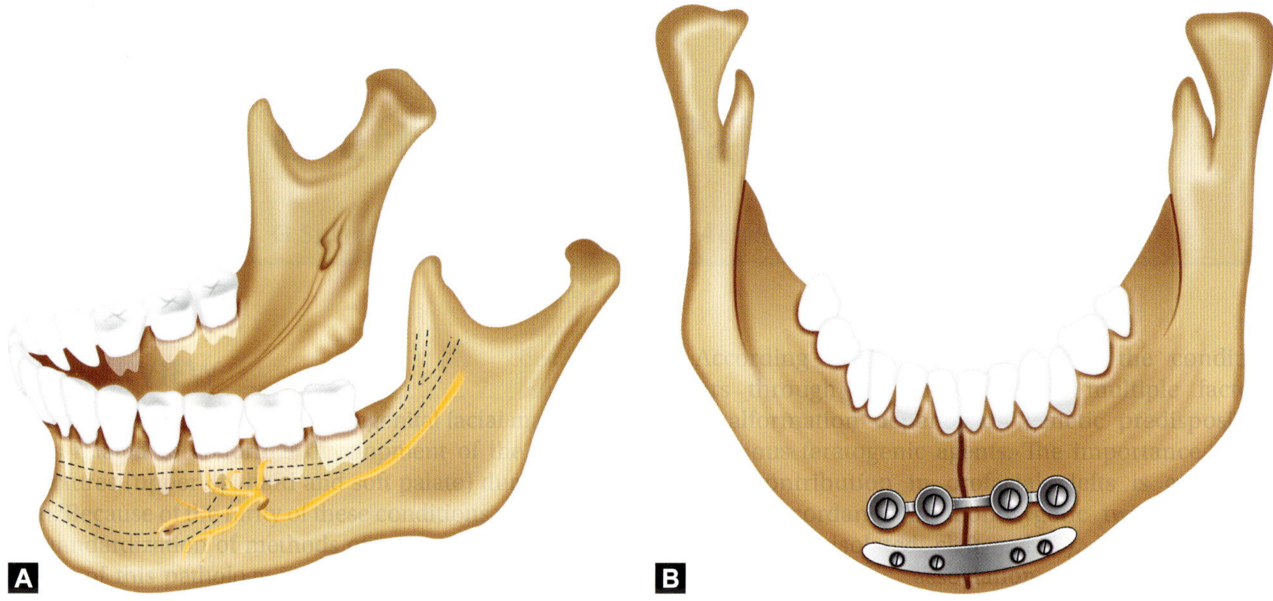

Figs 6A and B: (A) Champy's line; (B) Mini hole plate fixation along the Champy's line

- Behind the mental foramen, only one plate should be applied, immediately below the dental root and above the inferior alveolar nerve.
- Between the two canines and in front of mental foramen, another plate near the lower border of mandible is applied in addition to the upper plate.

Technique

These miniplates are around 0.9 mm thick and 6 mm wide. The difference between holes is standardized. The screws available are 5–15 mm in length. The diameter of the screws is 2 mm; screws usually used in mandible are 6 mm or 8 mm. The screws are of self-tapping type.

- The plate is bent first so as to be adapted to bone.
- Plate is placed on mandible, keeping in mind that there are two holes on either side of fracture line.
- In case of simple fractures, miniplate is used.
- In case of complex, comminuted fractures and infected fractures, reconstruction plate is used.
- 1.5 mm drill bit is used to create a hole almost perpendicular to the plate.
- Eccentric drilling or repeated insertion of drill produces unfavorable hole, thus diminishing the grip of the screw.
- During drilling, continuous liquid cooling is necessary to avoid thermal necrosis and the early loosening of screws
- A give away indicates penetration of drill in a cortical bone
- Soft tissue in-between the fracture line should be removed as it does not allow proper alignment. Also, there is a risk of nonhealing of fracture, if soft tissue is placed between fractured fragments.
- Use of drill sleeve, while drilling, provides protection to soft tissue.
- Drill bit used should be 0.5 mm less than the screw size. For example, if screw or plate of 2 mm is used, then 1.5 mm drill bit should be used to make hole.
- Damage to mental nerve, tooth root, inferior alveolar canal should be avoided.
- A space of about 5 mm should be kept between two plates.
- Then, screw is inserted near the fracture site and gradually tightened.
- This same procedure is carried out for insertion of screw in all the holes of plates.

The inferior alveolar nerve region is considered as the neutral zone of the mandible. Avoid plate and screw fixation in this area since it can cause damage to the nerve.

Principle

The authors follow Champy's principle of osteosynthesis. For example, in simple symphysis and parasymphysis fracture, they use two mini-hole plate (four holes)—one at upper border and the other on lower border to combat torsional and rotational force with one hole on either side of fracture (Figs 7A to D).

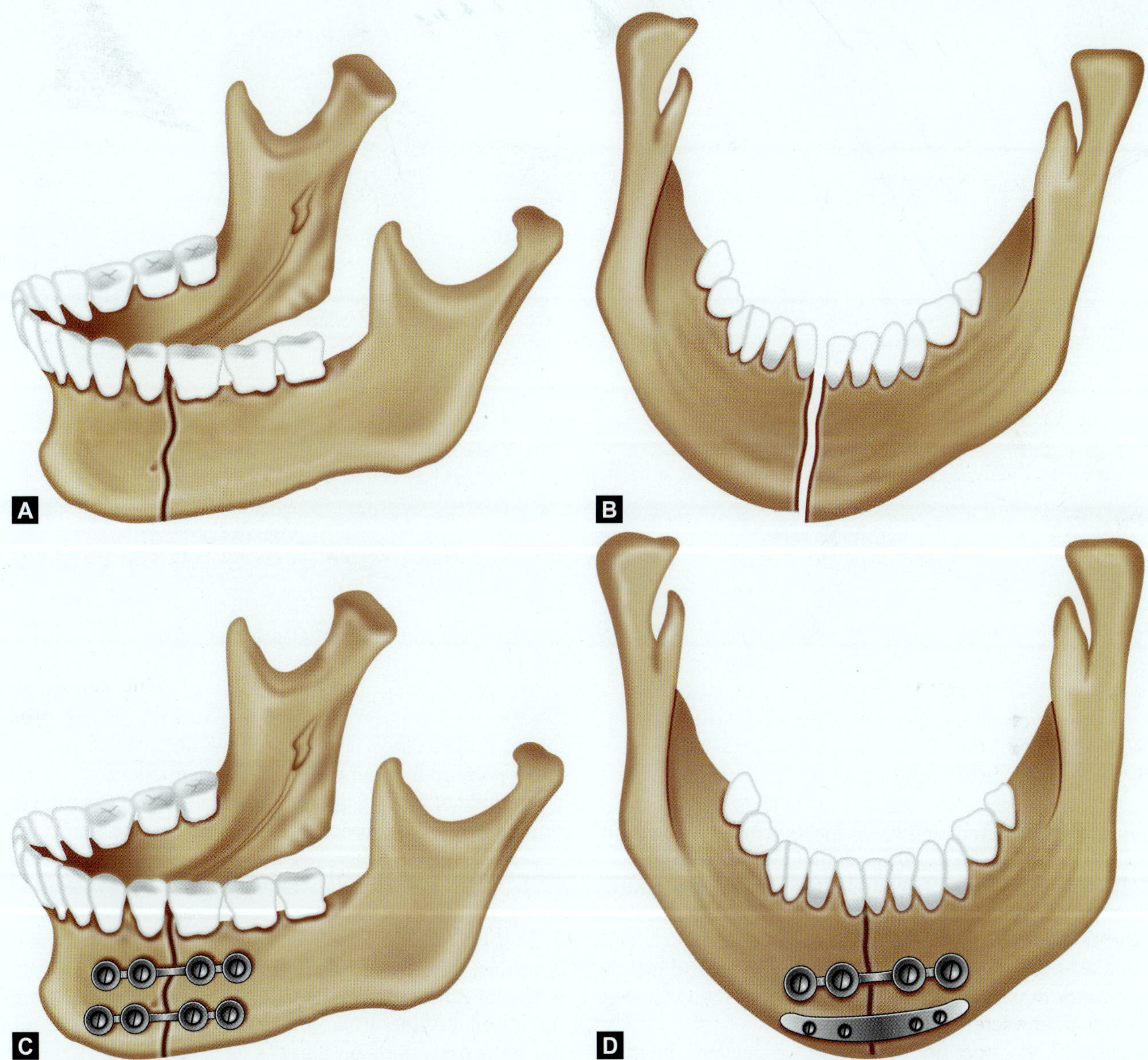

Figs 7A to D: (A) Parasymphysis fracture; (B) Symphysis fracture; (C) Four-hole plate, one at superior border and one at inferior border; (D) Four-hole plate one at superior border and one at inferior border

Fracture of Angle and Ramus

- A single monocortical miniplate applied on the external oblique line is enough for simple angle fracture
- Fracture between canine and angle (body) can be stabilized by superior border plating along the Champy's line as shown in (Figs 8A and B).

Complex Symphysis and Parasymphysis Fracture

Figures 9A to D show fractures in the parasymphysis area.

Complex Angle and Body Fracture

Figures 10A to D show angle and body fractures.

Condylar Fracture

These can be treated either by conservative approach or surgically, depending upon the amount of displacement. Conservative approach is advocated in condylar fractures which are without any displacement, condylar fractures with little displacement, and slight overriding in young children or subcondylar fractures which are slightly displaced.

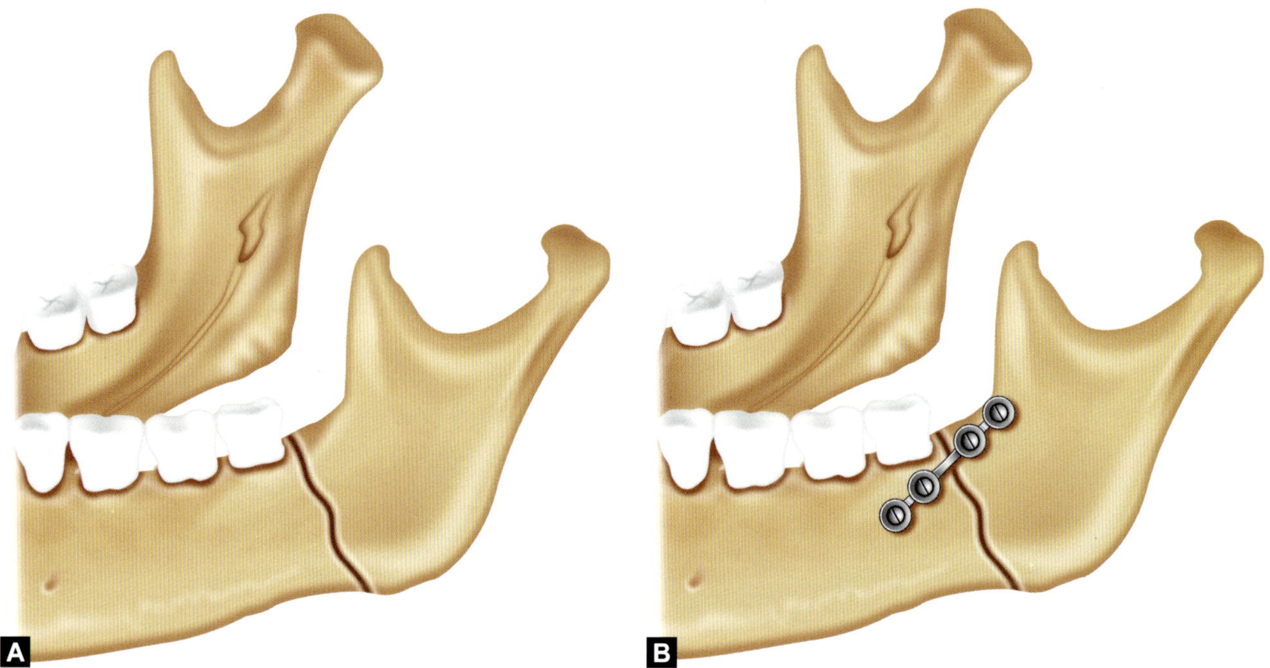

Figs 8A and B: (A) Fracture of angle; (B) Single mini-hole plate fixation at external ridge

Open Reduction

In grossly displaced condylar fracture, where reduction cannot be achieved by conventional method and there is a fear of future derangement or ankylosis, an open reduction is indicated.

The indications are

- Cases of condylar fracture with vertical overriding
- Cases in which normal occlusion cannot be achieved by manipulation or traction
- Cases of gross displacement, especially bilateral condylar fracture
- Cases in which condylar fractures interfere with jaw movement
- Cases in which condyles are partially fused in a wrong position.

The condyle is surgically approached by preauricular, submandibular or retromandibular approach. The fracture is reduced and fixed by either interosseous wiring or by monocortical miniplates.

Fracture of Coronoid Process

This account for 1% of fractures; most of the coronoid fractures do not require any treatment. Cases in which coronoid hinders the opening of mouth, treatment is advised. This coronoid fragment is fixed by interosseous wiring or by miniplate. If reduction is not possible and function is impaired, coronoid process is removed.

Alternative Surgical Approaches

Transparotid Approach

A vertical incision through skin and subcutaneous tissue is made, extending from just below the ear lobe to the mandibular angle. It should be parallel to the posterior border of the mandible (Fig. 11).

- Dissection: The subcutaneous tissue is undermined, exposing the superficial musculoaponeurotic system (SMAS). A vertical incision is made through the SMAS into the parotid gland.
- Blunt dissection of the parotid gland: The parotid gland is bluntly dissected parallel to the direction of the facial nerve branches and till the posterior border of the mandible. The dissection should be anterior to the retromandibular vein. Branches of the facial nerve may be found during the dissection. A nerve stimulator may be helpful to identify them. They should be mobilized and protected. Once the posterior border of the mandible is reached, an incision is made through the pterygomasseteric sling.

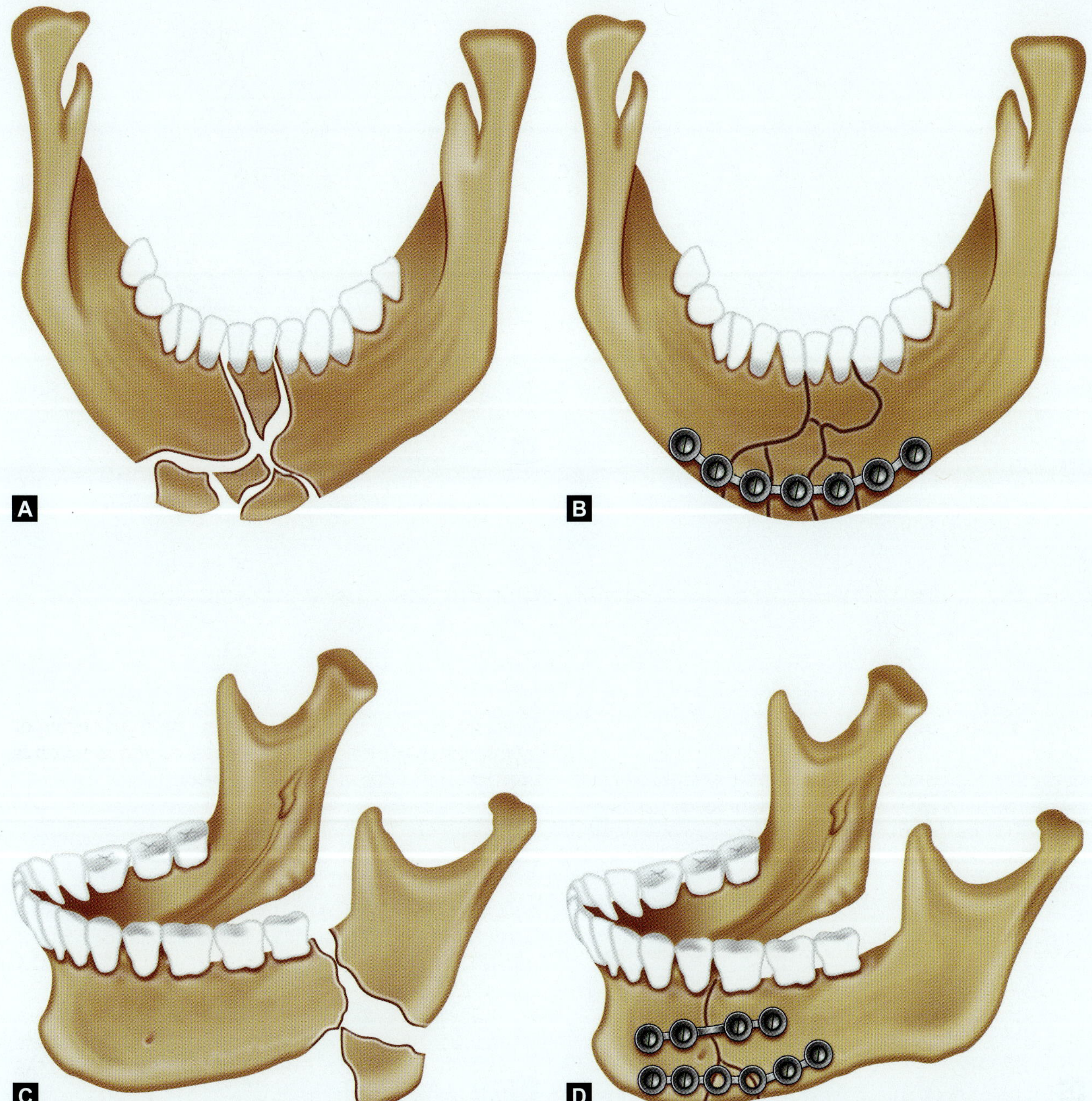

Figs 9A to D: (A) Comminuted fracture of parasymphysis; (B) Reconstruction plate (load-bearing osteosynthesis) at the inferior border to neutralize the tension and the compression force; (C) Basal triangle fracture of parasymphysis area and; (D) Reconstruction plate (load-bearing osteosynthesis) at an inferior border plus miniplate (load-sharing osteosynthesis) at the superior border

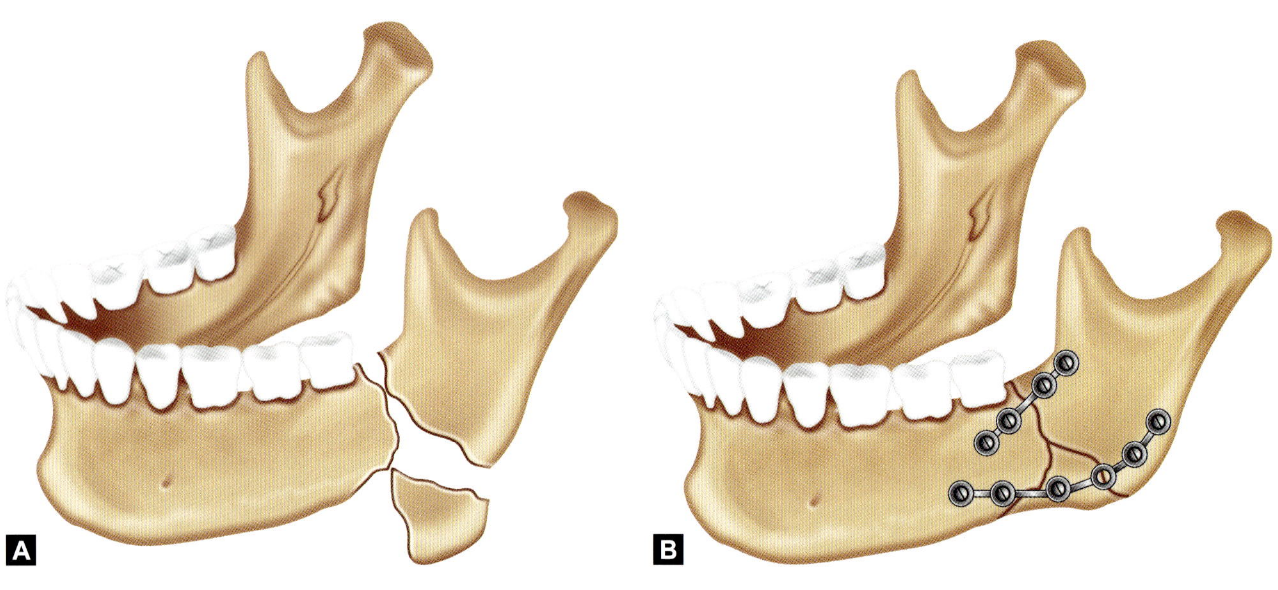

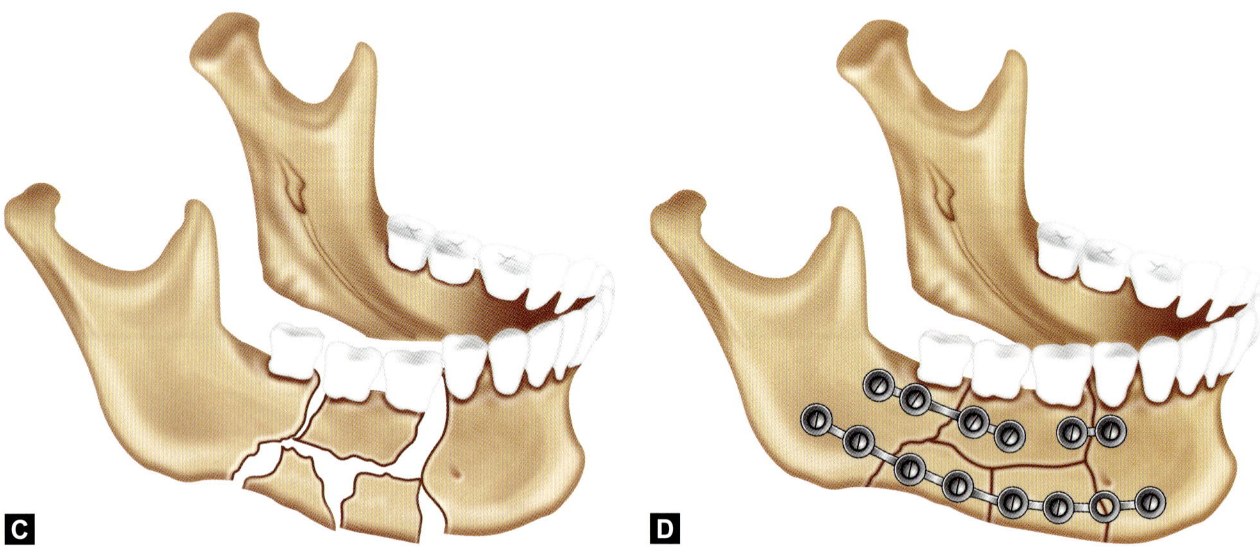

Figs 10A to D: (A) Basal triangle fracture of angle; (B) Miniplate (load-sharing osteosynthesis) at external oblique line plus reconstruction plate (load-bearing osteosynthesis) at inferior border; (C) Comminuted body fracture; (D) Reconstruction plate at lower border plus mini-hole plate at upper border

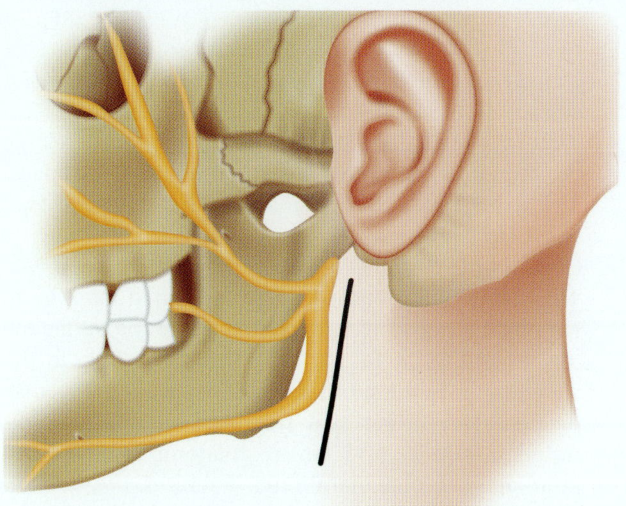

Fig. 11: Transparotid approach skin incision

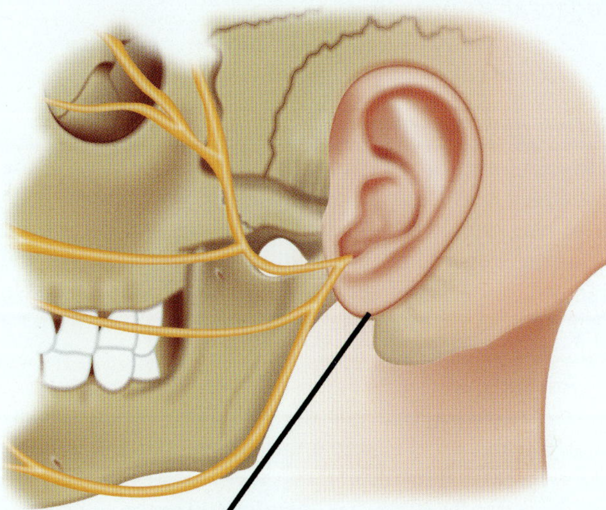

Fig. 12: Retroparotid approach

- Subperiosteal dissection of the mandibular ramus: A periosteal elevator is used to strip the masseter muscle from the ramus. Further dissection, superiorly along the posterior border, exposes the condylar process.
- Wound closure: The wound is closed in layers. Any dead space formation is avoided. The parotid gland capsule must be closed tightly to prevent salivary fistula. The SMAS is resuspended.

Retroparotid Approach

A frequently used alternative to the transparotid approach is one in which the parotid gland is lifted rather than dissected through. This requires the incision to be placed more posteriorly which means that exposure of the mandible is limited. Rather than approaching the mandible directly over the ramus, it is approached more posteriorly (Fig. 12).

- Skin incision: An oblique incision through skin and subcutaneous tissue is made, extending from the mastoid process to a point just below the angle of the mandible. The subcutaneous tissue is undermined, exposing the SMAS. An oblique incision is made through the SMAS. The posterior aspect of the parotid gland is identified and dissection continues behind the gland. The gland is lifted off the masseter muscle and retracted anteriorly.
- Dissection: Once the posterior border of the mandible has been reached, an incision is made through the pterygomasseteric sling.
- Subperiosteal dissection of the mandibular ramus: A periosteal elevator is used to strip the masseter muscle from the ramus. Further dissection, superiorly along the posterior border, exposes the condylar process.
- Wound closure: The wound is reapproximated in layers for anatomic realignment and avoidance of dead space.

The SMAS is resuspended. A suction drain may be placed.

The Various Modification of Preauricular Incision

Rowe modification

- Preauricular incision with temporal extension.
- An incision is angled from the point of the attachment of helix upwards and forward at 45°, lying within the hair-bearing area over the temporal region.
- This incision allows an extensive flap to be raised and avoid traction injury to upper branches of facial nerve.
- Reverse sigmoid-shaped incision gives the most satisfactory result by helping to disguise the final scars.

Blair and Ivy

- Preauricular incision with an inverted hockey stick incision over the zygomatic arch.
- It gives easy access and better stability along with facilitated exposure of arch along with the condylar arc.

Alkayat-Bramley preauricular incision

- Alkayat-Bramley preauricular incision along with a curved temporal extension (question mark shape) is advocated mainly for TMJ ankylosis, as it gives a wide area of exposure and also facilitates elevation of temporal flap for reconstructive purpose.

Endaural Approach

- This approach gives good scar but poor access, so rarely used.

Submental Approach

The submental approach is used to treat fractures of the anterior mandibular body and symphysis. These fractures can usually be approached and treated intraorally. However, depending on the difficulty or severity of the fracture, and/or the presence of a laceration, suitable an extraoral approach via the submental route may be indicated.

- Advantages
  - Lingual surface of the mandible can be easily inspected to ensure optimum reduction of fracture in this segment.
  - No major structures encountered in this area
  - Scar is not that visible.
- Variations in incision (Fig. 13)
  - Following curvature of anterior mandible
  - Hidden in submental skin crease.
- Dissection: The incision is carried through the skin and subcutaneous tissues to the platysma muscle. The platysma muscle must be divided. There may be a natural separation of the muscle in the midline region. Additionally, the platysma muscle becomes very thin in this region. Dissection is carried out to the inferior border of the mandible. The periosteum is incised sharply and the flap is elevated to expose the anterior surface of the symphysis.
- Wound closure: The wound is closed in layers to realign the anatomic structures and to eliminate dead space. The periosteum and platysma muscle should be closed in different layers.
- Option—bilateral extension/submental extension: The submental incision can be extended laterally to encompass both the right and left mandible by degloving the entire lateral surface of the mandible in the same way as in the submandibular approach. This may be necessary in complex fractures, such as comminuted, atrophic, and severe bilateral fractures. To approach complex mandibular fractures, the surgeon essentially combines a right and left submandibular incision with a submental one.

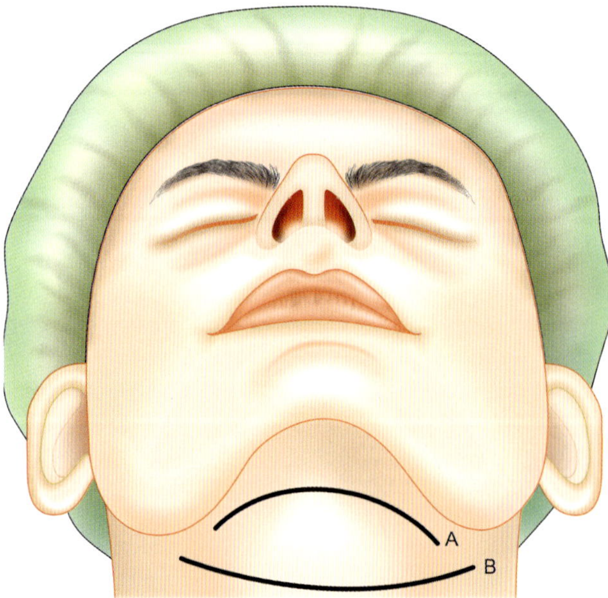

Fig. 13: Variations in incision. (A) Following curvature of anterior mandible; (B) Hidden in submental skin crease

Retromandibular Approaches

In 1967, Hinds and Girotti first described this approach (Fig. 14).

- Skin incision: Incision is made 3 cm above the submandibular incision. The incision is carried curving behind the angle of mandible;
  2% lidocaine with adrenaline can be used for vasoconstriction effect.
- Subplatysmal flap elevation: Superior subplatysmal dissection would expose the underlying marginal mandibular branch of the facial nerve (cranial nerve VII). By ligating and dividing the facial artery and vein and then retracting the vessels superiorly, the marginal mandibular branch of the facial nerve remains included in the superior flap and is thus protected. Divide the pterygomasseteric sling and incise the periosteum at the inferior border to expose the fracture site. This exposes the body and angle region.
- Wound closure: For wound closure, the pterygomasseteric sling is closed. The wound is closed in layers. A drain may be used if necessary.

Alternative Method of Intermaxillary Fixation

Alternative Way of Fixing Arch Bar

Wiring technique

- Gilmer method: This is the simplest way to establish intermaxillary fixation. This technique is simple and effective but has a disadvantage that mouth cannot be opened for inspection of the fracture side without removal of wire fixation. The method consists

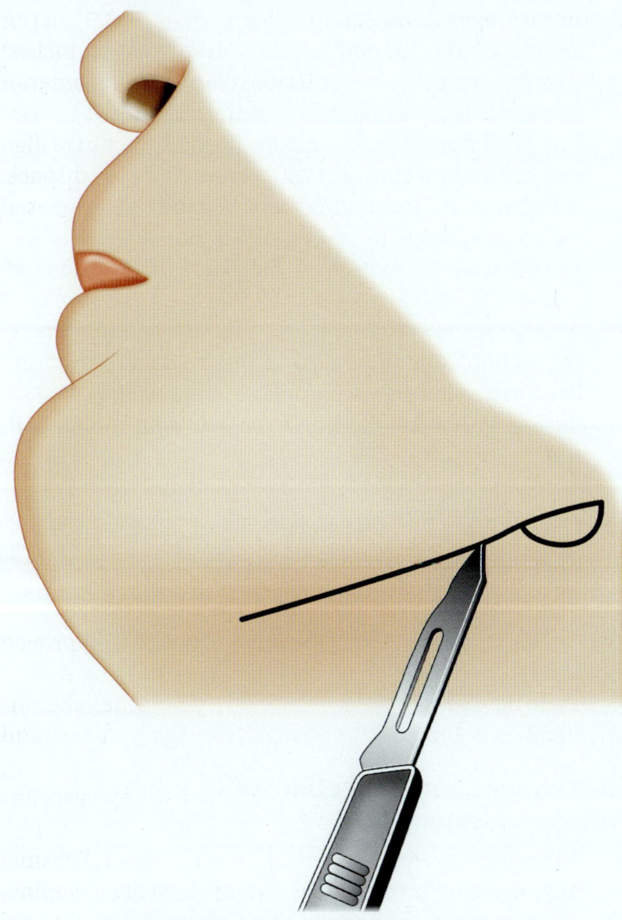

Fig. 14: Retromandibular approach

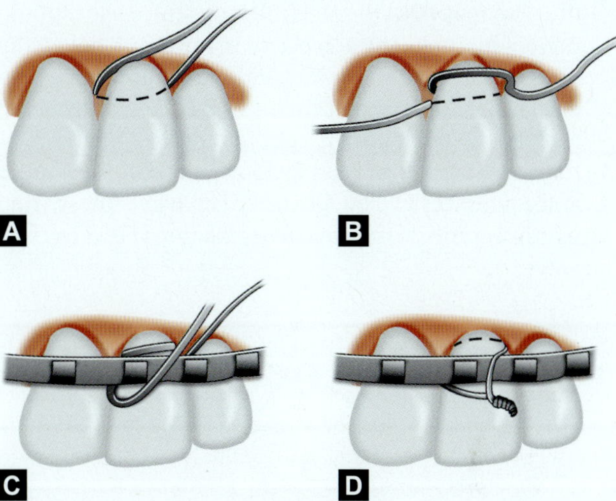

Figs 15A to D: (A) Passage of wire; (B) An extra loop is passed; (C) The wire is passed above and below the arch bar and; (D) The wire is tightened

of passing wire ligatures around neck of available teeth and twisting them in a clockwise direction until the wire is tightened around its tooth. After adequate number of wires have been placed, upper and lower teeth are brought into the occlusion and the wires are twisted one upper to one lower wire. A stainless steel (24-gauge or 26-gauge) gauge wires are usually applied (Figs 15 and 16).

- Eyelet method: This method of fixation has the advantage that jaws may be opened for inspection by removal of only the intermaxillary ligatures. This method consists of twisting a 20 cm length of 24-gauge or 26-gauge wire around an instrument to establish a loop. Both ends of the wire are passed through the interproximal space from the outer surface. One end of the wire is passed around the anterior tooth and the other one around the posterior tooth. One end of

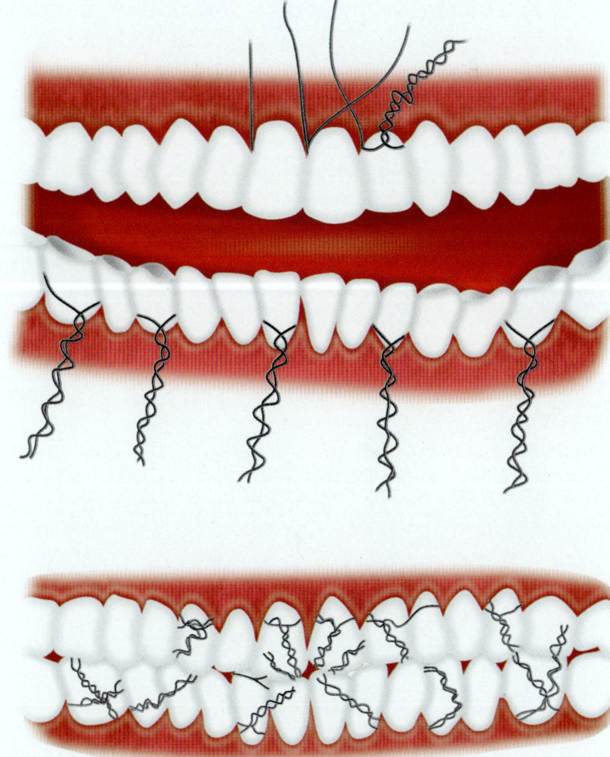

Fig. 16: Gilmers method of fixation

the wire may pass through the loop. The eyelet should project in upper jaw above and in lower jaw below the horizontal twist to prevent ends from impinging on each other. After establishment of sufficient number of eyelets, the teeth are brought into occlusion and ligatures are passed in loop fashion between one upper and one lower eyelet. The inter-jaw wires are twisted tightly to provide intermaxillary fixation (Fig. 17).

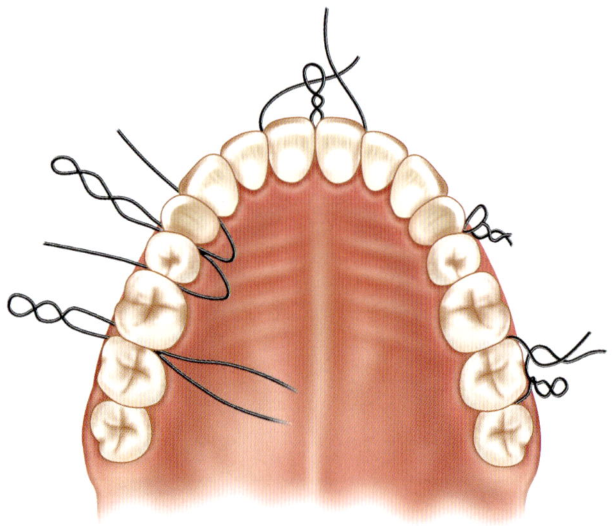

Fig. 17: Eyelet method of fixation

Intermaxillary fixation screw technique

- Intermaxillary fixation screws were introduced as labour saving device. Intermaxillary fixation screws provide a rapid method of immobilization of teeth in a good dentition, in uncomplicated fractures. The number and position of these screws is based on type of fracture, the location of fracture, and the surgeon's preference. Screw must be positioned superior to the maxillary tooth roots and inferior to the mandible tooth root (Fig. 18).
- Disadvantage is minimal, and a focused point of force application to maintain good intermaxillary fixation. The focus point of force applied may result in malocclusion by leaving the posterior dentition in an open bite.

SPECIAL INSTRUMENTS USED FOR THE SURGERY

Instruments for Gaining Surgical Access

- Scalpel
- Blade handle
- Blade.

Instruments for Reflection of Mucoperiosteum Flap

- Periosteal elevator
- Freys elevator or mastoid elevator can be used.

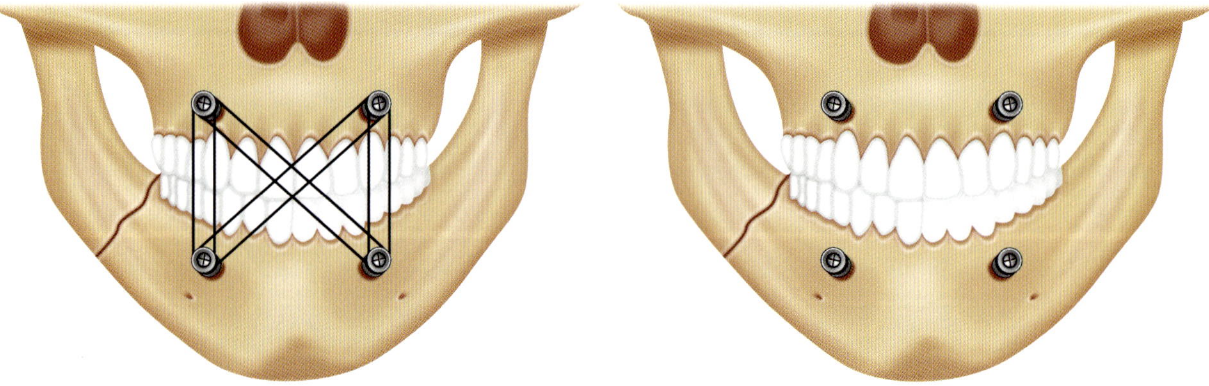

Fig. 18: Intermaxillary fixation screw technique

Instruments for Retraction

- C-shape retractor
- Cat paw retractors
- Langerbeck right angle retractor
- Chin retractors
- Tongue depressor.

These instruments are usually available in the authors' operation theaters.

Instrument for Drilling Holes

- Drill bits; use 1.5 mm drill bit to drill a hole for 2-mm screws; drill bit size should be 0.5 mm less than the diameter of screw to be used
- Drill machine with hand piece.

Implants for Mandible and Instruments that Need to Fix Them

Mini Hole Plates

Miniplates are available in various shapes and lengths, but can only be used with non-locking screws. For mandible, 2.5 mm or 2 mm plates are usually used (Fig. 19).

Reconstruction Plates

These are available in various sizes: 8 holes, 10 holes, 12 holes and 16 holes plates. Usually 2 mm reconstruction plates are used (Fig. 20).

Screw Driver and Screws

Screw driver is usually used depending on screw. For example, 2 mm screw driver is used for 2 mm screws. They are available in 1.5 mm, 2 mm, and 2.5 mm sizes (Fig. 21).

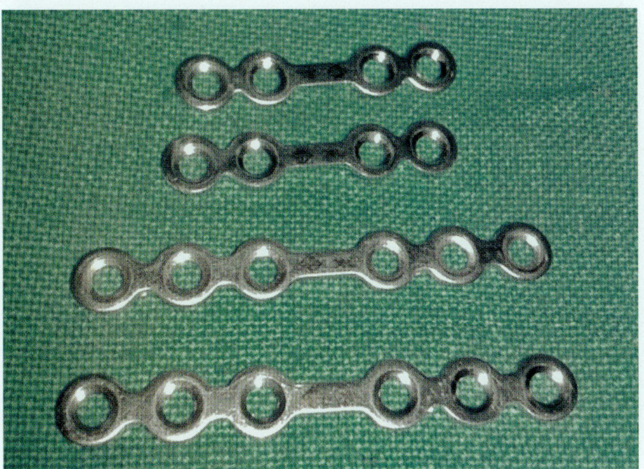

Fig. 19: Mini-hole plates

Instrument Used for Intermaxillary Fixation

- Erich arch bar—its standard arch bar is used
- No. 26 reel wire
- Cutter
- Long arteries
- Twister.

COMPLICATIONS

Serious complications, arising as a result of mandible fracture, are rare as fractures are treated competently nowadays. Minor complications are more common than the major ones. The complications are divided into early complications and late complications. The authors encounter more of late complications than early ones.

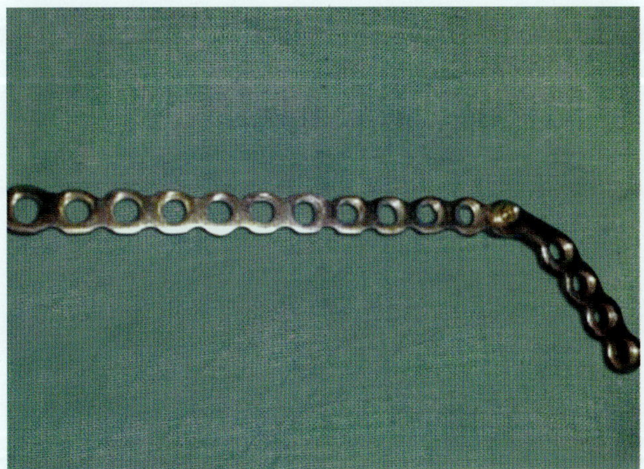

Fig. 20: Reconstruction plate

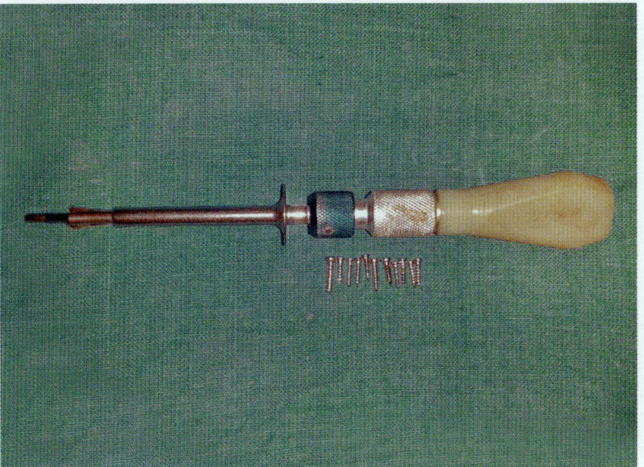

Fig. 21: Screw driver with screw of different sizes

Early Complications

Infection

Most common early complication is infection. Infected fractures usually demonstrate one or more of the following signs/symptoms:
- Swelling
- Erythema
- Trismus
- Pain
- Purulent discharge.

Infection occurring in fractures usually results from one or more of the following etiology:
- Microorganisms
- Fracture instability
- Devital tissues (teeth, bone, etc.).

The treatment of infected fractures involves:
- Incision and drainage of abscesses,
- Irrigations of the wounds as necessary
- Systemic antibiotics
- Removal of devital teeth/bone
- Removal of any loose internal fixation devices
- Restabilization of fracture
- Stronger and longer plates need to be applied
- Function should be permitted after the infection is cleared
- Bone grafting should be considered in a case of big gap in a fracture.

Late Complications

Fixation Failure

This is the commonest late complication. Implant failure includes plate fracture and screw head fracture and extrusion, kenacort and hylinese—kenacort and hyaluronic acid of screws. Fixation failure results in fracture mobility that can subsequently lead to infection, nonunion and/or malunion.

Fixation fails by a number of mechanisms which include:
1. Insufficient amount of fixation
2. Fracture of the plate
3. Loosening of the screws
4. Devitalization of bone around screws.

Insufficient amount of fixation: Left mandibular angle fracture was treated using a malleable miniplate 2.0 at the inferior border of the mandible. This is insufficient fixation for this fracture. In such a case, the patient needs to be operated upon again to fix a correct plate.

Malunion/malocclusion
- *Etiology*: Malunions occur due to one of several reasons:
  - Inadequate occlusal reduction during surgery
  - Inadequate osseous reduction during surgery
  - No osseous reduction (e.g. condyle fractures)
  - Imprecise application of internal fixation devices
  - Inadequate stability (lack of rigidity).
- *Treatment*: The treatment of a malunion must involve:
  - Identification of the cause and treatment
  - Orthodontic reference
  - Osteotomies as necessary (refracture, standard osteotomies, combinations).

Limitation of Opening of Mouth

Prolong immobilization of mandible and intermaxillary fixation can result in weakening of muscles of mastication. Substantial hemorrhage within muscle leads to organized hematoma with early scar tissue formation. All this leads to decreased mouth opening.
- Treatment
  - Physiotherapy may accelerate the recovery period
  - Simple jaw exercises should be employed
  - Occasionally, manipulation of mandible under anesthesia may assist the breakdown of scar tissue within muscle.

Scar

- Etiology
  - Contamination of wound with dirt, especially tar products
  - Improper technique of suturing
  - Associated infection
  - Tendency of patient.
- Treatment
  - Wait and watch for first year as they may soften and fed away
  - Massage of the scar
  - Pressure bandage
  - Application of lanoline
  - Infiltration of injection of kenacort and hylaronic acid
  - Surgical revision if possible.

CHAPTER

110 Faciomaxillary Fractures

Arunesh Gupta, Akshay P Deshpande, Dipesh J Malviya

INTRODUCTION

Faciomaxillary fractures are of two types: (1) mandible fractures and (2) maxilla fractures, of which three predominant types are mentioned.

1. Le Fort I
2. Le Fort II
3. Le Fort III

MANDIBLE FRACTURES

INDICATIONS

The indications for open reduction and internal fixation are as follows.

- Malocclusion
- Displaced fracture
- Unfavorable fracture
- Submental nerve compression

PREOPERATIVE EVALUATION

Clinical Examination (Figs 1 and 2)

- Oral cavity
  - Mouth opening
- Occlusion
  - Segmental mobility of mandibular arch
  - Dentoalveolar fracture
  - Teeth loss
  - Loose teeth
  - Associated maxillary fracture

External Examination (Fig. 3)

- Swelling
- Bruises
- Wounds
- Exposed bone
- Sensation in the region of mental nerve

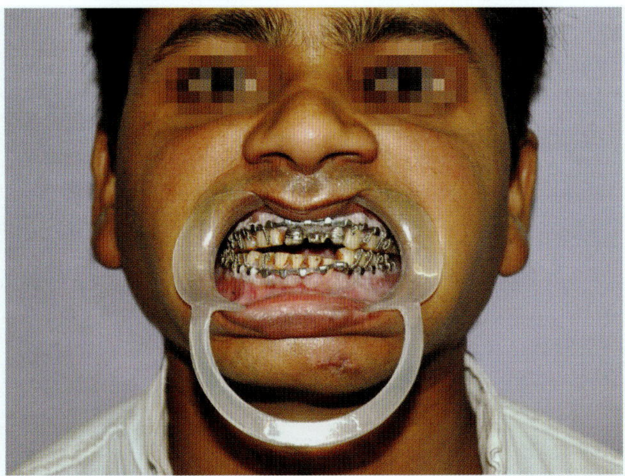

Fig. 1: Patient of fracture mandible showing malocclusion with anterior open bite

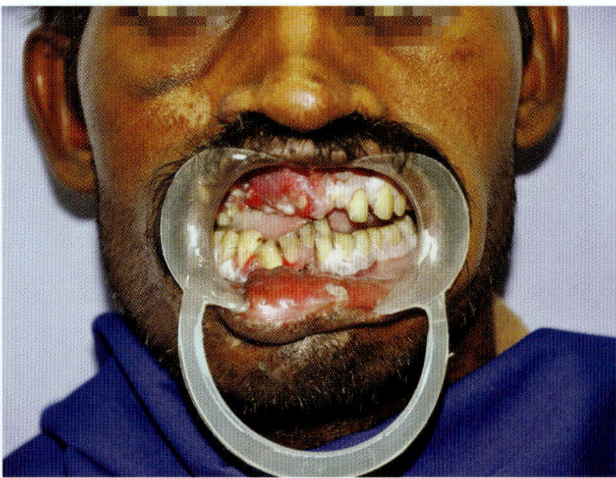

Fig. 2: Fracture mandible, right maxilla and dentoalveolar fracture with teeth loss

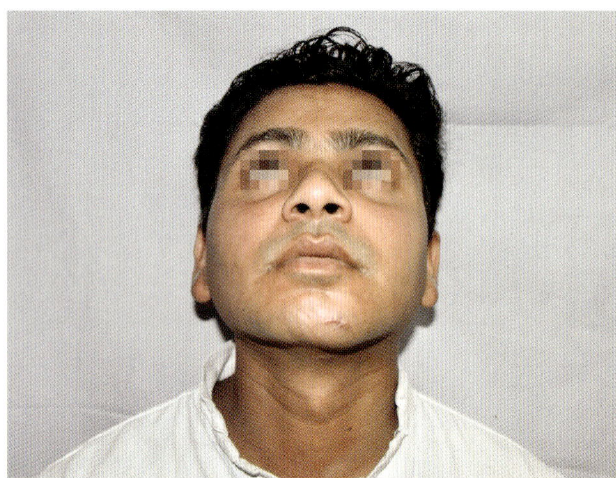

Fig. 3: Deformity over chin and scar of injury

Specific Investigations

1. Orthopantogram
2. CT scan of face with three-dimensional reconstruction (Figs 4A to C).

CLASSIFICATION OF MANDIBLE FRACTURES

Mandibular fractures can be classified as;

Simple

- Linear fracture

Complex

- Comminuted fracture
- Compound fracture

Classification on the Basis of Region

- Symphysis and parasymphysis
- Body
- Angle and ramus
- Condylar process and head

Classification on the Basis of Other Associated Injuries to

- Face
- Head and neck
- Other areas of the body

SPECIFIC ANESTHETIC CONSIDERATIONS

- Mouth opening
- Loose teeth
- Nasomaxillary fractures
- Active intraoral and intranasal bleed
- Nasal intubation (Fig. 5)

SURGICAL STEPS

Arch Bar Insertion (Figs 6A and B)

This method is a gold standard for achieving maxillary mandibular fixation (MMF).

Maxillary Mandibular Fixation (Figs 7A to D)

It is done when normal occlusion is achieved.

Other Methods of the Maxillary Mandibular Fixation

- Gilmer method
- Eyelet method
- Suspension wiring
- Circummandibular wiring.

Approach

- *Intraoral approach*: Incision is taken at lower gingivobuccal sulcus at the site of fracture with preserving strip of mucosa on gingival side to facilitate closure at the end of procedure (Figs 8A to C).

  This method is used for (i) symphysis and parasymphysis, (ii) body, and (iii) angle and ramus.
- *Extraoral approach*: This approach is used, when there is (i) existing laceration over the site of fracture, (ii) comminuted fracture requiring the application of reconstruction plate, (iii) angle and ramus fracture, and (iv) condylar process and head fracture.

Different types of incisions used are:

- *Submental incision*: It is used for symphyseal and parasymphyseal fractures.
- *Submandibular or Risdon's incision*: It is used for body, angle, ramus and low subcondylar fractures.
- *Retromandibular incision*: It is used for ramus and condylar fractures.
- *Preauricular incision*: It is used for condylar and head fractures.

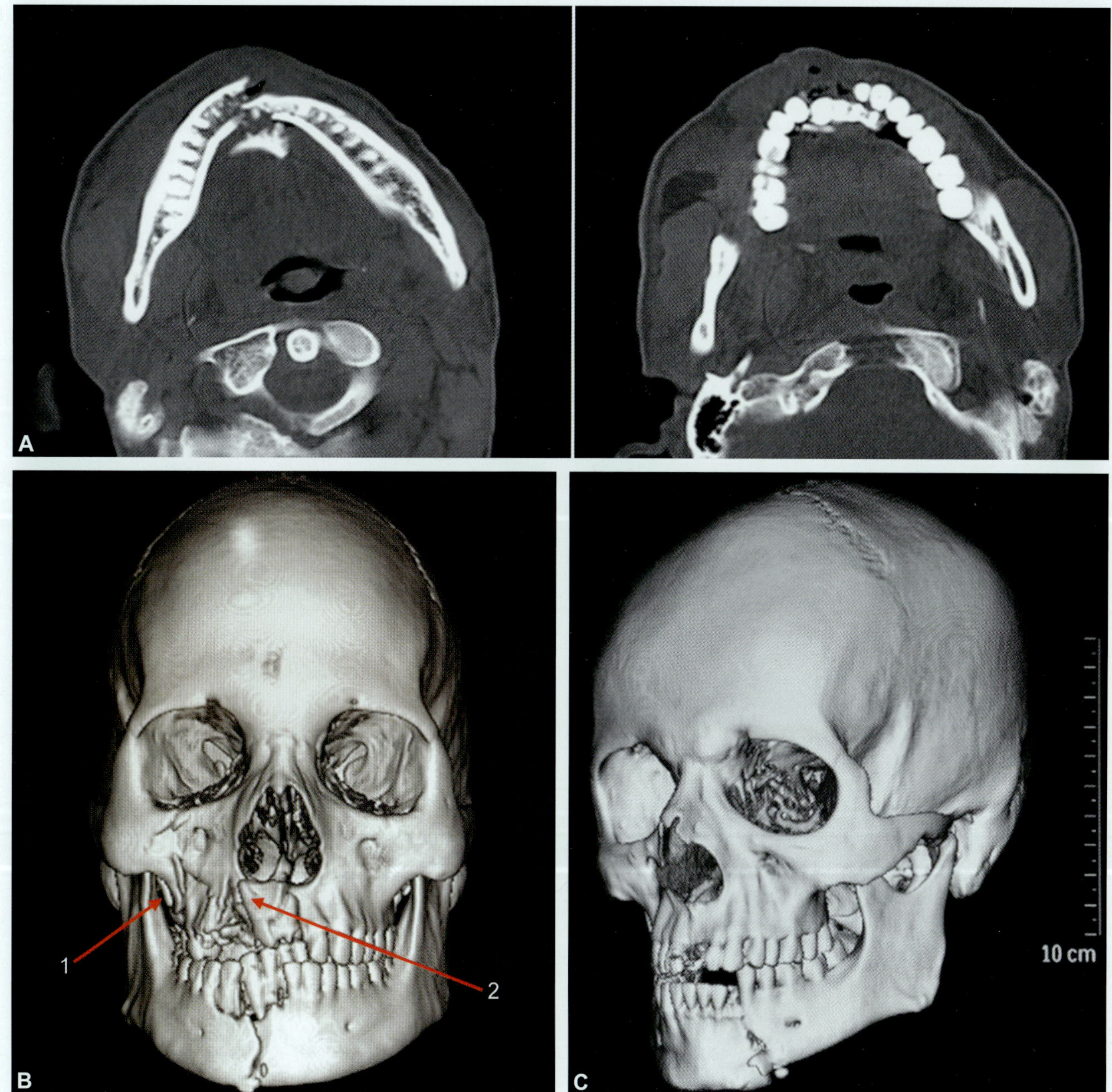

Figs 4A to C: (A) CT scan axial sections showing displaced fracture in symphyseal region and dentoalveolar fracture; (B) 3-D CT-Fracture of symphyseal region of mandible and right maxilla involving zygomaticomaxillary (1) and nasomaxillary (2) buttresses; (C) 3-D CT-Fracture of left parasymphyseal region of mandible

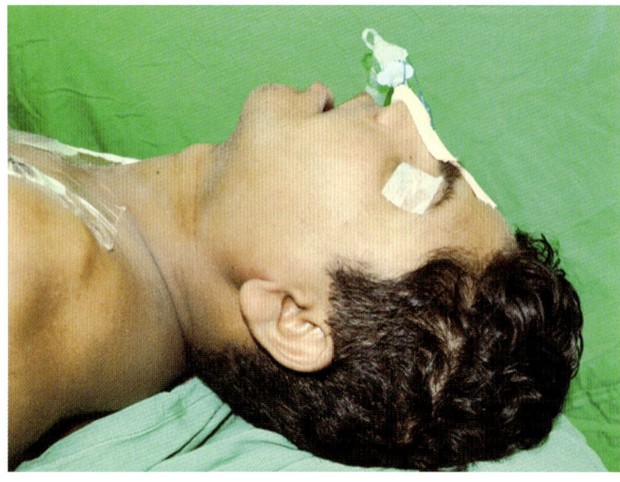

Fig. 5: Patient position—Head in extension with nasal intubation

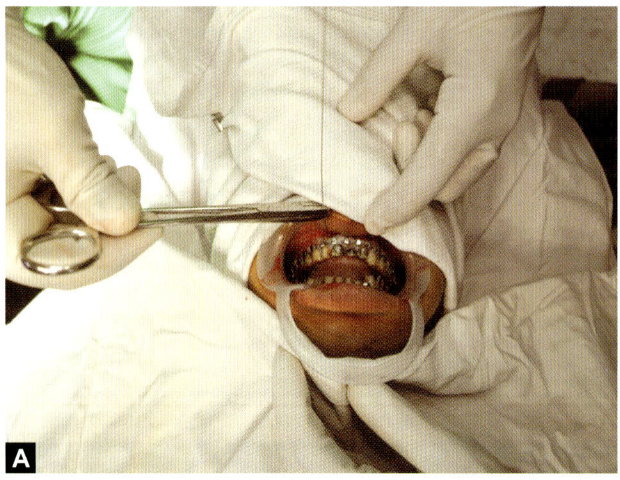

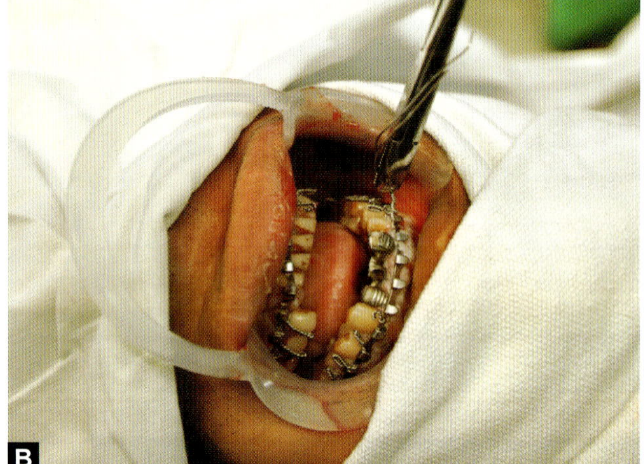

Figs 6A and B: Arch bar insertion. (A) Insertion of No. 24 stainless steel (S.S.) wire around tooth and arch bar; (B) SS wire is twisted clockwise to tighten and its cut edges are inverted to avoid injury to buccal mucosa

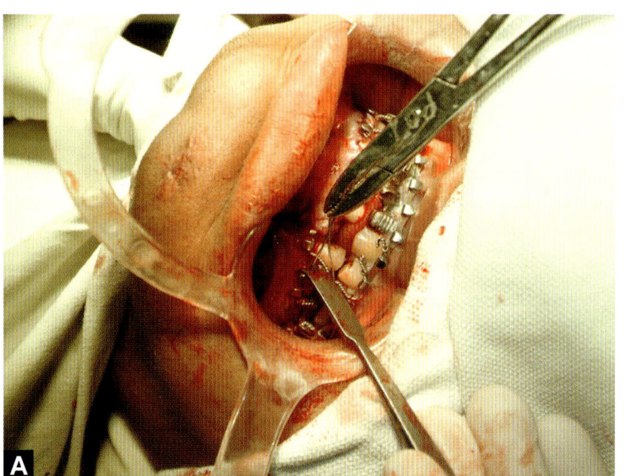

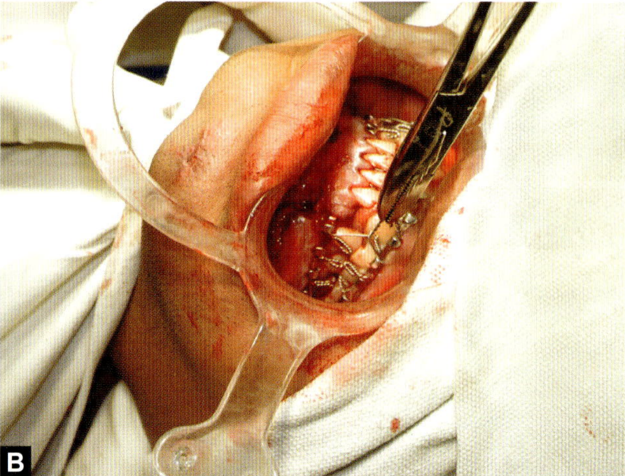

Figs 7A and B

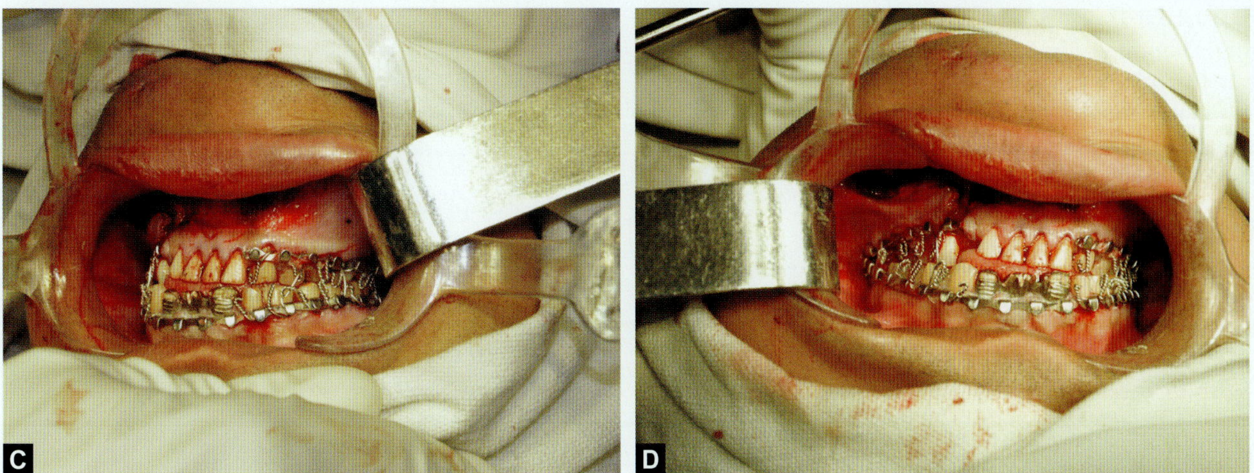

Figs 7A to D: Maxillary Mandibular fixation. (A) Loop of SS wire placed over 3 lugs each on upper and lower arch bar; (B) Wire loop tightened to achieve occlusion of teeth; (C) Occlusion on right side; (D) Occlusion on left side

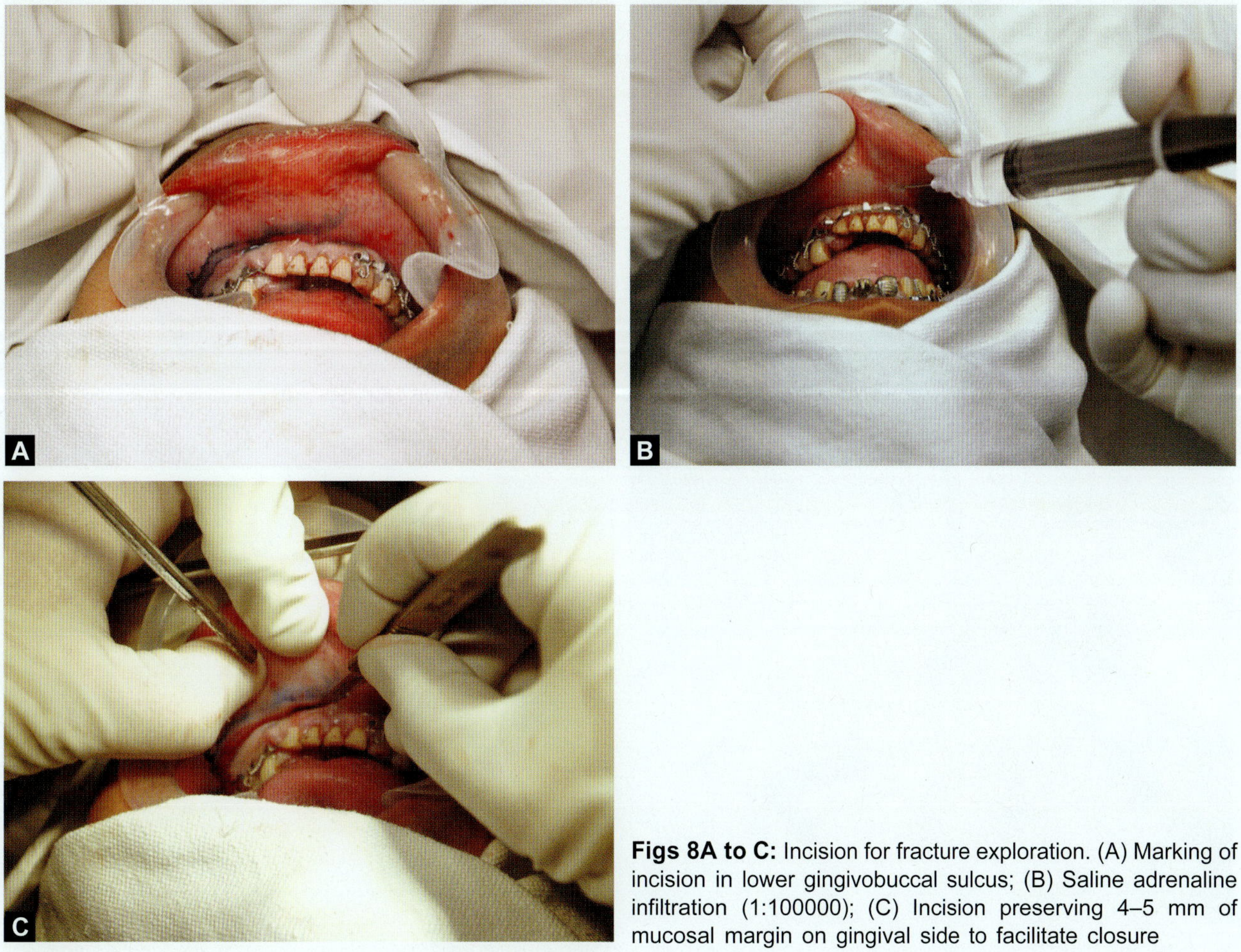

Figs 8A to C: Incision for fracture exploration. (A) Marking of incision in lower gingivobuccal sulcus; (B) Saline adrenaline infiltration (1:100000); (C) Incision preserving 4–5 mm of mucosal margin on gingival side to facilitate closure

Exposure (Figs 9A to D)

After taking incision, fracture fragments are exposed taking care to avoid injury to the surrounding vital structures, i.e. submental nerve, facial vessels. Periosteum over fracture fragments is stripped. Any granulation tissue/loose bony piece between the fracture fragments is removed.

Reduction (Fig. 10)

Fracture fragments are reduced manually with the bone holding forceps or stainless steel wire passed through fragments. After the reduction, occlusion is confirmed.

Selection of Implants

Symphysis and Parasymphysis (Fig. 11)

- Two miniplates
- Titanium screws

Body

- Two miniplates
- Titanium screws

Angle and Ramus

- One miniplate

Condylar Process and Head

- One miniplate

Comminuted Fractures

- Reconstruction plate

Plate Contouring and Placement

Plate is contoured, according to the location of fracture fragments.

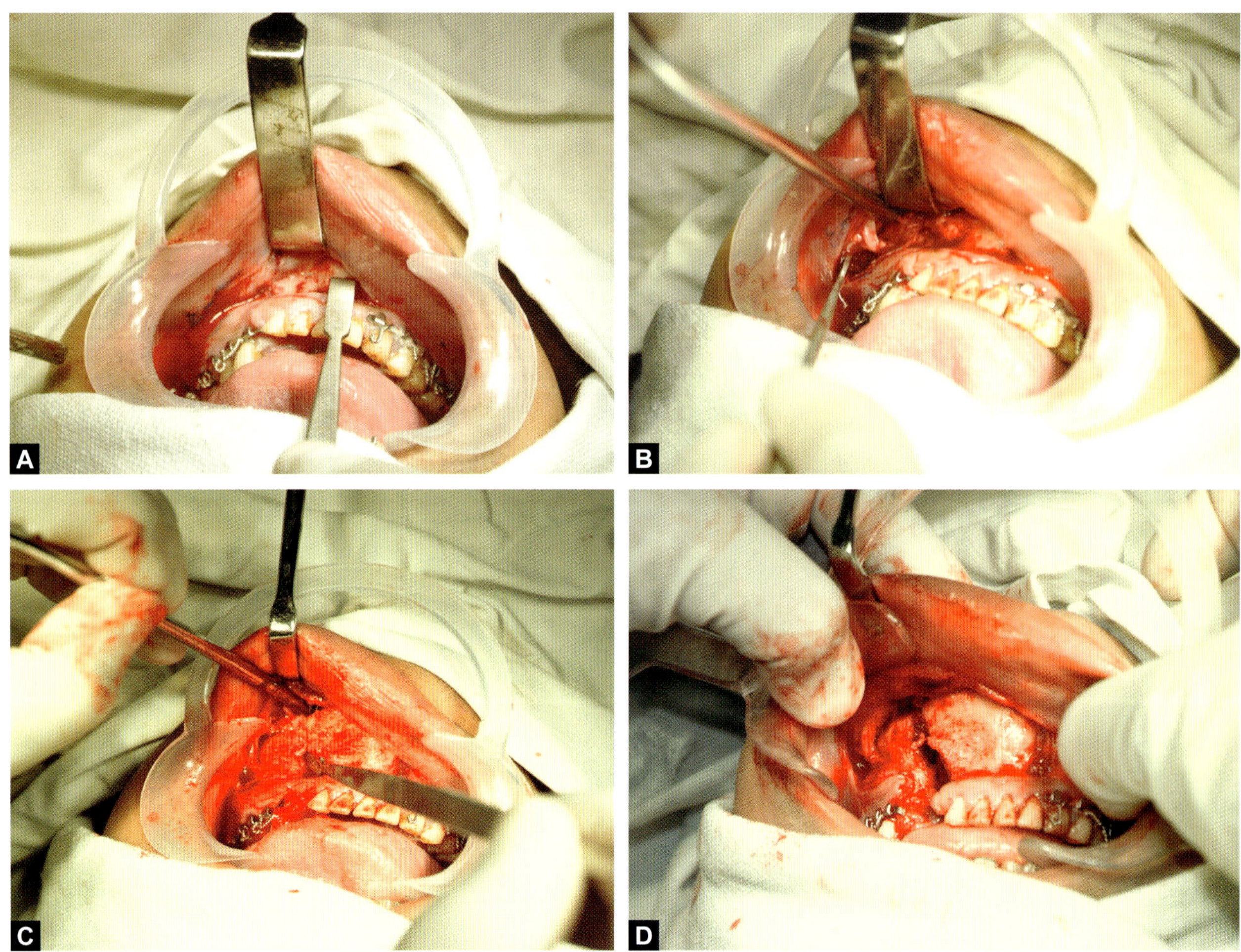

Figs 9A to D: Exposure of fracture. (A) Periosteum incised and elevated with periosteum elevator; (B) Mental nerve identified and preserved; (C) Exposed fracture; (D) All callus removed and fracture fragments rocked to achieve reduction

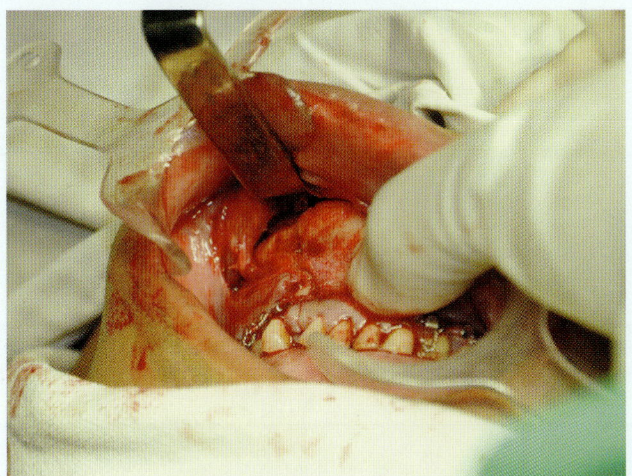

Fig. 10: Reduced fracture

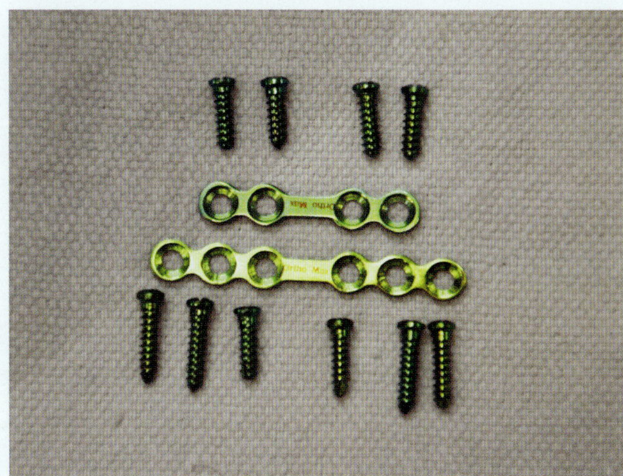

Fig. 11: Titanium mini plates (2.5 mm diameter), 4 hole and 6 hole along with screws (Courtesy of Orthomax)

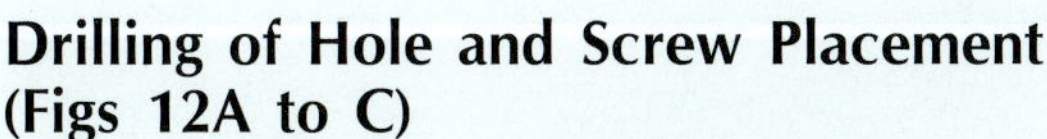

Drilling of Hole and Screw Placement (Figs 12A to C)

Holes are drilled with micromotor drill. Size of drill bit is 0.5 mm, smaller than that of plate. Screw mounts and screw driver are used to place screws.

Confirmation of Reduction and Occlusion (Fig. 12D)

After the fracture fixation, again reduction of fragments and occlusion is confirmed.

Closure (Fig. 12E)

Intraoral closure should be watertight. It is done with delayed absorbable sutures in horizontal mattress fashion. If external approach is used then wound is closed in two layers i.e. dermis with absorbable sutures and skin with non absorbable sutures.

MODIFICATIONS

Transbuccal Approach

It is used for angle, posterior part of the body and ramus, and lower subcondylar fractures combined with an intraoral approach.

Endoscopic Approach

It is used for condylar and head fractures combined with transbuccal incision.

COMPLICATIONS

The complications can be divided into early and late.

Early

- Hemorrhage
- Carotid injury
- Facial nerve injury
- Infection
- Avascular necrosis
- Osteitis/osteomyelitis

Late

- Temporomandibular joints ankylosis
- Nonunion
- Malunion
- Malocclusion
- Increased facial width
- Implant failure

SPECIAL INSTRUMENTS (FIGS 13A TO D)

Following special instruments are used.

- Cheek retractor
- Howarth periosteal elevator
- Bone holding forceps
- Micromotor drill machine
- Transbuccal trocar with cannula set
- Screw mounts and screw driver

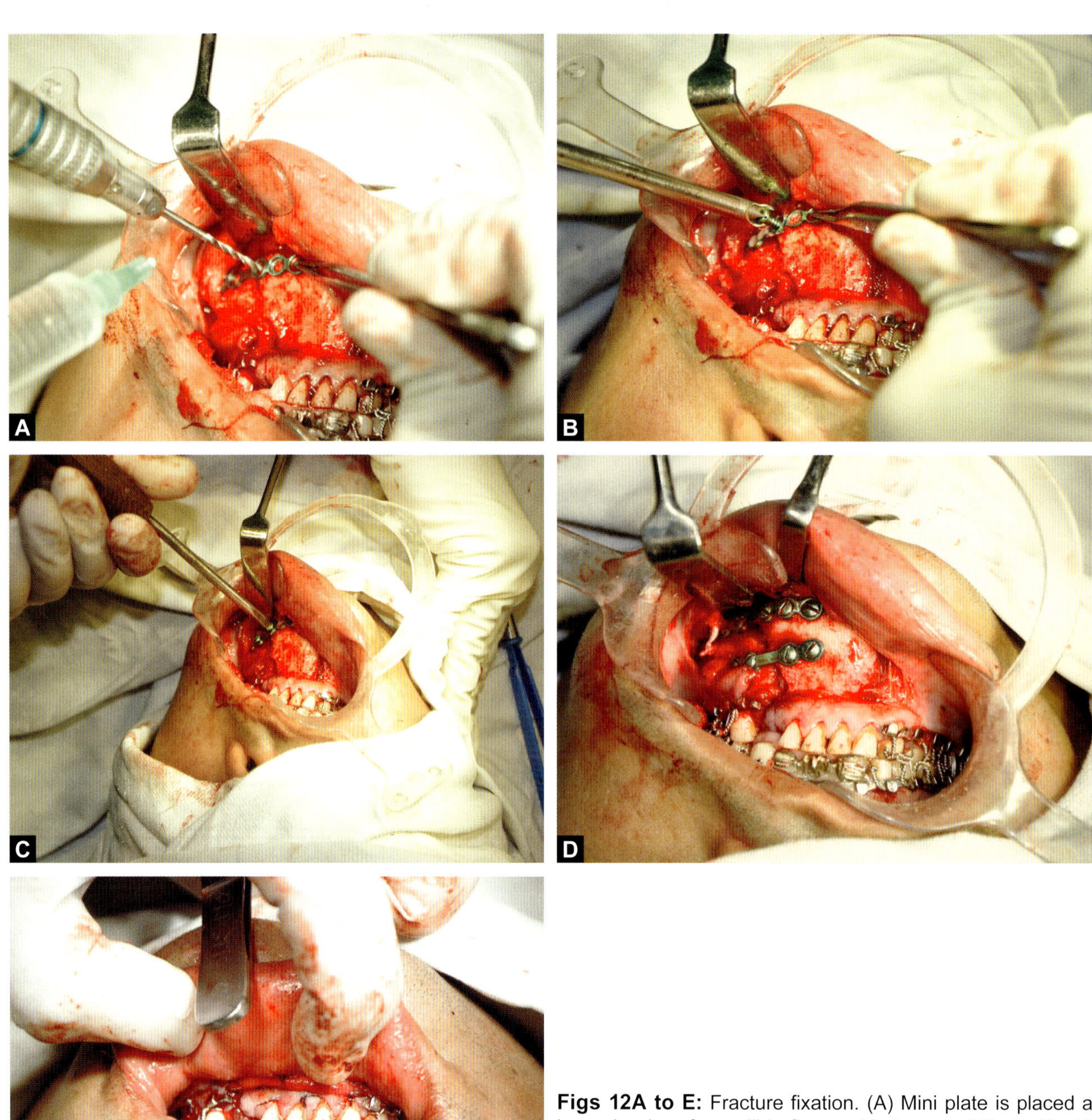

Figs 12A to E: Fracture fixation. (A) Mini plate is placed at lower border of mandible first and holes are drilled with drill bit (2 mm diameter); (B) Screw (2.5 mm diameter) is inserted using Sheath in holes near to fracture fragment; (C) Screws tightened with screw driver; (D) Similarly mini plate is applied near upper border and fixed. And simultaneously occlusion is confirmed; (E) Lower gingivobuccal incision closed in water tight fashion with absorbable horizontal mattress sutures

OTHER FIXATION TECHNIQUES

Maxillary Mandibular Fixation Only

- In simple, favorable and minimally displaced fractures
- Intracapsular condylar head fractures with minimal displacement

Lag Screw Technique

- Used for symphyseal fractures

External Fixator

- For infected, multiple fractures

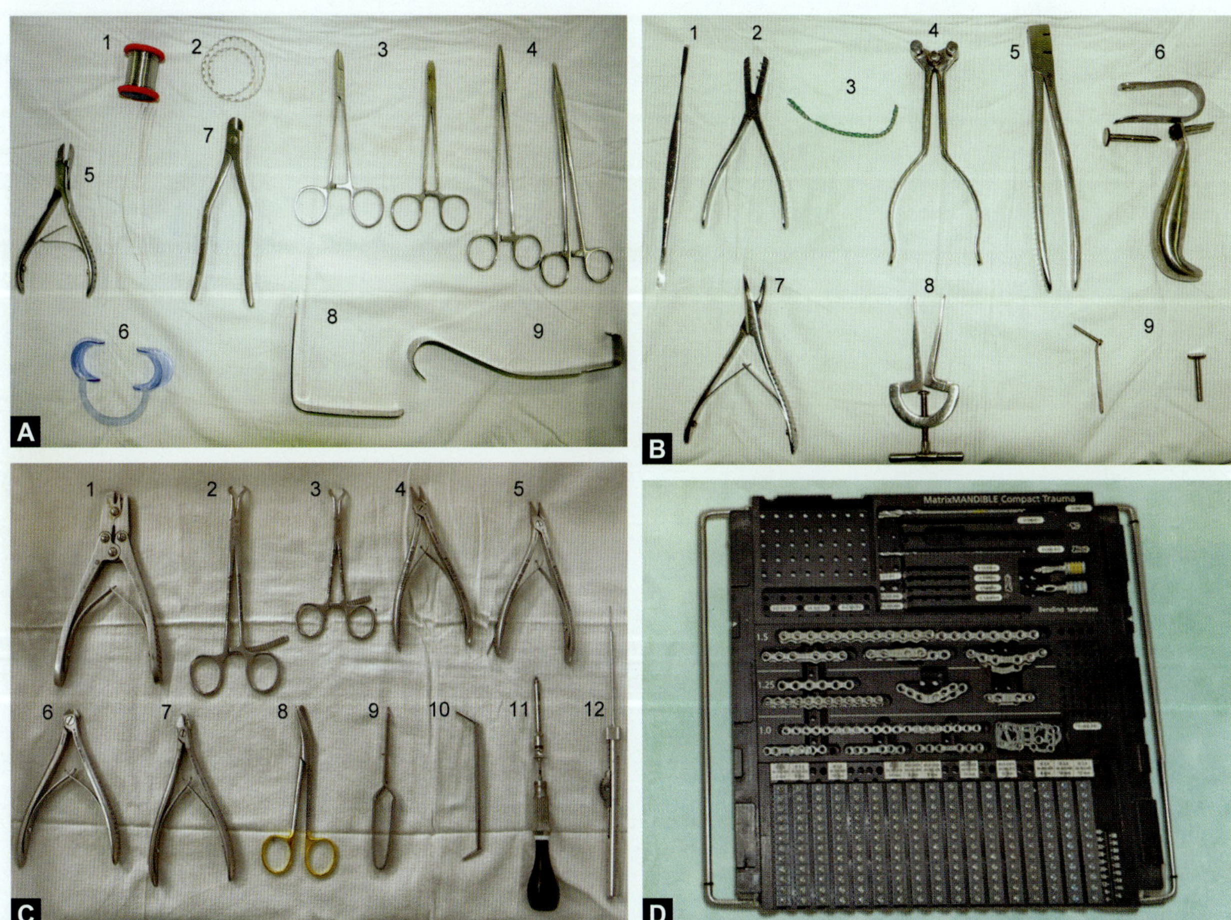

Figs 13A to D: Instruments required for open reduction and internal fixation of faciomaxillary fractures

(A) Instruments for Maxillary Mandibular fixation (*Courtesy* of Orthomax)

1. Stainless steel (SS) wire; 2. Arch bar; 3. Wire twister; 4. Long wire twister; 5. SS wire cutter; 6. Cheek retractor (plastic); 7. Arch bar cutter; 8. Tongue Depressor; 9. Metallic cheek retractor;

(B) Instruments for plate contouring and transbuccal approach (*Courtesy* of Orthomax)

1. Howarth periosteum elevator; 2. Plate holder; 3. Reconstruction plate; 4. Plate bender; 5. Plate cutter; 6. Transbuccal set with trochar; 7. Plate plier 8. Jaw stretcher; 9. Drill bit sheath

(C) Instruments for wire and plate cutting screw driver (*Courtesy* of AO foundation)

1. Plate cutter; 2. Bone holding forceps; 3. Plate plier; 4. SS Wire cutter; 5. Arch bar cutter 6. Thick scissor for cutting SS wire; 7. Plate holding forceps; 8. Drill bit sheath 9. Screw driver 10. Screw gauze

(D) Set of plates and screws with different shape and dimensions (*Courtesy* of AO foundation)

CHAPTER

111 Orbital Floor Fracture

Rajesh R Yadav, Girish Surlikar, PV Dhond

INTRODUCTION

Management of orbital floor fracture is usually accomplished through transconjunctival and subciliary incision. Authors hereby would discuss a new way to approach orbital floor fractures by endoscope.

ENDOSCOPIC REPAIR OF ORBITAL FLOOR FRACTURE

Advantages

- This approach provides adequate visualization and magnification
- The endoscopic approach obviates the need for an eyelid incision and thereby avoids potential lid complication like lid malposition such as ectropion and entropion, which occur with conventional incision
- Posterior orbit cannot be visualized properly due to angle of attack and prolapsed orbital fat and thereby, there is possibility of improper implant placement resulting into inadequate restoration of orbital volume and enophthalmos. Using endoscopic approach, the angle of inclination offers a more direct view of posterior orbit, thereby reduces a risk of poorly positioned implant.

INDICATIONS FOR ORBITAL FLOOR REPAIR

- Persistent diplopia after 10–14 days of trauma with a positive forced duction test and radiologic confirmation of an orbital floor fracture with entrapment of the inferior rectus or the perimuscular tissues surrounding the inferior rectus.

  Diplopia may be present initially after trauma but may resolve as the neuropraxia and/or orbital edema subsides.

  A subclass of orbital fracture with entrapment is called white-eye fracture in children. These patients need to be treated early.
- Enophthalmos of greater than 2 mm persisting for 10–14 days after trauma is cosmetically significant and therefore an indication for surgery. Orbital edema that is present initially may mask any enophthalmos. Therefore, measurements must be rechecked once the orbital edema has subsided.
- Fractures involving one-third or more of the orbit need to be repaired. If left unattended, these fractures tend to result in significant enophthalmos.

When surgery is indicated, it is usually best performed as close to 2 weeks from the trauma date as possible. This allows the swelling to subside and a more accurate examination of the orbit to be performed.

Indications for Endoscopic Repair of Orbital Floor Fracture

- Patient with trap door fracture and medial blowout fracture are excellent candidates for endoscopic repair (Figs 1A and B).

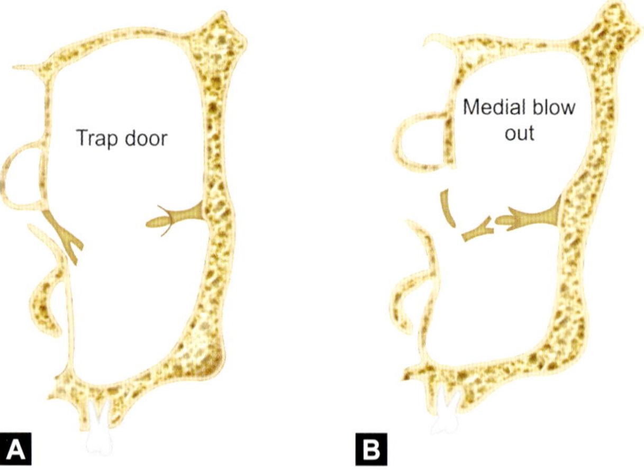

Figs 1A and B: (A) This figure is showing trap door fracture where fracture segment is hinged at one end; (B) This figure is showing medial blowout fracture where fracture is extending to medial wall but not extending beyond inferior orbital nerve

Limitations

Fractures extending lateral to infraorbital nerve or involving lamina papyracea are more difficult to repair endoscopically and these require open approach.

PREOPERATIVE EVALUATION

- Short history of mode of injury should be taken
- Ophthalmic evaluation should be undertaken to avoid any visual loss from optic neuropathy, retinal detachment or hyphema
- Computed tomography (CT) scan orbit needs to be done to see the extent of floor injury and accompanying injuries. A cut of 1 mm is required. Prolapsed fat and entrapment of muscle should be seen
- Head injury and spine injury should be ruled out. Patient needs to be hemodynamically stable prior to surgery.

SURGICAL STEPS

Repair is normally done in general anesthesia. Patient is placed in supine position (head high position of around 30°).

The forced duction test should be performed to determine ocular motility immediately after general anesthesia is induced.

Two percent lignocaine with adrenaline is infiltrated sublabially.

A 4 cm incision is made in gingivobuccal sulcus (Fig. 2), ensuring adequate mucosal stump at the alveolar end, so that suturing is convenient.

Incision is deepened through the periosteum to reach the anterior wall of maxilla. The periosteum is elevated exposing the anterior wall of maxilla up to the level of infraorbital nerve (Fig. 3).

Care is taken to avoid excessive traction or trauma to nerve. With the help of osteotome and Kerrison punch, appropriate sized window is created in thin wall of maxilla (Fig. 4).

Lip is retracted and a cottonoid/patty soaked in 4% lignocaine and adrenaline is placed in maxillary sinus for decongestion of mucosa. Then the endoscope is introduced to inspect the orbital floor. Any defect in orbital floor is analyzed for size, location, soft tissue prolapse and entrapment. Any entrapped tissue is made free and is reduced back to orbit with the help of freer elevator.

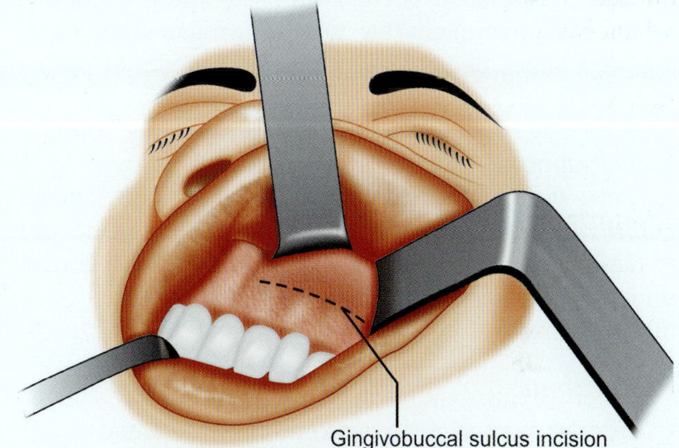

Fig. 2: Gingivobuccal sulcus incision

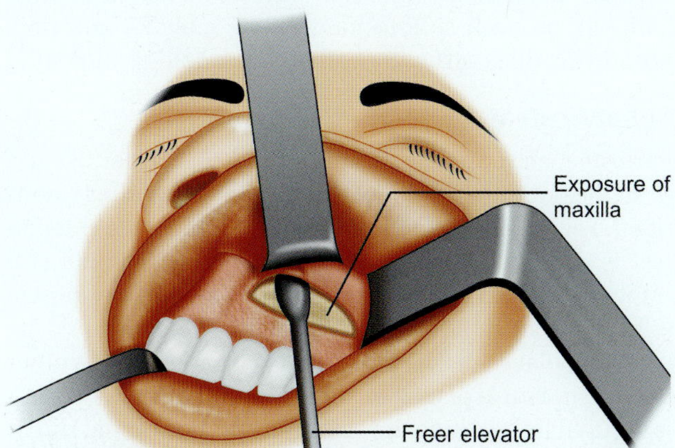

Fig. 3: Periosteum elevated and anterior wall of maxilla expose till the level of inferior orbital nerve

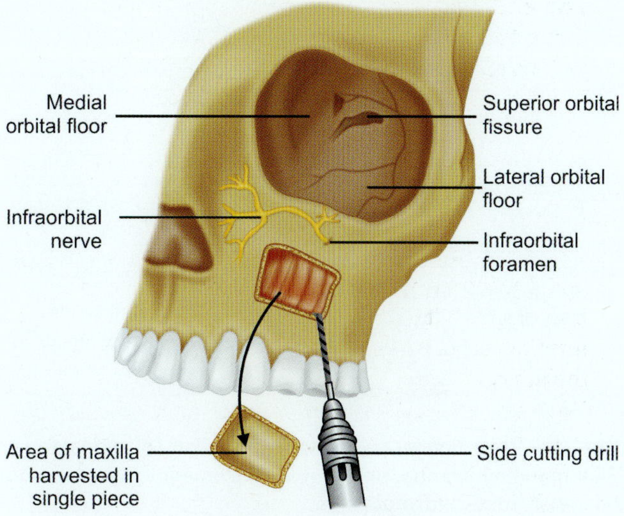

Fig. 4: This figure is showing creation of window on anterior wall of maxilla

Hinge Fracture

Any hinge fracture after replacement of soft tissues to orbit is then allowed to snap back into a place maintaining the reduction. Excessive medial dissection is avoided as this may destabilize the hinge and may require placement of implant.

Medial Blowout Fracture

- Elevate the mucosa around defect and expose the edge.
- Orbital content is reduced and all comminuted fragments of bone are removed.
- Size of defect is assessed and suitable implant is trimmed to size, which is 1 mm bigger than size of defect.

Implant is inserted over the stable posterior edge and is directed toward anterior edge with the help of freer elevator and suction implant (Fig. 5). During the manipulation, constant check needs to be kept that implant at posterior end is not shifted and remains at the same position. Anterior edge and the posterior edge form the primary area of support.

Pulse test (gentle external pressure is applied at globe and the pulsations are observed through the endoscope) is performed to see whether implant is stable. Forced duction test is performed again to check any restriction of movement.

Precautions

- Injuries to maxillary mucosa should be avoided
- Injuries to infraorbital nerve should be avoided
- No bony fragment is pushed into orbital cavity
- Any bone fragment or mucosa overhanging at area of maxillary ostium should be removed to prevent infection.

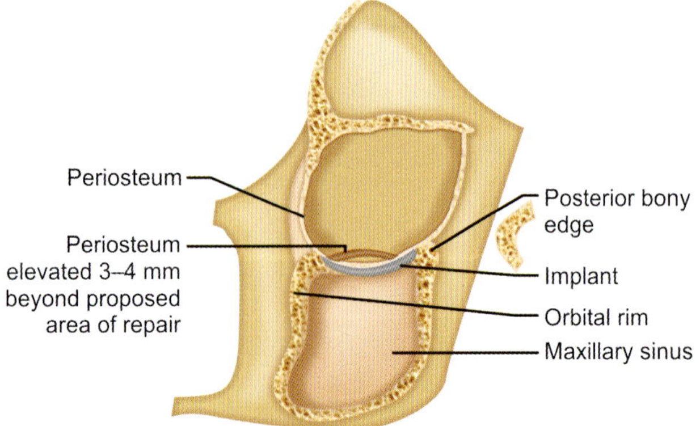

Fig. 5: This figure is showing elevation of periosteum 3–4 mm beyond the defect and placement of implant on posterior edge and orbital rim

Bone chip of anterior wall can be fixed again or kept open. Wound is closed in layers by 3.0 vicryl.

Failure to repair the fracture endoscopically will necessitate an alternative approach—subciliary and transconjuctival approach.

Subciliary Approach

Skin Incision

Two percent lignocaine with adrenaline is injected in lower lid. Few millimeters below the eye lashes, parallel to lid margin incision is made by No. 15 blade. The incision is carried through the skin layer only. The underlying orbicular muscle should become apparent immediately below skin incision.

Dissection

Initial dissection is superficial to orbicularis for few millimeters. The dissection is then deepened by dividing orbicularis oculi muscle. Raising skin-muscle flap and the dissection plane is made between the muscle and the septum orbitale (Figs 6A to D).

Precaution must be taken that septum is not breached so that prolapse of fat is prevented.

The suborbicular flap is extended downward till the anterior edge of the infraorbital rim is reached.

Periosteal Incision over the Infraorbital Rim

The skin-muscle flap is retracted inferiorly over the anterior edge of the infraorbital rim along its whole horizontal extent (Fig. 7).

A periosteum incision is made from anterior to inferior orbital rim to avoid orbital septum damage which is inserted on superior margin of inferior orbital rim.

Incision on septum can cause scarring, leading to vertical shortening of the lid. Periosteal edge is marked with silk on each side to identify the edge for suturing. Identifying these structures otherwise would be difficult.

Subperiosteal Dissection of Orbit

Periosteal elevators are then used to strip the periosteum from the underlying floor of orbit, and fracture site is identified. Fat, muscle is freed from defect and forced traction test is done to check for any entrapment. Suitable size implant of appropriate material (that can prevent muscle adherence and give proper contour to floor) should be used and placed on the posterior edge of defect. The other end of implant is placed on anterior orbital ridge. Implant is secured by inserting the screw on anterior orbital rim or by glue.

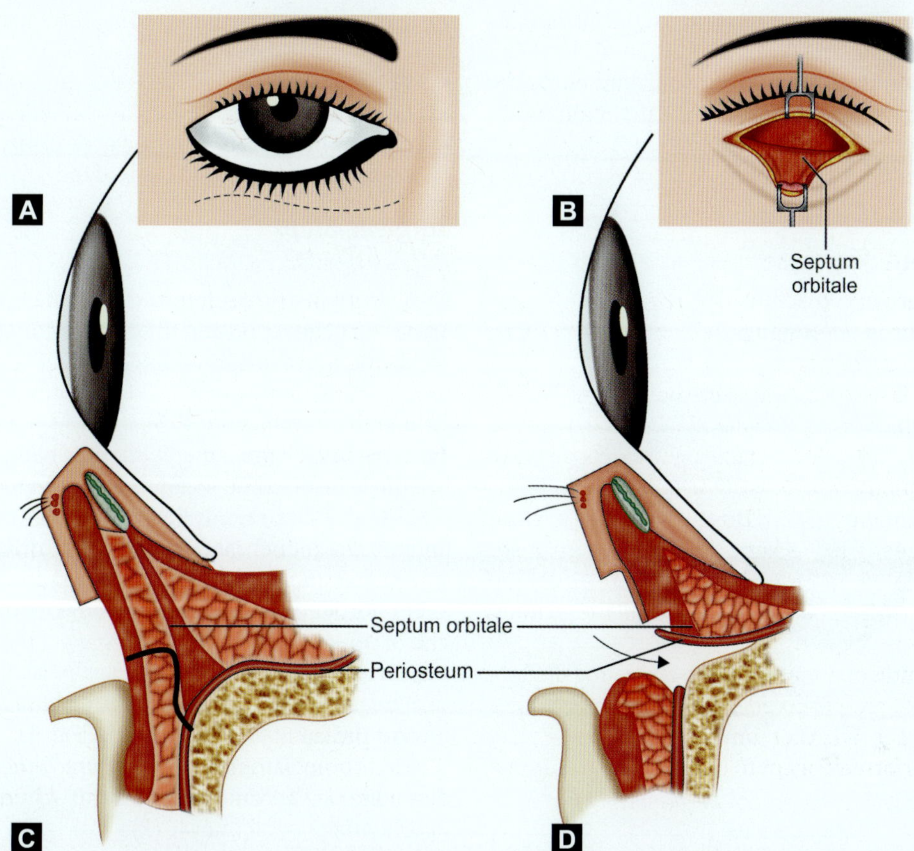

Figs 6A to D: (A) Subciliary incision extending from punctum to lateral canthus; (B) Skin and orbicularis oculi flap elevated without injuring septum orbitale; (C) Skin and orbicularis oculi flap elevated till infraorbital rim; (D) Incision on periosteum is taken to expose orbital floor

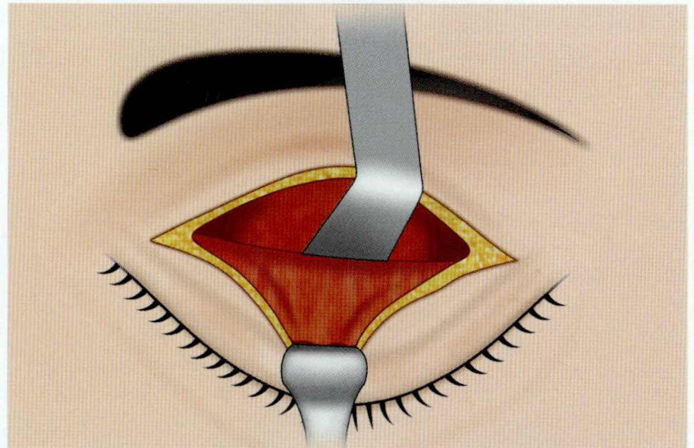

Fig. 7: Globe is retracted with malleable retractor applying minimal pressure on globe to expose orbital floor

Closure

Closure is performed in two or three layers: (1) periosteum—the periosteum is redraped over the bony surfaces and closed with resorbable interrupted sutures, (2) muscle (optional) and (3) skin—the skin wound is closed with a 6.0 nonresorbable or fast-resorbing suture. Either running or interrupted sutures can be used.

Care should be taken not to damage the:

- Palpebral anatomical structures
- Lacrimal drainage systems
- Ocular muscles
- Neural structures.

Care should be given following the open treatment of orbital fractures.

Evaluation of the patient's vision is performed as soon as they are out of anesthesia and then undertaken at regular intervals until they are discharged from the hospital.

Transconjunctival Approach

Advantages

- No scar seen
- Lower incidence of ectropion
- Less changes of lid shortening.

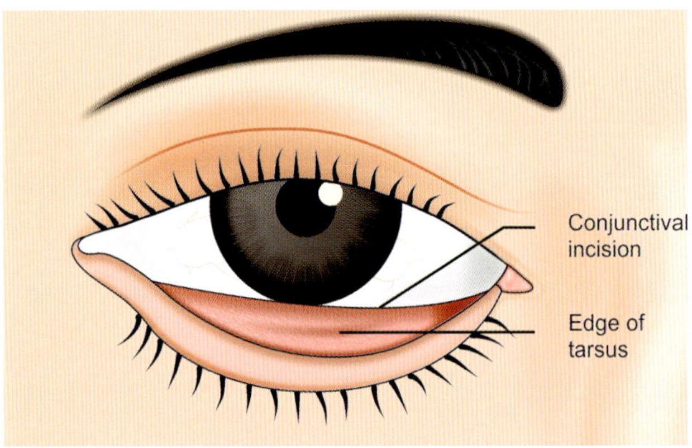

Fig. 8: Conjunctival incision below the lower border of the tarsus

Disadvantages

- Restricted access
- Limited extension
- Greater degree of operative dexterity is required, if complications have to be avoided.

Surgical Steps

Cornea protector is placed over the eye to protect cornea, globe from instrument, retractor or drill. Traction sutures are taken in lower lid and inferior conjunctival fornices for retraction and eversion of lower lid.

Infiltration and Incision

Two percent lignocaine with adrenaline is infiltrated. Needle is inserted between the conjunctiva and the tarsal plate and subsequently inserted again through the skin deep to the palpebral portion of the orbicularis oculi but superficial to septum. Conjunctival incision below the lower border of tarsus is taken on the medial aspect and in line of punctum (Fig. 8).

For the incision, scissors, scalpels or electrocautery can be used. Lower eyelid retractors are undermined toward the inner angle of the lids (Fig. 9).

Fat compartment and septum are identified, and dissection is carried out anterior to septum and posterior to orbicularis oculi muscle (Fig. 10).

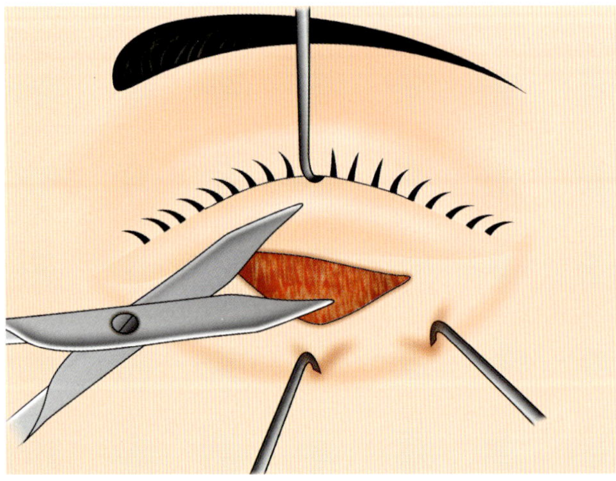

Fig. 9: Lower eyelid retractor is transacted and a dissection plane is established in front of the orbital septum

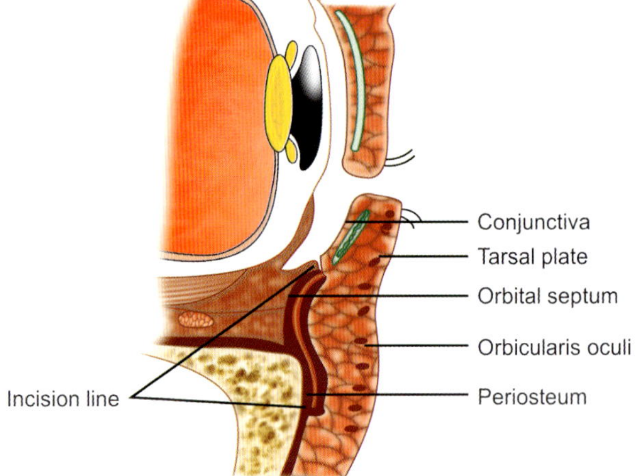

Fig. 10: This figure shows two incisions—first incision, few millimeters below tarsal plate and second incision on periosteum few millimeters anterior to rim

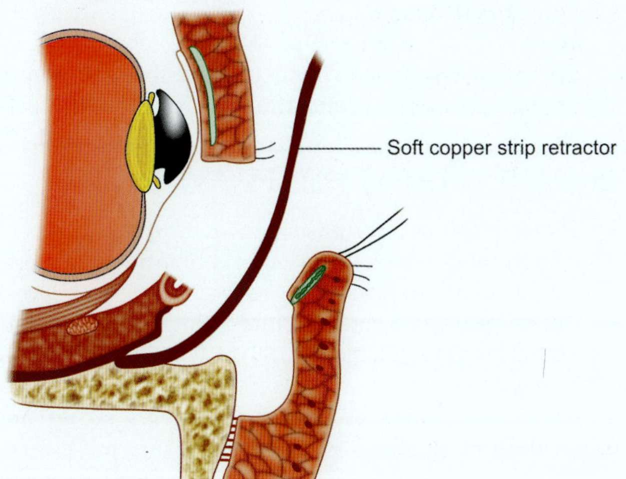

Fig. 11: Orbital content is elevated with malleable copper retractor to expose orbital floor

The dissection is carried out till infraorbital rim is reached (Fig. 11). Further steps are same as subciliary incision.

Wound Closure

Wound is closed in layers. First the periosteum over the periorbital rim is closed and then conjunctival layers are closed with 6.0 vicryl. The conjunctival flaps must be aligned accurately.

Postoperative Positioning

Keeping the patient's head in an upright position, both preoperatively and postoperatively may significantly improve periorbital edema and pain.

Nose-blowing

To prevent orbital emphysema, nose-blowing should be avoided for at least 10 days following orbital fracture repair.

Wound Care

Remove sutures from skin after approximately 5 days, if nonresorbable sutures have been used. Apply ice packs (may be effective in a short-term to minimize edema). Avoid sun exposure and tanning to skin incisions for several months.

Clinical Follow-Up

The patient needs to be examined and reassessed regularly.

MODIFICATIONS/SUGGESTIONS

Surgeons use titanium implant as it is safe, with less chances of infection and displacement of implant (when it is handled, contoured and secured accurately). Surgeons secure the implant either by placing a screw or by applying glue.

Titanium Meshes/Implant

Advantages

- Easy availability
- Good stability
- Can be well contoured
- Radio-opacity
- Spaces within the mesh to allow dissipation of fluids
- No donor site needed
- Tissue incorporation may occur.

Disadvantages

- Expensive
- Possibility of injury by sharp edges if not properly trimmed.

COMPLICATIONS

- *Infraorbital paresthesia*: This occurs due to stretching of nerve during retraction. It normally improves in 2–3 weeks
- *Maxillary sinusitis*: These complications may occur due to endoscopic repair
- Eyelid malposition like entropion
- Eye lid laxity
- *Scleral show*: These complications occur due to subciliary approach. These conditions improve in 3–4 weeks
- *Lagophthalmos*: This occurs due to conjunctival approach. It resolves eventually.

SPECIAL INSTRUMENTS (FIG. 12)

- *Corneal shield*: This is to protect cornea, globe from instrument, retractor or drill
- *Copper malleable retractors of various sizes and shapes*: These are used to retract the orbital globe away from floor without exerting too much pressure on the globe
- Suitable implant
- Fine scissors for dissection

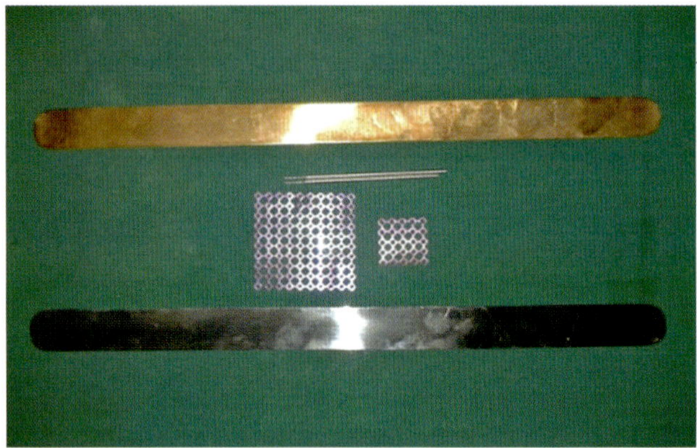

Fig. 12: Copper malleable retractor on either side, titanium mesh of various shape and size and drill bit

- Fine tipped forceps
- Glue
- 1.5 mm × 6 mm screw and 1 mm drill bit to secure implant at anterior orbital rim.

OTHER TREATMENTS AVAILABLE

- *Antral packing*: Antrum is packed with 3-6 meter of ribbon gauge which is soaked in antibiotic and a lubricant. It is kept in place for 3 weeks.
- *Antral balloons*: A special antral balloon is used preferably; if it's not available then 30 mL Foley's catheter can be used.

These procedures are blind procedures so do not assure desired results.

Index

Page numbers followed by *f* refer to figure and *t* refer to table

D

E

F

V

W

X

Z